The Final FRCA
Constructed Response Questions

This up-to-date study guide for the Final FRCA CRQ comprises questions based on every topic examined in the Royal College of Anaesthetists' Final written exam from the past 12 years. It therefore covers the areas of the syllabus that are key to exam success, offering factual learning and the opportunity to practise CRQ-style questions, with chapters that reflect the RCoA syllabus format to help organise learning.

The inclusion of diagrams and additional commentary ensure that that this book will help candidates to learn rather than just providing a list of suggested model answers. Advice is offered about revision approaches, best sources of learning for the examination, and guidance on structuring answers, which will support exam success in all parts of the Final FRCA. This resource will save hours of work for anaesthetists preparing for the Final FRCA.

Elizabeth Combeer BSc, MBBS, MRCP, FRCA, MA, is an anaesthetic consultant at Frimley Health NHS Foundation Trust and runs the FRCA teaching programme at Frimley Park Hospital. Her close involvement with trainees preparing for the FRCA exams means that she understands the requirements and level of knowledge needed to pass this assessment.

Mitul Patel MBBS, BSc, FRCA, is an anaesthetic registrar in South London with an interest in medical education.

MasterPass Series

The Final FRCR: Self-Assessment
Amanda Rabone, Benedict Thomson, Nicky Dineen, Vincent Helyar, Aidan Shaw

Geriatric Medicine: 300 Specialist Certificate Exam Questions
Shibley Rahman, Henry Woodford

Surgical and Anaesthetic Instruments for OSCEs: A Practical Study Guide
Kelvin Yan

Clinical Cases for the FRCA: Key Topics Mapped to the RCoA Curriculum
Alisha Allana

Spine Surgery Vivas for the FRCS (Tr & Orth)
Kelechi Eseonu, Nicolas Beresford-Cleary

MCQs, MEQs and OSPEs in Occupational Medicine: A Revision Aid
Ken Addley

ENT OSCEs: A guide to your first ENT job and passing the MRCS (ENT) OSCE, 3E
Peter Kullar, Joseph Manjaly, Livy Kenyon

The Final FFICM Structured Oral Examination Study Guide
Eryl Davies

ENT Vivas: A Guide to Passing the Intercollegiate FRCS (ORL-HNS) Viva Examination
Adnan Darr, Karan Jolly, Jameel Muzaffar

Plastic Surgery Vivas for the FRCS (Plast): An Essential Guide
Monica Fawzy

Clinical Consultation Skills in Medicine: A Primer for MRCP PACES
Ernest Suresh

Neurosurgery Second Edition: The Essential Guide to the Oral and Clinical Neurosurgical Exam
Vivian Elwell, Ramez Kirollos, Syed Al-Haddad, Peter Bodkin

Sport and Exercise Medicine: An Essential Guide
David Eastwood, Dane Vishnubala

Refraction and Retinoscopy: How to Pass the Refraction Certificate, Second Edition
Jonathan Park, Leo Feinberg, David Jones

The Final FRCA Constructed Response Questions: A Practical Study Guide, Second Edition
Elizabeth Combeer, Mitul Patel

For more information about this series please visit: www.routledge.com/MasterPass/book-series/ CRCMASPASS

The Final FRCA
Constructed Response Questions
A Practical Study Guide

Second Edition

Elizabeth Combeer and Mitul Patel
Illustrations by Paul Hatton

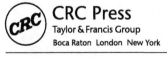

CRC Press
Taylor & Francis Group
Boca Raton London New York

CRC Press is an imprint of the
Taylor & Francis Group, an **informa** business

Second edition published 2024
by CRC Press
2385 NW Executive Center Drive, Suite 320, Boca Raton, FL 33431

and by CRC Press
4 Park Square, Milton Park, Abingdon, Oxon, OX14 4RN

CRC Press is an imprint of Taylor & Francis Group, LLC

© 2024 Elizabeth Combeer, Mitul Patel

First edition published by CRC Press 2019

ISBN: 978-1-032-48327-6 (hbk)
ISBN: 978-1-032-44524-3 (pbk)
ISBN: 978-1-003-38849-4 (ebk)

DOI: 10.1201/9781003388494

Typeset in Gill Sans
by Apex CoVantage, LLC

CONTENTS

ABBREVIATIONS

A-a	Alveolar-arterial	**CNS**	Central nervous system
AAA	Abdominal aortic aneurysm	**COETT**	Cuffed oral endotracheal tube
AAGBI	Association of Anaesthetists of Great Britain and Ireland	**COPD**	Chronic obstructive pulmonary disease
ABG	Arterial blood gas	**COVID**	Disease due to severe acute respiratory syndrome coronavirus 2
ACE	Angiotensin-converting enzyme		
AChR	Acetylcholine receptor	**COX**	Cyclic oxygenase
ACT	Activated clotting time	**CPAP**	Continuous positive airway pressure
ADP	Adenosine diphosphate		
AKI	Acute kidney injury	**CPB**	Cardiopulmonary bypass
ALS	Adult life support	**CPET**	Cardiopulmonary exercise testing
ALT	Alanine transaminase	**CPOC**	Centre for Perioperative Care
APL	Adjustable pressure limiting	**CPP**	Cerebral perfusion pressure
AT	Anaerobic threshold	**CPR**	Cardiopulmonary resuscitation
ATP	Adenosine triphosphate	**CRP**	C-reactive protein
APRV	Airway pressure release ventilation	**CRPS**	Complex regional pain syndrome
ARDS	Acute respiratory distress syndrome	**CRQ**	Constructed response question
		CSE	Combined spinal and epidural
ASA	American Society of Anesthesiologists	**CSF**	Cerebrospinal fluid
		CT	Computed tomography
AVPU	Alert, voice, pain, unresponsive	**CTPA**	Computed tomography pulmonary angiogram
BJA	*British Journal of Anaesthesia*		
BNF	*British National Formulary*	**CVC**	Central venous catheter
BP	Blood pressure	**CVP**	Central venous pressure
bpm	Beats per minute	**CXR**	Chest radiograph
BMI	Body mass index	**2,3 DPG**	2,3 Diphosphoglycerate
BNP	Brain natriuretic peptide	**DAPT**	Dual antiplatelet therapy
BSA	Body surface area	**DAS**	Difficult Airway Society
CABG	Coronary artery bypass graft	**DES**	Drug-eluting stent
cAMP	Cyclic adenosine monophosphate	**DIC**	Disseminated intravascular coagulation
CAPD	Continuous ambulatory peritoneal dialysis		
		DLCO	Diffusing capacity of the lungs for carbon monoxide
CBG	Capillary blood glucose		
CBT	Cognitive behavioural therapy	**DKA**	Diabetic ketoacidosis
CEACCP	*Continuing Education in Anaesthesia, Critical Care and Pain*	**DOP**	Delta opioid receptor
		DVT	Deep vein thrombosis
CICO	Can't intubate, can't oxygenate	**EBV**	Epstein-Barr virus
CK	Creatine kinase	**ECG**	Electrocardiogram
CKD	Chronic kidney disease	**Echo**	Echocardiogram
CMR	Cardiac MRI	**ECMO**	Extracorporeal membrane oxygenation
CMRO$_2$	Cerebral metabolic rate of oxygen		
CMV	Cytomegalovirus	**ED**	Emergency department

EEG	Electroencephalogram	**Iu**	International units
eGFR	Estimated glomerular filtration rate	**iv**	Intravenous
EMG	Electromyogram	**IVC**	Inferior vena cava
ENT	Ear, nose and throat	**ivi**	Intravenous infusion
ERAS	Enhanced recovery after surgery	**JAK**	Janus kinase
ERCP	Endoscopic retrograde cholangiopancreatography	**JVP**	Jugular venous pressure
		KOP	Kappa opioid receptor
ESR	Erythrocyte sedimentation rate	**LMA**	Laryngeal mask airway
ESRF	End-stage renal failure	**LMWH**	Low molecular weight heparin
etCO₂	End-tidal carbon dioxide	**LocSSIP**	Local safety standard for invasive procedure
ETT	Endotracheal tube		
EVAR	Endovascular aneurysm repair	**LVEDP**	Left ventricular end-diastolic pressure
FEV₁	Forced expiratory volume in 1 second		
		LVEF	Left ventricular ejection fraction
FiO₂	Fraction of inspired oxygen	**M&M**	Morbidity and mortality
FRC	Functional residual capacity	**MAC**	Minimum alveolar concentration
FRCA	Fellowship of the Royal College of Anaesthetists	**MAP**	Mean arterial pressure
		MCV	Mean corpuscular volume
GA	General anaesthetic	**MDT**	Multidisciplinary team
GBS	Guillain-Barré syndrome	**MEOWS**	Modified Early Obstetric Warning Score
GIRFT	Getting It Right First Time		
GMC	General Medical Council	**MHRA**	Medicines and Healthcare Products Regulatory Agency
GCS	Glasgow Coma Scale		
GGT	Gamma-glutamyl transferase	**MEP**	Motor evoked potential
GORD	Gastro-oesophageal reflux disease	**MI**	Myocardial infarction
GPAS	Guidelines for the provision of anaesthetic services	**MIBG**	Meta-iodobenzylguanidine nuclear medicine scan
		MOP	Mu opioid receptor
GTN	Glyceryl trinitrate	**MRI**	Magnetic resonance imaging
5HT₃	Serotonin (5-hydroxytryptamine)	**MRSA**	Methicillin-resistant *Staphylococcus aureus*
HbAlc	Glycosylated haemoglobin		
HDU	High dependency unit	**MSSA**	Methicillin-sensitive *Staphylococcus aureus*
HELLP	Haemolysis, elevated liver enzymes and low platelets syndrome		
		NAP	National Audit Project (of the Royal College of Anaesthetists)
HFNO	High-flow nasal oxygen		
HFOV	High-frequency oscillatory ventilation	**NCEPOD**	National Confidential Enquiry into Patient Outcome and Death
HIV	Human immunodeficiency virus		
HOCM	Hypertrophic obstructive cardiomyopathy	**NHS**	National Health Service
		NICE	National Institute for Health and Care Excellence
HSV	Herpes simplex virus		
IASP	International Association for the Study of Pain	**NICU**	Neonatal intensive care unit
		NIV	Noninvasive ventilation
ICD	Implantable cardiac defibrillator	**NMBD**	Neuromuscular blocking drug
ICP	Intracranial pressure	**NMDA**	N-methyl-D-aspartate glutamate receptor
ICU	Intensive care unit		
ID	Internal diameter	**NPSA**	National Patient Safety Agency
IR	Interventional radiology	**NSAIDs**	Nonsteroidal anti-inflammatory drugs
INR	International normalised ratio		
IQ	Intelligence quotient	**NYHA**	New York Heart Association
ITP	Immune thrombocytopenic purpura	**OAA**	Obstetric Anaesthetists' Association

ODP	Operating Department Practitioner	**S1Q3T3**	S wave in lead 1, Q wave and inverted T wave in lead 3
OSA	Obstructive sleep apnoea	**SLE**	Systemic lupus erythematosus
OSCE	Objective structured clinical examination	**SNRI**	Serotonin-noradrenaline reuptake inhibitor
PACU	Post-anaesthetic care unit	**SSRI**	Selective serotonin reuptake inhibitor
PaO₂	Partial pressure of oxygen in arterial blood	**SvO₂**	Mixed venous oxygen saturations
PaCO₂	Partial pressure of carbon dioxide in arterial blood	**SVR**	Systemic vascular resistance
PCA	Patient-controlled analgesia	**SVRI**	Systemic vascular resistance index
PCEA	Patient-controlled epidural analgesia	**TAP**	Transversus abdominis plane
PCI	Percutaneous coronary intervention	**TBSA**	Total body surface area
		TCA	Tricyclic antidepressant
PCR	Polymerase chain reaction	**TCI**	Target-controlled infusion
PCT	Percutaneous tracheostomy	**TEG**	Thromboelastrography
PEA	Pulseless electrical activity	**TENS**	Transcutaneous electrical nerve stimulation
PEEP	Positive end-expiratory pressure	**TIA**	Transient ischaemic attack
PEG	Percutaneous endoscopic gastrostomy	**TIVA**	Total intravenous anaesthesia
PEJ	Percutaneous endoscopic jejunostomy	**TNF**	Tumour necrosis factor
		TSH	Thyroid-stimulating hormone
PET	Positron emission tomography	**TURP**	Transurethral resection of the prostate
POETTS	Perioperative Exercise Testing and Training Society	**VAE**	Venous air embolism
PONV	Postoperative nausea and vomiting	**VAP**	Ventilator associated pneumonia
PPI	Proton pump inhibitor	**VATER**	Syndrome of vertebral, cardiac, renal and limb anomalies, tracheo-oesophageal fistula and anal atresia
PRES	Posterior reversible encephalopathy syndrome		
ROTEM	Rotational thromboelastometry	**vCJD**	Variant Creutzfeldt-Jakob disease
RQ	Respiratory quotient	**VCO₂**	Carbon dioxide production
RSI	Rapid sequence induction	**VF**	Ventricular fibrillation
SAD	Supraglottic airway device	**VO₂ max**	Maximal oxygen consumption
SALG	Safe Anaesthesia Liaison Group	**VRIII**	Variable rate intravenous insulin infusion
SAQ	Short answer question	**VT**	Ventricular tachycardia
SBP	Systolic blood pressure	**VTE**	Venous thromboembolism
SGLT-2	Sodium-glucose co-transporter-2	**V/Q**	Ventilation: perfusion
SIADH	Syndrome of inappropriate antidiuretic hormone	**vWF**	von Willebrand factor
		WHO	World Health Organization

PASSING THE FINAL CRQ

These are my top tips for approaching the Final CRQ. They are based on what I find myself saying repeatedly at weekly teaching with the trainees at Frimley.

Print a copy of the syllabus

Both core and intermediate-level syllabuses are tested in the Final. I know these are dauntingly large documents, but it really is important that you understand the breadth of what you need to learn, and looking at these helps you direct your reading. Revision for subspecialties such as burns, cardiothoracics, neuro, paediatrics and obstetrics can largely be covered by searching for CEACCP or BJA Education articles that relate to the specified learning objectives. In this way, you will be learning the College-approved facts on the subject. There is also a very strong link between topics addressed in the exam and topics that have featured in these articles within the preceding two years. Every time you do some revision that relates to something on the syllabus, cross it off. Remember that a broad understanding is more important than learning a few topics in great detail.

Three types of questions

There are three main types of questions in the Final CRQ. Firstly, there are those that relate to new guidance or reports (such as National Audit Projects or National Institute for Health and Care Excellence guidance). Secondly, there are the questions that test knowledge of the manner of anaesthesia provision for specific operations or in particular situations. The third group assesses knowledge of how particular patient conditions impact on anaesthesia management. Sometimes, they mix all of these in together. Very often, questioning on facts seemingly very specific to the Primary FRCA are thrown into the mix as well, so ignore the basic sciences at your peril!

Questions relating to new guidance or reports

Questions based on these topics tend to feature within two years of their publication. Search the likely websites (Royal College of Anaesthetists, Difficult Airway Society, Obstetric Anaesthetists' Association, National Institute for Health and Care Excellence, Association of Anaesthetists) and be aware of new national guidelines that are implemented in your place of work. Also, be aware of topical causes of medical error, such as new additions to the list of never events that are relevant to anaesthesia and statements and alerts from the Safe Anaesthesia Liaison Group. Think about the impact of these guidelines at the organisational level, not just at the point of delivery of anaesthesia.

Questions relating to the anaesthetic management of a specific operation or situation

This includes questions about nerve blocks as well. Specific nerve blocks have peaks of popularity and the timing of inclusion of questions about them in the CRQ reflects this. Remember to learn the specific complications of such blocks, not just "bleeding, infection, nerve damage." It is by listing the specific complications that you demonstrate that you actually know the relevant anatomy.

When considering the anaesthetic management of any operation, think in terms of preoperative, intraoperative and postoperative. Preoperatively, consider history, examination and investigations. However, in no section of the exam should you ever state that you would "take a full history, examine the patient and request ECG, FBC and U&E." Instead, you need to take a much more targeted approach, especially in the CRQ. Specify why you are asking this question in this particular patient, what you are seeking in the examination of this particular patient, or what investigation anomalies may be found in this particular patient. Intraoperatively, consider mode of anaesthesia, airway management, positioning and its impact, likely duration and its impact, need for warming, thromboprophylaxis, particular needs for monitoring, risk of bleeding and any special issues relating to this type of surgery. This is all as you would in real life. Following the alphabet (see next section) may help you here. Postoperatively, think of where the patient is going to be cared for, any ongoing need for oxygen or ventilatory support and how you will manage pain, nausea and thromboprophylaxis. Start to practise this systematic way of thinking in advance of every case you do, such that you could write a shopping list and recipe for any case you are involved in. It will help you when you get to the viva too.

Questions relating to particular patient conditions and their impact on anaesthetic management

You may get a question about a medical condition you have never learned about or really considered. You will all be familiar with using an ABC approach to patient assessment or ABCDE for trauma management. I have just taken that alphabet a little further.

A: airway
B: respiratory
C: cardiovascular
D: neurological, both central and peripheral (disability)
E: endocrine
F: pharmacology
G: gastrointestinal
H: haematology
I: immunology, infection
J: cutaneomusculoskeletal (joints)
K: renal (kidneys)
L: hepatic (liver)
M: metabolic
N: nutrition
O: obstetric
P: psychological

Following this alphabet will help you dredge the depths of your brain for issues that relate to diabetes, rheumatoid arthritis or epidermolysis bullosa. I promise you. Obviously, not all elements of the alphabet are relevant every time, but get into the habit of using it well in advance of the exam.

Finish the paper

If you miss out a question, you will fail (although you don't need to pass all questions in order to pass the paper overall). Do not allow yourself to run out of time. If you run over by 10 minutes on a question you know well and are enjoying answering, you will find it very difficult to make up time elsewhere. You have 45 seconds for each mark.

One mark per line

The College have made it clear that you will not get more than one mark per line and so you are obliged to prioritise your answers. This reiterates the need to be specific in your approach rather than filling all the lines available with generic detail about how you would manage any anaesthetic or any emergency situation. The College have made it clear in their Reports that they want you to prioritise your answers so that they are as specific as possible to the question. Generic answers, even if true, may not get a mark.

Read the question

The Chairs' Reports will show you how often candidates run into difficulty for failing to read the question and they often say that all the information included in a question is there for a reason. Sometimes, two questions are asked within one section of a question – make sure you answer both bits. Abbreviations can cause confusion: ASD may mean autistic spectrum disorder or atrioseptal defect, but the College is always careful to specify what any abbreviation they use means. Another common error is failing to notice the change in the focus of a question. The first part may relate to children with autistic spectrum disorder, the second part may relate to management of any child for dental surgery, not just those with autistic spectrum disorder. Slow down and read carefully.

Abbreviations

Beware of using too many abbreviations yourself. Generally, if I have used an abbreviation, I define what I mean by it within that answer. Abbreviations that I have used without defining what they mean are listed in the front of the book and, I think, are commonly accepted.

Don't assume you don't know

Don't know the precise definition of cerebral palsy or autistic spectrum disorder? Visualise the people you have met affected by these conditions and describe them. Who: male, female, child, adult. When: lifelong, reversible, terminal. Why: genetic, infection related, trauma related. Keep calm and you will cobble together an answer that will gain you most of the marks available.

Improve your clinical knowledge

The Chairs' Reports have frequently commented on lack of knowledge impacting on answer quality. This is often clinical rather than book-based knowledge. It particularly affects subspecialties such as cardiothoracics and neurosurgery that not all candidates may have rotated through by the time they sit the exam. The College have advised that, currently (although this may change in the future), 6 of the 12 CRQs will be based on the mandatory units of training (neuro, cardiothoracics, intensive care medicine, paediatrics, pain medicine and obstetrics) with the rest from the other units. In the same way that a picture may be worth a thousand words, spending a day in cardiothoracic or neuro theatres will be invaluable. Trainees at my hospital have followed the College's advice and have arranged a couple of days' experience in these subspecialties and have found it very worthwhile. In the same way, you may need to be proactive in getting some experience in vascular surgery, the interventional radiology suite and magnetic resonance imaging. Failing that, there's nothing you can't find on YouTube.

Remember that you don't need to get many marks to pass

Recent Chairs' Reports have said that each paper contains an even proportion of difficult, moderately difficult and easy questions. The recent Reports have not specified how many points are needed to pass a question, but older Reports have said that the pass mark for difficult questions is 10–11/20, for moderately difficult 12–13/20 and for easy 14/20. You can therefore miss out great chunks of what is present on the model answer and still pass! This exam is within your grasp.

Practise past questions

Practising past questions is a fantastic way to revise for a number of reasons. Question topics commonly recur: if you encounter a question you have previously practised, you will be able to answer it more quickly and with less brain fatigue, leaving you more time and energy for other questions. Looking at past questions helps you to develop technique. Also, you will get a feel for the topics that the College considers important by looking at what they have previously included in the exam.

This book

The topics of 24 past papers are covered in this book. This reflects 16 SAQ papers, seven CRQ papers and the hybrid one in between. The SAQ papers are published on the College website and we have adapted them in this book into CRQ style. The real CRQs are not published on the website, but the Chairs' Reports make it clear what the topics and some of the subsections were and we have created subsections based on what we think are important areas of knowledge. For each question, the relevant section of the Chairs' (or Chair's, before September 2015) Report is reproduced (where available), followed by our answers. We have included diagrams and additional commentary (in italics) to ensure that this book helps you to learn rather than just being a list of suggested model answers. We have no way of knowing how close our questions or answers are to the College's model answers, but they are referenced and represent a summary of the key topics that the College perceive as important. All have taken much more time to produce than you will have available to you in the exam and are answered much more extensively than the few words that the College wants from you in your answers (see the example CRQ model answers on the RCoA website). You must remember this when you are considering what level of detail of recall is required. You would not, therefore, need to write this level of detail in order to gain a pass in the exam.

ACKNOWLEDGEMENTS

We are very grateful to those who have read and revised sections of this book: Dr Andy Combeer, Epsom and St Helier University Hospitals: Drs Elaine Hipwell, Tom Heinink, Rebecca Thorne, David Timbrell, Sabina Bachtold and John Bailes, who are colleagues at Frimley Park Hospital: Drs Dom Spray, Elaine Monahan and Michael Puntis of St George's Hospital, London: and Dr Rehana Iqbal of Mediclinic City Hospital, Dubai. Our thanks also to Paul Hatton, who has kindly produced the excellent diagrams for fun and because he believes in contributing to education. Thanks also to the Royal College of Anaesthetists for allowing us to reproduce the SAQ questions and excerpts from the Chairs' Reports.

A massive thank you to Dr Mitul Patel, who has shared the work of this edition with me and has been able to give me a much more current view of the exam. I really couldn't have done it without him. I am thankful to my junior colleagues at Frimley, past and present, who come to Thursday afternoon teaching and help me to try to stay up-to-date. Finally, thanks to my family for their support, especially to my husband, who has been incredibly patient in allowing me the time to write this and to our children, George, Lucy, Thomas and Edward, who would rather I don't get involved in book writing again.

Dr Elizabeth Combeer

I would like to thank the supervisors and consultant bodies across Kent, Surrey, Sussex, South London and Wessex deaneries who have been integral to my training and development and who have made pursuing a career in anaesthesia extremely enjoyable. A special thanks is reserved for Dr Elizabeth Combeer, whose fierce dedication to education is an inspiration and without whom this second edition would not have been possible.

I am forever grateful to my parents and family for their unwavering support. Finally, thank you to my wife for making me smile when the depths of physiology, pharmacology and physics succeeded in achieving the opposite.

Dr Mitul Patel

ANAESTHESIA FOR NEUROSURGERY, NEURORADIOLOGY AND NEUROCRITICAL CARE

1.1 September 2011 Spinal cord injury

a) List the characteristic sensory, motor and autonomic neurological changes that occur <u>immediately</u> following transection of the spinal cord at the fourth thoracic vertebra. (3 marks)

b) List the characteristic sensory, motor and autonomic neurological changes that occur three months after transection of the spinal cord at the fourth thoracic vertebra. (3 marks)

c) State three ventilatory changes associated with complete transection of the spinal cord at the fourth thoracic vertebra. (3 marks)

d) List two gastrointestinal complications of spinal cord injury. (2 marks)

e) Give two reasons why patients with a recent spinal cord injury have an increased risk of thromboembolic disease. (2 marks)

f) Give one reason for poor body temperature regulation associated with spinal cord injury. (1 mark)

g) List four advantages of a regional anaesthetic technique for a cystoscopy in a patient with a previous spinal cord injury. (4 marks)

h) Why and when may suxamethonium be contraindicated in a patient with spinal cord injury? (2 marks)

The College likes this topic – it tests your neuroanaesthesia knowledge but also some primary anatomy and physiology. There was no Chair's Report for this paper.

a) List the characteristic sensory, motor and autonomic neurological changes that occur <u>immediately</u> following transection of the spinal cord at the fourth thoracic vertebra. (3 marks)

b) List the characteristic sensory, motor and autonomic neurological changes that occur three months after transection of the spinal cord at the fourth thoracic vertebra. (3 marks)

I have presented all the answers together in a table for revision purposes. There is more information here than would be necessary to achieve the total of six marks attributed to these two questions.

	Immediate	Changes at three months
Sensory	• Complete sensory loss below the T4 dermatome, extending cranially if there is secondary neurological injury e.g. oedema affecting the spinal cord.	• Ongoing anaesthesia below the T4 dermatome, extending proximally if secondary neurological injury present. • Development of neuropathic pain at or below the T4 dermatome. • Nociceptive pain may develop related to musculoskeletal injury caused by changes in function e.g. wheelchair use, muscle weakness and muscle spasm.

(Continued)

DOI: 10.1201/9781003388494-1

(Continued)

	Immediate	Changes at three months
Motor	• Spinal shock: flaccid paralysis with areflexia affecting lower intercostals, trunk and lower limbs (as even monosynaptic reflexes are dependent on descending tonic facilitation).	• Ongoing paralysis below the T4 dermatome (or more proximally if secondary neurological injury present). • Hyper-reflexia with spasticity. Initially, upregulation of receptors facilitates reflexes, then new interneurones develop.
Autonomic	• Hypotension (neurogenic shock) due to interruption of sympathetic pathways leaving unopposed parasympathetic activity. • If secondary injury extends cranially to affect cardioaccelerator fibres (T1–T4 segments), then bradycardia and reduced myocardial contractility occur, further worsening hypotension. • Loss of temperature control due to anhidrosis and cutaneous dilatation below T4 dermatome. • Loss of bowel and bladder function. • Occasionally, priapism may occur.	• Autonomic dysreflexia: non-noxious stimuli below the level of the lesion cause disproportionate reflex sympathetic output, resulting in lower body and splanchnic vasoconstriction increasing blood pressure. Life-threatening hypertensive crisis may occur (with headache, flushing, nasal congestion, seizures, retinal haemorrhages, stroke and coma). Rising blood pressure stimulates (via baroreceptors) parasympathetic activity above the level of the lesion causing bradycardia and vasodilation, but this may be insufficient to reduce blood pressure to normal. The effect is worse in high cord lesions. Onset is variable, taking up to a year to develop. • Bowel, bladder and coital reflexes return but may remain impaired. Many patients require catheterisation.

c) **State three ventilatory changes associated with complete transection of the spinal cord at the fourth thoracic vertebra. (3 marks)**

The outcome is variable, as a patient with transection at T4 may have symptoms of a higher lesion due to secondary neurological injury.

- Loss of abdominal muscle contraction leads to weak forced expiration and impaired cough with retained secretions.
- Loss of innervation of lower intercostal muscles impairs the expansion of the chest wall and the vital capacity is reduced.
- Ventilation is worse in the sitting position. Abdominal contents pull down on the diaphragm, thus expanding expiratory intrathoracic volume and increasing residual volume. Volume for expansion in inspiration is therefore reduced and an increased proportion of minute ventilation therefore used on ventilating dead space, resulting in V/Q mismatch and atelectasis.
- Loss of abdominal wall and intercostal muscle tone results in inefficient ventilation: the diaphragm contracts, pushes abdominal contents down and out due to loss of abdominal wall tone and the chest wall is pulled in.

d) **List two gastrointestinal complications of spinal cord injury. (2 marks)**

- Reduced gastrointestinal motility: delayed gastric emptying (aspiration risk), paralytic ileus, constipation, pseudo-obstruction.
- Increased risk of gall stones and their complications (thought to relate to altered motility of gastrointestinal structures causing slower transit of bile out of the gall bladder, altered enterohepatic circulation and metabolic changes causing altered bile lipids).
- Prone to stress ulceration due to unopposed vagal activity causing increased gastric acid production.

e) Give two reasons why patients with a recent spinal cord injury have an increased risk of thromboembolic disease. (2 marks)

The risk of death from pulmonary embolism is high in patients with spinal cord injury, contributed to by their increased risk of thromboembolic disease but also their inability to detect the limb changes that are associated with deep vein thrombosis which would prompt anticoagulant treatment. They are also at increased risk of ischaemic heart disease, partly due to their long-term prothrombotic state but also due to inability to undertake exercise. You will see that all three components of Virchow's triad are represented in the answer below.

- Immobility causing venous stasis.
- Loss of calf muscle pump activity causing venous stasis.
- Thrombogenic effect of the stress response of trauma.
- Inflammatory response of trauma causing endothelial damage.
- Use of venous lines.
- Associated surgery causing an increase in stress response.

f) Give one reason for poor body temperature regulation associated with spinal cord injury. (1 mark)

- Vasodilation below the level of spinal cord injury.
- Inability to sweat below the level of spinal cord injury *(risk of hyperhidrosis above the level of the injury)*.
- Inability to shiver below the level of the spinal cord injury.
- Loss of sensation of cold or hot environment below level of spinal cord injury.
- Loss of movement.
- Decrease in muscle bulk and reduced metabolic rate.

g) List four advantages of a regional anaesthetic technique for a cystoscopy in a patient with a previous spinal cord injury. (4 marks)

- Reduces the risk of autonomic dysreflexia.
- Avoids the need for intubation of a patient who may have previously had a tracheostomy with its attendant complications e.g. tracheal stenosis.
- Avoids the deterioration in lung function associated with general anaesthesia, thus reducing the risk of postoperative respiratory complications.
- Avoids opioid use with associated respiratory depression in a patient with compromised respiratory function.
- Reduces the risk of aspiration associated with delayed gastric emptying.
- Avoidance of unopposed parasympathetic response to airway instrumentation (bradycardia, cardiac arrest).

h) Why and when may suxamethonium be contraindicated in a patient with spinal cord injury? (2 marks)

- Upregulation of nicotinic acetylcholine receptors in extrajunctional sites results in massive potassium release with suxamethonium use.
- This effect is seen between approximately 72 hours following injury and six months.

REFERENCES

Bonner S, Smith C. Initial management of acute spinal cord injury. *Contin Educ Anaesth Crit Care Pain.* 2013: 13: 224–231.

Petsas A, Drake J. Perioperative management for patients with a chronic spinal cord injury. *BJA Educ.* 2015: 15: 123–130.

1.2 September 2012 Raised intracranial pressure

a) State three symptoms of raised intracranial pressure (ICP) in an adult. (3 marks)
b) Describe three signs of raised ICP in an adult. (3 marks)
c) Give the upper limit (mmHg) of normal ICP in an adult. (1 mark)
d) List two invasive monitoring methods of ICP in a patient with traumatic brain injury. (2 marks)
e) List eight management goals that may be undertaken in the Emergency Department of a non-neurosurgical centre to initiate optimal treatment of a patient with traumatic brain injury. (8 marks)
f) Give two pharmacological options, with doses, that may be used to treat acute rises in intracranial pressure whilst preparing for definitive neurosurgical intervention. (2 marks)
g) Give one other temporising measure for management of acute rises in intracranial pressure. (1 mark)

The Chair's Report of the original SAQ commented that many candidates misread one of the subsections and the pass rate for the question was 56%. This is a common topic in the written exam, the viva and real life and should be one that you are comfortable with answering.

a) **State three symptoms of raised intracranial pressure (ICP) in an adult. (3 marks)**

- Headache: bursting, throbbing *(exacerbated by sneezing, exertion, recumbency, and the raised PaCO$_2$ associated with sleep).*
- Vomiting *(often accompanies the headache and so tends to be worse in the morning after waking).*
- Visual disturbance.

b) **Describe three signs of raised ICP in an adult. (3 marks)**

- Progressive reduction in consciousness due to caudal displacement of midbrain.
- Eye signs including papilloedema, fundal haemorrhages, pupillary dilatation, ptosis, impaired upward gaze (midbrain compression), and abducens palsy.
- Motor features including ataxia, abnormal posturing, focal neurological deficit, and seizure activity.
- Respiratory irregularity, Cheyne-Stokes breathing, neurogenic hyperventilation due to tonsillar herniation.
- Cushing's triad of hypertension with high pulse pressure, bradycardia, and associated irregular respiration *(indicative of brainstem ischaemia associated with herniation).*

c) **Give the upper limit (mmHg) of normal ICP in an adult. (1 mark)**

- 15 mmHg.

d) **List two invasive monitoring methods of ICP in a patient with traumatic brain injury. (2 marks)**

- Intraventricular catheter *(also referred to as an external ventricular drain – can be calibrated and can be used to therapeutically drain CSF).*
- Transducer pressure monitoring in subdural, intraparenchymal, subarachnoid or epidural space. *(Transducer may be a balloon, strain gauge, or fibreoptic tip. Once it is sited, there is no ability to recalibrate it. May not reflect variation of intracranial pressure in different parts of brain.)*

e) List eight management goals that may be undertaken in the Emergency Department of a non-neurosurgical centre to initiate optimal treatment of a patient with traumatic brain injury. (8 marks)

According to the Monro-Kellie doctrine, the cranium is a closed compartment and so has a fixed capacity. If there is an increase in one component of its contents (brain, CSF, blood in blood vessels, other) some compensation can occur by reducing the amount of one of the other components. Once these compensatory mechanisms are exhausted, ICP will rise, ultimately causing pressure on the brain and direct tissue damage. This typically occurs > 20 mmHg (the Brain Trauma Foundation guidelines advise initiating treatment > 22 mmHg to prevent mortality). As ICP rises, the cerebral perfusion pressure will decrease according to the equation:

$$CPP = MAP - ICP$$

This will cause ischaemic brain damage. Successful initial management of a brain injured patient help to manipulate the size of the components in the closed box and reduce the risk of secondary brain injury. In real life, or a question with a different approach, don't forget that this patient may have a cervical spine injury too.

- Tracheal intubation if GCS ≤ 8, if not maintaining adequate gas exchange, has lost protective laryngeal reflexes, is spontaneously hyperventilating, or has irregular respirations.
- Avoid hypoxia, aim PaO_2 > 13 kPa.
- Maintain $PaCO_2$ between 4.5 and 5.0 kPa.
- Maintain MAP > 80 mmHg replacing lost volume with non-hypotonic fluid, blood if indicated, and using vasopressor if required.
- Adequate sedation (and analgesia) to reduce $CMRO_2$.
- Muscle paralysis if needed to facilitate ventilation to desired PaO_2 and $PaCO_2$ and if patient not synchronising with ventilator.
- Facilitate venous drainage by 30–45 degree head-up tilt, avoidance of tight tube ties, avoidance of PEEP > 12 cmH_2O or high peak airway pressures while ensuring adequate gas exchange and adopting a lung protective strategy (*higher airway pressures may later be used if monitoring shows ICP remains normal and is PEEP insensitive*).
- Treatment of seizures.
- Maintenance of normoglycaemia, < 10 mmol/l.
- Maintenance of normothermia.
- Discuss with regional neurosurgical unit to arrange early transfer.

f) Give two pharmacological options, with doses, that may be used to treat acute rises in intracranial pressure whilst preparing for definitive neurosurgical intervention. (2 marks)

- Mannitol 0.25–1 g/kg.
- Hypertonic saline 3% 2 ml/kg.

g) Give one other temporising measure for management of acute rises in intracranial pressure. (1 mark)

- Hyperventilation to a $PaCO_2$ of 4–4.5 kPa.

REFERENCES

Dinsmore J. Traumatic brain injury: an evidence-based review of management. *Contin Educ Anaesth Crit Care Pain.* 2013; 13: 189–195.

Elwishi M, Dinsmore J. Monitoring the brain. *BJA Educ.* 2019: 19: 54–59.

National Institute for Health and Care Excellence. *Head injury: assessment and early management: CG176*, Last updated September 2019.

Picetti E et al. Early management of isolated severe traumatic brain injury patients in a hospital without neurosurgical capabilities: a consensus and clinical recommendations of the World Society of Emergency Medicine (WSES). *World J Emerg Surg.* 2023: 18: 5.

Robba C et al. Mechanical ventilation in patients with acute brain injury: recommendations of the European Society of Intensive Care Medicine consensus. *Intensive Care Med.* 2020: 46: 2397–2410.

Tameem A, Krovvidi H. Cerebral physiology. *Contin Educ Anaesth Crit Care Pain.* 2013: 13: 113–118.

Wiles M et al. Management of traumatic brain injury in the non-neurosurgical intensive care unit: a narrative review of current evidence. *Anaesthesia.* 2023: 78: 510–520.

1.3 March 2013 Acromegaly and trans-sphenoidal hypophysectomy

A 45-year-old male with acromegaly presents for an elective trans-sphenoidal hypophysectomy.
a) What is the cause of acromegaly in <u>this</u> patient? (1 mark)
b) Where is the pituitary gland located? (1 mark)
c) State the visual impairment characteristically associated with a large pituitary tumour. (1 mark)
d) Describe the blood supply to the pituitary gland. (2 marks)
e) List two hormones secreted by the posterior pituitary gland. (2 marks)
f) List six clinical features of acromegaly of relevance to the anaesthetist. (6 marks)
g) How do the surgical requirements for this procedure influence the conduct of the anaesthesia? (4 marks)
h) State three specific complications of trans-sphenoidal hypophysectomy. (3 marks)

The SAQ on this topic had a 57% pass rate, but the Chair's Report suggested "that many candidates had not had experience of managing these patients for this type of surgery. Some candidates quoted the prone position for surgical access!"

a) **What is the likely cause of acromegaly in <u>this</u> patient? (1 mark)**

Adenomas can be microadenomas or macroadenomas: macroadenomas may also present with raised ICP or visual field defects (bitemporal hemianopia). Rarely, growth hormone can be secreted from non-pituitary tumours – but these patients would not be having a trans-sphenoidal resection.

- Hypersecretion of growth hormone from a pituitary adenoma.

b) **Where is the pituitary gland located? (1 mark)**

- Sits in the sella turcica, which is the part of the sphenoid bone.

A little bit of revision about the anatomy and function of the pituitary (as I don't want you to be one of the people who think that it is best accessed from the back of the head).

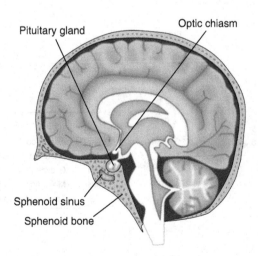

Sagittal section of the pituitary gland.

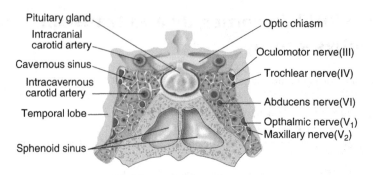

Coronal section of the pituitary gland.

c) State the visual impairment characteristically associated with a large pituitary tumour. (1 mark)

● Bitemporal hemianopia.

d) Describe the blood supply to the pituitary gland. (2 marks)

● The pituitary receives arterial supply from the hypophyseal and inferior hypophyseal arteries, which are branches of the internal carotid artery.
● The arteries anastomose with each other to form vascular plexuses around the gland and a portal circulation which connects to the dural venous sinuses and the hypothalamus.
● Venous drainage is into the cavernous and petrosal sinuses.

e) List two hormones secreted by the posterior pituitary. (2 marks)

● Anti-diuretic hormone (ADH)/vasopressin.
● Oxytocin.

Adenohypophysis or anterior pituitary: hypothalamus releases inhibitory or secretory factors, which travel via the portal system to the anterior pituitary, where they control the release of the anterior pituitary hormones.

Neurohypophysis or posterior pituitary: neurosecretory cells in the hypothalamus make oxytocin and vasopressin, which travel down axons to be released from the posterior pituitary.

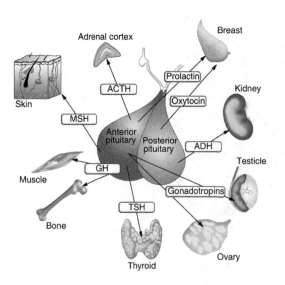

Pituitary gland hormones.

f) List six clinical features of acromegaly of relevance to the anaesthetist. (6 marks)

Now you are being asked about the features of acromegaly generally. Back to the alphabet.

Airway:

- Large lips, macroglossia, macrognathia, thickening of pharyngeal tissues, laryngeal stenosis. Possibility of difficult airway should be considered.

Respiratory:

- Obstructive sleep apnoea (OSA) with risk of hypoventilation and respiratory failure postoperatively.

Cardiovascular:

- Hypertension, left ventricular hypertrophy, cardiomyopathy with diastolic dysfunction, valvular regurgitation, ECG changes.
- Increased peripheral soft tissue deposition may make cannulation difficult.

Neurological:

- Raised ICP (obstruction of the third ventricle).
- Spinal cord compression. Meticulous care with padding and positioning required.
- Peripheral neuropathies due to impingement by soft tissue or bony overgrowth.

Endocrine:

- Diabetes mellitus. Blood glucose should be monitored and managed with insulin intraoperatively if necessary.

Gastrointestinal:

- Increased risk of colonic polyps and cancer – may necessitate surgery.

Cutaneomusculoskeletal:

- Osteoarthritis, bony overgrowth around joints, limited movement. Care with positioning and padding.

Renal:

- Renal dysfunction may impact on perioperative drug choices.

g) How do the surgical requirements for this procedure influence the conduct of the anaesthesia? (4 marks)

Even if you have never seen this operation before, you know something about the logistics of anaesthesia where the patient's head is distant from the anaesthetist from doing ENT surgery.

Surgical requirement	Conduct of anaesthesia
Use of operating microscope.	"Hypotensive" anaesthesia, intra-arterial monitoring, immobile patient (muscle relaxant or remifentanil infusion). Preparation of nasal mucosa with e.g. Moffat's solution or phenylephrine.
Periods of intense stimulation and periods of minimal stimulation.	Blood pressure may be very labile, necessitating intra-arterial monitoring. Remifentanil is ideal for management of periods of intense stimulation.
Supine position with head-up tilt.	Potential for air embolism. Ensure adequate intravenous filling.

(Continued)

(Continued)

Surgical requirement	Conduct of anaesthesia
Operation on head.	Airway under drapes, armoured tube, anaesthetist distant from airway, meticulous securing of tube, protection of eyes, nerve stimulator on leg, circuit extensions for breathing system and for intravenous fluids.
Risk of bleeding from internal carotid or cavernous sinus.	Intubate (anticipate difficult airway), throat pack, two group and save samples preoperatively.
Rapid emergence, need ability to assess neurology as soon as possible postoperatively.	Use of short-acting and rapidly reversible agents.
Suprasellar portion of tumour may need pushing into surgical field.	Lumbar drain with injection of saline or, less commonly, controlled ventilation to ensure high-normal $PaCO_2$.
Avoid postoperative surges in ICP, especially if CSF leak has occurred.	Smooth emergence, adequate reversal, adequate antiemetic, airway and CPAP for known OSA.

h) State three specific complications of trans-sphenoidal hypophysectomy. (3 marks)

- Surgical damage to anatomically related structures:
    - Cranial nerve III, IV, V, or VI palsy.
    - Visual field defects (proximity of optic chiasm).
    - Major haemorrhage.
    - CSF leak.
- Postoperative endocrine dysfunction:
    - Diabetes insipidus – may resolve spontaneously.
    - SIADH.
    - Hypopituitarism – steroid replacement with weaning regimen may be required.
- Pituitary apoplexy.
- Venous air embolus (rare, but theoretically possible due to sitting position).

REFERENCE

Menon R, Murphy P, Lindley A. Anaesthesia and pituitary disease. *Contin Educ Anaesth Crit Care Pain.* 2011: 11: 133–137.

1.4 September 2013 Posterior fossa surgery

A 34-year-old man is scheduled for a posterior fossa tumour excision.
a) Apart from the sitting position, give three patient positions that might be employed for this operation. (3 marks)
b) Venous air embolism is a complication of the sitting position. Give four other specific complications of the sitting position. (4 marks)
c) Give three abnormalities in routine intraoperative monitoring which may develop as a consequence of venous air embolism. (3 marks)
d) List three different monitoring techniques that can specifically detect the presence of venous air embolism during surgery and the features that would indicate the diagnosis for each monitor. (6 marks)
e) After calling for help and assessing the patient in a systematic manner, list four steps that can be undertaken to manage a significant venous air embolism in this patient. (4 marks)

The Chair's Report of the original SAQ stated that inexperience in anaesthesia for this type of surgery was apparent, with a 48.4% pass rate. This may be a type of surgery you do not see by the time of sitting your exam. However, the line of questioning about posterior fossa surgery, in either the written exam or the viva, will usually focus on the risks of positioning and diagnosis and management of venous air embolus, all of which are covered here.

a) **Apart from the sitting position, give three patient positions that might be employed for this operation. (3 marks)**

Search for images of the different positions for neurosurgery. It will really help you to retain the information about their associated complications. The sitting position is associated with significant risk but is good for access to midline lesions. Gravity assists venous and CSF drainage, thus improving the surgical field and facilitating access to deeper structures.

- Supine with head turned, supported by sandbags *(may be suitable for acoustic neuroma or cerebellopontine angle tumours)*.
- Prone *(as with the sitting position, this offers good access for midline structures)*.
- Lateral *(good access for lateral structures)*.
- Park bench *(modification of the lateral position with the patient semi-prone, head flexed to face the floor, offering greater access to the midline, avoiding the need for sitting or prone positioning)*.

b) **Venous air embolism is a complication of the sitting position. Give four other specific complications of the sitting position. (4 marks)**

These are all individual complications but have been grouped by body system to help you memorise them.

Airway:

- Endotracheal tube displacement.
- Jugular venous obstruction due to flexed neck causing laryngeal and tongue oedema with postoperative airway compromise.

Cardiovascular:

- Hypotension due to reduced venous return due to venous pooling in dependent areas.

Neurological:

- Cord or brainstem ischaemia due to head flexion and hypotension.
- Sciatic and femoral nerve damage from excessive hip flexion compounded by lower limb oedema due to dependent positioning.
- Pneumocephalus (delayed recovery, neurological deficit, confusion, headache).

Cutaneomusculoskeletal:

- Compartment syndrome.
- Lumbosacral pressure damage.

c) **Give three abnormalities in routine intraoperative monitoring which may develop as a consequence of venous air embolism. (3 marks)**

- Drop in SpO_2.
- Decrease in $etCO_2$.
- ST segment depression on ECG monitoring.
- Tachyarrhythmia.
- Hypotension.

d) **List three different monitoring techniques that can specifically detect the presence of venous air embolism during surgery and the features that would indicate the diagnosis for each monitor. (6 marks)**

In practice, precordial Doppler is used alongside gas exchange, invasive arterial and possibly central venous monitoring and, just as importantly, clinical suspicion.

Precordial Doppler:	Sound heard if air present in cardiac chambers *(this is the most sensitive noninvasive device).*
Transoesophageal echocardiography:	Air seen in right-sided cardiac chambers. *(In the presence of patent foramen ovale, it can detect air in the left heart also. Not necessarily suitable for long operations where the head is flexed.)*
Pulmonary artery or right atrial pressure:	Pulmonary artery pressure will rise with a significant air embolus and related right ventricular outflow tract obstruction can cause rise in right atrial pressure. *(Not routinely indicated for this purpose.)*
Oesophageal stethoscope:	"Mill wheel murmur". *(A large volume of air is required to cause the noise, at which point cardiovascular collapse may have occurred.)*
End-tidal nitrogen level:	Sudden rise in end-tidal nitrogen due to presence of nitrogen in the air embolus. *(More sensitive and specific for VAE than $etCO_2$ changes but not readily available.)*

e) **After calling for help and assessing the patient in a systematic manner, list four steps that can be undertaken to manage a significant venous air embolism in this patient. (4 marks)**

Each of the following is a separate step, but they have been grouped in order to assist with learning.

- Prevent further air entry:
  - Ask surgeon to flood site with saline and cover with wet packs.
  - Administer fluids especially if hypovolaemia thought to be contributory to air entrainment.
  - Lower the head of patient so that the surgical site is below the right atrium if possible.
  - Apply sustained positive airway pressure until these measures have been achieved.
- Reduce size of air embolism:
  - Administer 100% oxygen.
  - Stop nitrous oxide if it is being used.
  - Aspirate air from right atrium via central line if one is present.

- Overcome mechanical obstruction:
  - Left lateral or Trendelenburg positioning may help force bubble above the right ventricular outflow.
  - If the patient suffers cardiac arrest or severe haemodynamic compromise, chest compressions may assist in dispersing the bubble.
  - Inotropic support may be required.

REFERENCES

Association of Anaesthetists. *Quick Reference Handbook: 3–5 circulatory embolus v1*, 2018. https://anaesthetists.org/Home/Resources-publications/Safety-alerts/Anaesthesia-emergencies/Quick-Reference-Handbook-QRH/PDF-version. Accessed 21st March 2023.

Jagannathan S, Krovvidi H. Anaesthetic considerations for posterior fossa surgery. *Contin Educ Anaesth Crit Care Pain*. 2014: 14: 202–206.

1.5 March 2014 Stereotactic brain biopsy

A 64-year-old man is scheduled for a stereotactic brain biopsy. He is taking dual antiplatelet therapy (DAPT) following the insertion of a drug-eluting coronary artery stent six months previously.

a) Give three possible consequences of continuing antiplatelet medication in the perioperative period. (3 marks)
b) Give two possible consequences of premature cessation of DAPT in order to facilitate brain biopsy in this patient. (2 marks)
c) List four patient factors that will increase the risk of an ischaemic event following premature cessation of DAPT in this patient. (4 marks)
d) Give three approaches that may mitigate patient risk if a decision is made to stop DAPT in order to facilitate the stereotactic brain biopsy. (3 marks)
e) List four specific contraindications to stereotactic brain biopsy under sedation. (4 marks)
f) List four specific complications of stereotactic brain biopsy under sedation. (4 marks)

The Chair's Report following the original SAQ commented that "candidates misread or misinterpreted the question [and] did not appreciate that the management of antiplatelet therapy requires a balance of risks in a patient for whom intraoperative bleeding could be a critical event. Many candidates mentioned stent thrombosis and intracranial/extracranial haemorrhage but did not explain why these events would be important even though the question specifically asks for these details." The pass rate was 32.9%.

a) **Give three possible consequences of continuing antiplatelet medication in the perioperative period. (3 marks)**

- Significant extracranial bleeding.
- Intraparenchymal haemorrhage with limited ability to access the source and therefore control it.
- Haematoma development with pressure effect on brain resulting in specific neurological deficits or raised intracranial pressure.

b) **Give two possible consequences of premature cessation of DAPT in order to facilitate brain biopsy in this patient. (2 marks)**

- Risk of stent thrombosis which carries a high mortality risk.
- Risk of myocardial infarction or ischaemia as a consequence of pre-existing coronary artery disease.
- Rebound increase in tendency to thrombosis following cessation of ADP receptor antagonist.

c) **List four patient factors that will increase the risk of an ischaemic event following premature cessation of DAPT in this patient. (4 marks)**

- Cigarette smoking.
- Diabetes mellitus.
- Congestive heart failure/LVEF < 30%.
- Having had PCI prior to the PCI six months previously.
- Previous MI.
- MI as the indication for PCI and DES.

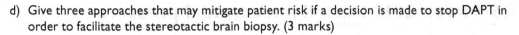

d) Give three approaches that may mitigate patient risk if a decision is made to stop DAPT in order to facilitate the stereotactic brain biopsy. (3 marks)

- Perform brain biopsy in a centre with on-site 24-hour interventional cardiology support to attempt to mitigate the severity of any thrombosis that occurs.
- Consideration of bridging with a short-acting GP IIb/IIIa inhibitor, starting within 24 hours of stopping ADP receptor blocker.
- Consideration of bridging with short acting, reversible $P2Y_{12}$ receptor antagonist, cangrelor.
- Consideration of continuing aspirin in the perioperative period if high risk of stent thrombosis and neurosurgeon deems the biopsy low risk for bleeding.

e) List four possible specific contraindications to stereotactic brain biopsy under sedation. (4 marks)

- Patient unable to comply with instruction e.g. learning disability, dementia, poor hearing.
- Patient refusal.
- Patient movement disorder, inability to lie still, inability to lie flat.
- Chronic cough.
- Significant sleep apnoea.
- Difficult airway.
- Patient anxiety or claustrophobia.

f) List four specific complications of stereotactic brain biopsy under sedation. (4 marks)

- Loss of airway and difficulties with access due to the use of a frame.
- Patient obtundation and therefore rise in $PaCO_2$ and decrease in PaO_2, which may cause increase in intracranial pressure and potential implications for the biopsy.
- Patient movement making biopsy not feasible or causing complications.
- Patient pain due to inadequate topicalisation of scalp or inadequate analgesia.
- Risk of nausea and vomiting due to e.g. opioid analgesia, stress.

REFERENCES

Barron T et al. Management of antithrombotic therapy in patients undergoing invasive procedures. *N Engl J Med*. 2013: 368: 2113–2124.

Burnand C, Sebastian J. Anaesthesia for awake craniotomy. *Contin Educ Anaesth Crit Care Pain*. 2014: 14: 6–11.

Dorairaj I, Hancock S. Anaesthesia for interventional neuroradiology. *Contin Educ Anaesth Crit Care Pain*. 2008: 8: 86–89.

Ramalingam G, Jones N, Besser M. Platelet for anaesthetists: part 2: pharmacology. *BJA Educ*. 2016: 16: 140–145.

Valgimigli M et al. 2017 ESC focused update on dual antiplatelet therapy in coronary artery disease developed in collaboration with EACTS: the task force for dual antiplatelet therapy in coronary artery disease of the European Society of Cardiology (ESC) and the European Association for Cardiothoracic Surgery (EACTS). *Eur Heart J*. 2018: 39: 213–260.

1.6 March 2015 Raised intracranial pressure

A 54-year-old patient is admitted to the emergency department following a traumatic brain injury. A CT scan reveals only cerebral oedema.

a) What is secondary brain injury and when is it likely to occur? (2 marks)
b) Outline four physiological and cellular changes associated with secondary brain injury. (4 marks)
c) List four indications for immediate intubation of this patient. (4 marks)
d) Give three respiratory goals for minimising the risk of secondary brain injury in this patient. (3 marks)
e) Give two cardiovascular goals for minimising the risk of secondary brain injury in this patient. (2 marks)
f) Give three other measures undertaken to minimise the risk of secondary brain injury in this patient. (3 marks)
g) Give two methods of managing acute rises in intracranial pressure whilst awaiting transfer to a neurosurgical centre. (2 marks)

The Chair's Report of the original SAQ commented that the 8.3% pass rate was "disturbing". They said, "Management of head injury not requiring neurosurgery is common to most intensive care units. Many candidates were unable to define secondary injury or give an appropriate time frame. Most were unaware of the pathophysiological cellular mechanisms and focused solely on the Monro-Kellie doctrine. Overall knowledge of NICE guidelines was superficial and most candidates did not define the physiological goals for therapy in enough detail. Treatment options were too narrow in scope although the information given was usually sensible. Examiners were left with the overall impression that many candidates have little theoretical knowledge or practical experience of care of the brain injured patient."

a) What is secondary brain injury and when is it likely to occur? (2 marks)

Primary brain injury occurs due to the initial insult and depends on the nature, intensity, and duration of impact. Macroscopically, it may involve fracture, contusion, haematoma, cerebral oedema, and diffuse brain injury. Microscopically it will involve cell wall disruption and increased membrane permeability disrupting ionic haemostasis.

- Primary brain injury causes a series of metabolic, inflammatory and vascular processes that may lead to secondary tissue damage beyond the initial injury site over the subsequent hours to days. It may be mediated by cerebral oedema, localised tissue hypoxia, excitotoxicity, or metabolic dysfunction. Additionally, systemic complications of traumatic brain injury may result in cardiovascular dysfunction causing further damage due to cerebral hypoperfusion and hypoxia.

b) Outline four physiological and cellular changes associated with secondary brain injury. (4 marks)

- Raised intracranial pressure in association with systemic hypotension may cause reduced cerebral perfusion pressure which can result in cerebral hypoperfusion with tissue ischaemia and inadequate substrate delivery.
- Local tissue damage causes excessive release of excitatory neurotransmitters (excitotoxicity), resulting in calcium influx to cells, cell oedema, and death.
- Injured cells release inflammatory mediators (platelet activating factor, leukotrienes, reactive oxygen species) that affect the blood brain barrier and increase blood vessel permeability, resulting in vasogenic oedema, raising ICP further.
- Impaired cell membrane function leads to accumulation of intracellular water and cytotoxic oedema. This increases intracerebral pressure and worsens tissue perfusion causing worsening injury.

- Impaired cerebral autoregulation may cause increased cerebral blood flow and vasogenic oedema with subsequent raised ICP.
- Hypoxia, hypotension, hyper- or hypocapnia and hyper- or hypoglycaemia will exacerbate secondary brain injury, worsen ability to autoregulate, cause direct changes to brain tissue size and therefore impact on ICP and perfusion, thus perpetuating a downward vicious cycle.
- Seizures will cause a significant increase in cerebral metabolism leading to ischaemia, cellular dysfunction and increased ICP. Generalised tonic-clonic seizures will also raise metabolic rate and, if ventilation is not increased, lead to raised $PaCO_2$ causing further increases in ICP.

c) List four indications for immediate intubation of this patient. (4 marks)

The information required for these next subsections is similar to that required in the question from September 2012. This answer is based on NICE CG176, which was originally published in 2014 and then featured in the exam a year later. However, even if you haven't read the guidance, I believe that anyone who has managed brain injured patients in the emergency department should know this answer.

- Coma, GCS ≤ 8.
- Loss or impairment of laryngeal reflexes.
- Ventilatory insufficiency (PaO_2 < 13 kPa, $PaCO_2$ > 6 kPa).
- Spontaneous hyperventilation causing $PaCO_2$ < 4 kPa.
- Irregular respirations.

d) Give three respiratory goals for minimising the risk of secondary brain injury in this patient. (3 marks)

- Target PaO_2 greater than 13 kPa.
- Target $PaCO_2$ 4.5–5.0 kPa.
- Avoiding excessive PEEP (aim < 12 cmH_2O) and high mean airway pressures whilst maintaining adequate ventilation and ensuring lung protective strategy.

e) Give two cardiovascular goals for minimising the risk of secondary brain injury in this patient. (2 marks)

- Maintain MAP > 80 mmHg replacing lost volume with non-hypotonic fluid, blood if indicated, and using vasopressor if needed.
- Facilitate venous drainage by 30–45 degree head-up tilt, avoidance of tight tube ties, avoidance of excessive PEEP or mean airway pressures (while ensuring adequate gas exchange and adopting a lung protective strategy), use of NMBD if coughing or straining on tube.

f) Give three other measures undertaken to minimise the risk of secondary brain injury in this patient. (3 marks)

Different guidelines have given slightly different target ranges for glycaemic control over the years depending on the evidence they have referenced, which depends on precisely how those studies were structured and what the limits of the control and intervention arms of the studies were. It currently seems that the target for any patient with a compromised brain should be < 10 mmol/l whilst avoiding hypoglycaemia. Very tight blood glucose control is associated with hypoglycaemic episodes, which are damaging to the already compromised brain.

- Adequate sedation (and analgesia) to reduce $CMRO_2$.
- Treatment of seizures.
- Maintenance of normoglycaemia, < 10 mmol/l.
- Maintenance of normothermia.
- Muscle paralysis if needed to facilitate ventilation to desired PaO_2 and $PaCO_2$ and if patient not synchronising with ventilator.

g) Give two methods of managing acute rises in intracranial pressure whilst awaiting transfer to a neurosurgical centre. (2 marks)

- Hyperventilation to a $PaCO_2$ of 4–4.5 kPa.
- Osmotherapy with mannitol 0.25–1 g/kg.
- Osmotherapy with hypertonic saline 3% 2 ml/kg.

REFERENCES

Brain Trauma Foundation TBI Guidelines. *Guidelines for the management of severe traumatic brain injury*, 4th edition, 2016. http://braintrauma.org/uploads/07/04/Guidelines_for_the_Management_of_Severe_Traumatic.97250__2_.pdf. Accessed 21st March 2023.

Dinsmore J. Traumatic brain injury: an evidence-based review of management. *Contin Educ Anaesth Crit Care Pain*. 2013: 13: 189–195.

Nathanson M et al. Guidelines for safe transfer of the brain-injured patient: trauma and stroke: guidelines from the Association of Anaesthetists and the Neuro Anaesthesia and Critical Care Society. *Anaesthesia*. 2020: 75: 234–246.

National Institute for Health and Care Excellence. *Head injury: assessment and early management: CG176*, Last updated September 2019.

Picetti E et al. Early management of isolated severe traumatic brain injury patients in a hospital without neurosurgical capabilities: a consensus and clinical recommendations of the World Society of Emergency Medicine (WSES). *World J Emerg Surg*. 2023: 18: 5.

Wiles M et al. Management of traumatic brain injury in the non-neurosurgical intensive care unit: a narrative review of current evidence. *Anaesthesia*. 2023: 78: 510–520.

1.7 September 2015 Spinal cord injury

A 19-year-old patient has suffered a complete transection of the spinal cord at the first thoracic vertebral level due to a fall but has no other injuries.

a) Outline the sequence of neurological effects that may develop in the first three months following injury. (6 marks)
b) Which disturbances of the cardiovascular, respiratory and gastrointestinal systems may subsequently occur? (8 marks)
c) When and why may suxamethonium be contraindicated in this patient? (2 marks)
d) Give the advantages of a regional anaesthetic technique for a patient having elective lower limb surgery two years after a high thoracic spine transection. (4 marks)

As this is a repeated topic, I have reproduced the SAQ here in its original format. The Chairs' Report stated that "This question had the highest correlation with overall performance; i.e. candidates who did well in this question performed well overall in the SAQ. The examiners commented that part (d), about the advantages of regional anaesthesia for elective lower limb surgery, was not well answered. Candidates tended to give general answers such as 'avoids the need for general anaesthesia' or 'maintains cardiovascular stability' rather than specific advantages such as 'reduces the risk of autonomic dysreflexia' or 'avoids postoperative respiratory inadequacy due to general anaesthesia.'" The pass rate was 49.4%. The knowledge required for this question is the same as that required for the question on spinal cord injury in September 2011. If candidates had prepared themselves by addressing the topics covered in past papers, more than half would have passed.

1.8 March 2016 Acromegaly and trans-sphenoidal hypophysectomy

A 54-year-old male with acromegaly presents for a trans-sphenoidal hypophysectomy.
a) What is acromegaly? (2 marks)
b) List the clinical features of acromegaly which are of relevance to the anaesthetist. (8 marks)
c) What other clinical presentations of a pituitary adenoma may be encountered? (2 marks)
d) What specific considerations, including surgical factors, may influence the conduct of anaesthesia in this patient? (8 marks)

Another repeated topic and so the SAQ is reproduced as it appeared in the exam. The Chairs' Report said that "this question was answered well despite it having been adjudged to be hard. However, few candidates either knew that acromegaly was a multisystem disease or could list the other possible clinical presentations of a pituitary adenoma e.g. mass effects. Candidates who performed poorly in part (d) failed to describe the specific issues when anaesthetising a patient for this procedure and focused more on general neuroanaesthetic principles. This is a common mistake that has occurred in many questions across many exams. This question also correlated well with overall performance." The pass rate was 58.8%. A score of only 10–11/20 was required to pass this "hard" question. It was very similar to that from March 2013 with only parts (a) and (c) being different and so answers to those parts are given below for the sake of learning.

a) What is acromegaly? (2 marks)

- Acromegaly is the condition that results from excessive growth hormone secretion after the growth plates have fused.
- In this patient and 90% of cases, it results from hypersecretion from a pituitary adenoma.
- Occasionally, it may result from an ectopic pituitary adenoma near, but not in, the sella turcica.
- Rarely, it results from secretion of growth hormone releasing hormone or growth hormone by lung, pancreatic or adrenal tumours.

c) What other clinical presentations of a pituitary adenoma may be encountered? (2 marks)

Non-secretory presentation:

- Local pressure effects causing visual disturbance (bitemporal hemianopia), headache.
- Raised intracranial pressure, cranial nerve palsies, and hydrocephalus due to third ventricle outflow blockage.

Hypersecretory presentation:

- Cushing's disease; hypersecretion of adrenocorticotrophic hormone (ACTH) resulting in fatigue, truncal obesity, striae, moon face, buffalo hump, hypertension, glucose intolerance, depression, anxiety.
- Hyperpituitarism; hypersecretion of any or all anterior pituitary hormones.

Hyposecretory presentation:

- Pituitary apoplexy; internal haemorrhage of the adenoma, or when the adenoma outgrows its blood supply, causing tissue necrosis and swelling. There is consequent loss of anterior pituitary hormones. Symptoms include visual loss, sudden-onset headache, cardiovascular instability.
- Central diabetes insipidus; a macroadenoma may cause damage to posterior pituitary blood supply, thus (rarely) causing diabetes insipidus with polyuria and polydipsia.

- Pituitary-related hypothyroidism; generally less severe than hypothyroidism of thyroid origin.
- Adrenocortical insufficiency; again, not as severe as adrenocortical insufficiency of adrenal origin.

REFERENCE

Menon R, Murphy P, Lindley A. Anaesthesia and pituitary disease. *Contin Educ Anaesth Crit Care Pain.* 2011: 11: 133–137.

1.9 September 2016 Guillain-Barré syndrome

a) What is Guillain-Barré syndrome (GBS)? (1 mark)
b) State the underlying pathophysiology of GBS. (1 mark)
c) List two possible triggers for GBS. (2 marks)
d) List four clinical features of GBS. (4 marks)
e) List three investigations that may be used to support the diagnosis and the findings for each which may indicate GBS. (6 marks)
f) List six specific considerations when anaesthetising a patient recovering from GBS. (6 marks)

The Chairs' Report of the SAQ on this topic stated that it "was surprisingly poorly answered, with some candidates becoming confused between Guillain-Barré syndrome and myasthenia gravis . . . some candidates lost marks by not mentioning the findings of investigations . . . [and] answered with regard to general principles of intraoperative management of a critically ill patient, rather than the measures specific to a patient recovering from GBS." The pass rate was 53.3%.

a) What is Guillain-Barré syndrome (GBS)? (1 mark)

Don't get your neurological disorders all mixed up – there are two great BJA Education articles that succinctly summarise the different disorders and their main implications for anaesthesia.

- Acute, immune-mediated, pre-junctional, ascending demyelinating (most commonly) polyneuropathy affecting sensory, motor, and autonomic nerves.

b) State the underlying pathophysiology of GBS. (1 mark)

GBS is also called acute inflammatory demyelinating polyradiculoneuropathy, ADIP, but this is only the most common subtype – there are a variety of clinical presentations and a more severe disease course with less certain recovery is caused by damage to the axons themselves instead of the myelin sheath.

- Autoantibody damage to myelin sheath or, less commonly, axon of nerves (associated with antiganglioside or other anti-glycolipid antibodies).

c) List two possible triggers for GBS. (2 marks)

- Gastrointestinal (especially campylobacter) or respiratory infection, which may be bacterial, viral (influenza, COVID-19, Zika, CMV, EBV, HIV), or protozoal.
- Vaccination.

d) List four clinical features of GBS. (4 marks)

Whenever you are describing a neurological condition, be clear in your mind whether it is upper or lower motor neurone; whether it affects motor, sensory or autonomic nerves; and whether the defect is of the axon, myelin sheath or neuromuscular junction. The presentation is variable depending upon the subtype.

- Acute onset of symptoms and signs. Recovery is variable, ranging from full recovery to prolonged disability, to relapsing and remitting form.
- Motor features: typically ascending symmetrical weakness (flaccid, areflexic paralysis), may ascend to involve respiratory muscles causing respiratory failure and also to cause facial nerve palsies with bulbar weakness and ophthalmoplegia.
- Sensory features: ascending sensory impairment associated with pain and paraesthesia.
- Autonomic features: arrhythmias, labile BP, urinary retention, paralytic ileus, hyperhidrosis, sudden death.
- Miller Fisher syndrome: this variant is typified by ataxia, areflexia, ophthalmoplegia +/– respiratory and limb weakness.

e) List three investigations that may be used to support the diagnosis and the findings for each which may indicate GBS. (6 marks)

Blood tests are routinely performed for any critically ill patient. You may see alterations reflective of the trigger cause and possibly raised ESR and CRP. Serology for known trigger pathogens may also be seen. The patient may have a positive stool culture for campylobacter. An ABG may show the development of respiratory failure and respiratory function tests will show why. A CT brain should be checked to rule out other causes. However, the tests that I would list here are the ones that have greater specificity for GBS.

- MRI of the spine: selective anterior spinal nerve root enhancement with gadolinium.
- Lumbar puncture: normal cell count and glucose, elevated protein levels (although even this may be normal early in the disease).
- Nerve conduction studies: depends on the subtype, the majority show demyelinating pattern (reduction in conduction velocity), some show axonal loss (reduction in compound action potential size).
- Antiganglioside (otherwise called antiglycolipid) antibodies may be positive especially if an axonal variant.

f) List six specific considerations when anaesthetising a patient recovering from GBS. (6 marks)

Back to the alphabet to help organise your thoughts. Pick the ones that are most important to get your 6 marks.

Airway:

- Bulbar weakness, poor cough, increased risk of aspiration. Intubation required – consider need for rapid sequence induction.
- May still have tracheostomy in situ if still requiring ventilatory support or assistance with secretion clearance.

Respiratory:

- Increased risk of pneumonia secondary to aspiration and poor ventilatory function. Make full assessment of this – history, nature of secretions, temperature, chest auscultation. Treat as required, delay non-urgent surgery if necessary.
- Significantly reduced ventilatory capacity, assess likelihood of requiring noninvasive or invasive ventilation postoperatively.

Cardiovascular:

- Autonomic instability, labile BP (with sensitivity to commonly used vasoactive drugs), risk of arrhythmia. Invasive monitoring indicated including cardiac output monitoring to guide fluid administration (ensure full circulation as dehydration will exacerbate lability).
- Prolonged illness with multiple cannulations, access may be tricky.

Neurological:

- Neuropathic pain common – may already be on antineuropathic drugs +/− opioid analgesia. Need to plan postoperative pain relief, involve acute pain team.

Pharmacology:

- Suxamethonium: contraindicated due to risk of hyperkalaemia due to upregulation of extrajunctional nicotinic receptors.
- Non-depolarising neuromuscular blocking drugs: increased sensitivity, prolonged paralysis may result, reduced dose should be used.

- Opioids: increased sensitivity to respiratory depressant effect in the presence of existing respiratory compromise, may already be taking opioids and so dose adjustments may be necessary.

Haematology:

- Risk of deep vein thrombosis due to prolonged immobility – continuation of thromboembolic deterrent stockings, consideration of use of pneumatic compression devices and pharmacological prophylaxis (check timing if planning neuraxial technique).

Cutaneomusculoskeletal:

- Prolonged illness may be associated with weight loss – care with positioning and padding.

Renal:

- Check renal function – may dictate drug choices.

REFERENCES

Marsh S, Ross N, Pittard A. Neuromuscular disorders and anaesthesia: part I: generic anaesthetic management. *Contin Educ Anaesth Crit Care Pain.* 2011: 11: 115–118.

Marsh S, Pittard A. Neuromuscular disorders and anaesthesia: part 2: specific neuromuscular disorders. *Contin Educ Anaesth Crit Care Pain.* 2011: 11: 119–123.

1.10 September 2017 Spinal cord injury

A 19-year-old patient has suffered a complete transection of the spinal cord at the sixth cervical vertebral level due to a fall, but has no other injuries.

a) Explain the sequence of neurological effects that may develop in the first three months following injury. (6 marks)

b) What disturbances of the cardiovascular (3 marks), respiratory (3 marks) and gastrointestinal (2 marks) systems may occur after three months?

c) List the advantages of choosing a regional anaesthetic technique if this patient is subsequently listed for lower limb surgery. (4 marks)

d) When, and why, may suxamethonium be contraindicated in this patient? (2 marks)

The Chairs acknowledged that this SAQ (reproduced here as it appeared in the exam) had been used before and was answered better on this occasion with a pass rate of 49.3%. "It was considered to be of moderate difficulty. Most marks were lost in part (a), with some candidates being unable to give a coherent explanation of the sequence of neurological events following a spinal cord injury." The SAQ was very similar to those from September 2011 and September 2015, except that the level of the injury is now at the sixth cervical vertebra. Be especially careful to read every word of familiar-looking questions. Cord transection at this level may result in secondary neurological injury to a few segments higher and so at least partial phrenic nerve loss must be considered. Such a patient may require noninvasive ventilation for at least part of the day. Higher cord injuries with complete loss of the phrenic nerve may necessitate long-term ventilation via tracheostomy.

1.11 March 2018 Acromegaly and trans-sphenoidal hypophysectomy

A 54-year-old male with acromegaly presents for a trans-sphenoidal hypophysectomy.

a) What is acromegaly? (2 marks)

b) List the clinical features of acromegaly which are of relevance to the anaesthetist. (8 marks)

c) What other clinical presentations of a pituitary adenoma may be encountered? (2 marks)

d) What specific considerations, including surgical factors, may influence the conduct of anaesthesia in this patient? (8 marks)

This question, reproduced in its original SAQ format, was identical to that from March 2016. The Chairs said that the pass rate was 48.7%: "Again, a previously used question, and as such, disappointingly poorly answered. Candidates did not give enough specific information in the management section, concentrating instead on generic anaesthetic considerations. This probably reflects lack of experience in this area of neurosurgery and lack of appreciation of the challenges of the procedure." More likely, it reflects a failure to learn topics that have previously featured in the Final FRCA.

1.12 September 2018 Guillain-Barré syndrome

A 68-year-old man is referred to the neuro-intensive care unit with suspected Guillain-Barré syndrome (GBS).
a) What is GBS and what are its causes? (3 marks)
b) List the clinical features (6 marks) and investigations/findings (2 marks) that can be used to aid the diagnosis.
c) What are the problems associated with anaesthetising a patient with GBS? (7 marks)
d) What specific treatments are available? (2 marks)

The Chairs' Report of this SAQ (reproduced here in its original format) stated that "Despite a respectable pass rate [56.9%], candidates . . . lacked some knowledge on this subject. The feeling of the examiners was that there was little focus on the answer and [they] feel that time may have been wasted. Very few people knew the correct definition of Guillain-Barré syndrome, nor the correct use of muscle relaxants in these patients." The only change from the SAQ in September 2016 was part (d), which I have answered below.

d) What specific treatments are available? (2 marks)

- Intravenous immunoglobulin.
- Plasma exchange.

REFERENCES

Hughes RAC, Brassington R, Gunn A, van Doorn PA. Corticosteroids for Guillain-Barré syndrome. *Cochrane Database Syst Rev.* 2016: (10): Article No. CD001446.
Richards K, Cohen A. Guillain-Barré: syndrome. *BJA CEPD Rev.* 2003: 3: 46–49.
Verboon C et al. Treatment dilemmas in Guillain-Barré syndrome. *J Neurol Neurosurg Psychiatry.* 2017: 88: 346–352.

1.13 March 2019 Acute stroke

a) Give an imaging modality recommended by The National Institute for Health and Care Excellence (NICE) for the diagnosis and evaluation of management options of acute stroke. (1 mark)

b) List four specific treatments that can be considered for patients with acute thrombotic ischaemic stroke. (4 marks)

c) What is the potential consequence of severe hypertension in patients with acute ischaemic stroke? (1 mark)

d) Give the levels that systolic and diastolic blood pressure should be below if thrombolysis is being considered for treatment of acute ischaemic stroke. (2 marks)

e) A patient has had a large hemispheric infarction following a stroke. Outline your ongoing management of this patient following admission to critical care. (12 marks)

The Chairs' Report following the SAQ on this topic gave a pass rate of 63.4% and stated that it "was well answered with candidates exhibiting good knowledge. Poorer candidates tended to discuss general ICU management and failed to consider the specific neurocritical care interventions." Don't panic when you read "NICE recommendation" in a question – the guideline is only really needed for three marks which you may know due to your clinical experience anyway. The remainder of the question can be tackled by being organised and applying your knowledge of physiology and neurocritical care.

a) **Give an imaging modality recommended by The National Institute for Health and Care Excellence (NICE) for the diagnosis and evaluation of management options of acute stroke. (1 mark)**

- Non-enhanced CT brain within 24 hours of symptom onset.
- (CT contrast angiography then recommended if thrombectomy might be indicated and CT perfusion imaging or MR equivalent if thrombectomy may be indicated beyond 6 hours of symptom onset.)

b) **List four specific treatments that can be considered for patients with acute thrombotic ischaemic stroke. (4 marks)**

- Thrombolysis: alteplase (within 4.5 hours of stroke onset).
- Antiplatelets: aspirin (300 mg within 24 hours and continuing for two weeks, followed by 75 mg daily) or alternative antiplatelet if aspirin intolerant.
- Anticoagulants: heparin initially and then warfarin aiming for INR 2–3 (reserved for patients with stroke due to cerebral venous sinus thrombosis).
- Thrombectomy: in patients with confirmed anterior circulation occlusion (within six hours of symptom onset).
- Carotid endarterectomy: in patients with non-disabling stroke (TIA) and 50–99% carotid artery stenosis on Doppler examination.

c) **What is the potential consequence of severe hypertension in patients with acute ischaemic stroke? (1 mark)**

- Haemorrhagic transformation (may be fatal due to sudden rise in ICP and risk is increased if thrombolysis has been given).

d) **Give the levels that systolic and diastolic blood pressure should be below if thrombolysis is being considered for treatment of acute ischaemic stroke. (2 marks)**

- Systolic < 185 mmHg.
- Diastolic < 110 mmHg.

e) A patient has had a large hemispheric infarction following a stroke. Outline your ongoing management of this patient following admission to critical care. (12 marks)

The mortality following a large hemispheric infarction is up to 80% and the priority is to restore perfusion to the ischaemic penumbra through thrombolysis or endovascular thrombectomy. This question does not state whether these reperfusion techniques have been employed. After admission to critical care, it will be important to maintain cerebral perfusion whilst avoiding secondary brain injury and any reperfusion injury. Meticulous supportive care should be provided and the patient closely monitored for malignant middle cerebral artery syndrome (rapidly deteriorating neurological function due to significant cerebral oedema), haemorrhagic conversion and consideration of decompressive craniectomy. Longer-term management will involve discussions with the family regarding potential for major disability or death and involvement of the MDT, including palliative care, where appropriate.

Airway:

- Endotracheal intubation for GCS ≤8, failure to maintain acceptable oxygenation or normocapnia, or bulbar dysfunction.

Respiratory:

- Target PaO_2 greater than 13 kPa.
- Target $PaCO_2$ 4.5–5.0 kPa.

Cardiovascular:

- Invasive BP monitoring, maintain MAP > 85 mmHg and address any hypovolaemia.
- Maintain BP < 185/100 mmHg for the first 24 hours if patient has had thrombolysis or thrombectomy.
- Maintain systolic BP < 220 mmHg in patients ineligible for thrombolysis or thrombectomy to reduce risk of haemorrhagic transformation.
- Facilitate venous drainage: 30-degree head-up tilt, avoidance of tight tube ties, avoidance of excessive PEEP (ideally < 12 mmHg) or mean airway pressures (while ensuring adequate gas exchange, and adopting a lung protective strategy), use of NMBD if coughing or straining on tube.

Neurological:

- Treat seizures.
- Maintain blood glucose 4–11 mmol/l.
- Treat pyrexia (which raises $CMRO_2$).
- Consideration of invasive ICP monitoring targeting < 20 mmHg to help ensure cerebral perfusion pressure > 60 mmHg.
- Sedate adequately to reduce $CMRO_2$.
- Osmotherapy (mannitol or hypertonic saline) if cerebral oedema or risk of impending herniation.
- Consideration of decompressive hemicraniectomy in patients under 60 years old with significant GCS drop, large infarct or evolving cerebral oedema.
- Serial assessments of neurology via sedation holds, guided by ICP monitoring and clinical condition.
- Commencement of aspirin once satisfied that haemorrhagic transformation has not occurred.

General ICU care:

- Gastric protection with PPI.
- Enteral feeding.
- VTE prophylaxis with intermittent pneumatic compression devices (risk of haemorrhagic transformation with LMWH).

REFERENCES

Dinsmore J, Elwishi M, Kailainathan P. Anaesthesia for endovascular thrombectomy. *BJA Educ.* 2018: 18: 291–299.

National Institute for Health and Care Excellence. *Stroke and transient ischaemic attack in over 16s: diagnosis and initial management: NG128*, Published 2019, updated April 2022.

Redgrave J, Ellis H, Eapen G. Interventional therapies in stroke management: anaesthetic and critical care implications. *BJA Educ.* 2017: 17: 42–47.

1.14 March 2020 Subarachnoid haemorrhage

A 63-year-old patient is admitted to the Emergency Department with a history suggestive of subarachnoid haemorrhage and a GCS of 10.
a) List three presenting features of subarachnoid haemorrhage. (3 marks)
b) List three congenital conditions that are associated with an increased risk of subarachnoid aneurysm development. (3 marks)
c) List three other risk factors for subarachnoid bleeding. (3 marks)
d) List two imaging modalities that are used in the diagnosis of subarachnoid haemorrhage. (2 marks)
e) Give the upper and lower range of acceptable systolic blood pressure values in a patient presenting with subarachnoid haemorrhage. (2 marks)
f) What grade of severity is this patient's subarachnoid haemorrhage according to the World Federation of Neurosurgeons Scale (WFNS)? (1 mark)
g) List three neurological complications following acute subarachnoid haemorrhage. (3 marks)
h) List three specific complications associated with endovascular coiling following subarachnoid haemorrhage. (3 marks)

The Chairs said that the pass rate for the CRQ on this topic was 74% and that this "is a common question in all parts of the exam. Reassuringly, this was well answered by most candidates."

a) **List three presenting features of subarachnoid haemorrhage. (3 marks)**

- Sudden onset ("thunderclap"), occipital, severe headache.
- Signs of meningism due to blood in the subarachnoid space – headache, vomiting, neck stiffness, photophobia.
- Reducing consciousness level.
- Development of focal neurology.
- Seizures.
- Cardiac arrest.

b) **List three congenital conditions that are associated with an increased risk of subarachnoid aneurysm development. (3 marks)**

Aneurysms tend to arise from the vessels of the circle of Willis close to bifurcations.

- Autosomal dominant polycystic kidney disease.
- Ehlers-Danlos type 4.
- Familial intracerebral aneurysm disease.
- Pseudoxanthoma elasticum.
- Marfan's syndrome.
- Hereditary haemorrhagic telangiectasia.
- Arteriovenous malformations.

c) **List three other risk factors for subarachnoid bleeding. (3 marks)**

- Poorly controlled hypertension.
- Cigarette smoking.
- Cocaine use.
- Excessive alcohol use.
- Trauma.
- Arteriosclerosis.
- Increased size of existing aneurysm.

d) **List two imaging modalities that are used in the diagnosis of subarachnoid haemorrhage. (2 marks)**

- Non-contrast CT brain (*first-line investigation, highly sensitive for diagnosing subarachnoid blood. Will also diagnose complications e.g. cerebral oedema and hydrocephalus. If a CT brain is negative but subarachnoid haemorrhage is still strongly suspected, a lumbar puncture looking for red blood cells, bilirubin, and xanthochromia is indicated*).
- CT angiogram (*identifies site of aneurysm*).
- Digital subtraction angiography (*may be used if CT angiogram is negative – radio-opaque structures are removed from the image to enhance the view of the blood vessels*).
- MRI brain (*less commonly used due to logistics involved*).

e) **Give the upper and lower range of acceptable systolic blood pressure values in a patient presenting with subarachnoid haemorrhage. (2 marks)**

Your management of the patient more generally will be according to the principles of management of any brain injured patient aiming to limit the impact of the primary brain injury and minimise the development of secondary brain injury. Autoregulation is lost after acute subarachnoid haemorrhage and cerebral perfusion becomes MAP-dependent. Hypertension should therefore be avoided in patients with unsecured aneurysms to prevent excessive transmural pressure.

- Systolic blood pressure < 160 mmHg.
- Systolic blood pressure > 100 mmHg (or MAP >80 mmHg).

f) **What grade of severity is this patient's subarachnoid haemorrhage according to the World Federation of Neurosurgeons Scale (WFNS)? (1 mark)**

The WFNS scale is commonly used and provides a means of communicating severity and predicting morbidity, disability, and death after subarachnoid haemorrhage: grade 1 – GCS 15; grade 2 – GCS 13–14 without motor deficit; grade 3 – GCS 13–14 with motor deficit; grade 4 – GCS 7–12; and grade 5 – GCS <7.

- Grade 4.

g) **List three neurological complications following acute subarachnoid haemorrhage. (3 marks)**

The following could all be suspected in a patient with new neurological deterioration after presenting with subarachnoid haemorrhage.

- Re-bleeding resulting in further brain injury.
- Delayed cerebral ischaemia or vasospasm (*routine nimodipine for 21 days following subarachnoid haemorrhage reduces these risks and systemic hypertension, with euvolaemia, may be used to increase cerebral perfusion in patients with vasospasm and a secured aneurysm*).
- Hydrocephalus.
- Seizures.
- Cerebral oedema.
- Death according to neurological criteria.

h) **List three specific complications associated with endovascular coiling following subarachnoid haemorrhage. (3 marks)**

Most aneurysms are now managed neuroradiologically instead of with neurosurgical clipping. As well as coiling, where metal coils are deployed within the aneurysmal sac to occlude it, stents can be used to seal the coiled aneurysm off from its parent artery or to divert blood flow from the sac. Stents will necessitate long-term antiplatelet therapy.

- Complications related to vascular access (normally femoral or radial) including haemorrhage, infection, pseudoaneurysm formation.
- Intracranial vessel injury.
- Aneurysmal rupture.
- Cerebral vascular occlusion resulting in ischaemia due to thrombus, embolus (dislodgement from the aneurysmal sac), vasospasm, misplaced catheter or coils.
- Failure to adequately coil the aneurysm.

REFERENCES

Luoma A, Reddy U. Acute management of aneurysmal subarachnoid haemorrhage. *Contin Educ Anaesth Crit Care Pain.* 2013: 13: 52–58.

Patel S, Reddy U. Anaesthesia for interventional neuroradiology. *BJA Educ.* 2016: 16: 147–152.

1.15 September 2020 Raised intracranial pressure

A 40-year-old patient is admitted to neuro-intensive care following a traumatic brain injury.
a) Define the normal range for intracranial pressure (ICP) in adults and children. (2 marks)
b) Describe the normal appearance of the ICP waveforms. (3 marks)
c) State the equation of cerebral perfusion pressure. (1 mark)
d) List two indications for ICP monitoring following traumatic brain injury. (2 marks)
e) List two invasive monitoring methods of ICP in a patient with traumatic brain injury. (2 marks)
f) At what level is an intracranial pressure monitor zeroed? (1 mark)
g) Give the pressure above which management should be undertaken to lower ICP. (1 mark)
h) List two physiological parameters for which the measurement of jugular venous oxygen saturations ($SjvO_2$) may be used as a surrogate. (2 marks)
i) Describe the correct positioning of a catheter for jugular venous oxygen saturation monitoring and state why malposition will cause error. (2 marks)
j) Give two factors which may cause low $SjvO_2$ and two factors which may cause raised $SjvO_2$. (4 marks)

The original CRQ had the highest overall pass rate for the paper (88.1%). The Chairs said that "The knowledge-based components of this question were answered well. Candidates performed poorly on the components relating to jugular venous oxygen saturation. Most notably on the last section which required the physiological and pathophysiological causes of a low jugular venous oxygen saturation."

a) Define the normal range for intracranial pressure (ICP) in adults and children. (2 marks)

- Adults 10–15 mmHg.
- Older children 5–15 mmHg, infants 3–4 mmHg.

b) Describe the normal appearance of the ICP waveforms. (3 marks)

The normal ICP waveform is triphasic and analysis of the waveform appearance, alongside the ICP value, can help to assess if cerebral compliance is changing.

- P1 "percussion wave" – waveform transmitted by arterial pulsation.
- P2 "tidal wave" – a reflection of P1 so representing intracranial compliance. If brain compliance decreases, P2 will rise and may become higher than or merge with P1.
- P3 "dicrotic wave" – due aortic valve closure (the lowest wave of the three).

c) State the equation of cerebral perfusion pressure. (1 mark)

Sometimes CVP is substituted for ICP if the CVP is greater than ICP. In these circumstances, a negative pressure gradient results such that no venous outflow occurs until ICP exceeds CVP and venous flow starts again.

- CPP = MAP − ICP

d) List two indications for ICP monitoring following traumatic brain injury. (2 marks)

- All patients with traumatic brain injury GCS ≤ 8 and abnormal CT brain scan.
- Patients with severe traumatic brain injury and normal CT brain scan if they have ≥ 2 of the following:
  — Age > 40 years.
  — Motor posturing.
  — SBP < 90 mmHg.

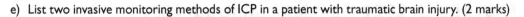

e) List two invasive monitoring methods of ICP in a patient with traumatic brain injury. (2 marks)

- Intraventricular catheter *(also referred to as an external ventricular drain – can be calibrated and can be used to therapeutically drain CSF).*
- Transducer pressure monitoring in subdural, intraparenchymal, subarachnoid, or epidural space. *(Transducer may be a balloon, strain gauge, or fibreoptic tip. Once it is sited, there is no ability to recalibrate it. May not reflect variation of intracranial pressure in different parts of brain.)*

f) At what level is an intracranial pressure monitor zeroed? (1 mark)

- The foramen of Monro, which correlates with the external acoustic meatus in the supine patient with head in neutral position.

g) Give the pressure above which management should be undertaken to lower ICP. (1 mark)

- 22 mmHg.

h) List two physiological parameters for which the measurement of jugular venous oxygen saturations ($SjvO_2$) may be used as a surrogate. (2 marks)

- Cerebral oxygenation.
- Cerebral blood flow.

i) Describe the correct positioning of a catheter for jugular venous oxygen saturation monitoring and state why malposition will cause error. (2 marks)

- A catheter is inserted in a retrograde direction in the internal jugular vein to the jugular bulb, usually on the dominant side (determined by compressing each internal jugular vein and seeing which causes the greatest rise in ICP), and the tip checked at C1/2 intervertebral level on lateral C-spine X-ray.
- Poor positioning will result in admixture from extracranial blood and therefore error.

j) Give two factors which may cause low $SjvO_2$ and two factors which may cause raised $SjvO_2$. (4 marks)

Normal values are between 55 and 75%. Like with measuring mixed venous oxygen saturations when assessing systemic oxygen delivery, it is a question of supply and demand.

Low values:

- Reduction in oxygen delivery: raised ICP, cerebral ischaemia, hypoxia, profound hypocarbia.
- Increased cerebral oxygen demand: seizures, pyrexia.

High values:

- Reduction in cerebral oxygen consumption: coma, hypothermia, cerebral infarction.
- Increased oxygen delivery: hypercapnia, vasodilation.

REFERENCES

Brain Trauma Foundation TBI Guidelines. *Guidelines for the management of severe traumatic brain injury*, 4th edition, 2016. http://braintrauma.org/uploads/07/04/Guidelines_for_the_ Management_of_Severe_Traumatic.97250__2_.pdf. Accessed 21st March 2023.

Dinsmore J. Traumatic brain injury: an evidence-based review of management. *Contin Educ Anaesth Crit Care Pain*. 2013: 13: 189–195.

Elwishi M, Dinsmore J. Monitoring the brain. *BJA Educ*. 2019: 19: 54–59.

1.16 March 2021 Cervical spine surgery

A 45-year-old patient presents for cervical spine surgery. The neurosurgeons have requested prone positioning and neurophysiological monitoring.
a) Describe the arterial supply to the spinal cord. (3 marks)
b) Give three forms of neurophysiological monitoring that may be used during cervical spine surgery. (3 marks)
c) List two ways in which the use of neurophysiological monitoring may require alteration in anaesthetic technique. (2 marks)
d) Give three physiological approaches to minimising the risk of neurological injury during cervical spine surgery. (3 marks)
e) Give three surgical complications of cervical spinal surgery. (3 marks)
f) State six potential complications of general anaesthesia in the prone position. (6 marks)

The original CRQ was well answered, with a pass rate of 80%. The Chairs said that candidates gave "very comprehensive answers. Marks were dropped on the initial sections and less than half the candidates knew the blood supply to the spinal cord. Very few candidates scored full marks on the complications of the prone position."

a) Describe the arterial supply to the spinal cord. (3 marks)

This is core knowledge that is often examined as part of questions on spinal, cardiothoracic, and aortic vascular surgery, during which spinal cord ischaemia may occur as a complication.

- Anterior spinal artery, formed by the union of the two vertebral arteries at the foramen magnum, supplies the anterior 2/3 of the cord (spinothalamic and corticospinal tracts).
- Two posterior spinal arteries are formed from each of the vertebral arteries or the posterior inferior cerebellar arteries, and supply the posterior 1/3 of the cord (dorsal columns).
- Segmental arterial supply. Numerous paired branches perfuse the spinal cord along its length, arising from vertebral, deep cervical, intercostal, aortic and pelvic vessels. The arteria radicularis magna/artery of Adamkiewicz is the biggest segmental artery and forms a major supply to the lumbosacral spinal cord, arising at a variable vertebral level between T8–L4, but typically at T12–L1. It usually originates from an intercostal or, less commonly, a lumbar artery.

b) Give three forms of neurophysiological monitoring that may be used during cervical spine surgery. (3 marks)

Neurophysiological monitoring for spinal cord ischaemia is important in patients undergoing spinal surgery. For this answer you only need to list the different types, but I have included a bit more information as this is also a common viva topic. Spinal cord ischaemia generally causes reduced amplitude and increased latency of measured evoked potentials.

	Description	Other notes
Somatosensory evoked potential	*Peripheral sensory nerves (usually ulnar/ median/posterior tibial) are stimulated and electrodes placed on the scalp to record cortical response.*	*Mainly tests the integrity of dorsal column +/- spinothalamic tracts.*
Motor evoked potential	*Motor cortex is stimulated and electrodes on peripheral muscles record impulses.*	*Mainly tests the integrity of corticospinal tracts. Risks include biting and tongue damage, scalp burns, seizures.*

	Description	Other notes
Electromyography	Needle electrodes placed into a specific muscle group to detect surgical irritation or damage of a particular nerve.	Complete transection of the nerve will result in loss of signal.
EEG	Topical scalp electrodes give information about depth of anaesthesia and cerebral blood flow.	

c) **List two ways in which the use of neurophysiological monitoring may require alteration in anaesthetic technique. (2 marks)**

- Volatile agents reduce the amplitude of motor evoked potentials – TIVA is therefore more commonly used.
- Neuromuscular block results in loss of MEP and EMG signal and therefore should be avoided.
- Ketamine can increase the amplitude of motor and sensory evoked potentials and may be used to enhance low-amplitude, poorly defined MEP responses.
- Alpha-2 agonists may reduce motor evoked potentials and may therefore be unhelpful during monitored surgery.

d) **Give three physiological approaches to minimising the risk of neurological injury during cervical spine surgery. (3 marks)**

Physiological prevention of <u>any</u> neurological injury (be it spinal cord, cerebral or peripheral nerve) relates to maintenance of oxygen delivery and perfusion.

- Optimal ventilation to avoid hypoxia and hypercapnia.
- Maintenance of MAP in order to ensure spinal cord perfusion pressure.
- Replacement of any significant blood loss.
- Maintenance of normal acid-base status.
- Maintenance of normothermia.

e) **Give three surgical complications of cervical spinal surgery. (3 marks)**

Cervical spine surgery can be performed via a posterior approach, as is the case for the patient in this question, but may also be undertaken via an anterior approach. The approach and the level of surgery, would dictate some of the important surgical complications – go back to your anatomy and think what is nearby.

- Spinal cord or nerve root injury due to direct injury, local haematoma, or metalwork migration.
- Bleeding or haematoma resulting in postoperative airway compromise.
- Infection leading to discitis, meningitis, or cerebral abscess.
- Dural tear and CSF leak.
- Damage to local structures – anterior approach surgery may cause damage to the oesophagus, trachea, vertebral and carotid arteries, recurrent laryngeal and hypoglossal nerves, and the sympathetic chain. Posterior approach surgery may cause damage to the vertebral arteries.

f) **State six potential complications of general anaesthesia in the prone position. (6 marks)**

This is a common viva question too – be systematic in your approach and go by organ system:

Airway:

- Accidental extubation.
- Airway and tongue oedema leading to postoperative airway obstruction.

Respiratory:

- In obese patients, lung expansion may be reduced by failure to accommodate the abdomen within the pre-cut shape of the Montreal mattress.
- (Generally, prone positioning may improve V/Q matching – see intensive care medicine chapter.)

Cardiovascular:

- Abdominal pressure may cause IVC compression reducing venous return and cardiac output.
- Loss of intravenous access on turning the patient.

Neurological:

- Abnormal neck flexion or extension may result in impaired cerebral perfusion and venous drainage.
- Peripheral neuropathies affecting brachial plexus, ulnar nerve at elbow, and common peroneal nerve.
- Central retinal artery occlusion due to pressure on eye, corneal abrasion, ischaemic optic neuropathy.

Gastrointestinal:

- Increased intra-abdominal pressure if care not taken to ensure accommodation of abdomen in cut-out of Montreal mattress resulting in gastric acid reflux with consequent oral and eye irritation.

Cutaneomusculoskeletal:

- Direct pressure effects to face, pinna, breasts, genitalia, femoral triangle.

REFERENCES

Felix B, Sturgess J. Anaesthesia in the prone position. *Contin Educ Anaesth Crit Care Pain.* 2014: 14: 291–297.
Hunningher A, Calder I. Cervical spine surgery. *Contin Educ Anaesth Crit Care Pain.* 2007: 7: 81–84.
Levin D, Strantzas S, Steinberg B. Intraoperative neuromonitoring in paediatric spinal surgery. *BJA Educ.* 2019: 19: 165–171.
Nowicki R. Anaesthesia for major spinal surgery. *Contin Educ Anaes Crit Care Pain.* 2014: 14: 147–152.
Yee T, Swong K, Park P. Complications of anterior cervical spine surgery: a systematic review of the literature. *J Spine Surg.* 2020: 6: 302–322.

1.17 March 2021 Awake craniotomy

a) List two indications for an awake craniotomy. (2 marks)
b) Give two surgical contraindications to awake craniotomy. (2 marks)
c) Give two examples of anaesthetic technique for an awake craniotomy. (2 marks)
d) Give three advantages and one disadvantage of using dexmedetomidine for sedation as part of an awake craniotomy technique. (4 marks)
e) An intraoperative seizure occurs. What immediate management should take place? (2 marks)
f) Give two drugs, with doses, that can be given to terminate seizures intraoperatively. (2 marks)
g) Give two effects of using such drugs on the surgery. (2 marks)
h) What are four specific intraoperative complications that may occur during awake craniotomy? (4 marks)

The Chairs' Report of the original CRQ stated that "Candidates answered this question poorly and this may reflect a lack of experience in neuro-anaesthesia. Knowledge of pharmacology was again poor. Not many candidates knew about the role of dexmedetomidine in this context. Section (f) asked about drugs used to terminate an intraoperative seizure. Very few candidates knew what drugs to give for a seizure, but those who did frequently didn't know the correct doses. It is important to read the question and answer what is asked: the last section of this question asked for specific intraoperative complications, yet most candidates gave general complications." It is a common criticism in Chairs' Reports that candidates give answers that are too general. The pass rate was 40.9%. I would encourage reading the referenced CEACCP article as awake craniotomies are generally rare and many candidates are unlikely to witness one even if they have completed their neuroanaesthesia module.

Scalp blocks come hand in hand with awake craniotomy and are a popular viva question. The sensory innervation of the scalp is as follows:

- *Posterior to the auricle:*
  - *Branches of the cervical plexus (lesser occipital, greater auricular), and the greater occipital nerve.*
- *Anterior scalp:*
  - *Branches of VI – supraorbital and supratrochlear.*
- *Lateral scalp:*
  - *Zygomaticotemporal nerve (branch of V2).*
  - *Auriculotemporal nerve (branch of V3).*

a) List two indications for an awake craniotomy. (2 marks)

This is generally to perform surgery whilst maintaining real-time neurological assessment of the impact on surrounding brain:

- Tumour excision from an area within or close to functionally important cortex.
- Epilepsy surgery.
- Deep brain stimulation surgery.
- Resection of vascular lesions from vessels supplying functionally important areas of the brain.

b) Give two surgical contraindications to awake craniotomy. (2 marks)

Read the question – it asks for <u>surgical</u> contraindications. The general contraindications are as follows:

Absolute; patient refusal, inability to lay still/flat, inability to co-operate due to confusion, anxiety, low GCS, or learning disability.

Relative; morbid obesity, severe sleep apnoea, anticipated difficult intubation, uncontrollable seizures, chronic cough, young age.

- Highly vascular lesions.
- Significant dural involvement (this will cause pain during resection).
- Low occipital lobe lesions – patients may be unable to tolerate positioning for surgical access.

c) Give two examples of anaesthetic technique for an awake craniotomy. (2 marks)

The term "awake" craniotomy means that the patient is fully awake during cortical mapping and lesion resection but may be sedated or asleep for other parts of the operation. Local anaesthesia with scalp blocks may be used for all methods.

- Local anaesthesia with sedation:
  - Scalp blocks are performed.
  - Conscious sedation is maintained with target-controlled infusions of propofol and/or remifentanil and sedation deepened for the stimulating parts of the operation (Mayfield pins, skin incision, removal of bone flap and dura).
- General anaesthesia ("asleep/awake/asleep")
  - Patient is anaesthetised and an airway (supraglottic or endotracheal tube) is placed. Maintenance may include TIVA.
  - When mapping needs to commence, anaesthesia is reduced and the patient is woken up and the airway removed.
  - Patient can be anaesthetised again and an airway reinserted after mapping is complete.

d) Give three advantages and one disadvantage of using dexmedetomidine for sedation as part of an awake craniotomy technique. (4 marks)

Dexmedetomidine is an alpha-2 agonist (similar to clonidine) which can be used as an infusion for conscious sedation:

Advantages:

- Analgesic properties.
- Minimal respiratory depression.
- Minimal effects on ICP.
- Sedative and anxiolytic properties.
- Minimal effect on interictal epileptiform activities (IEAs) – the presence and location of these IEAs can be used to localise an epileptogenic focus and guide surgical resection.

Disadvantages:

- Bradycardia and hypotension.
- User unfamiliarity.

e) An intraoperative seizure occurs. What immediate management should take place? (2 marks)

Seizures may occur during cortical mapping, the awake phase of the surgery.

- Irrigation of brain tissue with ice-cold saline.
- Declare emergency, ask surgeons to stop, call for help.
- Rapid and succinct A to E assessment, apply 100% oxygen, airway management with SAD (head may be fixed in head pins, distant to ventilator, so insertion of an SAD is usually easier to manage than intubation).

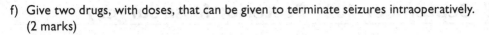

f) **Give two drugs, with doses, that can be given to terminate seizures intraoperatively. (2 marks)**

If irrigation of the surgical field fails, then proceed to pharmacological management.

- Propofol: 10–30 mg titrated to effect.
- Midazolam: 2–5 mg titrated to effect.
- Thiopentone: 25–50 mg titrated to effect.

g) **Give two possible effects of using drugs to terminate seizures on the ongoing surgery. (2 marks)**

Electrocorticography (ECoG) refers to placement of EEG electrodes on the cortex to detect interictal epileptiform activity to guide localisation of target in epilepsy surgery.

- May cause significant sedation with need to secure airway, delaying the "awake" phase of surgery and potentially leading to delayed wake up postoperatively.
- Interference with neurophysiological monitoring:
  — Thiopentone activates interictal epileptiform activity (IEA).
  — Benzodiazepines suppress IEA.
  — Propofol has a variable effect on IEA.
  — Most intravenous anaesthetics and benzodiazepines suppress ECoG activity.

h) **List four other specific intraoperative complications that may occur during awake craniotomy. (4 marks)**

There is a very long list of possible complications, but I have restricted this list to the ones that are more specific to awake craniotomy.

Airway and respiratory:

- Alveolar hypoventilation due to sedation, airway obstruction or apnoea with head immobilised.
- Hypoxia and hypercapnia (leading to poor surgical conditions with brain swelling).
- Failure to resite airway device, laryngospasm.
- Aspiration.

Circulation:

- Difficult to manage hypotension due to sitting position and venous pooling.

Disability:

- Patient intolerance of the procedure due to pain from semi-seated position with immobilised head, catheter irritation, seizures, and need to convert to general anaesthesia.
- Ineffective local anaesthesia leading to technique failure.
- Venous air embolus.
- Focal neurological deficit.

REFERENCES

Burnand C, Sebastian J. Anaesthesia for awake craniotomy. *Contin Educ Anaesth Crit Care Pain.* 2014: 14: 6–11.

Larkin C, O'Brien D, Maheshwari D. Anaesthesia for epilepsy surgery. *BJA Educ.* 2019: 19: 383–389.

1.18 September 2021 Posterior fossa surgery

A 55-year-old presents for posterior fossa surgery. The neurosurgeons require the sitting position for surgical access.

a) List three structures contained within the posterior fossa. (3 marks)
b) Describe three neurological features that you would specifically assess for prior to posterior fossa surgery in the sitting position. (3 marks)
c) List two other positions that may be suitable for posterior fossa surgery. (2 marks)
d) List two absolute contraindications to the sitting position for craniotomy. (2 marks)
e) List three complications due to the sitting position for craniotomy. (3 marks)
f) Give two ways in which the risk of development of venous air embolus can be minimised during the sitting position for craniotomy. (2 marks)
g) After calling for help and assessing the patient in a systematic manner, list four steps that can be undertaken to manage a significant venous air embolism in this patient. (4 marks)
h) What is the most sensitive noninvasive monitoring technique for the detection of venous air embolus? (1 mark)

There was no Chairs' Report for this exam sitting as this was the CRQ paper that was withdrawn following difficulties with the online exam platform.

a) **List three structures contained within the posterior fossa. (3 marks)**

The posterior fossa is posterior to the petrous part of the temporal bone and its inferior boundary is largely formed by the occipital and temporal bones. Its contents are clearly more numerous than this, but these are the main anatomical features.

- Brainstem, which leaves the posterior fossa via the foramen magnum.
- Cerebellum and aqueduct of Sylvius.
- Vertebral and basilar arteries.
- Cranial nerves VI, VII, VIII, IX, X, XI, XII.
- Venous sinuses – sigmoid, transverse, and occipital.

b) **Describe three neurological features that you would specifically assess for prior to posterior fossa surgery in the sitting position. (3 marks)**

Leading on from (a), it would be important to assess the neurological functions pertinent to the structures in the posterior fossa as they could be already compromised by the disease process or be damaged by surgery.

- Cerebellar function: co-ordination, posture, and gait *(the acronym DANISH was often used in medical school OSCEs, meaning dysdiadochokinesis, ataxia, nystagmus, intention tremor, slurred speech, hypotonia).*
- Cranial nerve function: in particular bulbar weakness can lead to loss of airway protection and the need for postoperative ventilation.
- Raised ICP: reduced level of consciousness, headache, or vomiting. This may be the result of the pathology or due to the development of hydrocephalus.

c) **List two other positions that may be suitable for posterior fossa surgery. (2 marks)**

- Supine with head turned, supported by sandbags *(may be suitable for acoustic neuroma or cerebellopontine angle tumours).*
- Prone *(like the sitting position, this offers good access for midline structures).*
- Lateral *(good access for lateral structures).*
- Park bench *(modification of the lateral position with the patient semi-prone, head flexed to face the floor, offering greater access to the midline, avoiding the need for sitting or prone positioning).*

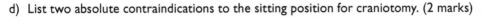

d) List two absolute contraindications to the sitting position for craniotomy. (2 marks)

- Ventriculo-atrial shunt: shunt blockage could occur in the context of venous air embolism, leading to raised ICP.
- Right-to-left heart shunt: venous air passing to the left side of the circulation can potentially lead to stroke.

I also list the relative contraindications below:

- *Patent foramen ovale.*
- *Uncontrolled hypertension.*
- *Severe autonomic neuropathy.*
- *Extremes of age.*

e) List three complications due to the sitting position for craniotomy. (3 marks)

These are all individual complications but have been grouped by body system to help you memorise them.

Airway:

- Endotracheal tube displacement.
- Jugular venous obstruction due to flexed neck causing laryngeal and tongue oedema with postoperative airway compromise.

Cardiovascular:

- Venous air embolism.
- Hypotension due to reduced venous return due to venous pooling in dependent areas.

Neurological:

- Cord or brainstem ischaemia due to head flexion and hypotension.
- Sciatic and femoral nerve damage from excessive hip flexion compounded by lower limb oedema due to dependent positioning.
- Pneumocephalus (delayed recovery, neurological deficit, confusion, headache).

Cutaneomusculoskeletal:

- Compartment syndrome.
- Lumbosacral pressure damage.

f) Give two ways in which the risk of development of venous air embolus can be minimised during the sitting position for craniotomy. (2 marks)

Venous air embolus occurs when there is entrainment of air into the venous system due to the presence of open venous sinuses which are at negative pressure in relation to the heart. With this in mind, there are several ways to reduce the risk:

- Positioning: if sitting position is absolutely necessary, then Trendelenburg tilt or leg elevation may help to reduce the risk.
- Reduce venous hypotension by avoiding dehydration and hypotension.
- Surgical technique: minimise open veins, attention to haemostasis.

g) **After calling for help and assessing the patient in a systematic manner, list four steps that can be undertaken to manage a significant venous air embolism in this patient. (4 marks)**

Each of the following is a separate step, but they have been grouped in order to assist with learning.

- Prevent further air entry:
  - Ask surgeon to flood site with saline and cover with wet packs.
  - Administer fluids especially if hypovolaemia thought to be contributory to air entrainment.
  - Lower the head of patient so that the surgical site is below the right atrium if possible.
  - Apply sustained positive airway pressure until these measures have been achieved.

- Reduce size of air embolism:
  - Administer 100% oxygen.
  - Stop nitrous oxide if it is being used.
  - Aspirate air from right atrium via central line if one is present.

- Overcome mechanical obstruction:
  - Left lateral or Trendelenburg positioning may help force bubble above the right ventricular outflow.
  - If the patient suffers cardiac arrest or severe haemodynamic compromise, chest compressions may assist in dispersing the bubble.
  - Inotropic support may be required.

h) **What is the most sensitive noninvasive monitoring technique for the detection of venous air embolus? (1 mark)**

- Precordial Doppler.

REFERENCES

Association of Anaesthetists. *Quick Reference Handbook: 3–5 circulatory embolus v1*, 2018. https://anaesthetists.org/Home/Resources-publications/Safety-alerts/Anaesthesia-emergencies/Quick-Reference-Handbook-QRH/PDF-version. Accessed 21st March 2023.

Jagannathan S, Krovvidi H. Anaesthetic considerations for posterior fossa surgery. *Contin Educ Anaesth Crit Care Pain*. 2014: 14: 202–206.

1.19 March 2022 Guillain-Barré syndrome

The CRQ in March 2022 covered very much the same content as the SAQs from September 2016 and September 2018. The only new line of questioning was about the degree of respiratory muscle weakness that would warrant consideration of intubation in a patient with GBS. The Chairs' Report of the original CRQ stated that the pass rate was 66.1% and that "This proved to be a straightforward question for the majority of candidates. Part (g) was generally answered well but some candidates discussed the general principles of the intraoperative management of a critically ill patient as opposed to the measures specific to a patient recovering from Guillain-Barré." That is almost identical to the Report after the September 2018 SAQ, reiterating the need to learn from past topics, questions and candidate performance.

a) Give the forced vital capacity (FVC) (ml/kg), maximum inspiratory pressure (cmH$_2$O) and maximum expiratory pressure (cmH$_2$O) values that would warrant consideration of intubation in a patient with GBS. (3 marks)

GBS causing respiratory muscle weakness may lead to hypoventilation and respiratory failure, warranting intubation and ventilation. FVC is commonly monitored on wards to predict the requirement of mechanical ventilation due to respiratory muscle weakness. There is a range of values in the literature, but these ones fit nicely into the 20/30/40 rule and so are easier to remember. Other considerations for intubation would be the patient's ability to protect their own airway in the context of bulbar weakness and rapidly dropping FVC, or inspiratory or expiratory pressures.

*   FVC 20 ml/kg.
*   Maximal inspiratory pressure (PI max) < 30 cmH$_2$O (this is a measure of inspiratory muscle strength).
*   Maximal expiratory pressure (PE max) < 40 cmH$_2$O (this is a measure of forced expiratory muscle strength).

REFERENCES

Harms M. Inpatient management of Guillain-Barré. *Neurohospitalist*. 2011: 1: 78–84.
Lawn N et al. Anticipating mechanical ventilation in Guillain-Barré syndrome. *Arch Neurol*. 2001: 58: 893–898.

1.20 September 2022 Hydrocephalus

a) What is the normal adult volume (ml) of cerebrospinal fluid (CSF)? (1 mark)
b) Where is CSF absorbed? (1 mark)
c) State four non-congenital causes of hydrocephalus. (4 marks)
d) List three clinical features of acute hydrocephalus. (3 marks)
e) Describe how you would zero and commence use of an external ventricular drain (EVD). (3 marks)
f) List four complications associated with an EVD. (4 marks)
g) List four specific anaesthetic considerations for a patient with an indwelling ventricular shunt for hydrocephalus presenting for general surgery. (4 marks)

The pass rate for the original CRQ was 89.8% with the Chairs saying it "was the highest in the paper and was generally answered well. This proved to be a straightforward question for the majority of candidates."

a) **What is the normal adult volume (ml) of cerebrospinal fluid (CSF)? (1 mark)**

- 150 ml.

b) **Where is CSF absorbed? (1 mark)**

- Via the subarachnoid granulations to the cranial venous sinuses.

CSF is produced in the ependymal cells of the choroid plexus. The rate is independent of CPP and ICP until ICP has risen to such a level that CSF production is inhibited. From here its passage is as follows:

- *Into the third ventricle via the foramen of Monro.*
- *From the third to the fourth ventricle via the aqueduct of Sylvius.*
- *From the fourth ventricle via the foramina of <u>L</u>uschka <u>L</u>aterally into the subarachnoid space, or <u>M</u>agendie <u>M</u>edially towards the spinal cord.*

c) **State four non-congenital causes of hydrocephalus. (4 marks)**

I have included some congenital causes in the table below for completeness. "Communicating" and "non-communicating" refer to whether the cause of hydrocephalus is related to an abnormality in CSF flow – there is usually an obstruction to flow in "non-communicating" causes. Sub-arachnoid haemorrhage initially causes communicating hydrocephalus as subarachnoid blood interferes with reabsorption at the granulations. Further rises in ICP or midline shift can subsequently cause non-communicating hydrocephalus too.

	Non-congenital	Congenital
Communicating:	After subarachnoid or intracerebral haemorrhage. Choroid plexus papilloma. Following intracerebral infection.	*Achondroplasia.* *Craniofacial or skull base abnormalities associated with syndromes.*
Non-communicating:	Intracerebral tumour. Post-inflammatory adhesions. Cerebellar haematoma or infarct.	*Aqueduct stenosis.* *Chiari malformations.* *Dandy-Walker malformation.*

d) **List three clinical features of acute hydrocephalus. (3 marks)**

The <u>acute</u> features are a mixture of generalised features of raised ICP and the effects of raised ICP on specific cranial nerves.

- Headache.
- Impaired conscious level.

- Vomiting.
- Seizures.
- Diplopia or ophthalmoplegia
- Bulging fontanelle in infants

e) Describe how you would zero and commence use of an external ventricular drain (EVD). (3 marks)

Even if you have not done this before, you will have zeroed an arterial line transducer and would be able to gain marks by applying the principles of measuring a gauge pressure. An EVD consists of a catheter (placed in the lateral ventricle) connected to a burette within which CSF rises to reach a set pressure beyond which the remaining CSF fills a drainage bag below the burette.

- Adjust the height of the pressure scale so that the zero mark is level with the foramen of Monro (external acoustic meatus in supine position with head in neutral position, between the eyebrows in a patient in lateral position).
- The CSF collection chamber is positioned in relation to the pressure scale depending upon the desired ICP, allowing CSF in excess of a certain pressure to be collected and delivered to a drainage bag.
- The system must be rezeroed if the patient's position changes.
- Clamping of drain e.g. during transport, should be avoided particularly in patients who are dependent on CSF drainage to avoid deleterious rises in ICP.

f) List four complications associated with an EVD. (4 marks)

Again, even if you have no experience with EVDs, just think what it is – a foreign body placed into the brain.

- Failure of EVD to control hydrocephalus or ICP.
- Intracerebral haemorrhage.
- Seizures.
- Excessive CSF drainage (> 20 ml/h) can lead to ventricular collapse or subdural haemorrhage.
- Catheter complications – blockage, displacement, kinking.
- Catheter infection. *(Antibiotic prophylaxis is usual but infections may occur in up to 20% and requires prolonged therapy with intravenous antibiotics and sometimes intrathecal antibiotics. Use of silver- or antibiotic-coated catheters is common practice.)*

g) List four specific anaesthetic considerations for a patient with an indwelling ventricular shunt for hydrocephalus presenting for general surgery. (4 marks)

Indwelling ventricular shunts for hydrocephalus may include ventriculo-peritoneal (VP), ventriculo-atrial (VA), ventriculo-pleural, and lumbar-peritoneal shunts. They are used in patients with a longer-term tendency to hydrocephalus with subcutaneous tunnelling of the distal end of the catheter to its drainage site. The major considerations when patients with a pre-existing shunt have other surgery are related to avoiding shunt damage and infection.

- Assessment for any signs of raised ICP before and after surgery.
- Consider transfer to neurosurgical centre of patients with a VP shunt with significant intrabdominal infection.
- Care with regional anaesthesia for upper limb surgery as most shunts are tunnelled behind the ear or behind the posterior border of sternocleidomastoid.
- Care with positioning to prevent external pressure on the tunnelled part of the shunt.
- Minimisation of duration and pressure of laparoscopic surgery (although shunts now have one-way pressure valve) and visualisation by surgeon at the end of procedure that tip of shunt is still draining.

- Avoidance of internal jugular (and possibly subclavian) access for patients with indwelling VA shunts – use an alternative venous access site.
- IPPV can cause blockage of an indwelling ventriculo-pleural shunt – consider this in a slow to wake patient.
- Lower respiratory tract infection in a patient with a ventriculo-pleural shunt should be avoided – postoperative physio and incentive spirometry may be useful.

REFERENCES

Krovvidi H, Flint G, Williams A. Perioperative management of hydrocephalus. *BJA Educ.* 2018: 18: 140–146.

Whitney P, Sturgess J. Anaesthetic considerations for patients with neurosurgical implants. *BJA Educ.* 2016: 16: 230–235.

1.21 February 2023 Spinal cord injury

A patient with previous spinal cord injury presents for elective cystoscopy and ureteroscopy. They have a history of autonomic dysreflexia.

a) At what level of spinal cord injury is autonomic dysreflexia more common and why? (2 marks)
b) List two cardiovascular effects of autonomic dysreflexia. (2 marks)
c) List two other features of autonomic dysreflexia. (2 marks)
d) List two common triggers for the development of acute autonomic dysreflexia. (2 marks)
e) Other than the need for appropriate consent and an anaesthetist present on standby, list three conditions that must be met for surgery to take place without anaesthesia. (3 marks)
f) List three drugs that may be used in the acute management of the hypertension of autonomic dysreflexia. (3 marks)
g) Give two reasons why a reduced dose of induction agent may be required when providing general anaesthesia for a patient with spinal cord injury. (2 marks)
h) List three benefits of spinal anaesthesia over general anaesthesia for cystoscopy in a patient with autonomic dysreflexia. (3 marks)
i) How long after a spinal cord injury can suxamethonium be safely used? (1 mark)

The Chairs' Report acknowledged that "this topic has appeared in various guises in the Final FRCA for many years," and indeed, it is the fourth time spinal cord injury has been examined over the time period covered by this book, this time with a pass rate of 53%. This question focussed more specifically on autonomic dysreflexia, rather than the global principles of anaesthetising a patient with previous spinal cord injury, with the majority of content relating to the BJA Education article referenced. The article contains a lot of practical information about managing patients with spinal cord injury for a range of commonly required procedures and it would be sensible to read it as it may form the subject of a question on spinal cord injury in the future. Subsections (h) and (i) have been covered in the answer to the question from September 2011.

a) **At what level of spinal cord injury is autonomic dysreflexia more common and why? (2 marks)**

Patients with complete lesions are also more susceptible to a profound response.

- Above T6.
- This is because vasoconstriction will include the large splanchnic circulation which will make a major contribution to the consequent hypertension and resulting symptoms.

b) **List two cardiovascular effects of autonomic dysreflexia. (2 marks)**

Remember the pathophysiology of autonomic dysreflexia: a dysregulated sympathetic response occurs in response to stimulation below the level of the injury due to loss of descending inhibition from higher centres. A compensatory parasympathetic response occurs but is limited in effect to above the level of the injury.

- Hypertensive crisis which may lead to myocardial ischaemia, arrhythmia, heart failure, or haemorrhagic stroke.
- Bradycardia or other bradyarrhythmia.

c) **List two other features of autonomic dysreflexia. (2 marks)**

- Hypertension may lead to severe headache, cerebral oedema with reduction in GCS, retinal haemorrhages, cerebral haemorrhage, seizures, death.
- Flushing.
- Nasal congestion.
- Sweating.

- Piloerection.
- Pallor.

d) List two common triggers for the development of acute autonomic dysreflexia. (2 marks)

- Urinary retention or blocked urinary catheter *(may account for up to 80% of cases)*.
- Constipation.

Other triggers include pressure ulcers, uterine contractions, sexual activity, acute abdominal pathology, urinary tract infection, and skeletal fractures.

e) Other than the need for appropriate consent and an anaesthetist present on standby, list three conditions that must be met for surgery to take place without anaesthesia. (3 marks)

- Surgical site below the level of the spinal cord lesion.
- Complete spinal cord injury.
- Absence of previous autonomic dysreflexia.
- Absence of muscle spasms or dystonia.

f) List three drugs that may be used in the acute management of the hypertension of autonomic dysreflexia. (3 marks)

This escalating list is taken from the 2008 Royal College of Physicians guidance for the management of autonomic dysreflexia which is featured in the BJA Education article referenced. Before pharmacological management is initiated, it advises to sit the patient up, remove tight clothing and support stockings, ensure the bladder is empty (by catheterising, flushing an existing catheter, or emptying the bladder if intraoperative), and exclusion and management of constipation with a rectal examination.

- Sublingual GTN (may need to escalate to intravenous GTN).
- Sublingual nifedipine.
- Intravenous hydralazine.
- Intravenous diazoxide.
- Intravenous magnesium.
- Intravenous phentolamine.

g) Give two reasons why a reduced dose of induction agent may be required when providing general anaesthesia for a patient with spinal cord injury. (2 marks)

- Altered pharmacokinetics due to reduced blood volume and muscle mass.
- Possibility of absent sympathetic response to hypotension resulting in risk of profound hypotension with cerebral and myocardial hypoperfusion if normal doses used.

REFERENCES

Petsas A, Drake J. Perioperative management for patients with a chronic spinal cord injury. *BJA Educ.* 2015: 15: 123–130.

Royal College of Physicians British Society of Rehabilitation Medicine, Multidisciplinary Association of Spinal Cord Injury Professionals, British Association of Spinal Cord Injury Professionals, British Association of Spinal Injury Specialists and Spinal Injuries Association. *A series of evidence-based guidelines for clinical management: guideline number 9: chronic spinal cord injury: management of patients in acute hospital settings.* London: Royal College of Physicians, 2008.

2

CARDIOTHORACIC ANAESTHESIA AND CARDIOTHORACIC CRITICAL CARE

2.1 September 2012 Endoscopic thoracic sympathectomy

a) List three indications for endoscopic thoracic sympathectomy (ETS). (3 marks)
b) Describe the sympathetic nerve supply to the upper limb. (3 marks)
c) Outline three general implications of managing a patient for ETS under general anaesthesia. (3 marks)
d) State three complications due to patient positioning that may occur during ETS under general anaesthesia. (3 marks)
e) Outline three options for airway management for ETS under general anaesthesia. (3 marks)
f) State three intraoperative complications that may be encountered during ETS. (3 marks)
g) State two postoperative complications that may occur following ETS. (2 marks)

The Chair's Report following the original SAQ found it to be "universally answered badly", with a 26.5% pass rate, and went on to comment that "clearly, most candidates had never anaesthetised a patient for the procedure nor had any knowledge about the procedure despite [it] being part of the syllabus. Knowledge of the effects of one-lung anaesthesia, effects of a capnothorax and indications for a sympathectomy were relevant in the answer. The pass mark had been adjusted to reflect the level of difficulty ('hard'). These ten key facts would have been sufficient for a pass (there were 23 in the model answer):

a) Indications for transthoracic sympathectomy

- *Hyperhidrosis*
- *Chronic pain/upper limb regional pain syndrome*

b) General implications

- *Large-bore IV access*
- *Potential for major haemorrhage*
- *May need arterial line*
- *Airway implications*
- *May need double lumen tube*

c) Intraoperative problems

- *Hypotension from capnothorax*
- *Hypoxia*
- *Postoperative problems*
- *May have residual pneumothorax*
- *May be painful*

The mean score was 7.7/20. The question was a strong discriminator.
Whilst the question appeared difficult, most of the answers required a systematic approach."

DOI: 10.1201/9781003388494-2

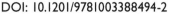

The level of detail from the Chair's Report is very useful here: it is reassuring to see that the majority of marks can be gained by writing sensible things like ensuring large-bore intravenous access and that a double lumen tube may be required. The topic was addressed in a CEACCP article from three years previously. Make sure you make use of these articles as they are so often the basis of a question.

a) List three indications for endoscopic thoracic sympathectomy (ETS). (3 marks)

- Palmar, axillary, or craniofacial hyperhidrosis.
- Chronic regional pain syndromes of the upper limb.
- Facial blushing.
- Chronic angina pectoris, unmanageable by pharmacological or cardiac intervention *(very unusual indication now)*.

b) Describe the sympathetic nerve supply to the upper limb. (3 marks)

Sympathetic nerve supply to the eye, head and neck, and upper limb is a common viva anatomy topic too. Even if you don't know the details, go back to the basics of the autonomic nervous system – preganglionic, ganglion, postganglionic.

- Preganglionic sympathetic fibres originate from spinal nerves T1–T4/5.
- Synapse in the superior, middle cervical, and inferior (stellate) cervical ganglia.
- Postganglionic fibres travel to effector cells.

c) Outline three general implications of managing a patient for ETS under general anaesthesia. (3 marks)

Patients having hyperhidrosis surgery are predominantly young and fit, but may also be older with comorbidities especially if the indication is for refractory angina pectoris; consider the need for additional assessment and investigation preoperatively. Complications are rare but can be catastrophic. Ensure the patient has full understanding of risks versus benefits.

- Occasionally, conversion from laparoscopic to open surgery is necessary: prep and drape ready for thoracotomy.
- Risk of major haemorrhage: ensure large-bore intravenous access and two group and save samples for rapid blood issue.
- Periods of hypoxia are common: shunt due to one-lung ventilation, atelectasis, and failure to fully inflate the first lung before proceeding with surgery on the second side.
- Periods of hypotension due to capnothorax likely: consider invasive blood pressure monitoring or more frequent noninvasive monitoring.

d) State three complications due to patient positioning that may occur during ETS under general anaesthesia. (3 marks)

I have grouped the risks depending on the different positioning options for ease of learning.

- Usually supine, reverse Trendelenburg, arms abducted: risk of brachial plexus injury.
- Sometimes prone: risk of facial or eye damage, dislodgement of airway, difficulty with ventilation, brachial plexus traction and injury.
- Sometimes lateral positioning: potential difficulty with ventilation, dislodgement of airway, damage to pressure points such as common peroneal nerve.

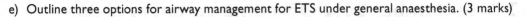

e) Outline three options for airway management for ETS under general anaesthesia. (3 marks)

During ETS there is a need to achieve collapse of one lung followed by the other for bilateral surgery. Options include the following:

- One-lung ventilation via double lumen tube.
- One-lung ventilation via endotracheal tube with bronchial blocker.
- Endotracheal tube with intrathoracic carbon dioxide insufflation.
- Laryngeal mask airway with intrathoracic carbon dioxide insufflation.

f) State three intraoperative complications that may be encountered during ETS. (3 marks)

Each of these are a different point, but I have grouped them for ease of learning and recall.

Airway:

- Malposition of double lumen tube or bronchial blocker may cause hypoxia.

Respiratory:

- One-lung ventilation causes shunt and, therefore, hypoxia. Efforts to improve this may actually worsen hypoxia (oxygen insufflation or CPAP to the deflated lung may reduce hypoxic pulmonary vasoconstriction, PEEP to the ventilated lung may increase resistance to blood flow to the ventilated side).
- With bilateral surgery, atelectasis of the reinflated lung may cause significant hypoxia when operating on the second side. Consider reinflation under direct vision.

Cardiovascular:

- Hypotension due to capnothorax, rarely cardiac arrest due to rapid insufflation.
- Cardiac arrhythmia induced by intrathoracic diathermy.
- Rarely, bleeding due to inadvertent damage to blood vessels on port insertion. May be catastrophic.

g) State two postoperative complications that may occur following ETS. (2 marks)

- Ongoing hypoxia due to atelectasis and residual pneumothorax.
- Risk of acute lung injury in the days following operation especially if protective one-lung ventilation not used.
- Chest pain during the immediate postoperative period requiring intravenous morphine – may necessitate overnight stay.
- Compensatory hyperhidrosis.

REFERENCES

Martin A, Telford R. Anaesthesia for endoscopic thoracic sympathectomy. *Contin Educ Anaesth Crit Care Pain.* 2009: 9: 52–55.

National Institute for Health and Care Excellence. *Endoscopic thoracic sympathectomy for primary facial blushing: IPG480.* May 2014a.

National Institute for Health and Care Excellence. *Endoscopic thoracic sympathectomy for primary hyperhidrosis of the upper limb: IPG487.* May 2014b.

Obeso Carillo GA, Cañizares Carretero MÁ, Padín Barreiro L, Soro García J, Blanco Tuimil L. Nonintubated bilateral single port thoracoscopic sympathectomy in the context of an outpatient program, the least invasive management for hyperhidrosis surgery. *Ann Transl Med.* 2015: 3: 357.

2.2 September 2012 Off-pump coronary artery bypass surgery

a) List two vessels which are commonly harvested for use in coronary artery bypass graft surgery. (2 marks)

b) List six theoretical advantages of "off-pump" coronary artery bypass grafting (OPCAB) compared to "on bypass" technique. (6 marks)

c) List five causes of haemodynamic instability during OPCAB. (5 marks)

d) List five strategies which can help to minimise haemodynamic instability during OPCAB. (5 marks)

e) List two methods that help to minimise perioperative hypothermia during OPCAB. (2 marks)

The Chair's Report following the original SAQ said that "Cardiothoracic anaesthesia is currently a mandatory unit of training, and as such, a question will feature in each SAQ paper. The Royal College recognises that candidates taking the exam at ST3 level may not have yet had significant experience of this sub-speciality, and for this reason, this question was designated as difficult. Nevertheless, it was felt that this question would be able to be answered by candidates using some basic principles. Many candidates answered (b) and (c) with on-pump rather than off-pump issues.

A pass would have been achieved by writing these 10 key points:

a) Theoretical advantages of OPCAB

- *Reduced platelet dysfunction*
- *Reduced neurological injury*

b) Causes of haemodynamic instability

- *Mechanical displacement of heart*
- *Arrhythmias*

d) Strategies to minimise haemodynamic instability

- *Avoid electrolyte disturbance*
- *Suspend surgical manipulation*

e) Minimising perioperative hypothermia (as with any anaesthetic)

- *Increase ambient theatre temperature*
- *Warm IV fluids*
- *Use hot-air warmers*

The only answers that were specific to OPCAB surgery were in (a); the other answers were generic. There were 24 key facts in the model answer. Factors contributing to poor performance were lack of knowledge, inexperience and failure to read the question. This question was the best discriminator in the paper."

This is from the same paper as the question on ETS — two cardiothoracic surgery questions in one paper. Once again, it was judged to be difficult; hence a score of 10–11/20 would have been needed to pass and, once again, a really useful report (albeit with a few typos) that shows that calm application of common sense can gain many marks.

a) **List two vessels which are commonly harvested for use in coronary artery bypass graft surgery. (2 marks)**

- Saphenous vein.
- Radial artery (in younger patients with non-calcified vessels).
- Internal mammary artery.

b) **List six theoretical advantages of "off-pump" coronary artery bypass grafting (OPCAB) compared to "on bypass" technique. (6 marks)**

Don't know anything about "off-pump" surgery? Basically, it means not using cardiopulmonary bypass (the pump) to facilitate heart surgery, operating on the beating heart instead. An immobilisation device is used to reduce movement of the area of myocardium being operated on at the time. Search for a video of off-pump surgery if you haven't seen it before. Think of all the issues that are associated with "on-pump" surgery and what might therefore be avoided by staying "off-pump."

- Reduced platelet dysfunction.
- Reduced consumption of clotting factors.
- Reduced risk of inappropriate fibrinolysis.
- Reduced risk of blood transfusion due to coagulation defects.
- Reduced risk of renal dysfunction.
- Reduced risk of SIRS.
- Reduced risk of direct aortic damage.
- Reduced risk of air emboli.
- Reduced risk of neurological dysfunction.
- Reduced risk of fluid overload/depletion.
- Reduced risk of electrolyte disturbance.
- Reduced hypothermia and its consequences on wound healing and coagulation.
- Earlier extubation, shorter/no ICU stay, reduced cost.
- Overall reduced morbidity and mortality.

c) **List five causes of haemodynamic instability during OPCAB. (5 marks)**

Think logically; the operation is being performed directly on a beating heart, which is still responsible for perfusion of the body at the time.

- Ischaemia due to vessel anastomosis (shunts may be used to minimise this).
- Manipulation of the heart for access to lateral and posterior aspects; lifting of heart vertically out of pericardial sac, ventricular filling must then happen vertically upwards, mitral and tricuspid annulus deformation resulting in reflux.
- Impaired filling due to immobilisation device.
- Arrhythmias induced by ischaemia, manipulation, reperfusion.
- Bleeding.

d) **List five strategies which can help to minimise haemodynamic instability during OPCAB. (5 marks)**

- Minimise heart manipulation, stop if major instability.
- Minimise periods of ischaemia, including through the use of shunts.
- Keep heart rate low/normal: this minimises oxygen requirement and reduces effect of periods of ischaemia.
- Monitor and treat electrolyte disturbances; keep potassium over 4.5 mmol/l and give magnesium routinely.
- Ensure that patient is adequately filled, guided by cardiac output monitoring.
- Good communication between the anaesthetist and the surgeon.

e) List two methods that help to minimise perioperative hypothermia during OPCAB. (2 marks)

Follow NICE guidance for prevention and management of hypothermia in adults having surgery.

- Ensure patient's temperature is normal before starting case, keep checking intraoperatively and targeting normal temperature.
- Minimise periods of leaving patient uncovered.
- Warmed intravenous fluids.
- Forced air warming blanket.
- Under body resistive heating mat.
- Raise ambient theatre temperature to a minimum of 21°C.
- Foil hat.

REFERENCES

Hett D. Anaesthesia for off-pump coronary artery surgery. *Contin Educ Anaesth Crit Care Pain.* 2006: 6: 60–62.

Møller CH, Steinbrüchel DA. Off-pump versus on-pump coronary artery bypass grafting. *Curr Cardiol Rep.* 2014: 16: 455.

National Institute for Health and Care Excellence. *Hypothermia: prevention and management in adults having surgery: CG65*, April 2008, updated December 2016.

2.3 March 2013 One-lung ventilation

a) List three absolute indications for one-lung ventilation (OLV). (3 marks)
b) List three relative indications for OLV. (3 marks)
c) Give two specific indications for placement of a right-sided double lumen tube. (2 marks)
d) List three disadvantages of using a double lumen tube for OLV. (3 marks)
e) How can the risks associated with lung resection be quantified preoperatively? (4 marks)
f) After calling for help and increasing FiO_2 to 1.0, list five steps that may improve hypoxaemia resulting from OLV. (5 marks)

The Chair's Report stated the original SAQ was designated as "easy," and this was matched by an 88.6% pass rate. They said that this topic "has been covered in previous SAQ exams (2006 and 2009) and was a very straightforward test of knowledge. Significant numbers of candidates scored 16/20 or higher."

a) List three absolute indications for one-lung ventilation (OLV). (3 marks)

- Isolation of a diseased lung to prevent contamination of a healthy lung e.g. empyema, massive haemorrhage.
- To control distribution of ventilation e.g. for bronchopleural fistula, major cyst or bullous disease, traumatic bronchial injury.
- Unilateral lung lavage for treatment of alveolar proteinosis, cystic fibrosis.

b) List three relative indications for OLV. (3 marks)

- Thoracic surgery (lobectomy, pneumonectomy, lung volume reduction surgery, video-assisted thoracoscopic surgery).
- Thoracic aortic aneurysm surgery.
- Oesophagectomy.
- Mediastinal mass surgery.
- Minimally invasive cardiac surgery.

c) Give two specific indications for placement of a right-sided double lumen tube. (2 marks)

Most procedures can be facilitated by a left-sided double lumen tube, which is easier to position. However, there are some indications where a right-sided tube may be necessary.

- Surgery involving the left main bronchus e.g. left pneumonectomy or lung transplant, left tracheobronchial disruption.
- Distortion of normal left main bronchus anatomy e.g. aneurysm of the descending thoracic aorta, tumour compressing the left main bronchus.

d) List three disadvantages of using a double lumen tube for OLV. (3 marks)

Once you have seen one or put one in, this will make a lot more sense!

- Significantly larger and more rigid compared to a standard endotracheal tube, increased risk of airway and oral trauma.
- Difficult to insert in patients with a difficult or distorted airway.
- Potential need for airway exchange to single lumen tube at end of case if ongoing postoperative ventilation is required.
- Movement or dislodgment of tube with subsequent failure of lung isolation.

e) How can the risks associated with lung resection be quantified preoperatively? (4 marks)

- Assessment of likelihood of postoperative dyspnoea by performing lung function tests and calculation of the predicted postoperative (PPO) FEV_1 and DLCO based on anatomic calculation (*i.e. calculating the predicted remaining FEV₁ and DLCO based on the preoperative measurements and the proportion of the 19 segments that are to be removed*), ventilation/perfusion scans, or CT evaluation (*PPO FEV₁ or DLCO less than 30% of predicted are at high risk of postoperative dyspnoea and need for long-term oxygen – formal functional assessment should be undertaken before proceeding*).

- Functional assessment for higher risk patients e.g. cardiopulmonary exercise testing (VO₂ peak being the most useful measure with < 10 ml O₂/kg/min being a contraindication, > 15 being "good physiological reserve" and > 20 being "safe" for pneumonectomy), stair climb, shuttle walk test or six-minute walk (*> 400 m being equivalent to a VO₂ peak of 15 ml O₂/kg/min*).
- Specific mortality risk prediction scores for lung surgery incorporating factors such as performance status, symptoms, age, sex, and comorbidities e.g. RESECT-90, Thoracoscore. Generally, poorly predictive of risk.
- Specific assessment of perioperative cardiac risk with risk prediction model e.g. Thoracic Revised Cardiac Risk Index.
- Assessment of pre-existing pulmonary hypertension with echocardiogram as this will be exacerbated by halving the pulmonary vasculature with pneumonectomy.

f) After calling for help and increasing FiO₂ to 1.0, list five steps that may improve hypoxaemia resulting from OLV. (5 marks)

Hypoxaemia during any anaesthetic is an emergency situation. You would alert the theatre team, request help, conduct a simultaneous assessment, and management should follow an ABC approach. This is how you may want to start your answer in a viva situation, before getting into the specific management that may resolve hypoxaemia specifically during OLV.

A:

- *Take over manual ventilation of patient to assess compliance.*
- *Check for obvious equipment failure such as disconnection.*
- *Check for double lumen tube or bronchial blocker dislodgement.*
- *Check for secretions or blood that may have occluded the tube.*

B:

- *Assess for compliance, capnography waveform, oxygen saturations.*
- *Auscultate the chest (if feasible whilst patient is draped) and consider bronchospasm, pneumothorax of ventilated lung, inadequate paralysis.*

C:

- *Assess for cardiovascular stability; check for sources of bleeding.*

- Bronchoscopy and repositioning of double lumen tube or bronchial blocker if position has slipped, and clearance of secretions as necessary.
- Ensure haemodynamic stability, giving fluids, vasopressors, or inotropes as appropriate.
- Perform recruitment manoeuvres to ventilated lung (*may cause transient hypotension and worsening hypoxaemia if more blood is diverted to the non-ventilated lung*).
- Increase PEEP to the ventilated, dependent (if in lateral position) lung to counteract the effect of mediastinal weight on functional residual capacity in the lateral decubitus position.
- Decrease PEEP to ventilated lung to reduce possible compression of pulmonary capillaries by excessive intra-alveolar pressure.
- CPAP to the non-ventilated lung to reduce the shunt effect caused by ongoing perfusion to the non-ventilated lung.
- Intermittent two-lung ventilation.
- If the surgery is for pneumonectomy, early clamping of pulmonary artery will resolve shunt issues.

REFERENCES

Ashok V, Francis J. A practical approach to adult one-lung ventilation. *BJA Educ.* 2018: 18: 69–74.

Brunelli A, Kim A, Berger K, Addrizzo-Harris D. Physiological evaluation of the patient with lung cancer being considered for resectional surgery: diagnosis and management of lung cancer, 3rd edition: American College of Chest Physicians evidence-based clinical practice guidelines. *Chest.* 2013: 143(5 suppl): e166S–e190S.

Mehrotra M, Jain A. *Single lung ventilation.* StatPearls Publishing, July 2022. www.ncbi.nlm.nih.gov/books/NBK538314/. Accessed 12th May 2023.

Ng A, Swanevelder J. Hypoxaemia during one-lung anaesthesia. *Contin Educ Anaesth Crit Care Pain.* 2010: 10: 117–122.

Ntima N, Lumb A. Pulmonary function tests in anaesthetic practice. *BJA Educ.* 2019: 19: 206–211.

Taylor M et al. Risk prediction for lung cancer surgery in the current era. *Video-Assist Thorac Surg.* 2022: 7: 21–47.

2.4 September 2013 Cardiac tamponade

You are asked to review a 65-year-old man on the cardiac intensive care unit who underwent coronary artery bypass surgery earlier in the day.

a) Which clinical signs suggest the development of acute cardiac tamponade? (8 marks)

b) List the investigations and their associated derangements that could confirm the diagnosis of acute cardiac tamponade. (3 marks)

c) What is the management of acute cardiac tamponade in this patient? (9 marks)

The Chair's Report following the original SAQ, reproduced here as it appeared in the exam, found a 57.6% pass rate and said it "was designated an 'easy' question by the exam board and was a good discriminator. The investigations and associated derangements were linked, and 1 mark was awarded for both correct answers. The management of acute pericardial tamponade was generally answered in a generic way (ABC, call for help etc.), but a number of candidates wasted time and effort on managing an anaesthetic in this situation. Many failed to monitor the clotting and administer blood products or reversing agents if indicated." Tamponade featured again in an SAQ in September 2016 and then in a CRQ in March 2022 and so will be addressed later in this chapter.

2.5 March 2014 Rigid bronchoscopy

A 71-year-old patient requires a rigid bronchoscopy for biopsy and possible laser resection of an endobronchial tumour.

a) List two possible options to maintain anaesthesia. (2 marks)
b) List four options to maintain gas exchange. (4 marks)
c) List three specific patient-safety considerations if laser is required. (3 marks)
d) Give three other considerations for safe laser use. (3 marks)
e) List four anaesthetic complications of rigid bronchoscopy. (4 marks)
f) List four surgical complications of rigid bronchoscopy. (4 marks)

The Chair's Report following the original SAQ stated that the "question proved discriminatory between candidates who gave a mature and thoughtful answer and those who did not understand the implications of 'tubeless' ENT/thoracic surgery. Weaker candidates proposed the use of laser-proof endotracheal tubes, and even double lumen endobronchial tubes and cardiac bypass, to facilitate gas exchange." The overall pass rate was 60.8%.

a) List two possible options to maintain anaesthesia. (2 marks)

In addition to general anaesthesia, topicalisation of the airway will help reduce the overall anaesthetic requirements, and immobility using NMBD or short-acting opioids may be required for resection.

- Volatile; connection of anaesthetic circuit to side port of rigid bronchoscope. *However, gas delivery may be intermittent as passage of tools via the bronchoscope will result in loss of seal at the proximal end. Unlike an endotracheal tube, the bronchoscope is not cuffed distally, and oxygen delivery must be paused during laser treatment.*
- Total intravenous anaesthesia can be used with any option for gas exchange management.

b) List four options to maintain gas exchange. (4 marks)

Apnoeic oxygenation utilising high-flow nasal oxygenation is generally not an option for rigid bronchoscopy in adults because the width of the bronchoscope normally occupies the entire airway, so there is no route for supraglottic oxygen to reach the distal airways. This would therefore only be useful in the shortest of cases using rigid bronchoscopy.

- High-frequency automated jet ventilation (e.g. Monsoon) attached at the jet ventilation port.
- Manual low-frequency jet ventilation (e.g. Sander's manual jet ventilator) attached at the jet ventilation port.
- Controlled ventilation via the anaesthetic circuit attached at the 22 mm side port of the bronchoscope. The oropharynx is packed with gauze, and silicone caps are used over the proximal bronchoscope openings (through which instruments may be passed) to reduce loss of gases.
- High-flow supplemental oxygen for apnoeic oxygenation via the 22 mm side port – a leak is necessary to avoid baro- or volutrauma with high flows. Not appropriate if laser to be used as results in excessive oxygen concentration in airway.
- Spontaneous ventilation via the anaesthetic circuit attached at the 22 mm side port with intermittent manual assistance, although this is unlikely to be sufficient for a prolonged case or if laser does become necessary as the patient will need to be still and therefore may be given NMBD or opioids.
- ECMO, infrequently used in cases where location of tumour means that alternative options for gas exchange are not feasible.

c) List three specific patient-safety considerations if laser is required. (3 marks)

- Maintain fraction of inspired oxygen as low as possible, certainly less than 0.4.
- Do not use nitrous oxide.
- Saline-soaked gauze in airway, over mouth, teeth.
- Goggles for patient.
- Ensure readiness for airway fire management (saline syringes to flood airway, self-inflating bag and mask or other method to ventilate with room air after initial removal of bronchoscope).
- Ensure that oxygen enriched pockets of gas are not allowed to develop during any breathing circuit or oxygen tubing disconnections e.g. under any drapes that are used.
- Ensure that all equipment that will be used to instrument the airway during the time the laser is to be used is laser-compatible, non-reflective, and that e.g. suction catheters are withdrawn before laser is activated.

d) Give three other general theatre considerations for safe laser use. (3 marks)

- Goggles for staff.
- Signage on doors.
- Theatre doors locked.
- Blinds down.
- Presence of laser-trained staff member, assurance of safe practice, avoiding accidental laser activation.
- Assurance of equipment maintenance.

e) List four anaesthetic complications of rigid bronchoscopy. (4 marks)

- Barotrauma associated with jet ventilation: pneumothorax, pneumomediastinum, pneumopericardium, pneumoperitoneum, subcutaneous emphysema.
- Awareness: secondary to intermittent anaesthesia delivery if inhalational technique used.
- Inadequate gas exchange: hypercapnia, hypoxia. Patient with existing lung pathology at higher risk.
- Laryngospasm, bronchospasm.
- Impaired venous return: high intrathoracic pressures associated with gas trapping, resulting in cardiovascular instability.
- Dysrhythmia and associated cardiovascular instability associated with jet ventilation.
- Airway contamination: ventilation without airway protection.

f) List four surgical complications of rigid bronchoscopy. (4 marks)

- Soft tissue trauma: lips, tongue, vocal cords, trachea, bronchi. Airway oedema may cause airway compromise or obstruction post-procedure.
- Dental damage.
- Major haemorrhage: associated with soft tissue damage, resection of lesion, or direct trauma to major blood vessel.
- Pneumothorax: due to resection or biopsy.
- Cervical spine damage: assess range of movement preoperatively. Consider radiological assessment if the patient has a risk factor such as rheumatoid arthritis.

REFERENCES

English J, Norris A, Bedforth N. Anaesthesia for airway surgery. *Contin Educ Anaesth Crit Care Pain*. 2006: 6: 28–31.

Evans E, Biro P, Bedforth N. Jet ventilation. *Contin Educ Anaesth Crit Care Pain*. 2007: 7: 2–5.

Galway U, Zura A, Wang M, Deeby M, Riter Q, Li T, Ruetzler K. Anesthetic considerations for rigid bronchoscopy: a narrative educational review. *Trends Anaesth Crit Care*. 2022: 43: 38–45.

Pathak V et al. Ventilation and anesthetic approaches for rigid bronchoscopy. *Ann Am Thorac Soc*. 2014: 11: 628–634.

Pearson K, McGuire B. Anaesthesia for laryngo-tracheal surgery, including tubeless field techniques. *BJA Educ*. 2017: 17: 242–248.

Roberts S, Thornington R. Paediatric bronchoscopy. *Contin Educ Anaesth Crit Care Pain*. 2005: 5: 41–44.

2.6 September 2014 Cardioplegia

a) What are the purposes (3 marks), typical composition (4 marks) and physiological actions (5 marks) of cardioplegia solutions?
b) By which routes can solutions of cardioplegia be administered? (2 marks)
c) What are the possible complications of cardioplegia solution administration? (6 marks)

The Chair's Report following this SAQ, reproduced here as it appeared in the exam, stated that cardioplegia was a "basic tool in cardiac anaesthesia" and that "it was evident from the answers which candidates had undertaken an attachment in this area of practice or had read an appropriate textbook. The importance of considering the mandatory units of training in preparation for the Final FRCA examination has been emphasised previously." The pass rate was just 16.5%. The topic was repeated in an SAQ in September 2019.

2.7 March 2015 Anticoagulation for cardiac surgery

A 67-year-old patient is to undergo coronary artery surgery on cardiopulmonary bypass (CPB).

a) What dose of heparin is used to achieve full anticoagulation for CPB, and how is it given? (2 marks)

b) Which laboratory and "point-of-care" tests determine the effectiveness of heparin anticoagulation in CPB patients? Give the advantages and/or disadvantages of each test. (10 marks)

c) What are the causes of inadequate anticoagulation in a patient whom it is believed has already received heparin? (5 marks)

d) Describe the possible adverse reactions to protamine. (3 marks)

The Chair's Report of the original SAQ, reproduced here as it appeared in the exam, stated (once again) that the "question proved straightforward to candidates who had rotated through a cardiac unit or had read a textbook on cardiothoracic anaesthesia. Many weak candidates neither had knowledge of the intraoperative dosing of heparin for bypass surgery nor aspects of appropriate monitoring. Again, inexperience was the predominating factor in success or failure in this item." The pass rate was 61.5%. The topic was then the subject of a CRQ in March 2020.

2.8 September 2015 Neurological complications after coronary artery bypass surgery

a) List four central neurological complications of coronary artery bypass surgery. (4 marks)
b) List four peripheral neurological complications of coronary artery bypass surgery. (4 marks)
c) List four patient risk factors for the development of central neurological complications due to coronary artery bypass surgery. (4 marks)
d) List three surgical risk factors for the development of central neurological complications after coronary artery bypass surgery. (3 marks)
e) Give one anaesthetic risk factor for the development of central neurological complications after coronary artery bypass surgery. (1 mark)
f) List four intraoperative approaches to minimising the risk of central neurological complications after coronary artery bypass surgery. (4 marks)

The Chairs' Report following the original SAQ stated that "Candidates who did well in this question tended to do well overall." The pass rate was 54.6%. "There was quite a spread of scores, with some candidates having a very clear idea of the answers and others seemingly not very much idea at all. Whether this reflects the fact that some candidates sitting the exam have no experience of cardiac anaesthesia is not clear."

a) **List four central neurological complications of coronary artery bypass surgery. (4 marks)**

It hasn't specified on-pump or off-pump surgery, so you should include the complications of both. Complications of prolonged surgery, surgery in an arteriopath, the issues related to going on-pump, and periods of hypotension should all be included as well as the specific complications caused by the different surgical approaches.

- Postoperative cognitive dysfunction, both short- and long-term, subtle behavioural or personality changes.
- Stroke, whether ischaemic, embolic (from existing patient thrombus or vessel lesions or as a result of CPB), or haemorrhagic.
- Transient ischaemic attack.
- Gas emboli.
- Ischaemic spinal cord injury.
- Delirium.

b) **List four peripheral neurological complications of coronary artery bypass surgery. (4 marks)**

- Brachial plexus injury; central line insertion, positioning, sternal retraction (rotation of first rib pushes clavicles into retroclavicular space putting traction on plexus) and internal mammary artery (IMA) harvesting (wider retraction necessary).
- Ulnar nerve injury; positioning associated with radial artery harvesting.
- Phrenic nerve injury (left phrenic nerve passes between lung and mediastinal pleura so at greater risk) with IMA harvesting.
- Recurrent laryngeal nerve injury; intubation (prolonged, with periods of hypotension), surgical dissection, especially of IMA.
- Saphenous nerve injury; damage occurring during saphenous vein harvesting due to close proximity at ankle.
- Intercostal nerve damage; minimally invasive direct coronary artery bypass (MIDCAB), where the incision is between the ribs rather than sternotomy.

c) List four patient risk factors for the development of central neurological complications due to coronary artery bypass surgery. (4 marks)

These factors are most significant.

- Age.
- Hypertension.
- Hypercholesterolaemia.
- History of stroke.
- Diabetes mellitus.
- Carotid stenosis.
- Preoperative cognitive dysfunction, including due to Alzheimer's, Parkinson's, and cerebral vascular disease.
- History of substance or alcohol misuse.
- Poor left ventricular function.

d) List three surgical risk factors for the development of central neurological complications after coronary artery bypass surgery. (3 marks)

- Duration of surgery (possibly relating to stress response, disruption of the blood-brain barrier, and altered autoregulation).
- Microemboli from diseased aorta when clamped, cannulated, or handled.
- Microemboli from cardiopulmonary bypass (CPB) circuit.
- Rapid rewarming after hypothermia can cause loss of autoregulation, resulting in cerebral oedema.
- Failure to maintain adequate cerebral perfusion pressure during CPB.

e) Give one anaesthetic risk factor for the development of central neurological complications after coronary artery bypass surgery. (1 mark)

Anaesthetic factors are the least significant contributors.

- Low intraoperative mean arterial pressure and so cerebral perfusion pressure.
- Prolonged deep hypnotic time.

f) List four intraoperative approaches to minimising the risk of central neurological complications after coronary artery bypass surgery. (4 marks)

- Minimally invasive techniques to reduce overall stress response.
- Adequate priming of CPB circuit, if used, and use of bubble traps and embolus filters.
- Surgical care to avoid disrupting aortic plaques on clamping and cannulation, use of ultrasound to check vessels before cannulation.
- Maintenance of haemodynamic stability to ensure adequate cerebral and cord perfusion pressure.
- Careful anticoagulation monitoring and management.
- Careful neck positioning, especially if there are risk factors that may already compromise blood supply to cervical cord.
- Optimal blood glucose management.
- Possibly avoiding excessive periods of excessively deep anaesthesia with the use of depth of anaesthesia monitoring.
- Monitoring and management of acid-base balance to avoid deleterious effects on brain autoregulation.
- If hypothermia induced, avoidance of fast rewarming which predisposes to cerebral oedema.
- Cerebral regional oximetry monitoring with appropriate management in response to decreases.

REFERENCES

Kapoor M. Neurological dysfunction after cardiac surgery and cardiac intensive care admission: a narrative review: part 1: the problem: nomenclature: delirium and postoperative neurocognitive disorder: and the role of cardiac surgery and anesthesia. *Ann Card Anaesth.* 2020a: 23: 383–390.

Kapoor M. Neurological dysfunction after cardiac surgery and cardiac intensive care admission: a narrative review: part 2: cognitive dysfunction after critical illness: potential contributors in surgery and intensive care: pathogenesis: and therapies to prevent/treat perioperative neurological dysfunction. *Ann Card Anaesth.* 2020b: 23: 391–400.

Miang Ying Tan A, Amoako D. Postoperative cognitive dysfunction after cardiac surgery. *Contin Educ Anaesth Crit Care Pain.* 2013: 13: 218–223.

Vu T, Smith J. An update on postoperative cognitive dysfunction following cardiac surgery. *Front Psychiatry.* 2022: 13: 884907.

2.9 March 2016 Aortic stenosis

A 70-year-old woman with aortic stenosis presents for an open aortic valve replacement (AVR).

a) What is the pathophysiology of worsening aortic stenosis? (8 marks)
b) Which specific cardiac investigations may be used in assessing the severity of this woman's disease? (3 marks)
c) Give values for the peak aortic flow velocity, mean pressure gradient and valve area that would indicate that this woman has severe aortic stenosis. (3 marks)
d) What would be your haemodynamic goals for the perioperative management of this patient? (6 marks)

The Chairs' Report following this SAQ, reproduced here as it appeared in the exam, surprisingly found that the "pass rate for this question [41.8%] was the second lowest overall. Aortic stenosis is a common condition, and its pathophysiology and management should be known to candidates sitting this exam. In part (a), many candidates simply gave the symptoms of aortic stenosis rather than describing the pathophysiology. This could have been due to not reading the question carefully enough but may also reflect lack of knowledge. As mentioned in previous reports, candidates should endeavour to arrange taster sessions in modules such as cardiac anaesthesia if they have not done them prior to sitting the SAQ paper." This question covered the same content as one from September 2019 in the perioperative medicine chapter, and you will find the details there, as well as in a question about TAVI from September 2022 in this chapter.

2.10 September 2016 Cardiac tamponade

You are asked to review a 65-year-old woman on the cardiac intensive care unit who has undergone coronary artery bypass surgery earlier in the day.

a) What clinical features might suggest the development of cardiac tamponade? (9 marks)
b) Describe specific investigations with their findings that could confirm the diagnosis of cardiac tamponade. (2 marks)
c) Outline the management of acute cardiac tamponade in this patient. (9 marks)

The Chairs' Report of the original SAQ, reproduced here as it was in the exam, reflected a pass rate of 81.4%, which was "the highest pass rate in the paper. It is an important topic and it is good to see that candidates are aware of the signs and symptoms and treatment options for this emergency." This question is virtually identical to the one that featured in the September 2013 paper except that part (a) asks for "clinical features," not signs, and part (b) asks for investigations to be "specific" and now only has 2 marks assigned to it. Perhaps, the 2013 cohort had the same difficulties that I did in terms of thinking of enough investigations that would realistically be useful in the likely time frame of acute tamponade.

2.11 March 2017 Off-pump coronary artery bypass surgery

a) What are the theoretical advantages of "off-pump" coronary artery bypass grafting (OPCAB) compared to an "on-bypass" technique? (7 marks)
b) What are the potential causes of haemodynamic instability during OPCAB? (5 marks)
c) Which strategies help to minimise this haemodynamic instability? (8 marks)

The Chairs' Report following the original SAQ, reproduced here as it appeared in the exam, said it was "encouraging that the pass rate for this question was high [60.4%]. Hopefully, this reflects the fact that candidates are ensuring that they get exposure to the subspecialty of cardiac anaesthesia prior to sitting the exam. Some candidates did not give enough detail in parts (b) and (c), concerning the causes and mitigation of haemodynamic instability during off-pump cardiac surgery, so they failed to score well. This question correlated well with overall performance: i.e. those candidates who scored well in this question did well in the exam overall."

Apart from some tiny tweaks to the wording, the only difference between this question and the one from September 2012 is that this question did not ask about temperature maintenance. Anyone who had bothered to look at past papers must have been delighted when this question came up again.

2.12 September 2017 Intra-aortic balloon pump

a) What is meant by counterpulsation in the context of an intra-aortic balloon pump (IABP)? (1 mark)

b) Briefly explain the effect of counterpulsation from an IABP on coronary blood flow and the left ventricle. (4 marks)

c) What are the indications for (6 marks) and contraindications to (3 marks) the use of an IABP in an adult?

d) List possible complications of an IABP. (6 marks)

This is the SAQ as it appeared in the exam paper. The Chairs said, "This question correlated well with overall performance and was generally well answered in the clinical sections (parts (c) and (d)). However, part (b), which required an explanation of the physiological effects of counter-pulsation, was answered poorly." IABP has been the subject of the cardiothoracic question in two further exam sittings covered by the time period of this book.

2.13 September 2018 One-lung ventilation

a) How can the risks associated with lung resection be quantified preoperatively? (6 marks)
b) What factors can lead to the development of high airway pressures during one-lung ventilation (OLV)? (6 marks)
c) How would you manage the development of hypoxaemia during OLV? (8 marks)

The Chairs' Report of the original SAQ, reproduced here as it appeared in the exam, said that this was "a common question in all parts of the exam and requires a good understanding of physiology. Reassuringly this was well answered by the majority of candidates and had a reasonable pass rate [58.4%]. Candidates particularly answered the section on one lung ventilation well." This SAQ covered the same content as that from March 2013, with just subsection (b) being new. There is a long list of possible reasons for raised airway pressures during OLV, some are generally applicable to ventilation of any patient and some specific to OLV. I have given a fairly full list below, but if this question were asked in a CRQ, it would be important to prioritise the issues that are most relevant to OLV to gain maximum marks.

b) What factors can lead to the development of high airway pressures during one-lung ventilation (OLV)? (6 marks)

- Mechanical factors:
  - Double lumen tube is narrower than a standard endotracheal tube.
  - Double lumen tube is more readily obstructed with secretions or blood due to the narrowness of its channels.
  - Double lumen tube malposition resulting in loss of airway patency or advancement into a more distal airway.
  - Inappropriate ventilation e.g. excessive tidal volumes, especially when considering that ventilation is of one lung only.
  - External compression of breathing circuit.

- Patient factors:
  - Atelectasis of ventilated lung which is exacerbated by dependent position if patient in lateral position for lung surgery.
  - Pre-existing lung disease which may be what has necessitated the surgery.
  - Obesity.
  - Failure to maintain adequate muscle relaxation.

- Acute events:
  - Simple or tension pneumothorax.
  - Anaphylaxis.
  - Bronchospasm.
  - Development of acute lung injury due to prolonged surgery or OLV.

2.14 March 2019 Dilated cardiomyopathy

a) List three possible ways in which a patient with dilated cardiomyopathy (DCM) may present. (3 marks)

b) Give four pharmacological (4 marks) and two non-pharmacological management options for a patient with DCM. (2 marks)

c) Give two predictors of poor outcome in patients with DCM undergoing surgery. (2 marks)

d) Give four haemodynamic goals when anaesthetising patients with DCM. (4 marks)

e) Give two anaesthetic approaches to achieving these goals. (2 marks)

f) List three monitoring techniques (beyond the standard basic monitoring requirements for anaesthesia), and the information that may be gained from them, that may help guide anaesthesia management to achieve the desired haemodynamic goals. (3 marks)

Cardiomyopathies are classified as dilated, hypertrophic, restrictive, arrhythmogenic right ventricular, and unclassified. Each of these may be genetic or acquired. Dilated cardiomyopathy is the presence of left ventricular dilatation and systolic dysfunction in the absence of abnormal loading conditions (e.g. hypertension or valvular disease). There may be similar right heart changes.

Genetic causes for dilated cardiomyopathy include autosomal dominant inheritance of defects in cardiac muscle structure, X-linked DCM, and X-linked muscular dystrophies such as Becker and Duchenne. Acquired causes of DCM include the consequences of viral myocarditis, drugs such as some chemotherapeutic agents, alcohol, tachycardiomyopathy, pregnancy-associated DCM, and nutritional defects such as thiamine.

As the left ventricle enlarges, the overlap between the actin and myosin filaments reduces, resulting in reduction of stroke volume. This stretch also results in valvular dysfunction. According to Laplace's law, the increased fluid content of the ventricle increases wall tension, impairing oxygen delivery and causing further cardiac muscle compromise and loss of function. The inefficient systole also results in the development of intracardiac thrombus.

The Chairs stated a pass rate of 67.6% but said that "Despite a respectable pass rate, many candidates demonstrated a lack of knowledge on this subject. The feeling of the examiners was that the question proved straightforward to those candidates who had rotated through a cardiac module. Many weaker candidates didn't have sufficient knowledge or clinical experience to discuss the practicalities of anaesthetising patients with dilated cardiomyopathy." There was a BJA Education article on cardiomyopathies and anaesthesia in 2017.

a) **List three possible ways in which a patient with dilated cardiomyopathy (DCM) may present. (3 marks)**

- Signs and symptoms of heart failure: shortness of breath, poor exercise tolerance, fatigue, ascites, peripheral oedema.
- Arrhythmias and their consequences.
- Embolic events.
- Sudden death.
- Screening including of family members after diagnosis of index case.

b) **Give four pharmacological (4 marks) and two non-pharmacological management options for a patient with DCM. (2 marks)**

Pharmacological:

- Beta-blockers.
- Aldosterone inhibitors.
- Diuretics.

- ACE inhibitors or angiotensin-2 receptor blockers.
- Anticoagulants.
- SGLT-2 inhibitors *(reduce cardiovascular events and hospitalisation for heart failure, mechanism unclear)*.
- Atrial natriuretic peptide *(currently only available for intravenous use)*.
- Angiotensin receptor-neprilysin inhibitor *(ANRi e.g. sacubitril-valsartan. Neprilysin breaks down endogenous peptides such as atrial natriuretic peptide and so inhibition of this promotes favourable effects in DCM. However, neprilysin also breaks down angiotensin-2 and inhibition of this effect would lead to vasoconstriction, unhelpful in the setting of DCM. The neprilysin inhibitor is therefore given in conjunction with an angiotensin-2 receptor blocker)*.

Non-pharmacological:

- Partial left ventriculectomy.
- Cardiac resynchronisation pacing therapy.
- Implantable cardiac defibrillator.
- Left ventricular assist device as a bridge to transplant.
- Heart transplant.

c) **Give two predictors of poor outcome in patients with DCM undergoing surgery. (2 marks)**

- LVEF < 20%.
- Elevated LVEDP.
- Left ventricular hypokinesia.
- Non-sustained VT.

d) **Give four haemodynamic goals when anaesthetising patients with DCM. (4 marks)**

This heart is struggling, and you don't want to do anything that makes it more difficult to eject blood.

- Avoid myocardial depression.
- Maintain adequate preload.
- Prevent increases in afterload.
- Avoid tachycardia and tachyarrhythmia.
- Prevent sudden hypotension *(this will impair coronary perfusion)*.

e) **Give two anaesthetic approaches to achieving these goals. (2 marks)**

- Perform surgery under peripheral nerve block only, if feasible, as this has minimal effect on haemodynamics.
- Use of central neuraxial block – reduction in afterload can improve cardiac output *(though too much will result in myocardial hypoperfusion)*.
- Slow intravenous induction (as circulation time will be impaired) to avoid overdosing of agents and excessive decrease in afterload and myocardial depression.
- Increased opioid component to intravenous anaesthetic technique or induction as these have less of an impact on haemodynamics and will reduce need for other anaesthetic agents.
- Balanced maintenance of anaesthesia as inhalational agents cause myocardial depression in high concentrations.

f) **List three monitoring techniques (beyond the standard basic monitoring requirements for anaesthesia), and the information that may be gained from them, that may help guide anaesthesia management to achieve the desired haemodynamic goals. (3 marks)**

- Transoesophageal echocardiography to provide a dynamic assessment of heart filling and cardiac output.
- Oesophageal Doppler to provide an algorithm-based assessment of stroke volume.

- Central venous catheterisation for assessment of cardiac preload.
- Invasive arterial blood pressure monitoring to give an algorithm-based assessment of stroke volume variation, assessment of acid-base, gas exchange, and electrolyte status, all of which might have deleterious impact on heart function, and beat-to-beat blood pressure monitoring to assist in rapid response to adverse changes.
- Depth of anaesthesia monitoring to give an indication of anaesthetic depth and so allow minimum necessary anaesthetic drug administration.
- Cerebral oxygenation monitoring to assess oxygen delivery and allow appropriate manipulation to reduce the risk of postoperative cognitive dysfunction.

REFERENCES

Elliott P et al. Classification of the cardiomyopathies: a position statement from the European Society of Cardiology working group on myocardial and pericardial diseases. *Eur Heart J.* 2008: 29: 270–276.

Mahmaljy H, Yelamanchili V, Singhal M. *Dilated cardiomyopathy.* StatPearls Publishing, February 2023. www.ncbi.nlm.nih.gov/books/NBK441911/. Accessed 12th May 2023.

Rasmi Ibrahim I, Sharma V. Cardiomyopathy and anaesthesia. *BJA Educ.* 2017: 17: 363–369.

Verdonschot J et al. Role of targeted therapy in dilated cardiomyopathy: the challenging road toward a personalized approach. *JAHA.* 2019: 8: e012514.

2.15 September 2019 Cardioplegia

a) List four purposes of cardioplegia solution use in cardiac surgery. (4 marks)
b) Give the typical composition of cardioplegia solution. (4 marks)
c) List the physiological effects of cardioplegia solution on the myocardium. (4 marks)
d) List two routes by which solutions of cardioplegia can be administered. (2 marks)
e) List six complications of cardioplegia solution administration. (6 marks)

The Chairs' Report following the original SAQ (this was the hybrid paper of six CRQs and six SAQs) said that "this question proved straightforward to candidates who had rotated through a cardiac module, with weaker candidates lacking sufficient knowledge or clinical experience of cardiac anaesthesia." The massively improved pass rate, 71.2%, compared to the very similar SAQ from September 2014 suggests that candidates made sure they had learned from past topics. I have changed the question minimally to make it into more of a CRQ format.

a) List four purposes of cardioplegia solution use in cardiac surgery. (4 marks)

Myocardial protection:

- Cardiac arrest in diastole and manipulation of the extracellular environment to minimise ongoing metabolic activity and its deleterious consequences during a period of suboptimal perfusion.
- Cooling of the heart.

Facilitation of surgery:

- Still, relaxed heart.
- Bloodless field.

b) Give the typical composition of cardioplegia solution. (4 marks)

c) List the physiological effects of cardioplegia solution on the myocardium. (4 marks)

Stay calm. There aren't many marks for each of these individual sections so I cannot imagine that they want a detailed list of the precise concentrations of the electrolytes in cardioplegia – there is a variety of solutions available, after all. However, they want you to demonstrate that you know what the point of its use is, and some aspects of how it works are closely tied up with its constituents, hence my presentation in tabulated form.

Typical composition	Physiological actions
High potassium concentration, approximately 20 mmol/l.	Arrest of heart in diastole – high extracellular potassium levels prevent repolarisation of myocytes, causing inactivation of the fast inward voltage sensitive sodium channels that are important in phase 0 of the action potential.
Calcium at a lower concentration than plasma.	Calcium is required to maintain cell membrane integrity, but keeping the concentration low reduces the amount of calcium available for contraction, thus avoiding myocardial activity.
Magnesium concentration exceeding normal plasma level.	Prevents magnesium loss from the cells, thus maintaining its role as enzymatic cofactor, and competes with calcium, thus reducing calcium-induced contraction.
Sodium and chloride usually at levels near those found in plasma.	Alternatively, low sodium concentration can be used as the mechanism to induce cardiac arrest.

(Continued)

(Continued)

Typical composition	Physiological actions
Bicarbonate, histidine, or other buffer.	To offset tendency to metabolic acidosis associated with ischaemia.
Mannitol.	To raise the osmolarity of the solution, thus reducing tissue oedema.
Other additives: Procaine. Blood.	Reduction of arrhythmia at reperfusion. Oxygen-carrying capacity.

d) List two routes by which solutions of cardioplegia can be administered. (2 marks)

- Anterograde: specialised cannula placed into ascending aorta or directly into coronary ostia *(dependent on adequate root pressure, good coronary perfusion, and competent aortic valve to reach all of the myocardium if not introduced directly into coronary ostia).*
- Retrograde: cannula into the coronary sinus.

e) List six complications of cardioplegia solution administration. (6 marks)

Remember to include the issues that may arise from the method of <u>administration</u> as well as from the cardioplegia itself, but avoid veering off into listing the risks of cardiopulmonary bypass.

- Direct vessel damage associated with the cannulation.
- Dislodgement of plaque on cannulation resulting in embolic stroke or myocardial infarction.
- Air bubbles in cardioplegia solution can cause air emboli in the coronary arteries or systemic circulation with consequent ischaemia.
- Failure to attain widespread cardiac perfusion with the cardioplegia, leaving areas of myocardium warm and active whilst ischaemic.
- Fluid overload.
- Haemodilution, anaemia.
- Myocardial oedema, haemorrhage and injury resulting from high infusing pressures.
- Postoperative electrolyte derangement with consequent risk of arrhythmia.
- Postoperative acid-base disturbance and dilution of clotting factors with negative impact on coagulation.

REFERENCES

Chambers D, Fallouh H. Cardioplegia and cardiac surgery: pharmacological arrest and cardioprotection during global ischemia and reperfusion. *Pharmacol Ther.* 2010: 127: 41–52.

Jameel S, Colah S, Klein A. Recent advances in cardiopulmonary bypass techniques. *Contin Educ Anaesth Crit Care Pain.* 2010: 10: 20–23.

Kunst G et al. 2019 EACTS/EACTA/EBCP guidelines on cardiopulmonary bypass in adult cardiac surgery. *BJA.* 2019: 123: 713–757.

Machin D, Allsager C. Principles of cardiopulmonary bypass. *Contin Educ Anaesth Crit Care Pain.* 2006: 6: 176–181.

Scott T, Swaneveder J. Perioperative myocardial protection. *Contin Educ Anaesth Crit Care Pain.* 2009: 9: 97–101.

2.16 March 2020 Anticoagulation for cardiac surgery

A 67-year-old patient is to undergo coronary artery surgery on cardiopulmonary bypass (CPB).
a) State the dose of heparin (IU/kg) used to achieve full anticoagulation for, and the target activated clotting time (ACT) prior to initiation of CPB. (2 marks)
b) State the primary mechanism of action of heparin. (1 mark)
c) List three other laboratory or "point-of-care" tests that may be used to determine the effectiveness of heparin anticoagulation in CPB patients, giving an advantage and disadvantage of each test. (9 marks)
d) List four causes of inadequate anticoagulation after heparin administration. (4 marks)
e) Give three possible adverse reactions to protamine. (4 marks)

The Chairs' Report of the original CRQ said that "Examiners were surprised at the lack of knowledge displayed in this question and particularly because this topic had come up in a recent paper. Part (b) was answered incorrectly by many. Most candidates mentioned inactivation of thrombin or activation of antithrombin III. Very few mentioned both inactivation of thrombin and factor Xa. In section (c), most candidates mentioned 3 or 4 tests correctly but very few managed to correctly give the advantage and disadvantage of each test."

a) State the dose of heparin (IU/kg) used to achieve full anticoagulation for, and the target activated clotting time (ACT) prior to initiation of CPB. (2 marks)

Check the baseline ACT. Give the heparin via a central venous cannula. Check the ACT after 3–5 minutes. It should be rechecked every 15–30 minutes during CPB.

- 300–400 IU/kg.
- ACT is 3 × baseline or greater than 480 s.

b) State the primary mechanism of action of heparin. (1 mark)

- Binds to antithrombin III to potentiate its inhibitory action on thrombin and factor Xa.

Low molecular weight heparins are smaller molecules with greater anti factor Xa activity and minimal (varies according to type of LMWH) thrombin inhibition.

c) List three other laboratory or "point-of-care" tests that may be used to determine the effectiveness of heparin anticoagulation in CPB patients, giving an advantage and disadvantage of each test. (9 marks)

I have included the advantages and disadvantages of ACT as well for completeness.

Test	Advantage	Disadvantage
Activated partial thromboplastin time (APTT), lab test.	Cheap.	Slow turnaround time which may result in less well-directed management.
Anti-Xa assay, lab test.	Correlates well with heparin activity.	Not widely used for this purpose, poor inter-laboratory correlation. Slow.
Activated clotting time (ACT), point-of-care test.	Rapid response. Cheap. Familiar.	Thrombocytopenia, antiplatelet agents, hypothermia, haemodilution and aprotinin may all prolong ACT so it lacks specificity. ACT has poor correlation with anti-Xa activity.

(Continued)

(Continued)

Test	Advantage	Disadvantage
Heparin concentration monitoring, point-of-care test.	Measuring of heparin concentration once haemodilution has occurred with CPB may be more appropriate to direct heparin administration than ACT, which is prolonged by commencing CPB (higher doses of heparin will be indicated when using this method).	Expensive, not widely available.
Thromboelastography (TEG), point-of-care test.	TEG gives a graphical representation of the ability of blood to clot. Optionally, heparinase can be added to the test to negate the effect of systemic heparin thus predicting the patient's coagulation state after heparin has been reversed – can therefore guide blood product replacement as well.	Cost of equipment. Training required for interpretation. Takes time for clot to evolve.

d) List four causes of inadequate anticoagulation after heparin administration. (4 marks)

Administration error:

- Wrong drug administered.
- Drug not given.
- CVC not patent.
- CVC not flushed after dose given.

Pharmacokinetic factors:

Heparin is highly protein bound, so an increase in the presence of plasma proteins reduces free, and therefore active, drug.

- Acutely ill patients.
- Malignancy.
- Peri- or postpartum.

Lack of antithrombin III *(can be treated by administration of fresh frozen plasma)*:

- Drug-induced; recent heparin use.
- Accelerated consumption; DIC, sepsis.
- Dilution; CPB.
- Decreased synthesis; liver cirrhosis.
- Increased excretion; protein-losing states.
- Familial; 1/2 000–20 000.

e) Give three possible adverse reactions to protamine. (4 marks)

As a result of the potential reactions, protamine is normally given as an infusion or slowly over the course of 15–20 minutes. The dose of protamine given is typically 1 mg per 100 IU of heparin administered.

- Arterial hypotension or reduced cardiac output.
- Pulmonary vasoconstriction.
- Anaphylaxis.
- Unbound protamine inhibits platelet reactivity, adhesion, and aggregation. An excessive dose therefore promotes bleeding.

REFERENCES

Kunst G et al. 2019 EACTS/EACTA/EBCP guidelines on cardiopulmonary bypass in adult cardiac surgery. *BJA*. 2019: 123: 713–757.

Machin D, Allsager C. Principles of cardiopulmonary bypass. *Contin Educ Anaesth Crit Care Pain*. 2006: 6: 176–181.

O'Carroll-Kuehn B, Meeran H. Management of coagulation during cardiopulmonary bypass. *BJA Educ*. 2007: 7: 195–198.

Srivastava A, Kelleher A. Point-of-care coagulation testing. *Contin Educ Anaesth Crit Care Pain*. 2013: 13: 12–16.

2.17 September 2020 Intra-aortic balloon pump

a) What is meant by counterpulsation in the context of an intra-aortic balloon pump (IABP)? (1 mark)
b) State the benefits of counterpulsation to oxygen delivery to the left ventricle. (2 marks)
c) State the effect of counterpulsation on the output from the left ventricle. (1 mark)
d) List four indications for the insertion of an IABP. (4 marks)
e) List three contraindications to insertion of an IABP. (3 marks)
f) Give the anatomical location at which the cephalad end of the balloon of the IABP should be placed. (1 mark)
g) List two methods for timing balloon inflation when using an IABP. (2 marks)
h) List two physiological consequences of mistimed inflation of an IABP. (2 marks)
i) List four other complications of insertion or use of an IABP. (4 marks)

The Chairs' Report of the original CRQ stated that the question was well answered, with a pass rate of 70.6%. They said the parts "that required factual recall were answered well but [the section] on applied physiology was the worst performing stem for this question."

a) **What is meant by counterpulsation in the context of an intra-aortic balloon pump (IABP)? (1 mark)**

- Inflation of the balloon in diastole and deflation just before systole.

b) **State the benefits of counterpulsation to oxygen delivery to the left ventricle. (2 marks)**

- Inflation forces blood proximally increasing the perfusion pressure of the coronary arteries (and therefore oxygen delivery to the myocardium).
- Deflation decreases afterload, reducing myocardial wall stress and reducing oxygen demand in systole.
- Endothelially derived nitric oxide release due to vascular stretch may result in coronary arteriolar dilatation, increasing blood flow and oxygen delivery.

c) **State the effect of counterpulsation on the output from the left ventricle. (1 mark)**

- Inflation forces blood distally and proximally (e.g. to cerebral vessels), therefore augmenting the apparent output from the left ventricle, with deflation decreasing afterload during systole to promote ejection.

d) **List four indications for the insertion of an IABP. (4 marks)**

- Acute heart failure with hypotension.
- Myocardial infarction with acute left ventricular failure.
- Myocardial infarction with acute mechanical complications causing shock e.g. acute mitral regurgitation due to papillary muscle rupture.
- Low cardiac output after CABG or failure to separate from CPB.
- As prophylaxis or adjunctive treatment in high-risk percutaneous coronary intervention.
- As a bridge to definitive treatment in patients with intractable angina or myocardial ischaemia, refractory heart failure, or intractable ventricular arrhythmias.

e) **List three contraindications to insertion of an IABP. (3 marks)**

- Moderate to severe aortic regurgitation or dissection.
- Chronic end-stage heart failure with no further treatment options.
- Uncontrolled sepsis.
- Uncontrolled bleeding diathesis.

- Aortic aneurysm or dissection.
- Severe untreated peripheral artery or aortic disease or reconstructive vascular surgery.
- Tachyarrhythmia *(at a rate that the IABP cannot synchronise with)*.

f) Give the anatomical location at which the cephalad end of the balloon of the IABP should be placed. (1 mark)

Fluoroscopic guidance is used to site the IABP, and position can be checked with this, with X-ray, on ultrasound, or with transoesophageal echo. The distal end of the balloon should lie above the origin of the renal arteries.

- In the descending thoracic aorta 2 to 3 cm distal to the origin of the left subclavian artery.

g) List two methods for timing balloon inflation when using an IABP. (2 marks)

The device can be set to augment every heartbeat or can trigger at a ratio which can be weaned with improvement of the patient's condition. During cardiac arrest, an IABP must be changed to pressure trigger mode as the ECG will no longer provide reliable triggering. Specifically during PEA, the IABP will give the false impression of a cardiac output due to the augmented IABP waveform.

- ECG triggered; balloon inflates with T wave, deflates with peak of R wave.
- Arterial pressure waveform triggered; balloon inflates with the dicrotic notch (closure of aortic valve), deflates just before upstroke of arterial pressure waveform (just before the aortic valve opens).

h) List two physiological consequences of mistimed inflation of an IABP. (2 marks)

Any mistiming can lead to haemodynamic instability, and this question is asking specifically for the underlying physiology. If you go back to the desired mechanism of an IABP (inflating during diastole and deflating at the onset of systole), then you can work out what happens when things go wrong.

- Early inflation (before aortic valve closes) causes increased left ventricular afterload, aortic regurgitation, and increased myocardial oxygen demand.
- Late inflation (after the dicrotic notch) causes suboptimal coronary artery perfusion due to inadequate counterpulsation.
- Early deflation (before onset of systole) causes suboptimal reduction in afterload, failing to improve myocardial oxygen demand.
- Late deflation (after onset of systole) causes an increase in afterload due to left ventricular ejection against inflated balloon and consequent increased myocardial oxygen demand.

i) List four other complications of insertion or use of an IABP. (4 marks)

Related to vascular access:

- Vascular injury causing bleeding, haematoma, false aneurysm, arteriovenous fistula.
- Infection.
- Poor perfusion to the limb distally, compartment syndrome.

Related to device use:

- Limb, cerebral, spinal cord, mesenteric or renal ischaemia due to incorrect placement.
- Aortic dissection.
- Cardiac tamponade.
- Thromboembolism.
- Thrombocytopaenia and haemolysis.
- Balloon rupture resulting in gas embolus *(the gas used is helium as its low density means that it is transferred rapidly from the machine to the balloon tip and back, and it is rapidly absorbed into the blood in the event of balloon rupture)*.

Related to systemic anticoagulation:

- Bleeding.

REFERENCES

Brand J, Mcdonald A, Dunning, J. Management of cardiac arrest following cardiac surgery. *BJA Educ.* 2018: 18: 16–22.

Khan T, Siddiqui A. *Intra-aortic balloon pump.* StatPearls Publishing, June 2022. www.ncbi.nlm.nih.gov/books/NBK542233/. Accessed 12th May 2023.

Krishna M, Zacharowski K. Principles of intra-aortic balloon pump counterpulsation. *Contin Educ Anaesth Crit Care Pain.* 2009: 9: 24–28.

MacKay E et al. Contemporary clinical niche for intra-aortic balloon counterpulsation in perioperative cardiovascular practice: an evidence-based review for the cardiovascular anesthesiologist. *J Cardiothorac Vasc Anesth.* 2017: 31: 309–320.

2.18 March 2021 Pneumonectomy

A 70-year-old male with 50 pack year smoking history with lung cancer presents for pneumonectomy.

a) List three other comorbidities this patient may have. (3 marks)
b) Give three preoperative physiological measurements used to assess for suitability for pneumonectomy. (3 marks)
c) List three contraindications to pneumonectomy for this patient. (3 marks)
d) List three other possible indications for pneumonectomy. (3 marks)
e) List two ways to optimise this patient preoperatively. (2 marks)
f) Describe how correct placement of a left-sided double lumen tube is performed clinically. (3 marks)
g) List three specific complications of pneumonectomy. (3 marks)

This Chairs' Report of the original CRQ commented on this being a "fairly common topic in the Final FRCA, so a pass rate of only 47.7% was disappointing. The question did correlate well with overall performance, however, no component was particularly well answered, with candidates consistently dropping one or two marks on each stem. In parts (b) and (c), physiological measurements and contraindications to pneumonectomy, we were looking for more detail than that offered by the candidates." This topic's appearance in the exam followed on from an article about pneumonectomy in BJA Education in 2019. It contained most of the knowledge necessary to pass. At the time of writing, this CRQ had not been re-examined. Past experiences would suggest it as a repeated topic in the near future due to the Chairs' disappointment with the pass rate!

a) List three other comorbidities this patient may have. (3 marks)

Formulate your answer in a structured way. Smoking is the most common cause of lung cancer, and so this patient is at risk of other smoking-related diseases so these are what I would focus on.

Respiratory:

- Chronic obstructive pulmonary disease, emphysema.

Cardiovascular:

- Ischaemic heart disease.
- Hypertension.
- Heart failure, including right heart failure as a consequence of lung disease.
- Peripheral vascular disease.

Neurological:

- Cerebrovascular disease.

Haematology:

- Anaemia as a result of malignancy.
- Polycythaemia as a result of severe COPD.

Nutritional:

- Poor nutritional status in association with malignancy.

b) **Give three preoperative physiological measurements used to assess for suitability for pneumonectomy. (3 marks)**

This is similar to the question asked in March 2013, but is asking what measurements from the tests are important rather than what tests.

- DLCO, used to predict PPO DLCO, which will give an indication of likelihood of postoperative dyspnoea.
- FEV_1, used to predict PPO FEV_1, which will give an indication of likelihood of postoperative dyspnoea.
  - PPO DLCO and $FEV_1 > 60\%$ indicates low risk and no further investigation is necessary.
  - PPO DLCO or FEV_1 30–60% should prompt low tech exercise test e.g. stair climb > 22 m altitude or shuttle walk > 400 m indicate low risk.
  - PPO DLCO and $FEV_1 < 30\%$ or failure of low tech exercise test should prompt consideration of cardiopulmonary exercise testing.
- VO_2 peak as a measure of cardiopulmonary reserve as measured by cardiopulmonary exercise testing, ideally > 20 ml O_2/kg/min (pneumonectomy contraindicated if < 10 ml O_2/kg/min or < 35% predicted).
- Pulmonary artery pressure, measured on echocardiography, as a measure of pre-existing pulmonary hypertension as this is likely to get worse after pneumonectomy.

c) **List three contraindications to pneumonectomy for this patient. (3 marks)**

- Non-suitability based on physiological testing.
- Pre-existing significant pulmonary hypertension.
- Severe valvular heart disease or poor ventricular function.
- Metastatic disease, subdiaphragmatic extension of the tumour, or nodes in contralateral hemithorax.

d) **List three other possible indications for pneumonectomy. (3 marks)**

- Traumatic injury with uncontrolled haemorrhage.
- Infective disorders:
  - Chronic tuberculosis.
  - Fungal infection (e.g. aspergilloma).
  - Abscess or empyema.
- Inflammatory lung disease.
- Congenital lung disease.

e) **List two ways to optimise this patient preoperatively. (2 marks)**

There is often very little time for patient optimisation for lung cancer surgery due to the risk of delay causing tumour progression and deterioration of respiratory function. However, the principles of enhanced recovery after surgery apply to pneumonectomy, and I would prioritise ones that are most specifically relevant to a patient with lung cancer.

- Smoking cessation. Even over a short time period this can return carbon monoxide levels to normal and reduce the effects of circulating nicotine.
- Optimisation of associated smoking-related lung disease (and concomitant infection) with medication and physiotherapy.
- Physical exercise training to improve lung function parameters and improve muscle mass.
- Nutritional optimisation to improve postoperative outcomes and wound healing.
- Management of any associated anaemia.
- Optimisation of any other comorbidities including diabetes, heart disease.

f) Describe how correct placement of a left-sided double lumen tube is performed clinically. (3 marks)

Bronchoscopy should be used to confirm placement. When checking a right-sided double lumen tube, it is important to visualise that the Murphy's eye has aligned with the right upper lobe bronchus. It is also important to check for any slippage after turning the patient into the lateral position.

- Check for bilateral chest movement and auscultation of breath sounds when both cuffs are inflated and both lumens of the double lumen tube are connected to the breathing circuit.
- Then, clamping of the tubing to the bronchial lumen and opening of the bronchoscopy cap on that side should result in only right chest movement and breath sounds.
- Then, after unclamping the tubing and replacing the cap on the bronchial lumen, the tubing to the tracheal lumen is clamped, and the bronchoscopy cap is opened, and chest movement and breath sounds should be on the left side only.

g) List three specific postoperative complications of pneumonectomy. (3 marks)

- Atrial tachyarrhythmias (up to 40% of patients may develop atrial fibrillation).
- Pulmonary hypertension with progressive right heart failure.
- Post-pneumonectomy pulmonary oedema; rare but with high mortality, due to lung injury and capillary leak in the remaining lung, presenting with respiratory failure in the first two to three days after surgery.
- Bronchopleural fistula due to breakdown of the bronchial stump (increased risk if need for prolonged postoperative ventilation, large-diameter stump, or if residual tumour in the stump).
- Cardiac herniation, a rare complication of right pneumonectomy, which has involved pericardial stripping. Presents with sudden cardiovascular collapse.
- Nerve damage e.g. phrenic or recurrent laryngeal.

REFERENCES

Beshara M, Bora V. *Pneumonectomy.* StatPearls Publishing, March 2023. www.ncbi.nlm.nih.gov/books/NBK555969/. Accessed 12th May 2023.

Brunelli A et al. Physiological evaluation of the patient with lung cancer being considered for resectional surgery: diagnosis and management of lung cancer, 3rd edition: American College of Chest Physicians evidence-based clinical practice guidelines. *Chest.* 2013: 143: e166S–e190S.

Hackett S et al. Anaesthesia for pneumonectomy. *BJA Educ.* 2019: 19: 297–304.

Li T, Yang M, Tseng A. Prehabilitation and rehabilitation for surgically treated lung cancer patients. *J Canc Res Pr.* 2017: 4: 89–94.

Rongyang L et al. The effect of enhanced recovery after surgery program on lung cancer surgery: a systematic review and meta-analysis. *J Thorac Dis.* 2021: 13: 3566–3586.

2.19 March 2022 Cardiac tamponade

You are asked to see a 54-year-old patient on Cardiac ICU who has undergone coronary artery bypass surgery earlier in the day.

a) List four clinical features that might suggest she has developed cardiac tamponade. (4 marks)
b) List three other causes of cardiac tamponade. (3 marks)
c) Name two echocardiographic (apart from pericardial effusion), two chest X-ray, two ECG, and one pulmonary artery catheter findings in cardiac tamponade. (7 marks)
d) State the surface landmark for needle insertion for pericardiocentesis. (1 mark)
e) List one complication of pericardiocentesis apart from pneumothorax. (1 mark)
f) List two haemodynamic goals when anaesthetising a patient with tamponade. (2 marks)
g) What are the immediate effects on the left ventricle of initiating IPPV during tamponade? (2 marks)

The Chairs' Report after the original CRQ stated that it "was considered to be one of the harder questions in the paper, therefore it was reassuring to see it answered well [pass rate 76.9%] and it correlated with overall performance in the paper. However, a lack of knowledge of basic sciences hindered the majority of candidates and as a result the last stem was answered poorly."

This question has a number of similarities with the SAQs on tamponade asked in September 2013 and 2016. The subsections repeated in all three years reflect key areas of knowledge – namely, clinical features, investigations, and physiology underlying cardiac tamponade.

a) List four clinical features that might suggest she has developed cardiac tamponade. (4 marks)

Cardiac tamponade is the decompensated phase of cardiac compression due to intrapericardial pressure. Hypotension, raised jugular venous pressure, and muffled heart sounds form the classic Beck's triad of features. However, post-cardiac surgery patients may have localised tamponade (e.g. due to localised haematoma) and not demonstrate all of these classic features, so a high index of suspicion is required.

- Hypotension or cardiogenic shock (or cardiac arrest).
- Raised jugular venous pressure/increasing central venous pressure measurements.
- Oliguria.
- Increasing vasopressor requirement.
- Sudden reduction or cessation of drain output postoperatively.
- Tachycardia.
- Dyspnoea.
- Muffled heart sounds.
- Pericardial rub *(soft sign, may be present as a result of surgery)*.
- Sharp chest pain *(although this may be due to the recent surgery and therefore is an unreliable feature in this context)*.
- Pulsus paradoxus: abnormally large reduction in systolic pressure during inspiration *(during spontaneous inspiration, the full right heart encroaches on the left and blood pools in the pulmonary vasculature, both of which reduce left heart filling, thus causing a decrease in systolic pressure. In tamponade, the effect is exacerbated, and the difference in pressure between the right and left heart is lost. Positive pressure ventilation results in a reversal of timings)*.
- Kussmaul's sign: rise/lack of fall of JVP with inspiration *(due to failure of the constricted right heart to accommodate the increase in venous return that occurs with the drop in intrathoracic pressure that accompanies spontaneous inspiration)*.

b) List three other causes of cardiac tamponade. (3 marks)

Any pericardial disease may cause tamponade, although acute causes of tamponade (largely due to haemorrhage) may be more immediately life threatening than insidious causes.

- Acute haemorrhagic tamponade; chest trauma (usually penetrating trauma), type A aortic dissection, iatrogenic following interventional cardiology procedures.
- Infectious pericarditis.
- Non-infectious pericarditis; idiopathic, autoimmune, uraemic, malignant.

c) Name two echocardiographic (apart from pericardial effusion), two chest X-ray, two ECG, and one pulmonary artery catheter findings in cardiac tamponade. (7 marks)

The following are some of the main features that may be seen with each investigation. Echocardiography is crucial in the investigation of tamponade and has high sensitivity in the diagnosis: effusions greater than 20 mm are considered significant.

Echocardiography:	Collapse of cardiac chambers. IVC dilatation due to right heart compression. Leftward shift of intraventricular septum during spontaneous ventilation (see *(g)* for explanation). Increased variation in intracardiac blood flow with respiration. "Swinging heart."
Chest X-ray:	Enlarged or globular appearance of cardiac silhouette. Evidence of heart failure, pulmonary oedema.
ECG:	Sinus tachycardia. Atrial arrhythmias. Low voltage QRS complexes *(due to attenuation of electrical impulses)*. Electrical alternans *(beat-to-beat variation in QRS amplitude and axis)*.
Pulmonary artery catheter:	Equalisation of the diastolic pressures in all heart chambers. Pulmonary capillary wedge pressure may be raised in patients with left heart compression.

d) State the surface landmark for needle insertion for pericardiocentesis. (1 mark)

Although the traditional blind approach to pericardiocentesis was the subxiphoid approach, the use of echocardiogram has meant that other needle entry points may be more appropriate in terms of targeting the biggest depth of pericardial fluid whilst avoiding visceral damage. Any of these answers are valid.

- 1–2 cm inferior to the left xiphochondral junction (subxiphoid).
- Fifth left intercostal space close to sternal margin (parasternal).
- 1–2 cm lateral to apex beat within fifth, sixth, or seventh intercostal space (apical).

e) List one complication of pericardiocentesis apart from pneumothorax. (1 mark)

- Laceration of ventricle, coronary vessel, intercostal vessel, or thoracic vessel with consequent haemorrhage.
- Puncture of abdominal viscera or peritoneal cavity.
- Pneumopericardium.
- Arrhythmias.
- Pericardial decompression syndrome; left ventricular dysfunction resulting in pulmonary oedema or cardiogenic shock.

f) List two haemodynamic goals when anaesthetising a patient with tamponade. (2 marks)

The patient in this question may need urgent decompressive sternotomy on the cardiac ICU as there will not be the time to return them to theatre if they are significantly compromised. Management therefore includes calling for senior anaesthetic support and cardiothoracic input, contacting theatre and the perfusionist if the patient will have to go back on bypass, and initiating the major haemorrhage protocol whilst simultaneously assessing and managing the patient from an A-to-E perspective. If they have arrested or are periarrest, an anaesthetic, as such, may not be required. The traditional teaching for tamponade was described as "fast, full and tight."

- Maintain preload by replacing lost volume.
- Maintain sinus rhythm; arrhythmia will have a very deleterious effect on left ventricular filling and further reduce cardiac output.
- Avoid bradycardia; stroke volume will be impaired so normal-high heart rate is required to maintain cardiac output.
- Maintain systemic vascular resistance (which will be high due to sympathetic response and may be compromised by most anaesthetic agents) to maintain coronary perfusion by avoiding vasodilatory drugs and using vasopressors as necessary.
- Maintain cardiac contractility by avoiding myocardial depressants.

g) What are the immediate effects on the left ventricle of initiating positive pressure ventilation during tamponade? (2 marks)

The right ventricle, which is normally a lower pressure system than the left, is compressed early in acute tamponade with consequent reduction in filling and is therefore at risk of right ventricular failure when initiating positive pressure ventilation. The aims of a ventilatory strategy in this situation would therefore be the use of the lowest possible ventilatory pressures whilst maintaining normoxia and normocapnia.

- Acute rise in intrathoracic pressure results in compression of pulmonary vasculature causing an acute rise in venous return to the left ventricle, shift of the interventricular septum towards the right, and increase in stroke volume.
- However, the rise in intrathoracic pressure causes a further reduction in venous return to the right heart which will consequently result in reduced preload to the left ventricle and ultimately a further reduction in cardiac output.

REFERENCES

De Carlini C, Maggiolini S. Pericardiocentesis in cardiac tamponade: indications and practical aspects. *eJ Cardiol Pract.* 2017: 15: 19.

Madhivathanan P, Corredor C, Smith A. Perioperative implications of pericardial effusions and cardiac tamponade. *BJA Educ.* 2020: 20: 226–234.

2.20 September 2022 Aortic stenosis

An 84-year-old patient with severe aortic stenosis presents for transcatheter aortic valve implantation (TAVI).
a) List three classical symptoms of aortic stenosis (AS). (3 marks)
b) Give the following echocardiographic values for severe AS: peak aortic flow velocity (m/s), mean transaortic pressure gradient (mmHg), and valve area (cm²). (3 marks)
c) List four factors that would favour a TAVI over a surgical aortic valve replacement. (4 marks)
d) State one absolute contraindication to TAVI. (1 mark)
e) State two options for anaesthesia in a patient presenting for a TAVI. (2 marks)
f) List four haemodynamic goals when anaesthetising a patient undergoing a TAVI. (4 marks)
g) List three causes of haemodynamic instability in a patient undergoing TAVI. (3 marks)

The Chairs' Report after the original CRQ stated that "aortic stenosis is a common condition and its pathophysiology and management should be known to candidates sitting this exam. This is a common topic in the Final FRCA exam and reassuringly it was well answered. The questions related to TAVI is where the majority of candidates dropped marks." Indeed, aortic stenosis has been addressed in the Final written paper before with both a cardiothoracic and a perioperative medicine slant. This is the first time that they have asked about TAVI and perhaps this is why candidates did not do so well on these subsections. However, note the time period between the two BJA Education articles on TAVI (referenced below) and this question. The pass rate was 67.9%. TAVI and interventional cardiology procedures are becoming increasingly common, and this may be reflected in topics for CRQs in the future.

a) **List three classical symptoms of aortic stenosis (AS). (3 marks)**

The development of symptoms indicates decompensation, with myocardial ischaemia and heart failure.

- Presyncope, syncope.
- Dyspnoea, heart failure.
- Angina.
- Sudden death.

b) **Give the following echocardiographic values for severe AS: peak aortic flow velocity (m/s), mean transaortic pressure gradient (mmHg), and valve area (cm²). (3 marks)**

It is now recognised that aortic stenosis may occur in the absence of elevated flow velocity or mean pressure gradient – it is the valve area that is the unifying diagnostic criterion. A failing left ventricle will be unable to generate significant velocity, which can lead to underestimation of severity if only velocity and pressure measurements are used. Sometimes overestimation of severity may occur if the cardiac output is insufficient to cause adequate valve opening of a relatively normal valve, resulting in the appearance of a small valve area (pseudostenosis).

- Peak aortic flow velocity > 4 m/s.
- Mean transaortic pressure gradient > 40 mmHg.
- Valve area < 1.0 cm² (equal to an indexed valve area of < 0.6 cm/m² BSA).

c) **List four factors that would favour a TAVI over a surgical aortic valve replacement. (4 marks)**

TAVI is being increasingly performed on younger patients with fewer comorbidities with recent evidence (PARTNER 2, PARTNER 3, and SURTAVI trials) showing that TAVI had no difference to open surgery in mortality and major morbidity in low and intermediate risk patients, and a lower risk of complications such as AF, AKI, and haemorrhage.

- Patient factors:
  — Increased age.
  — Severe comorbidities.

- Surgical factors:
  - Previous cardiac surgery.
  - Previous aortic valve replacement *(due to the increased risk associated with redo sternotomy).*
  - Favourable vascular access.
  - Heavily calcified aorta *(this may prevent safe aortic cross-clamping).*
  - Only aortic valve surgery required (other valves normal and normal coronary arteries).
  - Chest wall deformity.

d) State one absolute contraindication to TAVI. (1 mark)

Relative contraindications include severe patient comorbidities that would mean the procedure is unlikely to benefit the patient's quality of life or life expectancy, and anatomical factors which may make a TAVI more technically challenging, such as the aortic annulus size and the distance between the annulus and the coronary ostia.

- Infective endocarditis.

e) State two options for anaesthesia in a patient presenting for a TAVI. (2 marks)

These vary by institution, but the options for anaesthesia are the same as for any case! Oversedation should be avoided as hypoxia or hypercarbia could precipitate right heart failure.

- Local anaesthesia alone; this is becoming increasingly common with local anaesthesia administered by cardiologists to the vascular access site (usually femoral).
- Local anaesthesia with conscious sedation; this can be achieved by target-controlled infusion of propofol or intermittent bolus regimens of fentanyl or midazolam.
- General anaesthesia.

f) List four haemodynamic goals when anaesthetising a patient undergoing a TAVI. (4 marks)

- Maintenance of preload.
- Maintenance of sinus rhythm.
- Maintenance of normal heart rate.
- Maintenance of cardiac contractility.
- Maintenance of afterload/blood pressure.

g) List three causes of haemodynamic instability in a patient undergoing TAVI. (3 marks)

Other important complications include stroke, complications related to vascular access, and abnormal valve placement.

- Major haemorrhage due to iatrogenic injury to aortic root or annulus, or intrathoracic blood vessels.
- Arrhythmia due to damage to the AV node or bundle of His upon valve deployment.
- Cardiac ischaemia due to occlusion of the ostia by the implant.
- Rapid ventricular pacing at up to 200 bpm performed as part of the TAVI procedure to dramatically reduce cardiac output for up to ten seconds during valve deployment to prevent its migration.

REFERENCES

Charlesworth M, Williams B, Buch M. Advances in transcatheter aortic valve implantation: part 1: patient selection and preparation. *BJA Educ.* 2021a: 21: 232–237.

Charlesworth M, Williams B, Buch M. Advances in transcatheter aortic valve implantation: part 2: perioperative care. *BJA Educ.* 2021b: 21: 264–269.

Mahmaljy H, Tawney A, Young M. *Transcatheter aortic valve replacement.* StatPearls Publishing, November 2022. www.ncbi.nlm.nih.gov/books/NBK431075/. Accessed 12th May 2023.

2.21 February 2023 Intra-aortic balloon pump

This is the third time that intra-aortic balloon pump has been the focus of the cardiothoracic anaesthesia and critical care question of the exam during the time period covered by this book. Again, the main lines of questioning were on indications, contraindications, underlying physiology, and complications. The only brand-new question specifically asked about the gas used to inflate the balloon. If candidates had learned from the content of past questions, they would have easily had the knowledge required to pass this year's question, yet only 43.9% did, with the Chairs commenting that although "Some of the practicalities were well answered . . . the working principles and therefore the haemodynamic effects were not."

a) **State the gas used to inflate the balloon of the intra-aortic balloon pump and give one reason why this gas is used. (2 marks)**

- Helium.
- Low density means that flow will be laminar such that the gas is rapidly transferred from the IABP machine to the balloon tip.
- Rapid absorption into blood in event of balloon rupture.

REFERENCE

Krishna M, Zacharowski K. Principles of intra-aortic balloon pump counterpulsation. *Contin Educ Anaesth Crit Care Pain*. 2009: 9: 24–28.

3 AIRWAY MANAGEMENT

3.1 September 2011 Awake fibreoptic intubation

a) Complete the table below indicating which cranial nerves provide sensory innervation to structures encountered during awake nasal fibreoptic intubation. (3 marks)
b) List five techniques that may be employed as part of an overall strategy for airway topicalisation prior to awake nasal fibreoptic intubation. (5 marks)
c) State the maximum dose of lidocaine (mg/kg) that can be used for topicalisation of the airway prior to awake nasal fibreoptic intubation. (1 mark)
d) List five predictors of difficult airway that may indicate the need for awake fibreoptic intubation for securing of the airway. (5 marks)
e) State how tracheal tube placement should be confirmed prior to commencement of anaesthesia in a patient having an awake nasal fibreoptic intubation. (2 marks)
f) Patient refusal is a contraindication to awake fibreoptic intubation. List four other relative contraindications to awake fibreoptic intubation. (4 marks)

NAP4 was published in 2011, a comprehensive analysis of complications of airway management in a year in the UK. It became the basis of many subsequent Final SAQs. The summaries and the vignettes to the chapters are well worth reading even if you don't feel you could manage the whole report. The Difficult Airway Society has developed many guidelines on airway management after the findings of NAP4, and these too have been the basis of Final questions. They are essential reading for your exam as well as for clinical practice.

a) Complete the table below indicating which cranial nerves provide sensory innervation to structures encountered during awake nasal fibreoptic intubation. (3 marks)

Airway structure	Sensory innervation
Nasal air passages	Trigeminal nerve
Oropharynx	Glossopharyngeal nerve
Larynx	Vagus nerve

b) List five techniques that may be employed as part of an overall strategy for airway topicalisation prior to awake nasal fibreoptic intubation. (5 marks)

I have included a little more detail in my list below in case this question was part of a viva instead of a CRQ, but for a CRQ you would just have to list the options.

- Mucosal atomisation device use e.g. lidocaine to pharynx, larynx, trachea or co-phenylcaine to nostrils *(as effective from an analgesic perspective as cocaine topicalisation of the nose but without the cardiovascular complications).*
- Spray-as-you-go. Lidocaine spray to oropharyngeal structures followed by spray above and below cords via epidural catheter or working channel of fibreoptic bronchoscope.

DOI: 10.1201/9781003388494-3

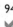

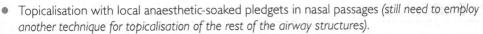

- Topicalisation with local anaesthetic-soaked pledgets in nasal passages *(still need to employ another technique for topicalisation of the rest of the airway structures)*.
- Nebulised local anaesthetic *(it can be difficult to keep within safe doses of local anaesthetic, requires patient to take good breaths, which is often not possible in patients requiring awake intubation)*.
- Individual nerve blocks e.g. glossopharyngeal nerve block, superior laryngeal nerve block *(risk of patient discomfort, especially in a patient who already has airway compromise, multiple blocks needed, expertise in unusually performed blocks required, associated with high plasma local anaesthetic levels)*.
- Cricothyroid puncture for translaryngeal block *(anaesthetises larynx only, risk of patient discomfort – however, if a cannula is used, it may be employed in a rescue oxygenation technique if required)*.

c) **State the maximum dose of lidocaine (mg/kg) that can be used for topicalisation of the airway prior to awake nasal fibreoptic intubation. (1 mark)**

- 9 mg/kg lean body weight.

d) **List five predictors of difficult airway that may indicate the need for awake fibreoptic intubation for securing of the airway. (5 marks)**

- Previous difficult airway for oxygenation or intubation.
- Head and neck pathology (including malignancy, previous surgery, or radiotherapy).
- Limited mouth opening (facial fractures, rheumatoid arthritis, dental abscess, scleroderma).
- Limited neck movement (rheumatoid arthritis, ankylosing spondylitis, previous cervical spine surgery or trauma).
- Obstructive sleep apnoea.
- Morbid obesity.
- Airway anatomy abnormality (thyroid, tongue, tonsillar or laryngeal tumours, Ludwig's angina, airway oedema or burns, retrognathia).
- Syndromes associated with difficult airway (Pierre-Robin, Treacher-Collins).

e) **State how tracheal tube placement should be confirmed prior to commencement of anaesthesia in a patient having an awake nasal fibreoptic intubation. (2 marks)**

- Visualisation of the tracheal lumen.
- Capnography trace consistent with tracheal intubation.

f) **Patient refusal is a contraindication to awake fibreoptic intubation. List four other relative contraindications to awake fibreoptic intubation. (4 marks)**

- Patient not able to comply with instruction (confusion, young age etc.).
- Local anaesthetic allergy.
- Operator inexperience.
- Significant laryngeal or subglottic stenosis or narrowing (fibreoptic intubation thus being unable to bypass the area of concern).
- Threat of airway obstruction.
- Airway bleeding or risk of significant airway bleeding due to e.g. vascular tumour.

REFERENCES

Ahmad I et al. Difficult Airway Society guidelines for awake tracheal intubation (ATI) in adults. *Anaesthesia.* 2019: 75: 509–528.

Cook T, Woodall N, Frerk C (eds.). *4th National Audit Project of the Royal College of Anaesthetists and the Difficult Airway Society: major complications of airway management in the United Kingdom.* London: The Royal College of Anaesthetists and Association of Anaesthetists of Great Britain and Ireland, 2011.

Leslie D, Stacey M. Awake intubation. *Contin Educ Anaesth Crit Care Pain.* 2015: 15: 64–67.

3.2 September 2011 Extubation

a) List four airway problems that may follow removal of a tracheal tube. (4 marks)
b) List four respiratory complications that may follow removal of a tracheal tube. (4 marks)
c) List two cardiovascular complications that may follow removal of a tracheal tube. (2 marks)
d) Complete the following table to give six patient-related factors or comorbidities that might contribute to a high-risk extubation. (6 marks)
e) List four surgical factors that may contribute to a high-risk extubation. (4 marks)

Of all the airway issues reported to NAP4, 1-in-6 complications occurred at emergence and 1-in-6 in recovery. NAP4-based topics have come up repeatedly in the exam, in airway questions and also in other subspecialty questions such as intensive care medicine. The Difficult Airway Society have produced guidelines to help structure the management of extubation. In the lead-up to the exam, it is important to stay up to date with publications and guidelines that are of relevance to anaesthesia.

a) List four airway problems that may follow removal of a tracheal tube. (4 marks)

- Sore throat, hoarseness.
- Foreign body causing obstruction: teeth, throat pack, blood clot.
- External compression of airway due to surgical site swelling or bleeding.
- Laryngospasm triggered by blood, secretions, or airway manipulation during light anaesthesia.
- Laryngeal oedema.
- Laryngeal trauma caused during intubation (e.g. bougie use), causing bleeding, swelling, tears.
- Vocal cord paralysis due to direct trauma/pressure.
- Vocal cord dysfunction.
- Tracheomalacia: erosion/softening of tracheal rings due to prolonged intubation, retrosternal thyroid, large thymus or tumour.
- Tracheal stenosis after prolonged intubation.

b) List four respiratory complications that may follow removal of a tracheal tube. (4 marks)

- Coughing.
- Mucociliary dysfunction.
- Diffusion hypoxia.
- Basal atelectasis causing ventilation/perfusion mismatch.
- Post-obstructive pulmonary oedema.
- Bronchospasm.
- Pulmonary aspiration.
- Respiratory failure due to any respiratory or airway complications.

c) List two cardiovascular complications that may follow removal of a tracheal tube. (2 marks)

- Catecholamine release causing tachycardia and hypertension.
- Catecholamine release causing tachycardia and increased systemic vascular resistance resulting in reduced ejection fraction or even acute heart failure in patient with coronary artery disease.
- Risk of silent or overt myocardial infarction due to increased myocardial oxygen demand (effect exacerbated if there is hypoxaemia due to other complications of extubation).

d) Complete the following table to give six patient-related factors or comorbidities that might contribute to a high-risk extubation. (6 marks)

	Patient-related factor or comorbidity
Airway:	• Dysmorphia. • Airway pathology e.g. tumour. • Obesity.
Respiratory:	• Asthma. • Obstructive sleep apnoea. • Chronic obstructive pulmonary disease. • Recent upper respiratory tract infection (especially in children). • Smoking.
Cardiovascular:	• Ischaemic heart disease. • Unstable arrhythmia.
Neurological:	• Posterior fossa tumour surgery. • Head injury. • Guillain-Barré syndrome. • Myasthenia gravis. • Multiple sclerosis.
Gastrointestinal:	• Full stomach. • Reflux. • Hiatus hernia.
Musculoskeletal:	• Muscular dystrophy. • Dystrophia myotonica. • Rheumatoid arthritis or ankylosing spondylitis affecting neck movement.

e) List four surgical factors that may contribute to a high-risk extubation. (4 marks)

- Site of surgery: airway, head, neck, thorax, posterior fossa, or cervical spine surgery.
- Surgery requiring use of double lumen tube.
- Prolonged duration of surgery.
- Trendelenberg or prone positioning risks development of laryngeal oedema.
- Intraoperative issues not directly related to airway: difficulty achieving adequate ventilation, hypothermia, significant blood loss, electrolyte imbalance, fluid shifts.

REFERENCES

Batuwitage B, Charters P. Postoperative management of the difficult airway. *BJA Educ.* 2017: 17: 235–241.

Cook T, Woodall N, Frerk C (eds.). *4th National Audit Project of the Royal College of Anaesthetists and the Difficult Airway Society: major complications of airway management in the United Kingdom.* London: The Royal College of Anaesthetists and Association of Anaesthetists of Great Britain and Ireland, 2011.

Popat M et al. Difficult Airway Society guidelines for the management of tracheal extubation. *Anaesthesia.* 2012: 67: 318–340.

3.3 March 2012 Tracheostomy

You have been called urgently to attend a ventilated patient on the ICU who has become acutely agitated, hypertensive and profoundly hypoxic. A percutaneous tracheostomy was performed 18 hours ago and is being weaned from ventilatory support.

a) List possible causes for this patient's acute hypoxia. (5 marks)
b) What clinical features support an airway problem? (8 marks)
c) How would you manage an airway problem in this patient? (7 marks)

This SAQ, reproduced here as it appeared in the exam, had a 76.6% pass rate. A CRQ on the topic of tracheostomy featured in September 2019 and so will be found later in this chapter. However, there were some useful learning points from the 2012 SAQ part (a) that were not addressed in the 2019 CRQ.

a) List possible causes for this patient's acute hypoxia. (5 marks)

Patient problems	Equipment problems
Pneumothorax.	Tracheostomy tube blocked with secretions or blood.
Haemothorax.	Dislodged tube.
Pneumomediastinum.	Cuff puncture or deflation or herniation over end of tube.
Haemomediastinum.	Cuff inflated with speaking valve in situ.
Surgical emphysema.	Ventilator circuit blockage or disconnection.
Atelectasis, inadequate ventilation due to overly rapid weaning.	Inappropriate ventilator settings.
Aspiration.	Inappropriately low fraction of inspired oxygen.

3.4 March 2019 Extubation

a) List four airway risk factors that may predict a difficult extubation. (4 marks)
b) List four general risk factors that may predict a difficult extubation. (4 marks)
c) List three patient factors that can be optimised prior to extubation. (3 marks)
d) List two non-patient factors that can be optimised prior to extubation. (2 marks)
e) List four strategies that you could employ to manage a high-risk extubation. (4 marks)
f) List three possible indications for exchanging an endotracheal tube for a supraglottic airway device to aid extubation. (3 marks)

The Chairs' Report for the SAQ on this topic in 2019 stated that it was a new question. There was some overlap with the question from 2011, but this one was very heavily based on the Difficult Airway Society extubation guidelines. Once again, sources that are useful in your clinical practice are useful for your exam prep. The pass rate for the question was 64.1%.

a) **List four airway risk factors that may predict a difficult extubation. (4 marks)**

- Known difficult airway.
- Airway deterioration (trauma, oedema or bleeding).
- Restricted airway access (e.g. mandibular wiring, halo brace).
- Obesity or obstructive sleep apnoea.
- Risk of aspiration.

b) **List four general risk factors that may predict a difficult extubation. (4 marks)**

- Cardiovascular comorbidity e.g. coronary artery disease or unstable arrhythmia.
- Respiratory comorbidity e.g. asthma, COPD, recent upper respiratory tract infection, smoking.
- Neurological comorbidity e.g. posterior fossa tumour surgery, head injury, Guillain-Barré, myasthenia gravis, multiple sclerosis.
- Metabolic disorder including complications from surgery or duration of anaesthesia such as fluid shifts, electrolyte imbalance, hypothermia, acid-base disturbance.
- Special surgical requirements e.g. need for smooth emergence following neurosurgery or flap surgery.

c) **List three patient factors that can be optimised prior to extubation. (3 marks)**

- Respiratory: ensure ventilatory adequacy, optimised gas exchange with supplementary oxygen to raise lung partial pressure of oxygen in case of difficulties at extubation.
- Cardiovascular: pharmacological correction of unstable blood pressure or rhythm, adequate fluid replacement.
- Metabolic: optimise acid-base balance, ensure coagulation status is acceptable, ensure normothermia.
- Neuromuscular: ensure adequate reversal from neuromuscular blockade through accelerometer or train of four monitoring, and reversal agent given (neostigmine with glycopyrrolate or sugammadex) in appropriate dose.

d) **List two non-patient factors that can be optimised prior to extubation. (2 marks)**

- Ensure extubation in appropriate location – operating theatre due to availability of staff and equipment, or ICU.
- Presence of skilled assistant.
- Monitoring as for intubation.

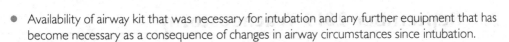

- Availability of airway kit that was necessary for intubation and any further equipment that has become necessary as a consequence of changes in airway circumstances since intubation.

e) **List four strategies that you could employ to manage a high-risk extubation. (4 marks)**

- Laryngeal mask exchange.
- Remifentanil technique.
- Airway exchange catheter.
- Postponement of extubation in order to achieve risk factor optimisation first.
- Tracheostomy.

f) **List three possible indications for exchanging an endotracheal tube for a supraglottic airway device to aid extubation. (3 marks)**

- Surgical requirement for minimising coughing and raised venous pressure at extubation e.g. after ocular surgery, neurosurgery, flap surgery.
- Avoidance of excessive catecholamine release at extubation resulting in risk of cerebrovascular consequences in at risk patients or myocardial ischaemia in patients with severe coronary artery disease.
- Reduction of airway stimulation in patients at risk of adverse respiratory consequences of extubation e.g. smokers, asthmatics.

REFERENCE

Popat M et al. Difficult Airway Society guidelines for the management of tracheal extubation. *Anaesthesia.* 2012: 67: 318–340.

3.5 September 2019 Tracheostomy

a) List three indications for tracheostomy insertion. (3 marks)
b) List three possible indications for surgical placement rather than percutaneous insertion of tracheostomy. (3 marks)
c) List four significant complications that may be encountered at the time of (surgical or percutaneous) tracheostomy insertion. (4 marks)
d) You are called urgently to review a patient on the intensive care unit who has a percutaneous tracheostomy to facilitate weaning from mechanical ventilation. The patient is awake and appears to be struggling to breathe. The nurse caring for him has applied high flow oxygen over the patient's mouth and tracheostomy. List three steps you would take to assess tracheostomy patency. (3 marks)
e) You have established that the tracheostomy tube is not patent, there is no bag movement of a Mapleson C circuit when attached to the tracheostomy, and no capnography trace. List your immediate actions. (3 marks)
f) You are unsuccessful with these manoeuvres, and the patient is becoming cyanosed. List four options to try to secure this patient's airway. (4 marks)

The Chairs' Report for the question on this topic said there was a 47.7% pass rate. It gave a very useful level of detail about the College's expectations from candidates in their CRQ answers, and I reproduce it here in its entirety: "The pass rate for this question was the lowest overall for this paper. It highlighted the fact that candidates have not adapted the way they answer questions in the new CRQ format. The CRQs are designed to elicit specific information and usually a short 1–3 word answer is required. The first three sections were answered as if they were SAQs, with candidates producing mini essays and failing to give specific details. In the other sections of this question, it was clear from the answers given that candidates had not adequately read the questions. For example, candidates failed to appreciate that section (d) related to the assessment of patency of the tracheostomy, section (e) related to the immediate management of a blocked tracheostomy and the last section related to management of worsening hypoxia. The answers to sections (d), (e) and (f) were muddled, with candidates repeating their answers in multiple sections. Tracheostomy care has been highlighted in numerous patient safety bulletins and therefore candidates should know this in more detail than was demonstrated in the September paper." I certainly haven't managed to restrict my answers to 1–3 words, but then I don't know the precise questions that the College asked, and I have added extra detail to help with understanding rather than just listing answers to be learnt by rote. From the way the Report refers to parts (d), (e) and (f) of the CRQ, it seems they wanted reproduction of the sequential steps of the National Tracheostomy Safety Project's emergency tracheostomy management guideline. It's a very fair ask of the candidates to be familiar with this guideline when you consider that anaesthetic trainees commonly care for patients with tracheostomies on the ICU. NAP4 reported a range of tracheostomy-related incidents that were frequently exacerbated by lack of capnography use, lack of availability of difficult airway kit, and an unstructured rescue strategy. It is important to note, however, that the emergency tracheostomy guidelines suggested by NAP4 in 2011 recommended an attempt at ventilation of a possibly blocked tracheostomy, but the current guidelines do not.

a) List three indications for tracheostomy insertion. (3 marks)

- Prolonged mechanical ventilation/to facilitate weaning from mechanical ventilation/to avoid complications of long-term intubation when weaning/to allow cessation of sedation and communication with the patient during wean from mechanical ventilation.
- Pulmonary hygiene in patients unable to clear secretions.
- Airway protection in patients with reduced airway reflexes e.g. neurological conditions resulting in bulbar dysfunction or reduced conscious level.
- As part of a surgical procedure e.g. head and neck cancer surgery including laryngectomy, or short term where immediate reintubation would be challenging e.g. after a maxillofacial free flap.

- Upper airway obstruction (emergency and elective) e.g. vocal cord palsy, trauma, burns, infection.

b) **List three possible indications for surgical placement rather than percutaneous insertion of tracheostomy. (3 marks)**

- When the tracheostomy is being performed as part of an operative procedure.
- Morbid obesity.
- Cervical instability.
- Challenging anatomy such as short neck, limited neck extension, tracheal deviation, concerns about aberrant vessels crossing the insertion site.

c) **List four significant complications that may be encountered at the time of (surgical or percutaneous) tracheostomy insertion. (4 marks)**

- Loss of airway (obstruction by blood, secretions, or foreign body, or dislodgement or misplacement of tracheostomy tube) with consequent hypoxia and hypoxic brain damage.
- Damage to airway (fracture of tracheal cartilages, damage to posterior wall of the trachea).
- Pneumothorax.
- Derecruitment with consequent hypoxia.
- Aspiration.
- Haemorrhage.
- Recurrent laryngeal nerve injury.

d) **You are called urgently to review a patient on the intensive care unit who has a percutaneous tracheostomy to facilitate weaning from mechanical ventilation. The patient is awake and appears to be struggling to breathe. The nurse caring for him has applied high flow oxygen over the patient's mouth and tracheostomy. List three steps you would take to assess tracheostomy patency. (3 marks)**

- Remove speaking valve or cap and the inner tube.
- Attempt to pass a suction catheter via the tracheostomy.
- Deflate cuff if unable to pass suction catheter.

e) **You have established that the tracheostomy tube is not patent, there is no bag movement of a Mapleson C circuit when attached to the tracheostomy, and no capnography trace. List your immediate actions. (3 marks)**

This patient has had a percutaneous tracheostomy and so has a connection between their mouth and lungs – if a patient has had a surgical tracheostomy as part of surgery for laryngectomy, this will not be the case, and airway rescue approaches will need to be modified accordingly.

- Remove tracheostomy tube and assess again for breathing – if not, call resuscitation team – commence CPR if no pulse or signs of life.
- Oral airway manoeuvres while covering stoma: bag-valve-mask, oral or nasal airway adjuncts, supraglottic airway device.
- Ventilation via stoma: paediatric face mask or LMA applied to stoma.

f) **You are unsuccessful with these manoeuvres, and the patient is becoming cyanosed. List four options to try to secure this patient's airway. (4 marks)**

- Oral intubation with uncut tube to advance beyond stoma.
- Attempt stomal intubation with small tracheostomy tube or size 6.0 cuffed endotracheal tube.
- Intubation of stoma with Aintree catheter and fibreoptic scope.
- Use of bougie or airway exchange catheter to facilitate stomal intubation.

REFERENCES

Batuwitage B, Webber S, Glossop A. Percutaneous tracheostomy. *Contin Educ Anaesth Crit Care Pain.* 2014: 14: 268–272.

Cook T, Woodall N, Frerk C (eds.). *4th National Audit Project of the Royal College of Anaesthetists and the Difficult Airway Society: major complications of airway management in the United Kingdom.* London: The Royal College of Anaesthetists and Association of Anaesthetists of Great Britain and Ireland, 2011.

Hashimoto D, Axtell A, Auchincloss H. Percutaneous tracheostomy. *N Engl J Med.* 2020: 383: e112.

Lewith H, Athanassoglou V. Update on management of tracheostomy. *BJA Educ.* 2019: 19: 370–376.

McGrath B, Bates L, Atkinson D, Moore J. Multidisciplinary guidelines for the management of tracheostomy and laryngectomy airway emergencies. *Anaesthesia.* 2012: 67: 1025–1041.

3.6 September 2020 Awake fibreoptic intubation

The focus of the CRQ on this topic was very much in line with that of the SAQ from September 2011, with the references detailed at the end of that question being very useful sources for further reading.

3.7 February 2023 Airway stenting

a) List three types of malignancy which may require tracheobronchial stenting as part of management. (3 marks)

b) List five airway concerns affecting patients requiring tracheobronchial stenting. (5 marks)

c) List two methods of ventilation provision for tracheobronchial stenting other than high frequency jet ventilation (HFJV). (2 marks)

d) List the three determinants of minute ventilation when using HFJV. (3 marks)

e) List four complications of HFJV. (4 marks)

f) List three possible reasons for stridor and respiratory distress in recovery after tracheobronchial stenting. (3 marks)

The Chairs acknowledged that this was thought to be a "difficult question" but "although the finer points of jet ventilation were not well answered, potential complications were well answered." This was a new topic, so you should not be at all surprised that there was a recent BJA Education article in which the majority of answers could be found. Even if you knew nothing about airway stent surgery, the crux of the question content lies with anaesthesia for bronchoscopy (which overlaps with paediatrics and thoracic surgery) and should be something you are familiar with.

The physiology of gas exchange when using jet ventilation can be summarised as below:

- *Low frequency (8–30 jets/minute) manual jet ventilation uses the concept of convective ventilation, or "bulk flow," whereby there is mass flow of air in and out of the lungs and gas exchange is determined by tidal volume, dead space volume and respiratory rate. This is similar to "normal" physiology.*

- *High frequency (120–300 jets/minute) jet ventilation is different as the tidal volumes are smaller than dead space and so other mechanisms must be responsible for achieving ventilation:*
  - *Laminar flow in smaller airways results in a fast-moving jet down the centre of the airway and slower moving air near the edges of the airways that moves out in the opposite direction.*
  - *Taylor dispersion (enhanced molecular diffusion) describes the acceleratory effect that the fast-moving central jet of gas in an airway has on the diffusion of the molecules of that gas (oxygen) down its concentration gradient, resulting in movement into alveoli.*
  - *Regional differences in compliance throughout the lung causes some lung units to fill with gas and subsequently empty more easily than others. This allows gas transfer between different lung units during high frequency jet ventilation, the Pendelluft principle. It results in an increased dead space as carbon dioxide from one lung unit may move to another, rather than be directly exhaled.*
  - *Myocardial contraction leads to physical movement of lung units in proximity to the heart, facilitating gas movement called cardiogenic mixing.*

a) List three types of malignancy which may require tracheobronchial stenting as part of management. (3 marks)

- Cancers of the respiratory tract causing airway narrowing:
  - Primary lung cancer.
  - Adenoid cystic carcinoma.
  - Carcinoid disease.
- Cancers that metastasise to the airway:
  - Breast.
  - Colorectal.

Chapter 3 AIRWAY MANAGEMENT

- Tracheal or bronchial compression due to extrinsic pressure from cancer of nearby structure:
  — Oesophageal cancer.
  — Thyroid cancer.
  — Lymphoma.

b) **List five airway concerns affecting patients requiring tracheobronchial stenting. (5 marks)**

- Risk of airway collapse and complete airway obstruction on induction of anaesthesia due to loss of intrinsic muscle tone.
- Risk of obstruction on supine positioning for anaesthesia depending on nature of obstruction (e.g. large mediastinal mass)
- Trauma to teeth, oropharynx, larynx associated with rigid bronchoscopy use, causing bleeding, obstruction of view, contamination of airway.
- Risk of airway damage associated with rigid bronchoscopy resulting in bleeding or barotrauma if jet ventilation used.
- Risk of airway contamination due to aspiration associated with rigid bronchoscopy technique.
- Risk of maldeployment of stent or acute migration resulting in obstruction of airway.
- Shared airway, limits anaesthetist's access to rescue if complications encountered.
- Risks of laryngo- or bronchospasm associated with airway instrumentation, which may result in complete airway obstruction.

c) **List two methods of ventilation provision for tracheobronchial stenting other than high frequency jet ventilation (HFJV). (2 marks)**

Airway stenting can either be performed by flexible bronchoscopy (which may be tolerated by the awake or sedated patient, or performed under general anaesthesia), or rigid bronchoscopy (which is highly stimulating and requires deep general anaesthesia and ventilation). Venovenous ECMO is a possible approach to facilitating gas exchange in selected patients with severe tracheal obstruction.

- Maintenance of spontaneous ventilation with e.g. transnasal humidified rapid-insufflation ventilatory exchange (THRIVE) for awake or sedated patients having the procedure using flexible bronchoscopy.
- Use of a supraglottic airway device with controlled or spontaneous intermittent ventilation, or endotracheal tube with intermittent controlled ventilation, for procedures using flexible bronchoscopy.
- Manual low-frequency jet ventilation e.g. Sander's manual jet ventilator attached at the jet ventilation port of a rigid bronchoscope.
- Intermittent controlled ventilation via the anaesthetic circuit attached at the 22 mm side port of the rigid bronchoscope.
- High flow supplemental oxygen for apnoeic oxygenation via the 22 mm side port – a leak is necessary to avoid baro- or volutrauma with high flows.

d) **List the three determinants of minute ventilation when using HFJV. (3 marks)**

- Frequency of jets.
- Driving pressure.
- Inspiratory time.

e) List four complications of HFJV. (4 marks)

- Gas embolism.
- Barotrauma resulting in pneumothorax, tension pneumothorax, pneumomediastinum, subcutaneous emphysema.
- Gas trapping and hyperinflation which may lead to reduced venous return, reduced cardiac output, hypotension, and cardiovascular collapse.
- Inadequate ventilation with hypoxia, hypercapnia, and respiratory acidosis.

f) List three possible reasons for stridor and respiratory distress in recovery after tracheobronchial stenting. (3 marks)

- Airway bleeding.
- Stent dislodgement or migration.
- Laryngeal oedema due to e.g. trauma from rigid bronchoscope.

REFERENCE

Barnwell N, Lenihan M. Anaesthesia for airway stenting. *BJA Educ.* 2022: 22: 160–166.
Evans E, Biro P. Jet ventilation. *BJA Educ.* 2007: 7: 2–5.

CRITICAL INCIDENTS

4.1 September 2012 Wrong-sided nerve block

a) List the implications for the patient of an inadvertent wrong-sided peripheral nerve block. (5 marks)
b) Summarise the recommendations of the "Stop Before You Block" campaign and list the factors that have been identified as contributing to the performance of a wrong-sided block. (9 marks)
c) Define the term "never event" as described by the National Patient Safety Agency and list three never events of relevance to anaesthetic or intensive care practice. (6 marks)

This is the original SAQ that appeared in September 2012. "Stop Before You Block" was introduced in 2011, so this was a topical question. The Chair was disappointed with the 40.5% pass rate and that "many candidates displayed a relative unfamiliarity with the 'Stop Before You Block' campaign. This is an important national patient safety initiative that was introduced recently to reduce the incidence of inadvertent wrong-sided nerve blocks. Many examinees left some sections unanswered. Some candidates could not adequately define the term 'never event' despite its topicality." The National Patient Safety Agency ceased to exist in 2012, the current home of never event publications being NHS Improvement. The topic that this question is based on has featured a further two times in the Final over the time frame of this book, and so you will see the answers later in the chapter.

DOI: 10.1201/9781003388494-4

4.2 September 2012 Aspiration under anaesthesia

The 4th National Audit Project (NAP4) was published in 2011.
a) Which factors are most likely to lead to an adverse airway event when using a supraglottic airway device (SAD)? (6 marks)
b) How would you recognise that a patient has regurgitated and aspirated gastric contents during an anaesthetic administered via an SAD? (6 marks)
c) How would you manage this patient? (8 marks)

One-fifth of all reports to NAP4 concerned aspiration, and it accounted for half of anaesthesia-related deaths. Those patients that survived frequently had a prolonged ICU stay. The Chair's Report of the SAQ, which I have reproduced here in its original form, said that there was a good pass rate of 78.4% and stated that the question was "generally well answered. There was significant variation in the knowledge detailed in the NAP4 relating to the safe use of supraglottic airways. The diagnosis and management of aspiration was of appropriate standard." Recurrent themes of risk are readily identified by reading the vignettes of the NAP4 study. This topic was the focus of another SAQ in 2016 and then a CRQ in 2022. However, pay attention to small changes in wording. Part (a), above, asks about adverse airway incidents, not just aspiration, and part (b) specifically asks how you would recognise that a patient has regurgitated and aspirated.

b) How would you recognise that a patient has regurgitated and aspirated gastric contents during an anaesthetic administered via an SAD? (6 marks)

Airway:

- Gastric contents visible in the oropharynx/tubing of SAD.

Breathing:

- Desaturation.
- Cyanosis.
- Bronchospasm.
- Increased airway pressures/reduced tidal volumes in ventilated patient.
- Abnormal auscultation.

Cardiovascular:

- Tachycardia.

REFERENCES

Cook T, Woodall N, Frerk C (eds.). *4th National Audit Project of the Royal College of Anaesthetists and the Difficult Airway Society: major complications of airway management in the United Kingdom.* London: The Royal College of Anaesthetists and Association of Anaesthetists of Great Britain and Ireland, 2011.
Robinson M, Davidson A. Aspiration under anaesthesia: risk assessment and decision-making. *Contin Educ Anaesth Crit Care Pain.* 2014: 14: 171–175.

4.3 March 2013 Awareness under anaesthesia

a) State and define the two types of unintentional awareness that may occur during general anaesthesia. (4 marks)
b) What factors may increase the likelihood of intraoperative awareness? (11 marks)
c) What monitoring techniques can be employed to reduce the risk of awareness during general anaesthesia? (5 marks)

The Chair's Report of the SAQ, reproduced here as it appeared in 2013, said that the pass rate was 79.8% and that it was considered an "easy" question, which would therefore have required a score of 14/20 or more in order to pass. They said it was "A straightforward and topical question (National Audit Project 5) that had been widely predicted by candidates and trainers! A question on awareness has featured in 1996, 1998, 2000 and 2006 papers." It was then re-examined in March 2016. Older papers talk about implicit and explicit awareness where the patient lacks recall of events in the former, but there is a negative psychological and behavioural impact on the individual consequently. This sort of awareness was not addressed by NAP5, which gave the definition of accidental awareness as "any instance of recall of intraoperative events during general anaesthesia, induction or emergence that occurs with administration of anaesthesia" and stated that it sought incidences of explicit awareness. Awareness associated with the experience of pain or paralysis appears to have a greater association with long-term negative psychological sequelae compared to awareness without.

REFERENCES

Hardman J, Aitkenhead A. Awareness during anaesthesia. *Contin Educ Anaes Crit Care Pain.* 2005: 5: 183–186.
Pandit J, Cook T. *The NAP5 steering panel: NAP5: accidental awareness during general anaesthesia.* London: The Royal College of Anaesthetists and Association of Anaesthetists of Great Britain and Ireland, 2014.

4.4 September 2013 Intra-arterial drug injection

a) List three patient factors that can predispose to patient harm following inadvertent intra-arterial (IA) drug injection. (3 marks)

b) List two organisational factors that may predispose to inadvertent IA drug injection. (2 marks)

c) List two drug features that increase the likelihood of severe extremity injury if injected IA. (2 marks)

d) Describe three mechanisms of injury following inadvertent IA injection. (3 marks)

e) List three acute clinical features of inadvertent IA injection. (3 marks)

f) Outline seven steps in the management of inadvertent IA injection. (7 marks)

The Chair's Report of the original SAQ stated that this "question was answered well [pass rate 71.9%] and proved to be a good discriminator. The factors that predispose to intra-arterial injection were broken down to patient factors, anatomical anomalies and the appreciation that some drugs are particularly harmful when injected intra-arterially. One candidate sadly misread the question and wrote about local anaesthetic toxicity, confusing the abbreviation (IA) with (LA). All abbreviations are explained before using them later in the question. This resulted in a 'poor fail' for that particular question but an overall pass for the paper. It should be pointed out that a poor fail in four or more questions is likely to result in an overall fail for the paper."

a) **List three patient factors that can predispose to patient harm following inadvertent intra-arterial (IA) drug injection. (3 marks)**

Take care to read the question. It doesn't just ask what factors are likely to lead to inadvertent intra-arterial injection, but what factors then increase the likelihood of this error causing harm. The factors below may result in failure to appreciate that a cannula is intra-arterial and so cause ongoing use for drug administration that is intended as intravenous.

- Unconscious so unable to indicate pain on injection.
- Hypotension or hypoxia, causing failure to recognise cannula as arterial.
- Anatomically anomalous artery accidentally cannulated, or thoracic outlet syndrome with loss of radial pulse on abduction or rotation of arm.

b) **List two organisational factors that may predispose to inadvertent IA drug injection. (2 marks)**

- Poor training resulting in failure to differentiate between the artery and vein prior to cannulation.
- Failure to check which line is being accessed, proximity between venous and arterial sampling ports.
- Failure to label line as arterial.

c) **List two drug features that increase the likelihood of severe extremity injury if injected IA. (2 marks)**

- Vasoactive drugs.
- Hyperosmolar drugs.
- Alkaline drugs that crystallise at physiological pH.

d) Describe three mechanisms of injury following inadvertent IA injection. (3 marks)

- Arterial spasm resulting in distal ischaemia; secondary to the drug itself or due to mediators released in response to drug.
- Chemical arteritis; direct tissue damage causing endothelial damage.
- Initiation of release of harmful endogenous substances e.g. thromboxane, which cause endothelial damage and activation of platelets resulting in thrombosis.
- Drug precipitation and crystal formation in distal microcirculation causing ischaemia and thrombosis.

e) List three acute clinical features of inadvertent IA injection. (3 marks)

- Failure of drug (that should have been administered intravenously) to have intended effect.
- Pain at and distal to the injection site.
- Pallor, cyanosis and coolness of limb, or redness and warmth.
- Paraesthesia.
- Loss of distal pulse.

f) Outline seven steps in the management of inadvertent IA injection. (7 marks)

- Stop injection.
- ABC assessment of patient, to include intravenous access and administration of drug by intended route if urgent.
- Keep cannula in situ for intra-arterial treatment but ensure no other use.
- IA iloprost.
- IA local anaesthetic treatment.
- Elevation of extremity to improve venous and lymphatic drainage.
- Anticoagulation or thrombolysis.
- Pain control.
- Involvement of vascular surgeons, radiology or plastics.
- Consideration of stellate ganglion or lower limb sympathetic block depending on site of error.
- Duty of Candour explanation and letter to patient and family.
- Incident reporting.

REFERENCES

Lake C, Christina Beecroft L. Extravasation injuries and accidental intra-arterial injection. *Contin Educ Anaesth Crit Care Pain.* 2010: 10: 109–113.

Lokoff A, Maynes J. The incidence, significance and management of accidental intra-arterial injection: a narrative review. *Can J Anaesth.* 2019: 66: 576–592.

4.5 March 2014 Drug errors

a) List two pieces of information from a patient preoperative assessment that may help to prevent intravenous drug administration errors. (2 marks)

b) Describe four behavioural factors which may contribute to anaesthetic intravenous drug administration errors. (4 marks)

c) List four environmental factors which may contribute to anaesthetic intravenous drug administration errors. (4 marks)

d) Outline four organisational strategies that might minimise intravenous drug administration errors. (4 marks)

e) List three important aspects of responding to an anaesthesia-related intravenous drug administration error after the episode of care has been completed. (3 marks)

f) List three never events pertinent to the administration of intravenous medications during anaesthetic care. (3 marks)

The original SAQ on intravenous drug errors was as follows:

a) Which human factors contribute to intravenous drug administration errors in theatre-based anaesthetic practice? (6 marks)

b) Outline the organisational strategies that might minimise intravenous drug administration errors. (14 marks)

The Chair's Report said that "Relatively few candidates had good insight into the factors associated with drug errors and were able to suggest strategies to reduce the incidence. The Safe Anaesthesia Liaison Group (SALG) has generated a number of publications specifically aimed at this subject matter and strong candidates had taken advantage of these." The pass rate was just 39.2%. Even if the candidates had not read the relevant SALG reports, they should have picked up knowledge relevant to answering the question from their attendance at M&M meetings. It is difficult to see how the SAQ could be converted into an CRQ with a definitive answer scheme, and I wonder if this is now a topic more suited to the viva. We have included it in our book as we have brought together ideas and suggestions from a range of publications.

a) **List two pieces of information from a patient preoperative assessment that may help to prevent intravenous drug administration errors. (2 marks)**

- Drug history.
- Allergy status.
- Past medical and anaesthetic history.
- Patient height and weight.

b) **Describe four behavioural factors which may contribute to anaesthetic intravenous drug administration errors. (4 marks)**

Human factors are consistently implicated in errors in healthcare and encompass behavioural, process-based, and environmental factors that predispose to human error.

Lack of knowledge:

- Unfamiliarity with a particular drug, its route of administration, dilution etc.

Human cognition:

- Human memory – cannot be relied upon to remember all infusion mix-ups, dose variations etc.
- Difficulty with complex calculations e.g. paediatrics, infusions.

Distraction:

- Needing to address other tasks whilst also drawing up drugs, prescribing drugs, calculating doses, giving drugs.
- Handling more than one medication at a time.

Stress, fatigue, excessive physical demands:

- Tiredness e.g. due to night work.
- Non-work emotional issues causing reduced work performance.
- Excessive workload e.g. high turnover list.

Lack of teamwork:

- Lack of double checking of drugs.
- Failure to feel able to voice lack of knowledge about a particular drug and its administration.
- Failure to implement a "no-blame culture," lack of encouragement of reporting, and learning from errors.
- Poor communication, poor handover e.g. failure of one member of a team to give explicit instructions to another about the administration of a particular drug or whether a drug has already been given.

c) **List four environmental factors which may contribute to anaesthetic intravenous drug administration errors. (4 marks)**

- Cluttered workspace.
- Low light levels.
- Drugs with similar packaging, changes in packaging without notice, unclear or too small labelling and lettering size.
- Multiple drugs drawn up, similar-sized syringes, lack of labelling.
- Distractions, noisy environment.
- Non-intravenous lines e.g. arterial or epidural, being used during the same operation as intravenous, failure to adequately label non-intravenous lines as such.
- Drugs intended for intravenous use stored together with local anaesthetic drugs.
- Multiple concentrations of same drug available for use, drugs in excessive and dangerous concentrations (requiring dilution) available in anaesthetic cart.

d) **Outline four organisational strategies that might minimise intravenous drug administration errors. (4 marks)**

There are multiple issues to discuss here. The subheadings are not important except to act as a prompt to your brain to think about things.

Processes:

- Standardisation of cross-checking, handover etc.
- Standardisation of infusions, diluents etc. and preprogramming of pumps.
- Availability of reference databases for doses, calculations, diluents.
- Standardisation of trays including keeping emergency drugs separate from drugs to be used for the particular patient, and non-intravenous drugs separate from intravenous.
- Regulations regarding what is drawn up, by whom, and at what stage in the care of a patient.
- Avoidance of distraction during drug preparation.

- Checklist to ensure prescription chart checked before administration of drugs by anaesthetist to avoid double-dosing or omitted doses.
- Investigation of possibility of pre-mixed infusions.
- Flushing all lines as standard before leaving theatre and recovery.
- Barcode scanning identification of drugs before use.

Physical environment:

- Availability of red barrelled syringes for use with neuromuscular blocking drugs.
- Standardisation of layout and contents of anaesthetic carts.
- Use of NR fit equipment to reduce risk of inadvertent intravenous injection of local anaesthetic drugs.
- Ensure intrathecal or epidural drugs are stored separately from intravenous drugs.
- Removal of non-essential, rarely used drugs from cart which have high injury risk if inadvertently given.
- Ensuring label availability at all times.
- Process for dealing with unused ampoules to prevent them from being returned to incorrect box (e.g. second-person check or discard altogether).
- Ensure adequate lighting levels.
- Sourcing of products with clear labelling, sufficiently large lettering etc., where possible.

Team working:

- Simulation sessions to highlight risks to all team members.
- Unusual drugs to be dealt with in the team briefing.
- Encouragement of working environment where any team member feels able to voice concern.
- Inclusion of pharmacist in team for notification of team members about changes in product appearance, education about new drugs for inclusion in anaesthetic carts etc.

e) **List three important aspects of responding to an anaesthesia-related intravenous drug administration error after the episode of care has been completed. (3 marks)**

- Open incident reporting of errors and near misses with no-blame culture, with fair root-cause analysis and feedback to individual involved.
- Discussion at morbidity and mortality meetings for education of all team members about pitfalls that may lead to error.
- Regular audit of collective reports and quality improvement interventions where specific failings have been identified.
- Communication with patient, following Duty of Candour statutory duty.
- Management of staff involved in error in accordance with NHS England "A Just Culture Guide."

f) **List three never events pertinent to the administration of intravenous medications during anaesthetic care. (3 marks)**

- Mis-selection of a strong potassium-containing solution.
- Wrong route administration of medication.
- Overdose of insulin due to abbreviations or incorrect device.
- Mis-selection of high-strength midazolam during conscious sedation.

REFERENCES

Glavin R. Drug errors: consequences, mechanisms and avoidance. *BJA*. 2010: 105: 76–82.

Litman R. How to prevent medication errors in the operating room? Take away the human factor. *BJA*. 2018: 120: 438–440.

Mackay E, Jenning J. Medicines safety in anaesthetic practice. *BJA Educ*. 2019: 19: 151–157.

Marshall S, Chrimes N. Medication handling: towards a practical, human-centred approach. *Anaesthesia*. 2018: 74: 280–284.

NHS England. *A just culture guide*. www.england.nhs.uk/wp-content/uploads/2021/02/NHS_0932_JC_Poster_A3.pdf. Accessed 6th May 2023.

Safe Anaesthesia Liaison Group. *Patient safety updates*. www.salg.ac.uk/salg-publications/patient-safety-update/

Toff N. Human factors in anaesthesia: lessons from aviation. *BJA*. 2010: 105: 21–25.

4.6 March 2015 Bronchospasm

a) List the factors that may have contributed to an increase in the prevalence of asthma in developed countries in the last 20 years. (5 marks)
b) What are the possible causes of acute bronchospasm during general anaesthesia in a patient with mild asthma? (5 marks)
c) Outline the immediate management of acute severe bronchospasm in an intubated patient during general anaesthesia. (10 marks)

This is the SAQ that appeared in March 2015. The Chair's Report said that the pass rate was 47.0% with 8.5% of candidates receiving a poor fail. They said, "The poor pass rate for this question is of concern as patients with asthma are regularly encountered in daily practice. The treatment of common coexisting medical disorders is specified in the syllabus for the CCT. In general, the management of acute bronchospasm was more thoroughly answered than the aetiology and causation sections. This was reflected in a lower poor fail rate compared to other questions, which is reassuring for patient safety under general anaesthesia." Bronchospasm was re-examined as a CRQ in March 2022, and so I have only given answers to the first part of the SAQ below.

a) **List the factors that may have contributed to an increase in the prevalence of asthma in developed countries in the last 20 years. (5 marks)**

There are a number of suggested theories that have not been proven.

- Better identification of cases, influenced by targets for asthma management in primary care.
- Hygiene hypothesis; cleaner environment associated with increased rates of allergy-associated asthma.
- Obesity; increases an individual's risk due to altered airway mechanics and chronic inflammatory state.
- Urbanisation.
- Asthma development following survival from premature birth.
- Increased use of drugs such as beta-blockers, NSAIDs, aspirin.

REFERENCE

Stanley D, Tunnicliffe W. Management of life-threatening asthma in adults. *Contin Educ Anaesth Crit Care Pain.* 2008: 8: 95–99.

4.7 March 2016 Awareness under anaesthesia

a) List two drug factors associated with an increased risk of accidental awareness under general anaesthesia (AAGA). (2 marks)
b) List five patient factors associated with an increased risk of AAGA. (5 marks)
c) List three surgical factors associated with an increased risk of AAGA. (3 marks)
d) List two organisational factors associated with an increased risk of AAGA. (2 marks)
e) List four types of monitoring that can be used to help reduce the incidence of AAGA. (4 marks)
f) List four possible consequences to the patient of an episode of AAGA. (4 marks)

The Chairs' Report of the original SAQ commented that "This question had the highest correlation with overall performance. Most candidates obviously had good knowledge of the recent NAP5 publication and this resulted in a relatively high pass rate [57.1%]. Candidates who presented their answers in an organised way tended to score more highly than those who did not, probably reflecting their greater knowledge. Again, some candidates disadvantaged themselves by not reading the question carefully."

Some key statistics from NAP5 executive summary:

- *Incidence of AAGA: approximately 1/19 000.*
- *Incidence of AAGA if NMBD used: 1/8 000.*
- *Incidence of AAGA if no NMBD used: 1/136 000.*
- *Incidence of AAGA in obstetrics: 1/670.*
- *Incidence of AAGA in cardiothoracics: 1/8 600.*
- *Drug factors: NMBD, thiopentone, TIVA.*
- *Patient factors: female gender, young adults, obesity, previous AAGA, possibly difficult airway.*
- *Surgical factors: obstetric, cardiac, thoracic, neurosurgical.*
- *Organisational: emergencies, junior anaesthetists, out of hours operating.*

The majority of the marks could have been obtained by reading the executive summary only.

a) **List two drug factors associated with an increased risk of accidental awareness under general anaesthesia (AAGA). (2 marks)**

- TIVA. *Results in a full range of human and equipment error issues; tissued cannula; pump failure; failure to switch the pump on; pump wrongly programmed; syringe switches; lack of training.*
- Neuromuscular blocking drug (NMBD). *93% of the episodes of awareness reported to NAP5 included use of NMBD with a range of possible underlying causes: failure to reverse; failure to monitor depth of block; human error causing syringe switches; failure to label syringes properly; mixed-up ampoules.*
- Thiopentone. *Implicated for a number of reasons, involvement in syringe swaps; reducing familiarity with its use; use in obstetrics and therefore confounded by other factors at play in obstetric anaesthesia; failure to dose based on body weight.*
- Rapid sequence induction. *Association with obstetric anaesthesia, emergency surgery, fixed drug dosing, intubation shortly after induction agents given.*

b) **List five patient factors associated with an increased risk of AAGA. (5 marks)**

- Female sex.
- Young adults.
- Difficult airway.
- Obesity; *difficulties with drug dosing and increased risk of difficult airway.*
- Previous awareness; *possible genetic component.*
- Sick, cardiovascularly compromised patients; *lower doses of anaesthetic agents given, transfers of critically ill patients.*

c) List three surgical factors associated with an increased risk of AAGA. (3 marks)

- Obstetrics, especially emergency caesarean: *anxiety, no premedication, no opioid used at induction, physiological changes of pregnancy may mask awareness, NMBD used, thiopentone commonly used, may underdose due to failure to take account of body weight, rapid sequence induction, emergency (increased risk of error), junior anaesthetist, out of hours, short period between intubation and commencement of surgery, not giving adequate time for drugs to work. Failed regional is a risk factor according to the reports submitted.*
- Cardiac: *not many cases in NAP5 but previously high level of awareness reported at start of cardiopulmonary bypass. May also relate to cardiac anaesthesia technique (low hypnotic dose, high opioid dose). May be less likely to report as patients are warned of waking in cardiac ICU with tube still in situ, and older patients may possibly be more tolerant.*
- Thoracics: *NMBD usually used; switching endotracheal tubes (single lumen to double lumen) and failing to maintain anaesthesia by volatile technique; rigid bronchoscopy with episodes of intense stimulation and intermittent interruption to anaesthesia administration if volatile used.*
- Neurosurgical.

d) List two organisational factors associated with an increased risk of AAGA. (2 marks)

- Out of hours.
- Junior anaesthetist.
- Emergency surgery.

e) List four types of monitoring that can be used to help reduce the incidence of AAGA. (4 marks)

Most of the monitoring that we use can help reduce the incidence of AAGA but, in order to get the four marks on the four lines, I would choose the ones that had been specifically discussed in the NAP5 report:

- Train-of-four monitoring.
- End-tidal anaesthetic gas (ETAG) monitoring.
- Monitors that specifically reflect depth of anaesthesia e.g. processed EEG monitors.
- Standard patient monitoring which may be reflective of sympathetic response to light anaesthesia and developing awareness e.g. heart rate, blood pressure, respiratory rate (if not paralysed).

A fuller answer, as you may discuss during a viva, might include the following:

Clinical monitoring:

- *Presence of the anaesthetist throughout the case.*
- *Response to voice, jaw thrust.*
- *Eyelash reflex.*
- *Eye position.*
- *Pupillary dilatation and reactivity to light.*
- *Sweating.*
- *Lacrimation.*
- *Tachypnoea.*
- *Movement.*
- *Retching on tube/LMA.*

General monitoring:

- *Full equipment checks and ongoing monitoring during anaesthesia (pumps, anaesthetic machine, vaporisers).*
- *Heart rate, respiratory rate and tidal volume (if not paralysed), blood pressure.*

- End-tidal anaesthetic gas (ETAG) monitoring.
- TIVA pump effect-site or plasma-site concentration.
- Train-of-four monitoring to ensure that neuromuscular blockade is reversible before ending anaesthesia.
- Patient weight for drug dosing.

Monitoring that specifically reflects depth of anaesthesia:

- Processed EEG monitors convert the frontal signal into a dimensionless number, 1–100 (100 = fully awake). BIS (target 40–60 for absence of postoperative recall), M-Entropy, and Narcotrend.
- Raw EEG (more rarely used).
- Isolated forearm technique (a technique used in research).
- Other specific monitors use somatosensory evoked or auditory evoked potentials as a measure of depth of anaesthesia.

f) List four possible consequences to the patient of an episode of AAGA. (4 marks)

Only four marks here, a brief explanation only is required. NAP5 reflected the importance of believing the patient, meeting with them face-to-face, expressing regret, and referral for formal psychological input if required. Patients were also reassured by experiencing what they perceived to be good care whilst aware, raising the importance of appropriate communication within the theatre and with the patient especially at times of light anaesthesia, times of risk of awareness, or during induction and emergence.

- There may be immediate or delayed recall (or no recall at all with implicit awareness).
- Experiences may be auditory or tactile; may include pain and awareness of paralysis.
- Response very varied, ranging from neutral feelings to extreme distress at the time and subsequently in the form of post-traumatic stress disorder with flashbacks, nightmares, anxiety and depression, with impact on personal, social, and work life.
- May cause avoidance of all medical settings, or specifically anaesthesia, and loss of trust of healthcare professionals.
- No recall may still cause long-term problems with e.g. unexplained anxiety due to implicit memory.

REFERENCE

Pandit J, Cook T. *The NAP5 steering panel: NAP5: accidental awareness during general anaesthesia.* London: The Royal College of Anaesthetists and Association of Anaesthetists of Great Britain and Ireland, 2014.

4.8 September 2016 Aspiration under anaesthesia

A 60-year-old man is having an elective knee arthroscopy and has just aspirated a significant amount of gastric fluid during anaesthesia. He has a supraglottic airway device in place and is breathing spontaneously. His inspired oxygen fraction is 1.0 and the pulse oximeter shows an oxygen saturation of 91%.

a) Describe your immediate management of this patient. (4 marks)

b) List the respiratory complications he could develop in the next 48 hours. (2 marks)

c) What are the possible preoperative risk factors for regurgitation and aspiration of gastric contents in this case? (6 marks)

d) Describe the strategies available to reduce the risk and impact of aspiration of gastric contents in any patient. (8 marks)

The Chairs reported a pass rate of 77.5% for this SAQ and said "This was adjudged to be an easy question and most candidates answered it well demonstrating good knowledge of how to manage such an emergency and of the recommendations of NAP 4. The few candidates who did less well wasted time describing general intraoperative safety measures that were not relevant to the scenario outlined." You can see that it is very similar to the question on aspiration from 2012. Many of the issues were then revisited in a CRQ in March 2022 where I have given answers.

4.9 March 2017 Wrong-sided nerve block

a) List the implications for the patient of an inadvertent wrong-sided peripheral nerve block. (5 marks)

b) Summarise the recommendations of the "Stop Before You Block" campaign (4 marks) and list the factors that have been identified as contributing to the performance of a wrong-sided block. (5 marks)

c) Define the term "never event" (2 marks) and list four drug-related never events. (4 marks)

Oh dear. A question almost identical to one from five years previously, and yet the pass rate was 39%. The Chairs said, "This question related to an important safety initiative. Candidates did not have adequate knowledge of the factors contributing to the performance of a wrong-side block such as distraction, the patient being lateral or prone, or a site mark being covered by blankets." The next time this topic was repeated was September 2019, which is where you will find the answers.

4.10 September 2017 Dental damage under anaesthesia

a) List four anaesthetic factors that may predispose to perioperative dental damage. (4 marks)
b) List five dental factors that predispose to perioperative dental damage. (5 marks)
c) You have anaesthetised a 22-year-old man and you notice a missing front tooth after intubation. State four aspects of your initial management of this situation. (4 marks)
d) Describe actions to be taken after dental damage under anaesthesia, after management of the acute situation. (3 marks)
e) Suggest four strategies to avoid dental damage in a patient deemed at high risk for dental damage under general anaesthesia. (4 marks)

The Chairs' Report for the SAQ on this topic said, "This question was thought to be easy and the pass rate was correspondingly high [68.3%]. Part (d) concerned the need to be open with patients when things go wrong (duty of candour) and was not as well answered as the parts relating to purely clinical matters. It is important to be aware of how to manage such situations as misunderstandings can lead to great distress for all parties. As mentioned previously, some candidates failed to read the question properly and lost marks in part (a) because they listed patient rather than anaesthetic factors that could predispose to dental damage."

a) List four anaesthetic factors that may predispose to perioperative dental damage. (4 marks)

I would not have considered limited mouth opening under anaesthetic factors, but it is included in the Safe Anaesthesia Liaison Group guidance on management of dental trauma during anaesthesia, the document that I assume was the basis of this question.

- LMA use.
- Laryngoscopy.
- Tracheal intubation; use of double lumen endotracheal tube.
- Forceful removal of airway, biting during emergence.
- Vigorous oropharyngeal suctioning.
- Difficult intubation.
- Limited mouth opening.

b) List five dental factors that predispose to perioperative dental damage. (5 marks)

- Primary teeth.
- Poor dental health.
- Crowns, fillings, and bridges.
- Patient age over 50 years.
- Prominent upper incisors.
- Isolated teeth.
- Previously traumatised teeth.

c) You have anaesthetised a 22-year-old man and you notice a missing front tooth after intubation. State four aspects of your initial management of this situation. (4 marks)

- Assess for possibility of airway compromise as a result: alert team, call for senior assistance, assess airway and ventilation. Check for obvious presence of tooth in airway, check oxygen saturations, auscultate chest, ensure airway pressures and volumes appropriate.
- Locate missing tooth: look for tooth in mouth with laryngoscope, assess with chest radiograph if not located, discuss with ENT regarding retrieval if found in lungs on X-ray.

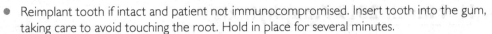

- Reimplant tooth if intact and patient not immunocompromised. Insert tooth into the gum, taking care to avoid touching the root. Hold in place for several minutes.
- Decision as to whether to proceed with surgery depends on urgency and possibility of further trauma to the mouth and teeth.
- If tooth cannot be reimplanted intraoperatively, it should be stored in saline or milk until urgent discussion with/assessment by dentist.

d) **Describe actions to be taken after dental damage under anaesthesia, after management of the acute situation. (3 marks)**

- Written referral to dentist (or on-site dental service if available) including details of damage and management at the time.
- Incident form.
- Discuss the dental damage with the patient and follow-up with letter in line with Duty of Candour statutory duty.
- Ensure adequate analgesia for management of dental damage, if required.

e) **Suggest four strategies to avoid dental damage in a patient deemed at high risk for dental damage under general anaesthesia. (4 marks)**

This subsection was not part of the original SAQ but preventative strategies are an important consideration in the management of all critical incidents.

- Avoid general anaesthesia if there is an appropriate alternative.
- Referral for preoperative dental treatment if poor dentition is assessed as a likely issue perioperatively.
- Stabilisation of a loose tooth preoperatively (with a suture or tie).
- Avoidance of laryngoscopy or airway instrumentation.
- Nasal fibreoptic intubation.
- Dental guards.
- Soft bite blocks during emergence, bite blocks on solid back teeth.

REFERENCES

Abeysundara L, Creedon A. Dental knowledge for anaesthetists. *BJA Educ.* 2016: 16: 362–368.
Milne A, Lockie J. Dental damage in anaesthesia. *Anaesth Intensive Care Med.* 2014: 15: 370–372.
Paolinelis G, Renton T, Djemal S, McDonnell N. *Dental trauma during anaesthesia.* King's Dental Unit with Safe Anaesthesia Liaison Group, 2012.

4.11 March 2019 Anaphylaxis

a) List the four most common triggers for perioperative anaphylaxis according to The Royal College of Anaesthetists' 6th National Audit Project (NAP6). (4 marks)

b) What is the estimated incidence of perioperative anaphylaxis? (1 mark)

c) Outline the pathophysiological processes underlying immunoglobulin E-mediated anaphylaxis. (3 marks)

d) Give the most common presenting feature of anaphylaxis in NAP6. (1 mark)

e) Give three other possible presenting features of perioperative anaphylaxis. (3 marks)

f) Give two indications for initiation of chest compressions in a case of suspected anaphylaxis. (2 marks)

g) Give four intravenous pharmacological options for treatment of hypotension associated with anaphylaxis in an adult, giving their bolus doses where applicable. (4 marks)

h) Give the timings of tryptase samples to be taken in the event of a suspected anaphylaxis. (2 marks)

The original question was an SAQ. The Chairs commented that the pass rate was 90.3%, "the highest on the paper. It is reassuring that candidates have sound knowledge of the management of anaphylaxis." The majority of marks for this question, both in its original SAQ form and my CRQ form, could have been gained by knowledge of the summary infographic about the NAP6 results and the guidance about anaphylaxis in the Association of Anaesthetists' Quick Reference Handbook.

a) List the four most common triggers for perioperative anaphylaxis according to The Royal College of Anaesthetists' 6th National Audit Project (NAP6). (4 marks)

- Antibiotics *(47%)*.
- Muscle relaxants *(33%)*.
- Chlorhexidine *(9%)*.
- Patent blue dye *(5%)*.

b) What is the estimated incidence of perioperative anaphylaxis? (1 mark)

- 1/10 000.

c) Outline the pathophysiological processes underlying immunoglobulin E-mediated anaphylaxis. (3 marks)

- Sensitisation: IgE antibodies develop against trigger agent.
- Re-exposure: allergen binds to and bridges between two IgEs bound to the cell membrane of mast cell or basophil.
- Signal transduction cascade results in release of preformed (e.g. histamine and tryptase) and newly made (leukotrienes, thromboxane A2, cytokines) inflammatory mediators.
- Resulting vasodilation, capillary leak, and bronchospasm cause the clinical effects.

d) Give the most common presenting feature of anaphylaxis in NAP6. (1 mark)

- Hypotension.

e) Give three other possible presenting features of perioperative anaphylaxis. (3 marks)

Bradycardia is thought to result from the Bezold-Jarisch reflex. Profound vasodilation associated with anaphylaxis results in poor venous return triggering a vagally mediated reflex which results in bradycardia to preserve diastolic filling.

- Bronchospasm.
- Tachycardia.

- Bradycardia.
- Angioedema.
- Cardiac arrest.
- Cutaneous flushing in association with another feature – often absent.

f) **Give two indications for initiation of chest compressions in a case of suspected anaphylaxis. (2 marks)**

- Cardiac arrest.
- Hypotension with systolic blood pressure < 50 mmHg.

g) **Give four intravenous pharmacological options for treatment of hypotension associated with anaphylaxis in an adult, giving their bolus doses where applicable. (4 marks)**

Hydrocortisone and chlorphenamine no longer have an acute role in the management of anaphylaxis.

- Crystalloid 20 ml/kg.
- Adrenaline 50 mcg.
- Glucagon 1 mg if beta blocked and unresponsive to adrenaline.
- Vasopressin 2 units.
- Metaraminol or noradrenaline if inadequate response to adrenaline.

h) **Give the timings of tryptase samples to be taken in the event of suspected anaphylaxis. (2 marks)**

The anaesthetist caring for the patient is responsible for liaising with the departmental lead for anaphylaxis for referring for immunological testing, reporting to the MHRA, informing the surgeon and the patient's GP, and informing the patient and advising them regarding alert bracelet use.

- As soon as patient is stable.
- One to two hours after the event.
- After 24 hours after the event.

REFERENCES

Association of Anaesthetists. *Quick Reference Handbook. 3.1 anaphylaxis*, updated April 2022. https://anaesthetists.org/Portals/0/PDFs/QRH/QRH_3-1_Anaphylaxis_v5.pdf? ver=2022-04-12-124225-493. Accessed 13th March 2023.

Dewachter P, Savic L. Perioperative anaphylaxis: pathophysiology, clinical presentation and management. *BJA Educ.* 2019: 19: 313–320.

Harper N, Cook T. *The NAP6 steering panel: NAP6: anaesthesia, surgery and life-threatening allergic reactions.* London: The Royal College of Anaesthetists and Association of Anaesthetists of Great Britain and Ireland, 2018.

4.12 September 2019 Wrong-sided nerve block

a) List five implications for the patient of an inadvertent wrong-sided peripheral nerve block. (5 marks)
b) State why the "Stop Before You Block" campaign was refreshed with the "Prep, Stop, Block" approach. (1 mark)
c) State four recommendations of the "Prep, Stop, Block" approach. (4 marks)
d) Apart from failure to engage with "Stop Before You Block," list five factors that have been identified as contributing to the performance of a wrong-sided block. (5 marks)
e) Define the term "never event." (1 mark)
f) List four drug-related never events. (4 marks)

The SAQ on this topic was almost identical to the two previous SAQs on "Stop Before You Block" and never events. The pass rate was 56.5% but, despite it being a repeated question, the Chairs commented that "weaker candidates showed similar failings. Candidates did not have adequate knowledge of the factors contributing to the performance of a wrong side block, such as distraction or the site mark being covered up. Drug-related, 'never' events are specific to certain medications and many candidates answered in far too general terms." Since 2019 the "Stop Before You Block" campaign has been updated with the three steps "Prep, Stop, Block," and my CRQ reflects this. Maybe time for a reappearance in the exam?

a) **List five implications for the patient of an inadvertent wrong-sided peripheral nerve block. (5 marks)**

- Potential adverse effects of unnecessary nerve block (including infection, bleeding, nerve damage, visceral damage).
- Bilateral block may be contraindicated (e.g. interscalene), resulting in cancellation of surgery, suboptimal pain relief, or experience of side effects of the alternative pain relief.
- Safe doses of local anaesthesia may be exceeded if correct side subsequently blocked.
- May result in wrong-sided surgery.
- Delayed discharge due to immobility if nerve blocks therefore undertaken on both legs.
- Loss of trust.

b) **State why the "Stop Before You Block" campaign was refreshed with the "Prep, Stop, Block" approach. (1 mark)**

- Failure of the campaign to result in reduction of wrong-sided nerve block rate.
- Local flexibility in application of "Stop Before You Block" contributing to its lack of success.

c) **State four recommendations of the "Prep, Stop, Block" approach. (4 marks)**

- Preparation: blocker prepares equipment and gives to assistant, then positions patient, scans, cleans the site, dons sterile gloves.
- Stop: just before block, blocker announces "Stop Before You Block" and with the assistant checks mark on patient with consent form and with patient if conscious.
- Block: assistant hands equipment to blocker for block to happen immediately.
- Process restarted if any delay to block or multiple blocks.

d) **Apart from failure to engage with "Stop Before You Block," list five factors that have been identified as contributing to the performance of a wrong-sided block. (5 marks)**

There are all sorts of things that may contribute to a wrong-sided block. These are the factors that have been documented, but if you hadn't read the "Stop Before You Block" campaign literature, you should still be able to have a good attempt at listing some issues that may increase the likelihood of error.

- Long duration since WHO sign-in.
- Patient being turned prone or lateral.
- Busy anaesthetic room; anaesthetist distracted.
- Lower limb blocks; arrow may not be immediately visible if patient covered for warmth or dignity.
- Anaesthetist not regularly performing blocks.
- Surgical mark absent or obscured.
- Distance between block and surgical site.
- More than one block being performed.
- Use of additional sticker to indicate block site.
- Changes to list.
- Inadequate supervision.
- Time pressures.
- Poor working culture.
- Wrong information from patient.

e) **Define the term "never event." (1 mark)**

According to their definition, it should be impossible for never events to happen – but unfortunately human error can still break down the supposed "strong systemic protective barriers," and so never events will not stop happening until aspects of equipment design change to prevent such occurrences.

- A serious incident that is wholly preventable because guidance or safety recommendations providing strong systemic protective barriers are available at a national level and should have been implemented by all healthcare providers.

f) **List four drug-related never events. (4 marks)**

- Mis-selection of a strong potassium-containing solution.
- Wrong route administration of medication.
- Overdose of insulin due to abbreviations or incorrect device.
- Overdose of methotrexate for non-cancer treatment.
- Mis-selection of high-strength midazolam during conscious sedation.
- Unintentional connection of patient requiring oxygen to an air flowmeter.

Below is the rest of the list of never events, as defined by NHS Improvement. A large proportion involve anaesthesia and drug administration. Some of them could be the basis of a future question. NHS Improvement categorises unintentional connection of a patient requiring oxygen to an air flowmeter as a general rather than drug-related never event. However, oxygen is a drug, or else we wouldn't be obliged to prescribe its use. Undetected oesophageal intubation has been temporarily suspended (for five years so far) from the never event list.

- *Wrong site surgery (includes wrong site block).*
- *Wrong implant/prosthesis.*
- *Retained foreign object post-operation.*
- *Failure to install functional collapsible shower or curtain rails.*

- *Falls from poorly restricted windows.*
- *Chest or neck entrapment in bedrails.*
- *Transfusion or transplantation of ABO-incompatible blood components or organs.*
- *Misplaced naso- or orogastric tube.*
- *Scalding of patients.*

REFERENCES

Adyanthaya S, Patil V. Never events: an anaesthetic perspective. *Contin Educ Anaesth Crit Care Pain.* 2014: 14: 197–201.

French J, Bedforth N, Townsley P. *Stop Before You Block supporting information.* http://salg.ac.uk/sites/default/files/SBYB-Supporting-Info.pdf. Accessed 27th June 2017.

Haslam N et al. 'Prep, stop, block': refreshing 'stop before you block' with new national guidance. *Anaesthesia.* 2021: 77: 372–375.

NHS Improvement. *Never events list 2018*, updated February 2021. www.england.nhs.uk/wp-content/uploads/2020/11/2018-Never-Events-List-updated-February-2021.pdf. Accessed 10th March 2023.

Torpor B et al. Best practices for safety and quality in peripheral regional anaesthesia. *BJA Educ.* 2020: 20: 341–347.

4.13 September 2019 Malignant hyperthermia

a) Explain the pathophysiology underlying malignant hyperthermia (MH). (2 marks)
b) List the two anaesthetic triggers for MH. (2 marks)
c) List three early clinical features of MH in an anaesthetised patient that should result in instigation of MH treatment. (3 marks)
d) List the three key elements of initial MH management once a suspected diagnosis has been made. (3 marks)
e) List five later onset features of MH which may require further treatment. (5 marks)
f) Give two methods for diagnosis of MH following recovery from a suspected episode. (2 marks)
g) List three patient groups who should be assessed for a possible increased risk of MH prior to elective anaesthesia. (3 marks)

The Chairs said of the original CRQ on this topic that it "was answered well, with one of the highest pass rates [80.3%]. Malignant hyperthermia, although uncommon, is a potentially life-threatening condition. It is therefore reassuring to see that candidates had a detailed appreciation of how to monitor and manage this condition." There is a definitive guideline on this condition from the Association of Anaesthetists which would offer significant scope for creation of questions on the topic with definitive answers.

a) Explain the pathophysiology underlying malignant hyperthermia (MH). (2 marks)

If you are ever asked about this in a viva, link your answer to the normal underlying physiology of excitation-contraction coupling. MH causes sustained skeletal muscle contraction and the multisystem morbidity that results can be easily explained when going back to basic physiology. Calcium binds to troponin C, which leads to actin-myosin cross-linking and muscular contraction, a process that uses ATP and results in carbon dioxide and heat production. Sustained contraction leads to ATP depletion (lactic acidosis), hyperthermia, and muscular rigidity (which may be observed clinically). Sarcomere integrity is lost, and intracellular contents leak out causing hyperkalaemia (with risk of arrhythmia) and rhabdomyolysis. Sustained acidosis, hyperthermia and rhabdomyolysis can lead to DIC. A stress response is triggered by the sympathetic nervous system, leading to tachycardia and worsening acidosis. Blood pressure may rise due to the sympathetic response or fall due to the presence of vasodilatory mediators.

- Mutation of ryanodine (or other calcium controlling) receptor.
- Trigger agent causes sustained released of calcium from the sarcoplasmic reticulum into the cytoplasm and therefore sustained muscle activity resulting in the features seen in MH e.g. hypercapnia, raised temperature etc.

b) List the two anaesthetic triggers for MH. (2 marks)

- Volatile anaesthetics – more potent volatiles give a quicker onset reaction.
- Suxamethonium.

c) List three early clinical features of MH in an anaesthetised patient that should result in instigation of MH treatment. (3 marks)

There are a range of features, but these three features that present early in the disease process should be enough to instigate management for MH. Muscle rigidity is a late sign and may signify irreversible disease.

- Unexplained, unexpected increase in heart rate.
- Unexplained, unexpected increase in $etCO_2$.
- Unexplained, unexpected increase in temperature.

d) List the three key elements of initial MH management once a suspected diagnosis has been made. (3 marks)

- Removal of trigger (*remove vaporisers, maximum gas flow, 100% oxygen, hyperventilate, charcoal filters, change soda lime and breathing circuit*).
- Patient cooling.
- Treatment with dantrolene 2.5 mg/kg bolus (*each vial reconstituted with 60 ml water. Further 1 mg/kg boluses every five minutes until etCO$_2$ < 6 kPa and core temperature < 38.5°C). Although there is no maximum limit for dantrolene dose, no response after 10 mg/kg is likely to have a poor outcome.*

e) List five later onset features of MH which may require further treatment. (5 marks)

- Acidosis.
- Hyperkalaemia.
- Arrhythmias.
- Myoglobinuria.
- Acute kidney injury.
- Disseminated intravascular coagulation.
- Compartment syndrome.
- Muscle rigidity.

f) Give two methods for diagnosis of MH following recovery from a suspected episode. (2 marks)

- DNA screening by blood test (*tests for known genetic associations with MH but has limited sensitivity*).
- Muscle biopsy with in vitro contracture test in response to trigger agents (*this must be done at the specialist MH referral unit in Leeds, more than four months after the suspected episode to allow time for muscle recovery, and only if the patient is over 10 years old*).

g) List three patient groups who should be assessed for a possible increased risk of MH prior to elective anaesthesia. (3 marks)

- Blood relatives of patients with known or suspected MH.
- Patients with a personal or family history of an episode which may be due to MH.
- Patients with a clinical myopathy with genetic aetiology implicated in MH susceptibility.
- Patients with a genetic variant in one of the genes implicated in MH susceptibility.
- Patients with a history of isolated or recurrent rhabdomyolysis of unknown cause.
- Patients with idiopathic hyperCKaemia.
- Patients with unexplained exertional heat illness.

REFERENCES

Gupta P, Bilmen J, Hopkins P. Anaesthetic management of a known or suspected malignant hyperthermia susceptible patient. *BJA Educ.* 2021: 21: 218–224.

Gupta P, Hopkins P. Diagnosis and management of malignant hyperthermia. *BJA Educ.* 2017: 17: 249–254.

Hopkins P et al. Guideline from the Association of Anaesthetists: malignant hyperthermia 2020. *Anaesthesia.* 2021: 76: 655–664.

4.14 March 2022 Aspiration under anaesthesia

You have anaesthetised a patient for elective knee arthroscopy using a supraglottic airway device (SAD). Thirty minutes into the procedure the patient starts to desaturate and has evidence of stomach contents in the tube of the SAD. You have declared an incident and applied 100% oxygen.

a) List three immediate actions you would take. (3 marks)
b) List two patient risk factors for aspiration under anaesthesia when using an SAD. (2 marks)
c) List two anaesthetic risk factors for aspiration when using an SAD. (2 marks)
d) List four respiratory complications that may develop over the next 48 hours. (4 marks)
e) List three approaches to reduce the volume and/or acidity of gastric contents preoperatively. (3 marks)
f) List two physiological mechanisms that help to protect against aspiration. (2 marks)
g) List two indications for performing point-of-care gastric USS. (2 marks)
h) Give the antral volumes (ml/kg) in the fasted and non-fasted patient, as estimated by point-of-care gastric USS. (2 marks)

The Chairs' Report of the CRQ on this topic stated that "This is an area of the syllabus that candidates would be expected to know. The question was deemed by the examiners to be one of the easier questions on the paper and this was reflected in a high pass rate," 69.4%. The question was essentially a repeat of the 2012 and 2016 SAQs but with some extra sections based around a recent BJA article on gastric ultrasound.

a) List three immediate actions you would take. (3 marks)

Make sure you read the question – you have already declared an incident (which I think includes calling for help and telling the theatre team) and applied 100% oxygen. It is difficult to know what three of a multitude of immediate actions the College would be looking for, but ABC so . . .

- Remove SAD.
- Suction patient's airway.
- Ventilate with 100% oxygen with bag-valve-mask.

I would probably then go on to deepen anaesthesia, if necessary, and give a neuromuscular blocking drug if I wasn't achieving good ventilation, and perform endotracheal intubation.

Once the immediate situation has been addressed, the ongoing management of the patient would be determined by your assessment of how compromised the patient is and may involve the following:

- *Early bronchoscopy if particulate matter has been aspirated – may be considered in theatre depending on severity of suspected aspiration.*
- *Decision to continue with surgery depends on circumstances.*
- *Extubation or ventilation on ICU, dependent on clinical condition.*
- *If extubated, extended recovery stay for observation of respiratory rate, oxygen saturations, other signs of respiratory distress.*
- *Chest X-ray.*
- *Maintenance of a high index of suspicion for aspiration pneumonia and treat early (antibiotics not routinely advocated).*
- *Discussion with patient and/or family followed up by written information of what symptoms should prompt the patient to seek medical help.*
- *Incident reporting.*

b) **List two patient risk factors for aspiration under anaesthesia when using an SAD. (2 marks)**

- Incompetent lower oesophageal sphincter: reflux or hiatus hernia, previous upper gastrointestinal surgery.
- Raised intra-abdominal pressure e.g. obesity, late pregnancy.
- Intra-abdominal pathology causing ileus or bowel obstruction.
- Conditions associated with delayed gastric emptying such as diabetes mellitus, chronic kidney disease, raised intracranial pressure, pain, pancreatitis, active labour.

c) **List two anaesthetic risk factors for aspiration when using an SAD. (2 marks)**

- Prolonged ventilation via SAD resulting in gastric insufflation.
- Poorly fitting SAD especially when positive pressure ventilation used.
- Light anaesthesia including at induction and emergence.
- First-generation SAD use.
- Junior anaesthetist working solo out of hours.

d) **List four respiratory complications that may develop over the next 48 hours. (4 marks)**

Pneumonia may develop consequent to these events but is likely to be later in the disease process.

- Hypoxia/type I respiratory failure.
- Atelectasis.
- Lobar collapse.
- Chemical pneumonitis.
- Acute respiratory distress syndrome.

e) **List three approaches to reduce the volume and/or acidity of gastric contents preoperatively. (3 marks)**

- Adherence to fasting guidelines.
- Nasogastric tube insertion and stomach drainage preoperatively.
- Premedication with prokinetic agents.
- Premedication with acid lowering medications; antacids, H_2 receptor antagonists, or proton pump inhibitors.

f) **List two physiological mechanisms that help to protect against aspiration. (2 marks)**

All of these are attenuated by loss of consciousness and most drugs used in anaesthesia:

- Lower oesophageal sphincter tone exceeding intragastric pressure prevents movement of stomach contents into the lower oesophagus. *Reinforced by the acute angle at the gastro-oesophageal junction and by the crura of the diaphragm. Its action is impaired by hiatus hernia which results in loss of reinforcement by the crura and the acute angle.*
- Upper oesophageal sphincter tone helps prevent reflux into pharynx. *Formed by cricopharyngeus, thyropharyngeus, the inferior constrictor, and cervical oesophagus.*
- Protective laryngeal reflexes including coughing, expiration, laryngospasm. *Reduced in the elderly.*

g) List two indications for performing point-of-care gastric USS. (2 marks)

Don't panic – even if you didn't know the first thing about gastric ultrasound, you would be able to guess some indications for it by thinking of patients in whom aspiration is a worry or where there might be difficulty in quantifying fasting status.

- Uncertain fasting status:
    — Cognitive dysfunction.
    — Language barrier.
    — Unclear history.
    — Paediatrics.
- Known or delayed gastric emptying:
    — Autonomic neuropathy (diabetes, Parkinson's, chronic kidney disease).
    — Acute pain.
    — Obesity.
    — Late pregnancy.
    — Systemic opioid use.

h) Give the antral volumes (ml/kg) in the fasted and non-fasted patient, as estimated by point-of-care gastric USS. (2 marks)

You could be forgiven for thinking this question is unfair, but you should already have got enough marks in this question to have passed it before even getting here! The typical stomach volume in an adult is about a litre.

- Fasted patient < 1.5 ml/kg
- Non-fasted patient > 1.5 ml/kg

REFERENCES

Cook T, Woodall N, Frerk C (eds.). *4th National Audit Project of the Royal College of Anaesthetists and the Difficult Airway Society: major complications of airway management in the United Kingdom.* London: The Royal College of Anaesthetists and Association of Anaesthetists of Great Britain and Ireland, 2011.

El-Boghdadly K, Wojcikiewicz T, Perlas A. Perioperative point-of-care gastric ultrasound. *BJA Educ.* 2019: 19: 219–226.

Robinson M, Davidson A. Aspiration under anaesthesia: risk assessment and decision-making. *Contin Educ Anaes Crit Care Pain.* 2014: 4: 171–175.

4.15 March 2022 Bronchospasm

A 54-year-old patient with a history of asthma has presented to pre-assessment prior to elective laparoscopic cholecystectomy.

a) List two characteristic findings of asthma on lung function testing. (2 marks)

b) Give two possible non-pharmacological reasons for poor asthma control in this patient. (2 marks)

c) List three steps that can help optimise the patient's asthma control preoperatively. (3 marks)

d) You are managing the patient intraoperatively, and their airway was secured with an endotracheal tube. During surgery, the peak airway pressure rises acutely. State four possible causes for this, apart from bronchospasm. (4 marks)

e) List three possible triggers of intraoperative bronchospasm in this case. (3 marks)

f) List three intravenous drugs and their bolus doses that you could use in the management of intraoperative bronchospasm in this patient. (3 marks)

g) List three immediate approaches to ventilation to avoid the risk of barotrauma. (3 marks)

The Chairs' Report for the CRQ on this topic gave a 61.9% pass rate and said, "This is a common question in all parts of the FRCA exam. It is an area of the curriculum that candidates would be expected to know and the initial scenario is one encountered by many trainees. Preoperative optimisation of the patient was the main area where candidates dropped marks but, in general, the aetiology and management of acute bronchospasm [were] well answered. This question shows the importance of getting to know your emergency guidelines."

a) List two characteristic findings of asthma on lung function testing. (2 marks)

Asthma is a reversible, obstructive airways disease – this is all you need to know to answer this question.

- Obstructive airways disease – reduced FEV_1 and reduced FEV_1/FVC ratio (< 70%).
- Reversibility of obstruction demonstrated by improvement in FEV_1 and FEV_1/FVC ratio after administration of bronchodilators.
- Variability in peak expiratory flow readings.
- Positive direct bronchial challenge test.

b) Give two possible non-pharmacological reasons for poor asthma control in this patient. (2 marks)

It is difficult to know whether "noncompliance" with medication or poor inhaler technique is classed as a pharmacological cause – I have not included them in the list below as there are plenty of other options to include for your two marks.

- Exposure to asthma triggers:
  - Housing conditions e.g. damp or mould, dust, pets.
  - Occupational exposure.
  - Cigarette smoking or second-hand exposure to cigarette smoke.
  - Allergic rhinitis resulting in seasonal variation in trigger exposure.
- Patient comorbidities:
  - Obesity.
  - Acid reflux.
  - Other lung disease.
  - Infective exacerbations of asthma.
- Incorrect diagnosis.

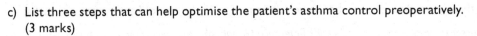

c) List three steps that can help optimise the patient's asthma control preoperatively. (3 marks)

- Reduce exposure to triggers, stop smoking.
- Encourage weight loss if obesity is a factor.
- Address any compliance or inhaler technique issues.
- Involve GP or respiratory physician in optimisation of pharmacological control as per NICE or BTS/SIGN guidelines.
- Breathing exercise programme.
- Treatment of reflux if this is a factor.

d) You are managing the patient intraoperatively and their airway was secured with an endotracheal tube. During surgery, the peak airway pressure rises acutely. State four possible causes for this, apart from bronchospasm. (4 marks)

Management and causes of a rise in airway pressure is addressed by the Association of Anaesthetists' Quick Reference Handbook.

- Equipment problem: kinking of breathing circuit or tube, patient biting on tube, blockage of tube with mucus plug or foreign body.
- Endobronchial migration of tube.
- Circulatory embolus.
- Aspiration.
- Pulmonary oedema.
- Pneumothorax.
- Insufflation of the abdomen for laparoscopic surgery.

e) List three possible triggers of intraoperative bronchospasm in this case. (3 marks)

- Pre-existing upper respiratory tract infection, poor asthma control, smoking.
- Airway irritation: cold inspired gases, airway secretions, airway suctioning, laryngoscopy, intubation, aspiration, carinal stimulation, or endobronchial intubation.
- Drugs causing histamine release, muscarinic block, or allergy.
- Vagal stimulation: peritoneal or visceral stretch etc.
- Light anaesthesia.

f) List three intravenous drugs and their bolus doses that you could use in the management of intraoperative bronchospasm in this patient. (3 marks)

Read the question – intravenous drugs only!

- Salbutamol 250 mcg.
- Adrenaline 10–100 mcg.
- Magnesium 2 g.
- Ketamine 20 mg.
- Aminophylline 5 mg/kg.
- Hydrocortisone 200 mg.

g) List three immediate approaches to ventilation to avoid the risk of barotrauma. (3 marks)

See the Association of Anaesthetists' Quick Reference Handbook approach to bronchospasm management. It also advises you to be alert to breath stacking but as this is not an approach to ventilation, I have not included it in the answer list.

- Increase expiratory time to allow complete exhalation.
- Use pressure control.
- Allow permissive hypercapnia.

REFERENCES

Association of Anaesthetists. *Quick Reference Handbook. 3.4 bronchospasm*, updated 2019 and *2.3 increased airway pressure*, 2018. https://anaesthetists.org/Home/Resources-publications/Safety-alerts/Anaesthesia-emergencies/Quick-Reference-Handbook-QRH/PDF-version. Accessed 13th March 2023.

Bali S, Seglani S, Challands, J. Perioperative management of the child with asthma. *BJA Educ.* 2022: 22: 402–410.

British Thoracic Society and Scottish Intercollegiate Guidelines Network. *SIGN 158: British guideline on the management of asthma*, 2019. www.brit-thoracic.org.uk/quality-improvement/guidelines/asthma/. Accessed 13th March 2023.

National Institute for Health and Care Excellence. *Asthma: diagnosis, monitoring and chronic asthma management: NG80*, Last updated March 2022. www.nice.org.uk/guidance/ng80/chapter/recommendations#self-management. Accessed 13th March 2023.

National Institute for Health and Care Excellence. *Clinical knowledge summary: when should I suspect asthma?* Last revised April 2022. https://cks.nice.org.uk/topics/asthma/diagnosis/diagnosis/. Accessed 13th March 2023.

Ntima N, Lumb A. Pulmonary function tests in anaesthetic practice. *BJA Educ.* 2019: 19: 206–211.

Stanley D, Tunnicliffe W. Management of life-threatening asthma in adults. *Contin Educ Anaesth Crit Care Pain.* 2008: 8: 95–99.

DAY SURGERY

5.1 September 2011 Diabetes mellitus

A 52-year-old man has been admitted for a tympanoplasty on the morning of surgery. He is a long-standing type I diabetic who has failed to attend the preoperative assessment clinic.
a) Give three specific issues that this patient's diabetes presents perioperatively. (3 marks)
b) List four perioperative complications associated with poor long-term diabetes control. (4 marks)
c) List four specific considerations for tympanoplasty in this patient. (4 marks)
d) Give three indications for the perioperative use of a variable rate intravenous insulin infusion (VRIII) for patients with type I diabetes. (3 marks)
e) List three prerequisites before a perioperative VRIII should be stopped in a patient with type I diabetes. (3 marks)
f) List three key causes of perioperative hyperglycaemia. (3 marks)

The SAQ on this topic appeared in the same year that "NHS Diabetes Guideline for the Perioperative Management of the Adult Patient with Diabetes" was first issued. In 2015, the AAGBI produced a guideline that aimed to tailor that advice to anaesthetists and to address some updates in recommendations. The CPOC guideline on perioperative care of diabetics, published 2021, was created in response to the issues raised regarding perioperative diabetes management in the NCEPOD enquiry and the need for a national, multidisciplinary standard. Diabetes care will always be topical as it is such a common disease, and its perioperative management is a source of such significant morbidity.

a) **Give three specific issues that this patient's diabetes presents perioperatively. (3 marks)**

The question asks for specific issues for this patient. The words to help you focus your thoughts are the following: 52 year old, long-standing, failed to attend, and admitted on the morning of surgery.

- Long-standing diabetes – high probability of micro- (retinopathy, neuropathy, nephropathy) and macrovascular (ischaemic heart disease, cerebrovascular disease) complications that have not been assessed for as did not attend preoperative assessment.
- Failure to attend preoperative assessment may be indicative of generalised poor compliance with medical management, which is associated with a greater burden of complications of diabetes.
- Failed to attend preoperative assessment so may not have had an assessment of recent diabetes control – HbA1c (glycosylated haemoglobin) > 69 mmol/mol is associated with increased risk of postoperative complications. Non-urgent surgery should be cancelled, and diabetes management optimised.
- Patient has not had instructions on alteration of insulin regimen and may now be at greater risk of perioperative hypo- or hyperglycaemia.

DOI: 10.1201/9781003388494-5

b) List four perioperative complications associated with poor long-term diabetes control. (4 marks)

Studies have shown variable outcomes, but these are the risks listed in the 2015 AAGBI guideline.

- 50% increase in mortality.
- More than doubling of risk of postoperative respiratory infections.
- Doubling of risk of surgical site infections.
- Threefold risk of urinary tract infections.
- Doubling of risk of perioperative myocardial infarction.
- Almost twofold increase in risk of perioperative acute kidney injury.
- Perioperative hypoglycaemia.
- Perioperative hyperglycaemia or ketoacidosis.

c) List four specific considerations for tympanoplasty in this patient. (4 marks)

- Local anaesthesia may be preferred to GA as it avoids loss of consciousness, which may make monitoring for hypoglycaemia easier in a diabetic patient.
- Facial nerve monitoring used during surgery – supraglottic airway device is often used to avoid need for NMBD but is contraindicated in the presence of gastroparesis associated with long-standing or poorly controlled diabetes.
- Tympanoplasty tends to be emetogenic, but it is important for this diabetic patient to avoid nausea and vomiting to facilitate return to normal oral intake and normal insulin regimen. Multimodal antiemesis and TIVA can be considered.
- Dexamethasone is relatively contraindicated as part of a multimodal approach to antiemesis as it worsens diabetic control.
- Oral analgesia usually sufficient for tympanoplasty, but NSAIDs may not be appropriate in a diabetic patient if they have renal complications.
- Hypotensive anaesthesia optimises surgical field but may be inappropriate in the presence of micro- and macrovascular comorbidities.
- Nitrous oxide should be avoided due to its emetogenic effect, which is unhelpful in a patient for whom a return to normal intake is so important, and also due to the risk of causing negative pressure in the middle ear after washout postoperatively with the risk of graft disruption.

d) Give three indications for the perioperative use of a variable rate intravenous insulin infusion (VRIII) for patients with type 1 diabetes. (3 marks)

Type 1 diabetics having planned surgery should have individualised advice about how to manage their insulin. Patients who take a long-acting insulin or mixed insulin will be advised to take a reduced dose on the morning of surgery (and then may safely miss a meal with hourly CBG monitoring) as they must always have a source of exogenous insulin to prevent catabolism, hyperglycaemia, and ketosis. During times of stress, such as surgery, the release of pro-catabolic hormones exacerbates this situation further.

- Patients who will miss more than one meal.
- Patients who have not taken their basal insulin.
- Poorly controlled diabetes with HbA1c > 69 mmol/mol.
- Patients with recurrent hyperglycaemias.
- Patients requiring emergency surgery who have a blood glucose > 10 mmol/l OR most type 1 diabetics needing emergency surgery.

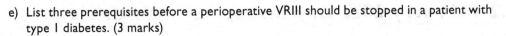

e) List three prerequisites before a perioperative VRIII should be stopped in a patient with type I diabetes. (3 marks)

- Ensure patient has returned to eating and drinking.
- Ensure CBG < 10 mmol/l.
- Ensure ketones < 0.6 mmol/l.
- Basal insulin should be given half an hour before cessation of VRIII.

f) List three key causes of perioperative hyperglycaemia. (3 marks)

- Hospital acquired diabetic ketoacidosis.
- Hyperosmolar hyperglycaemic state.
- Stress-induced hyperglycaemia.
- Insufficient medication e.g. incorrect omission of insulin, disconnection of VRIII, inappropriate prescription.
- Sepsis or infection.

REFERENCES

Association of Anaesthetists of Great Britain and Ireland. Peri-operative management of the surgical patient with diabetes 2015. *Anaesthesia*. 2015: 70: 1427–1440.

Centre for Perioperative Care. *Guideline for perioperative care for people with diabetes mellitus undergoing elective and emergency surgery*. London: Centre for Perioperative Care, 2021, updated December 2022.

Dhatariya K et al. NHS diabetes guideline for the perioperative management of the adult patient with diabetes. *Diabet Med*. 2012: 29: 420–433.

National Confidential Enquiry into Patient Outcome and Death. *Highs and lows*. London: National Confidential Enquiry into Patient Outcome and Death, 2018.

5.2 February 2023 Day case spinal anaesthesia

a) List two features of a local anaesthetic drug that make it ideal for use for day case spinal anaesthesia. (2 marks)

b) List four benefits of spinal anaesthesia for day case surgery. (4 marks)

c) Give one advantage and one disadvantage of unilateral spinal anaesthesia. (2 marks)

d) Complete the following table to give two drugs that can be used for spinal anaesthesia for day case surgery, stating for each a typical dose range, and giving the duration of surgical anaesthesia provided. (6 marks)

e) List three factors that may increase the risk of postoperative nausea and vomiting after spinal anaesthesia. (3 marks)

f) List three factors that increase the risk of urinary retention after spinal anaesthesia. (3 marks)

Although seemingly specific knowledge was tested in this CRQ, understanding the general principles of anaesthesia for day surgery and how spinal anaesthesia would impact these would allow you to have picked up most marks. The specific points regarding prilocaine and chloroprocaine were covered in a recent BJA Education article, once again highlighting their importance as a revision resource. The Chairs' Report said that this "was thought to be one of the easier questions" on the paper, but unfortunately the questions on "the finer points of local anaesthetic pharmacology were not well answered." The pass rate was 52.8%.

a) **List two features of a local anaesthetic drug that make it ideal for use for day case spinal anaesthesia. (2 marks)**

- Rapid onset of sensory and motor block.
- Short acting, with predictable offset.
- Minimal incidence of adverse effects.

b) **List four benefits of spinal anaesthesia for day case surgery. (4 marks)**

- Reduced postoperative pain and reduced need for rescue analgesia in recovery.
- Benefits of avoiding general anaesthesia:
  - Reduction in risk of postoperative nausea and vomiting.
  - Facilitation of day case surgery in patients with comorbidities such as obesity, OSA, lung disease.
  - Quicker return to oral intake, especially important in facilitating return to usual management regimen of diabetic patients.
  - Avoidance of psychoactive medications in the elderly may reduce risk of postoperative cognitive issues.
  - Avoidance of risks of airway management.
- Quicker time to discharge from recovery and discharge from hospital which may represent a cost saving.
- Some patients report improved satisfaction after awake surgery; involvement in care, able to ask questions and retain more information.
- Ability to present a choice of general anaesthesia or spinal anaesthesia to the patient, facilitates informed consent.

c) **Give one advantage and one disadvantage of unilateral spinal anaesthesia. (2 marks)**

Advantages:

- Increased patient satisfaction due to reduced numbness on nonoperative side.
- Earlier return to passing urine.
- Lower incidence of hypotension.

Disadvantages:

- Risk of wrong-sided block error is introduced.
- Increased anaesthesia time as patient will need to lie on one side for 10–15 minutes.

d) Complete the following table to give two drugs that can be used for spinal anaesthesia for day case surgery, stating for each a typical dose range, and giving the duration of surgical anaesthesia provided. (6 marks)

The two ideal drugs for spinal anaesthesia for day case surgery in widespread use are prilocaine and chloroprocaine. Lidocaine is now not licensed for day case spinal anaesthesia due to risks of neurotoxicity.

Drug	Dose	Duration of surgical anaesthesia
Hyperbaric 2% prilocaine	40–60 mg (2–3 ml)	Up to 90 minutes.
1% 2-chloroprocaine	40–50 mg (4–5 ml)	40 minutes (although doses in upper end of range may last up to 60 minutes, and some advocate a dose range up to 60 mg although this does not have MHRA approval).

e) List three factors that may increase the risk of postoperative nausea and vomiting after spinal anaesthesia. (3 marks)

- Hypotension associated with high block.
- Vagal hyperactivity associated with high block.
- Intrathecal opioid use (especially water soluble e.g. morphine)
- Inadequate block causing:
  - Intraoperative pain, stimulation, anxiety, and subsequent vagal response.
  - Intraoperative intravenous opioid supplementation.
  - Emergency conversion to general anaesthesia.

f) List three factors that increase the risk of urinary retention after spinal anaesthesia. (3 marks)

Some centres will have a day case surgery protocol that permits patients who have received spinal anaesthesia to be discharged before they have passed urine, but the safety of this approach is dependent on patient selection and education, and adequate access for help if there are subsequent problems. The risk of urinary retention may be influenced by the approach to the spinal anaesthetic itself, but patient and surgical factors also have a role.

- Drug factors:
  - Long-acting local anaesthetic (e.g. bupivacaine).
  - Intrathecal opioid administration.
  - Excessive perioperative intravenous fluids (> 500 ml) leading to bladder distension.
  - Administration of anticholinergics perioperatively (e.g. as treatment of bradycardia after high spinal).
- Patient factors:
  - Age > 70 years.
  - History of voiding difficulty or incontinence (including prostatic hypertrophy or neurogenic bladder).
- Surgical factors:
  - Type of surgery: urological, uro-gynaecological, inguinal hernia, perianal.

REFERENCES

Rattenbury R, Hertling A, Erskine R. Spinal anaesthesia for ambulatory surgery. *BJA Educ.* 2019: 19: 321–328.

Tweedie O et al. Spinal anaesthesia in day surgery: right drug, right patient, right procedure. *RA-UK handbook*, 2018. www.ra-uk.org/images/Covid_Webinar_2020/Spinal_Anaesthesia_in_Day_Surgery.pdf. Accessed 6th March 2023.

6.1 March 2012 Laparotomy for ovarian malignancy

A 52-year-old woman is due to undergo cytoreductive surgery and hyperthermic intraperitoneal chemotherapy (HIPEC) for ovarian cancer. She has completed three cycles of chemotherapy and will receive further chemotherapy postoperatively.

a) Give five reasons why this patient may be at increased risk of deep vein thrombosis. (5 marks)
b) Give four reasons for including a neuraxial technique in the anaesthetic management of this patient. (4 marks)
c) List five intraoperative complications of HIPEC that may affect the patient. (5 marks)
d) List four components of the Enhanced Recovery After Surgery (ERAS) Society guidelines for reducing the risk of surgical site infection after gynaecological oncology surgery. (4 marks)
e) Give two reasons for choosing TIVA-based anaesthesia rather than inhalational for this patient. (2 marks)

The question that originally featured as an SAQ in March 2012 concerned a 52-year-old woman having surgery for ovarian malignancy after three rounds of chemotherapy. Although she had a normal BMI, she had massive ascites. The question then asked for the "specific features of this case" that would affect the anaesthetist's pre-, intra- and postoperative approach. It would have required the candidate to think through all the body systems and how they might be impacted by such a disease process with her history of treatment and her ascites and then to consider how major and prolonged such surgery is. Following the alphabet helps to drag thoughts out of your brain. The same would be true for the CRQ I have made up here. Know nothing about HIPEC except that it is hot intraperitoneal chemotherapy? Think through a systems-based approach and you will start to get some facts down on paper.

a) **Give five reasons why this patient may be at increased risk of deep vein thrombosis. (5 marks)**

- Release of procoagulant factors by tumour.
- Presence of pelvic mass inhibiting venous return.
- Chemotherapy increases risk by endothelial damage and release of inflammatory mediators.
- Presence of long-term central venous catheter for previous chemotherapy.
- Prolonged surgery and hence immobility.
- Ovarian clear cell carcinoma is associated with a significantly raised risk of venous thromboembolism.

b) **Give four reasons for including a neuraxial technique in the anaesthetic management of this patient. (4 marks)**

- Major surgery and HIPEC increase pain scores – without neuraxial technique, the required opioid dose is likely to be high with significant impact of side effects (ileus, nausea, reduced respiratory function, drowsiness).

DOI: 10.1201/9781003388494-6

- Reduction in opioid use may reduce cancer progression.
- Local anaesthetic thought to have a directly positive impact on reducing risk of cancer recurrence.
- Neuraxial technique results in reduction of stress response thus attenuating the negative impact on patient immunity, possibly reducing risk of cancer progression.
- Reduction in thromboembolic risk postoperatively.

c) **List five intraoperative complications of HIPEC that may affect the patient. (5 marks)**

- Coagulopathy, with or without haemorrhage, consequent to the major surgery that has taken place.
- Electrolyte disturbance.
- Hyperthermia.
- Hyperglycaemia.
- Haemodynamic instability.
- Acute kidney injury.

d) **List four components of the Enhanced Recovery After Surgery (ERAS) Society guidelines for reducing the risk of surgical site infection after gynaecological oncology surgery. (4 marks)**

- Antimicrobial prophylaxis.
- Chlorhexidine-based skin preparation.
- Prevention of hypothermia.
- Avoidance of unnecessary drains or tubes.
- Avoidance of hyperglycaemia.

e) **Give two reasons for choosing TIVA-based anaesthesia rather than inhalational for this patient. (2 marks)**

- Use of short-acting agents supported by ERAS guidelines.
- Propofol may have a positive effect in reducing cancer recurrence.
- Propofol has an antiemetic effect.

REFERENCES

Durnford S, Boss, L, Bell J. Cytoreductive surgery and hyperthermic intraperitoneal chemotherapy. *BJA Educ.* 2021: 21: 187–193.

Evans M, Wigmore T, Kelliher L. The impact of anaesthetic technique upon outcome in oncological surgery. *BJA Educ.* 2019: 19: 14–20.

Morosan M, Popham P. Anaesthesia for gynaecological oncological surgery. *Contin Educ Anaesth Crit Care Pain.* 2014: 14: 63–68.

Nelson G et al. Guidelines for perioperative care in gynecologic/oncology: Enhanced Recovery After Surgery (ERAS) Society recommendations – 2019 update. *Int J Gynecol Cancer.* 2019: 0: 1–18.

6.2 September 2013 Laparoscopic Nissen's fundoplication

a) List five advantages of laparoscopic surgery compared to open surgery. (5 marks)
b) List two surgical risks specifically associated with laparoscopic surgery. (2 marks)
c) List four patient comorbidities which may contraindicate laparoscopic surgery. (4 marks)
d) List two possible complications related to positioning in a patient undergoing a laparoscopic Nissen's fundoplication. (2 marks)
e) List two possible respiratory consequences of pneumoperitoneum. (2 marks)
f) List three possible cardiovascular complications consequent to pneumoperitoneum. (3 marks)
g) List two possible neurological complications consequent to pneumoperitoneum. (2 marks)

The SAQ on this topic had a 72.5% pass rate. The Chair commented that it was a modification of a question on the effects of laparoscopy that had been used in a paper in 2006. This reiterates the need to focus on commonly occurring (in real life as well as the exam) issues in your revision. The Chair's Report commented that a "significant number of answers incorrectly referred to the effects of a Trendelenburg position raising intracranial and intraocular pressure" when being asked about Nissen's fundoplication. Remember, upper abdominal surgery tends to be performed in a head-up/reverse Trendelenburg position and lower abdominal or pelvic surgery in a head-down/Trendelenburg position.

a) **List five advantages of laparoscopic surgery compared to open surgery. (5 marks)**

- Reduced tissue damage results in reduced stress response to surgery.
- Reduced size of incisions results in lower pain scores postoperatively/reduced need for opioid-based analgesia with its side effects postoperatively.
- Reduced risk of surgical site and other postoperative infection.
- Faster postoperative recovery to normal activities.
- Reduced gut handling results in reduced risk of ileus with faster return to enteral feeding.
- Better visualisation of target structures compared to open surgery.
- Reduced blood loss.
- Reduced length of stay – some laparoscopic procedures undertaken as day cases e.g. laparoscopic cholecystectomy, others have shortened stay e.g. anterior resection.
- May be advantageous in obese patients compared to open surgery from the point of view of access and recovery.
- May be preferred option in patients with severe respiratory disease who would be unable to tolerate open surgery with large incision.

b) **List two surgical risks specifically associated with laparoscopic surgery. (2 marks)**

- Damage to organ by accidental injury on insertion of trocar or Veress needle.
- Haemorrhage due to accidental injury to vessel or organ by insertion of trocar or Veress needle.
- Accidental insufflation of vessel with carbon dioxide resulting in circulatory collapse due to gas embolus.
- Excessive pneumoperitoneum resulting in reduction in venous return and increase in systemic vascular resistance causing cardiovascular collapse.

c) **List four patient comorbidities which may contraindicate laparoscopic surgery. (4 marks)**

- Severe heart failure (where raised vascular resistance will result in further decrease in cardiac output).
- Right-to-left cardiac shunt (shunt may be increased by the necessary raised airway pressures and consequent right heart pressure).

- Raised intracranial pressure.
- Severe uncorrected hypovolaemia.
- Retinal detachment.

d) List two possible complications related to positioning in a patient undergoing a laparoscopic Nissen's fundoplication. (2 marks)

- Patient sliding on table, risk of falling.
- Reduced venous return causing hypotension with consequent organ effects e.g. myocardial ischaemia, cerebral ischaemia.
- Movement of patient in relation to tracheal tube, risk of accidental extubation.

e) List two possible respiratory consequences of pneumoperitoneum. (2 marks)

- Limited diaphragmatic excursion reduces pulmonary compliance, reducing functional residual capacity, affecting V/Q matching, resulting in hypoxaemia and hypercapnia.
- Atelectasis may result in respiratory compromise postoperatively.
- Raised airway pressures of ventilation to correct hypoxaemia and hypercapnia may result in barotrauma.

f) List three possible cardiovascular complications consequent to pneumoperitoneum. (3 marks)

- Compression of vena cava reduces venous return – compensation through increased heart rate but ultimately there will be reduction in cardiac output.
- Bradycardia.
- Compression of major arteries increases systemic vascular resistance, reduces cardiac output.
- Increased systemic vascular resistance increases myocardial wall tension and therefore risks ischaemia in susceptible patients.
- Atelectasis of lungs or the increased ventilatory pressures used to overcome lung changes will both further decrease venous return.
- Raised $PaCO_2$ will increase pulmonary artery pressure causing right heart failure in susceptible patients.
- Venous pooling increases risk of venous thromboembolism.

g) List two possible neurological complications consequent to pneumoperitoneum. (2 marks)

- Raised intrathoracic pressure reduces venous drainage and so increases intracranial pressure.
- Raised partial pressure of blood carbon dioxide from insufflated gas causes cerebral vasodilation and therefore raised intracranial pressure.
- Raised intracranial pressure may result in cerebral oedema.

REFERENCES

Carey B, Jones C, Fawcett W. Anaesthesia for minimally invasive abdominal and pelvic surgery. *BJA Educ.* 2019: 19: 254–260.

Hayden P, Cowman S. Anaesthesia for laparoscopic surgery. *Contin Educ Anaesth Crit Care Pain.* 2011: 11: 177–180.

6.3 March 2014 Phaeochromocytoma

a) List three characteristic symptoms of phaeochromocytoma. (3 marks)
b) List two specific biochemical investigations that may be used to confirm the presence of a phaeochromocytoma. (2 marks)
c) List three radiological investigations that may be used to confirm the location of a phaeochromocytoma after positive biochemical testing. (3 marks)
d) List four objectives of preoperative optimisation prior to surgery for phaeochromocytoma. (4 marks)
e) Complete the following table to give three classes of drugs that are commonly used in cardiovascular preoptimisation of patients undergoing surgery for phaeochromocytoma, the timing of initiation, and the rationale for their use. (6 marks)
f) Name a drug that may be used to treat catecholamine-resistant hypotension during surgery to remove a phaeochromocytoma, and state its mechanism of action. (2 marks)

Phaeochromocytomas are catecholamine-secreting neuroendocrine tumours usually arising from the adrenal medulla. Some are malignant (with risk of spread to the liver). Some are hereditary. Some are bilateral. When hereditary, they may be due to a specific autosomal dominant gene mutation, part of a multiple endocrine neoplastic (MEN) syndrome or in association with neuroectodermal dysplasia, for example, Von Hippel-Lindau or Von-Recklinghausen's. Catecholamine-secreting tumours can sometimes be found outside of the adrenal glands, in sympathetic ganglia, and these are called paragangliomas. Phaeochromocytomas predominantly secrete noradrenaline followed by adrenaline and then, to a much lesser extent, dopamine. Familial ones predominantly secrete adrenaline. They affect both genders and present mainly in the third to fifth decade of life. The Chair's Report for the SAQ on this topic stated that there was a 44.7% pass rate but that "some candidates confused the signs and symptoms of phaeochromocytoma with carcinoid syndrome."

a) List three characteristic symptoms of phaeochromocytoma. (3 marks)

- Headache.
- Palpitations/fast heart rate.
- Sweating.

These are the three classic symptoms. Patients may have very nonspecific symptoms such as anxiety, nausea, weight loss, tremor, abdominal pain due to vasoconstriction causing bowel ischaemia, and visual disturbance caused by papilloedema due to extreme hypertension. Others will be asymptomatic but diagnosed after an incidental finding of phaeochromocytoma on imaging or after the observation of raised blood pressure. Patients may present with hyperglycaemia due to the insulin-opposing effects of catecholamines.

b) List two specific biochemical investigations that may be used to confirm the presence of a phaeochromocytoma. (2 marks)

Phaeochromocytomas may secrete a mixture of adrenaline and noradrenaline and hence tests will assess levels of their breakdown products (superior to measuring the catecholamines themselves which have very short half-lives). Less frequently they will secrete dopamine and so tests of dopamine and its breakdown product homovanillic acid may also be performed.

- Plasma or urinary metanephrine.
- Plasma or urinary normetanephrine.
- Plasma or urinary dopamine.
- Plasma or urinary homovanillic acid.

c) List three radiological investigations that may be used to confirm the location of a phaeochromocytoma after positive biochemical testing. (3 marks)

- MRI.

- CT.
- MIBG scintigraphy (radioactive analogue of noradrenaline which is concentrated in phaeochromocytomas and paragangliomas and emissions detected on a gamma camera).
- PET scan (with tracer that binds to receptors on tumour cells).

d) List four objectives of preoperative optimisation prior to surgery for phaeochromocytoma. (4 marks)

- Blood pressure control.
- Correction of chronic circulating volume depletion.
- Heart rate and rhythm control.
- Optimisation of myocardial function.
- Reversal of glucose and electrolyte disturbances.

e) Complete the following table to give three classes of drugs that are commonly used in cardiovascular preoptimisation of patients undergoing surgery for phaeochromocytoma, the timing of initiation, and the rationale for their use. (6 marks)

Class of drug	Timing of initiation	Rationale for use
Non-selective α antagonist OR Selective α_1 antagonist.	1–2 weeks preoperatively but stopped 48 hours preoperatively to avoid intraoperative hypotension.	Vasodilation to reduce blood pressure and allow volume expansion. (Non-selective antagonist also blocks pre-synaptic α_2 receptors which results in loss of negative feedback on further catecholamine release and so can cause tachycardia via β_1 agonism as well as somnolence and headache from central α_2 agonism.)
β receptor antagonist, ideally selective β_1 receptor antagonists.	Commenced after α antagonist to avoid a hypertensive crisis caused by α-mediated vasoconstriction that may result from antagonism of β_2 mediated vasodilation. Selective antagonist therefore preferred.	Manage tachyarrhythmia.
Calcium channel antagonist.	After α blockade.	For hypertension control in patients inadequately controlled on α antagonist alone.

f) Name a drug that may be used to treat catecholamine-resistant hypotension during surgery to remove a phaeochromocytoma, and state its mechanism of action. (2 marks)

There is a risk of hypertension during surgery due to handling of the tumour, the surgical and anaesthetic triggers to catecholamine release, and the use of certain drugs. However, after tumour resection/clamping of its blood supply, there may be profound hypotension. This may be catecholamine-resistant due to receptor down regulation consequent to the previous time period of high circulating catecholamine levels.

- Vasopressin – systemic vasoconstriction via V1 receptor agonism and increased water reabsorption at the distal convoluted tubule and collecting duct via V2 receptor agonism.

REFERENCE

Connor D, Boumphrey S. Perioperative care of phaeochromocytoma. BJA Educ. 2016: 16: 153–158.

6.4 September 2014 Renal transplant

a) List three common causes of end-stage renal failure in the UK. (3 marks)
b) List four cardiovascular comorbidities that patients with end-stage renal failure are at risk of developing. (4 marks)
c) List two factors that may contribute to anaemia in patients with end-stage renal failure. (2 marks)
d) List three indications for dialysis prior to cadaveric renal transplant surgery. (3 marks)
e) List two aspects of management of the transplant organ aimed at reducing the risk of delayed graft function due to acute tubular necrosis. (2 marks)
f) List three intraoperative aspects of recipient patient management during cadaveric transplant aimed at optimising graft function. (3 marks)
g) Aside from regular paracetamol, list three options for part of a postoperative analgesic strategy following cadaveric renal transplantation. (3 marks)

The SAQ on this topic had a 59.1% pass rate. Remember that such a patient is affected by the original disease process that caused their renal failure, the multisystem effects of renal failure itself, the drugs used to manage renal failure, the access devices and multisystem consequences associated with their mode of dialysis, and the possibility of a previous, now failing, renal transplant with the associated antirejection medications.

a) **List three common causes of end-stage renal failure in the UK. (3 marks)**

- Diabetes.
- Hypertension.
- Glomerulonephritis.
- Chronic urinary tract infection.
- Outflow obstruction e.g. prostatic enlargement, kidney stones.
- Hereditary conditions e.g. polycystic kidney disease, Alport syndrome.
- Drug-related e.g. chronic NSAID use, chemotherapy.
- Cancers e.g. renal cancer, myeloma.
- Vascular disease.
- Autoimmune conditions e.g. scleroderma, SLE, IgA vasculitis.

b) **List four cardiovascular comorbidities that patients with end-stage renal failure are at risk of developing. (4 marks)**

- Hypertension.
- Accelerated ischaemic heart disease *(due to associated disease e.g. hypertension or diabetes, as well as factors related to CKD itself such as systemic inflammation, arterial calcification, endothelial dysfunction and dyslipidaemia).*
- Left ventricular hypertrophy with subsequent decompensation and failure *(increased afterload due to vascular calcification, increased preload due to increased circulating volume from fluid retention and presence of arteriovenous fistulae).*
- Uraemic cardiomyopathy *(myocardial fibrosis and collagen deposition).*
- Calcification and so reduced movement of cardiac valves.
- Arrhythmias related to electrolyte disturbances, left ventricular hypertrophy, cardiomyopathy.

c) List two factors that may contribute to anaemia in patients with end-stage renal failure. (2 marks)

- Anaemia due to lack of erythropoietin production.
- Blood loss from dialysis.
- Anaemia of chronic disease.
- Gastrointestinal losses due to gastritis and angiodysplasia associated with uraemia.

d) List three indications for dialysis prior to cadaveric renal transplant surgery. (3 marks)

- Hyperkalaemia.
- Fluid overload/pulmonary oedema.
- Uraemia.
- Acidosis.

e) List two aspects of management of the transplant organ aimed at reducing the risk of delayed graft function due to acute tubular necrosis. (2 marks)

- Minimisation of warm ischaemic time *(the duration that the organ remains at body temperature after its blood supply is stopped before it is actively cooled or reconnected to a blood supply)*.
- Minimisation of cold ischaemic time *(the time from cooling of an organ after its retrieval until rewarming after having its blood supply reconnected)*.

f) List three intraoperative aspects of recipient patient management during cadaveric transplant aimed at optimising graft function. (3 marks)

- Avoidance of hypotension; aim MAP > 90 mmHg or as guided by patient's usual blood pressure.
- Commencement of immunosuppressive induction intraoperatively.
- Avoidance of nephrotoxic drugs e.g. NSAIDs.
- Avoidance of hypovolaemia; consideration of cardiac output monitoring, aim CVP 12–14 cm H_2O if central access deemed necessary *(CVP monitoring used less commonly now)*.

g) Aside from regular paracetamol, list three options for part of a postoperative analgesic strategy following cadaveric renal transplantation. (3 marks)

- Transversus abdominis plane blocks.
- Local anaesthesia wound catheters.
- Opioid PCA using an opioid that does not accumulate in renal failure e.g. fentanyl or oxycodone.
- Epidural analgesia *(risk of hypotension and therefore impact on new graft function limits use of epidural in postoperative pain relief such that these are rarely now used)*.

REFERENCES

Aitken E et al. Renal transplantation: an update for anaesthetists. *Int J Anesthetic Anesthesiol.* 2016: 3: 052.

Jankowski J et al. Cardiovascular disease in chronic kidney disease: pathophysiological insights and therapeutic options. *Circulation.* 2021: 143: 1157–1172.

Mayhew D, Ridgway D, Hunter J. Update on the intraoperative management of adult cadaveric renal transplantation. *BJA Educ.* 2016: 16: 53–57.

Morkane C et al. Perioperative management of adult cadaveric and live donor renal transplantation in the UK: a survey of national practice. *Clin Kidney J.* 2019: 12: 880–887.

6.5 March 2015 Transurethral resection of prostate syndrome

A 75-year-old man is having a transurethral resection of the prostate (TURP) under spinal anaesthesia.
a) Which clinical features would make you suspect the patient has TURP syndrome? (6 marks)
b) List the intraoperative factors that may increase the risk of developing TURP syndrome. (7 marks)
c) How would you manage suspected TURP syndrome? (7 marks)

This is the SAQ that was asked in March 2015. The Chair's Report stated that the pass rate was 84.5%, "however weaker candidates did not mention CNS features and many had not read the question thoroughly and ignored the information that the patient had received neuraxial anaesthesia. Very few candidates mentioned repeated measurements of sodium and osmolality. This clinical problem is an old chestnut which all trainees should be able to manage safely and effectively." The topic appeared again in 2021 as a CRQ and covered a very similar range of aspects of the condition. You will find the answers there.

6.6 September 2015 Hodgkin's lymphoma

A 26-year-old patient with stage 4B Hodgkin's disease (spread to lymph nodes and other organs) requires an open splenectomy.

a) Give two possible airway concerns for this patient that may impact on your perioperative management. (2 marks)

b) Give two possible respiratory concerns for this patient that may impact on your perioperative management. (2 marks)

c) Give two possible cardiovascular concerns for this patient that may impact on your perioperative management. (2 marks)

d) Give three possible haematological concerns for this patient that may impact on your perioperative management. (3 marks)

e) Give two possible renal concerns for this patient that may impact on your perioperative management. (2 marks)

f) Give three options that may be used as part of the postoperative analgesia strategy for this patient and give a possible disadvantage of each. (6 marks)

g) List three vaccinations active against bacterial pathogens that the patient should receive. (3 marks)

The pass rate for the SAQ on this topic was just 38.8% with the Chairs' Report stating that "many examiners marking this question felt that either the candidates had not read the question as carefully as they should have done, or they lacked knowledge of the implications of Hodgkin's lymphoma and its treatment for anaesthesia. Rather than focusing on specific factors of importance, many candidates wrote about general problems when anaesthetising for a splenectomy. This was reflected in the pass rate."

In the SAQ that appeared in 2015, the first part of the question for ten marks was "list the specific factors that are of importance when planning your anaesthetic management." The style of CRQs is for questions to be broken down into many smaller subsections which is how I have changed it here. The knowledge you would need to pass remains the same.

Hodgkin's lymphoma:

- *Cancer of the lymphatic system therefore presenting with lymphadenopathy, splenomegaly, hepatomegaly.*
- *B symptoms: fever, night sweats, weight loss, itch, fatigue.*
- *Stages:*
  - *I: single lymph node involvement (or IE, single extralymphatic site).*
  - *II: two or more lymph nodes, same side of the diaphragm (or one lymph node plus contiguous extralymphatic site IIE).*
  - *III: lymph nodes on both sides of diaphragm, which may include the spleen (IIIS) and/or contiguous extralymphatic site (IIIE, IIIES).*
  - *IV: disseminated involvement of one or more extralymphatic organs e.g. liver.*
- *If B symptoms are absent, add A to the stage; if present, B. S denotes splenic involvement; X, bulky disease.*
- *Treatment is with chemo- and radiotherapy, targeted treatments, and antibody therapy.*

a) **Give two possible airway concerns for this patient that may impact on your perioperative management. (2 marks)**

- Mucositis from chemotherapy.
- Difficult airway due to oropharyngeal or cervical lymphadenopathy.
- Tracheal compression due to mediastinal lymph nodes (*may only become apparent upon anaesthetising the patient or on change of position*).

b) **Give two possible respiratory concerns for this patient that may impact on your perioperative management. (2 marks)**

This question, as with the original SAQ, does not give you the time scale of the patient's illness, and so they may have had a recurrence of disease after a period of remission, and so I would include concerns regarding the long-term effects of chemo- and radiotherapy in my answers.

- Risk of atelectasis and pneumonia due to bronchial or bronchiolar compression by lymph nodes.
- Risk of pulmonary toxicity if preceding bleomycin treatment – target oxygen saturations of 88–92%, minimising fraction of inspired oxygen where possible.
- Risk of radiation pneumonitis in the months following radiation treatment to the thorax or pulmonary fibrosis in the years following radiation treatment to the thorax.
- Pulmonary infiltration by Hodgkin's lymphoma.

c) **Give two possible cardiovascular concerns for this patient that may impact on your perioperative management. (2 marks)**

- Chemotherapy-induced heart damage, including cardiomyopathy, heart failure, myocarditis, pericarditis, arrhythmias.
- Radiation-induced heart damage, including cardiomyopathy, heart failure, valvular heart disease, arrhythmias, pericarditis and, in the longer term, accelerated ischaemic heart disease.
- Compression of major vessels or even heart due to mediastinal lymph nodes with risk of cardiovascular collapse under anaesthesia.
- Venous access may be difficult due to previous access for chemotherapy, and an access device may still be in situ.

d) **Give three possible haematological concerns for this patient that may impact on your perioperative management. (3 marks)**

This patient is having an open splenectomy which would imply that the spleen is significantly enlarged, and laparoscopic surgery is not feasible. An enlarged spleen due to lymphoma can result in hypersplenism which is overactivity of the spleen's usual function of removal of old blood cells and platelets. This patient may therefore be having the splenectomy to allow some correction of red and white blood counts to permit further chemotherapeutic treatment of their disease.

- Difficulties with cross match due to previous blood transfusions.
- Pancytopenia due to hypersplenism.
- Pancytopenia due to bone marrow disease.
- Pancytopenia due to chemotherapy, radiotherapy, antibody therapy or targeted drugs.
- Need for irradiated blood due to risk of transfusion-associated graft-versus-host disease.

e) **Give two possible renal concerns for this patient that may impact on your perioperative management. (2 marks)**

- Risk of lymphocytic infiltration or development of nephrotic syndrome resulting in acute or chronic kidney disease.
- Development of acute or chronic kidney disease due to chemotherapeutic treatment.

f) **Give three options that may be used as part of the postoperative analgesia strategy for this patient and give a possible disadvantage of each. (6 marks)**

- Oral analgesics: insufficient on their own. NSAIDs may be contraindicated in the presence of renal dysfunction; paracetamol dose may need adjusting in the presence of liver dysfunction; oral morphine may accumulate in the presence of renal dysfunction.
- Neuraxial analgesia: may be contraindicated due to thrombocytopaenia and even coagulation disturbance if there is liver involvement. Cardiovascular instability may occur as a high block would be required. High block may compromise respiratory function if the patient already has compromise due to mediastinal disease.
- Paravertebral block: avoids the cardiovascular instability that may result from an epidural but may still be contraindicated due to thrombocytopenia or disordered clotting.
- Patient-controlled analgesia (PCA): may need high doses to achieve adequate pain relief. Long-acting opioid such as morphine may accumulate in the presence of renal dysfunction, causing respiratory compromise and narcosis. Fentanyl or oxycodone PCA may be an alternative.
- Rectus sheath and transversus abdominis plane blocks: may be feasible at platelet levels where neuraxial analgesia would be contraindicated. These do not manage visceral pain but have a role in reducing analgesic requirements. Might not achieve cover of cephalad end of wound if midline laparotomy. Limited value if subcostal incision used.

g) **List three vaccinations active against bacterial pathogens that the patient should receive. (3 marks)**

The guidance regarding vaccinations for asplenic patients has changed since the time that this question appeared as an SAQ. Although it is encapsulated organisms to which such patients are vulnerable, vaccination against Haemophilus influenzae is no longer advocated by the "Green Book" due to the widespread uptake of the vaccine in the standard childhood schedule resulting in a very low prevalence of the disease. Asplenic patients should also be vaccinated against influenza and COVID as bacterial infections commonly follow viral ones. Ideally, the patient should have recovered some immune function after any treatments they have been having for their Hodgkin's, and two weeks should then be allowed to elapse before surgery to give time for an immune response to be mounted. However, it is uncertain how good a response a patient with active lymphoma will develop anyway.

- Pneumococcus.
- Meningitis B.
- Meningitis ACWY.

REFERENCES

Allan N, Siller C, Breen A. Anaesthetic implications of chemotherapy. *BJA Educ.* 2012: 12: 52–56.

Gent L, Blackie P. The spleen. *BJA Educ.* 2017: 17: 214–220.

Groenwold M, Olthof C, Bosch D. Anaesthesia after neoadjuvant chemotherapy, immunotherapy or radiotherapy. *BJA Educ.* 2022: 22: 12–19.

Ramsy M (ed.). *Immunisation against infection disease.* UK Health Security Agency and Department of Health and Social Care, 2021. Chapter 7.

6.7 March 2016 Laparoscopic Nissen's fundoplication

a) List and briefly state the reasons for the cardiovascular (7 marks) and respiratory (4 marks) effects of <u>laparoscopy</u> in the head-up position for a Nissen's fundoplication (anti-reflux procedure).

b) How may these effects be minimised? (9 marks)

Above is the SAQ that appeared in March 2016. It was virtually identical to that from September 2013 (and that was a repeat from 2006) except that here it asked specifically about cardiac and respiratory effects, not just adverse effects generally, and told the candidates what a Nissen's fundoplication was and reminded them that it took place in a head-up position, as this had caused some confusion in 2013. Despite the helpful pointers and the frequent appearance of this topic, the pass rate was only 54.5%. The Chairs said, "This question was judged to be of moderate difficulty. It would appear from their answers that many candidates had not seen a Nissen fundoplication and were unable to go back to first principles and talk about the effects of laparoscopy in the head-up position." As a moderately difficult question, a score of 12–13/20 would have been required to pass.

6.8 September 2016 Laparotomy for ovarian malignancy

A 52-year-old woman, who has completed three cycles of primary chemotherapy for ovarian malignancy, is to undergo an open laparotomy for surgical treatment of her disease. She has massive ascites. How do the <u>specific features</u> of this case affect your approach to the patient with regard to:

a) Preoperative assessment? (12 marks)
b) Intraoperative management? (8 marks)

This SAQ was very similar to one from March 2012 – the original version of that asked for pre-, intra- and postoperative considerations, but in 2016 the postoperative section was omitted – and as I have included a CRQ based on it previously, I have left it here in its SAQ format. As with cadaveric renal transplant and splenectomy for lymphoma, consider the issues relating to the disease process itself, the treatment of that disease and finally the operation the patient is to have. Despite the topic having been the focus of a question just four years previously, the pass rate was just 39.1% with the Chairs commenting that "candidates tended to talk about general principles of perioperative management rather than those issues that are specific to a patient having surgery as part of treatment for cancer such as possible bone marrow suppression or other organ damage due to chemo- or radiotherapy, cachexia, pleural or abdominal effusions and difficult venous access, to name but a few."

Here was my answer to the original March 2012 SAQ, which I have included here for more learning:

a) Preoperative assessment? (10 marks)

Airway:

- Massive ascites will increase risk of reflux and may require draining preoperatively.

Respiratory:

- Pleural effusion. Assess for likelihood: assess exercise tolerance, auscultate and percuss chest. However, the patient is likely to have recent imaging that will show effusions. Significant effusions can be drained preoperatively to improve lung function.
- Massively reduced functional residual capacity due to ascites. Affects V/Q matching and causes basal atelectasis. Consider need to drain preoperatively.

Cardiac:

- Assess for cardiotoxic effects of paclitaxel and cisplatin. Assess exercise tolerance, echo.
- Pericardial effusions. May be indicated by small complexes on ECG and detected on echo.
- Indwelling venous access may already be in situ for chemotherapy. Need to consider when deciding where to place lines for operation. Veins may be difficult to cannulate due to previous treatment and use.

Pharmacology:

- Paclitaxel and cisplatin cause bone marrow suppression (check full blood count), renal damage (check urea and electrolytes), liver dysfunction (check liver function tests and coagulation), and cardiotoxicity (request echo). Discuss with oncologist regarding any other effects of any chemotherapeutic agents that have been received.
- Diuretics may have been used to attempt to alleviate effusions and ascites: therefore, check for electrolyte imbalance that may need correcting.
- Antiemetics: may already be in use to manage nausea and vomiting associated with chemotherapy. Ensure uninterrupted treatment perioperatively.

- Opioids: may already have an opioid requirement which should be considered when planning postoperative analgesia.

Haematological:

- Risk of deep vein thrombosis (procoagulant factors released in cancer state, venous obstruction due to intra-abdominal mass and ascites). Some patients may have already been receiving prophylaxis. Perioperative prophylaxis plan needs addressing.
- Liver dysfunction may cause coagulopathy: check clotting, manage appropriately.
- Risk of significant bleeding with removal of many intra-abdominal and pelvic organs. Crossmatch is required preoperatively.

Immune, infection:

- Bone marrow suppression renders patient at greater risk of infection. Assess for possible infections preoperatively.

Renal:

- Risk of renal toxicity from chemotherapy. If there is renal impairment, consider impact on drugs to be used intraoperatively.

Liver:

- Risk of liver dysfunction from chemotherapy, from cholestasis secondary to massive ascites, and from malignant deposit. Check liver function tests. Consider impact on choice of drugs to be used.

Nutrition:

- Malnutrition and dehydration risk due to anorexia, chemotherapy, ascites. May need intravenous fluid preoperatively and dietician involvement from the outset.

b) Intraoperative management? (5 marks)

Airway:

- Intubate: major, prolonged, abdominal surgery, sometimes head-down position, risk of reflux from raised intra-abdominal pressure.

Respiratory:

- Reduced functional residual capacity due to ascites. Ensure thorough preoxygenation in head-up position.
- Capnography and arterial blood gas monitoring to target adequate ventilatory parameters, care with high airway pressures due to ascites (until abdomen opened).

Cardiac:

- Two large cannulae – risk of significant bleeding.
- Arterial line: beat-to-beat blood pressure monitoring and electrolyte monitoring useful in face of large fluid shifts.
- Cardiac output monitoring: massive fluid shifts due to further loss of ascites (this must be done slowly) and large amounts of tissue removal.

Neurological:

- Pain management: NSAIDs and paracetamol may be contraindicated if there is renal and liver dysfunction. May already be on opioids, so higher doses may be required. Avoid long-acting opioids in the presence of significant renal dysfunction. Consideration of epidural if clotting permits. Consideration of rectus sheath catheters for opioid-sparing effect.

Pharmacological:

- Increased volume of distribution for water-soluble drugs due to massive ascites e.g. thiopentone.

Haematological:

- Significant blood loss may occur due to ooze from many tissue surfaces. Monitor with near patient testing for haemoglobin and coagulation.
- Risk of DVT: automated intermittent leg compression devices intraoperatively.

Immune, infection:

- Bone marrow suppression renders patient at greater risk of infection. Scrupulous asepsis required.

Cutaneomusculoskeletal:

- Prolonged surgery, care with positioning and padding. Care if known bony metastases.

Renal:

- Catheterise to monitor urine output to assist with managing fluid balance in the presence of significant fluid shifts.
- Use of drugs whose metabolism is independent of renal function if patient has renal impairment e.g. remifentanil infusion, atracurium.
- Risk of liver dysfunction: consider drug suitability before giving.

Metabolic:

- Prolonged surgery: monitor temperature, use under body warming mattress, warmed fluids, insulating hat.
- Arterial blood gas analysis to monitor lactate and base excess in the presence of large fluid shifts.

c) Postoperative management? (5 marks)

Consideration of location of postoperative care: may need level 2 or 3 care if there has been significant blood loss or if there is significant preoperative or intraoperative organ dysfunction.

Respiratory:

- Postoperative oxygen especially if opioid PCA. May need additional respiratory support such as noninvasive ventilation.

Cardiac:

- Postoperative heart rate, blood pressure and cardiac output monitoring to guide ongoing fluids (reaccumulation of ascites may result in intravascular depletion).

Neurological:

- Pain management to be optimised by involving the acute pain management team. Oxycodone or fentanyl may be indicated if there is renal impairment.

Haematological:

- Risk of DVT: use of antiembolism stockings, low molecular weight heparin if no contraindications, early mobilisation.

Renal:

- Urine output monitoring to help guide ongoing fluid management.

Nutrition:

- Re-establish enteral nutrition as soon as possible or consideration of parenteral nutrition if this is likely to be delayed.

REFERENCE

Morosan M, Popham P. Anaesthesia for gynaecological oncological surgery. *Contin Educ Anaesth Crit Care Pain*. 2014: 14: 63–68.

6.9 March 2017 Renal transplant

A patient is to receive a cadaveric renal transplant.
a) Detail the aspects of your preoperative assessment specific to chronic kidney disease (CKD). (11 marks)
b) How can the function of the transplanted kidney be optimised intraoperatively? (3 marks)
c) How may this patient's postoperative pain be optimally managed? (3 marks)
d) Explain why some common postoperative analgesic drugs should be avoided or used with caution. (3 marks)

Bar just a few words, this SAQ was identical to the one from September 2014, similar to the CRQ from February 2023, and very similar to the SAQ about anaesthetising a patient with stage 4 CKD from March 2012 (see Perioperative Medicine chapter). Only 42.1% of candidates passed. Have I convinced you yet of the importance of looking at topics and questions that have previously featured in the exam? The Chairs said, "Renal transplantation is the most frequently undertaken form of transplant surgery, but it seemed that many candidates had not had any practical experience of it. This was particularly noticeable in the answers to part (b), improving the function of the transplanted kidney intraoperatively, and part (c), management of postoperative pain. However, even candidates who have never seen a renal transplant operation should know the principles of analgesic use in renal failure."

6.10 September 2017 Spleen and splenectomy

A 35-year-old woman presents for splenectomy for idiopathic/immune thrombocytopenic purpura, which is not controlled with medical management.

a) List three vaccinations active against bacterial pathogens that she should receive. (3 marks)
b) What is the optimal timing for these vaccinations? (1 mark)
c) List three perioperative haematological considerations for this patient. (3 marks)
d) List three immunological functions of the spleen in the adult. (3 marks)
e) Give two common reasons for splenomegaly in developed countries. (2 marks)
f) State two reasons for conservative management for traumatic splenic rupture. (2 marks)
g) State three factors that would be considered when deciding whether to conservatively manage a patient with splenic trauma. (3 marks)
h) List three obstetric diagnoses that may present in a clinically similar manner to splenic artery aneurysm rupture in late pregnancy. (3 marks)

When the SAQ on this topic appeared in 2017 it concerned just ITP, splenectomy for ITP, the immune function of the spleen, and splenic trauma. I have added the questions based on splenic artery rupture and splenomegaly to give some extra learning. Part (c) of the SAQ held most of the marks and wanted a generalised description of the preoperative considerations specifically related to the patient's condition. These are the types of questions that do not appear now in the CRQ format; instead, very specific points are questioned. The pass rate was just 34.4% (very similar to the pass rate of the last question about the spleen) and the Chairs' Report said, "The examiners considered this to be a difficult question, and this would seem to be confirmed by the pass rate. Most marks were available in section (c), which asked for preoperative considerations specifically related to the patient's condition. This would include such things as steroid dependence, anaemia or antibodies due to previous blood product transfusions. Many candidates answered in too generic a fashion, including only nonspecific considerations for anaesthesia for major surgery." The CRQ helps by focussing your answers, but only if you have enough knowledge.

a) List three vaccinations active against bacterial pathogens that she should receive. (3 marks)

This is the second time in just a few years that the College asked about vaccination for asplenic patients.

- Pneumococcus.
- Meningitis B.
- Meningitis ACWY.

b) What is the optimal timing for these vaccinations? (1 mark)

For patients that have had an emergency splenectomy, it is advised that two weeks should elapse after surgery before vaccinations are given.

- At least two weeks before surgery.
- Pneumococcus to be repeated every five years.

c) List three perioperative haematological considerations for this patient. (3 marks)

Splenectomy is undertaken to stop the splenic destruction of platelets. It is indicated if there is insufficient or non-sustained improvement with medical management. The patient may therefore have a very low platelet count preoperatively, and immunoglobulin infusions may be utilised to give a temporary boost. If the platelet count is critically low, there is a risk of spontaneous and catastrophic bleeding, and platelet transfusions may be required. Treatment of ITP traditionally involved immunosuppression mainly with oral corticosteroids, but a range of new drugs are now in use and in development with mechanisms of action that include stimulation of platelet production, reduction of

IgG (which is involved in the destruction of platelets) and interruption of the pathway of destruction of opsonised platelets.

- Platelet count may be very low, increasing risk of bleeding from surgical site and due to other minor traumas perioperatively such as cannulation and airway management. Platelet count may contraindicate neuraxial techniques.
- Cross match may be complicated by antibody development in response to previous blood product transfusions.
- Preoperative platelet count may be improved by steroid or immunoglobulin treatment.
- Perioperative platelet infusion may be necessary but ideally should be given after arterial supply to spleen has been surgically interrupted to avoid their sequestration and destruction.

d) List three immunological functions of the spleen in the adult. (3 marks)

- Synthesis of immune proteins (opsonins) that trigger phagocytosis of pathogens to which they are attached.
- Synthesis of chemicals such as cytokines that help regulate the immune response.
- Presentation of blood-borne antigens to lymphocytes.
- Macrophages remove antibody-coated blood cells and bacteria from the circulation.
- Storage of white blood cells that, upon stimulation, can be triggered to become a range of different types of specialised white blood cells involved in the immune response including T cells and antibody-producing B cells.

e) Give two common reasons for splenomegaly in developed countries. (2 marks)

- Infectious mononucleosis.
- Haematological malignancy.
- Portal hypertension due to liver disease.

f) State two reasons for conservative management for traumatic splenic rupture. (2 marks)

- Avoidance of major surgery with its attendant risks.
- Retention of splenic immunological function.

g) State three factors that would be considered when deciding whether to conservatively manage a patient with splenic trauma. (3 marks)

- Haemodynamic stability of patient.
- Grading of splenic injury on CT scanning, lower grades being more amenable to conservative management.
- Local availability of radiological interventions for angioembolisation if necessary.
- Need for laparotomy for any other associated injury.

h) List three obstetric diagnoses that may present in a clinically similar manner to splenic artery aneurysm rupture in late pregnancy. (3 marks)

Approximately 95% of splenic artery aneurysm ruptures occur in pregnancy, especially the third trimester. They more commonly affect multigravid women. As they may present nonspecifically with abdominal pain and shock, it is an important diagnosis to bear in mind as it is associated with a very high fetal and maternal death rate.

- Uterine rupture.
- Placental abruption.
- Amniotic fluid embolism.

REFERENCES

Bronte V, Pittet M. The spleen in local and systemic regulation of immunity. *Immunity*. 2013: 39: 806–818.

Davies J et al. British committee for standards in haematology guideline: update of guidelines for the prevention and treatment of infection in patients with an absent or dysfunctional spleen. *Clin Med*. 2002: 2: 440–443.

Gent L, Blackie P. The spleen. *BJA Educ*. 2017: 17: 214–220.

Hildebrand D et al. Modern management of splenic trauma. *BMJ*. 2014: 348: 27–31.

Provan D, Semple J. Recent advances in the mechanisms and treatment of immune thrombocytopenia. *EBioMedicine*. 2022: 76.

Ramsy M (ed.). *Immunisation against infection disease*. UK Health Security Agency and Department of Health and Social Care, 2021. Chapter 7.

The Royal College of Obstetricians and Gynaecologists. *Maternal collapse in pregnancy and the puerperium: green-top guideline no. 56*, December 2019.

6.11 March 2018 Phaeochromocytoma

This question was essentially a repeat from 2014 except for a small subsection at the end worth 2 marks, reproduced below. Sadly the pass rate did not improve, being just 39.3% on this occasion. The Chairs said, "This was a surprisingly poorly answered question, having the lowest pass rate of the exam. Some people did not read the question or, more likely, confused phaechromocytoma with carcinoid syndrome. It was clear to the examiners that most candidates had never seen the condition, but more worryingly would not be able to manage it in an acute situation."

a) How would you assess the adequacy of cardiovascular optimisation preoperatively? (2 marks)

- Normotension.
- Absence of postural hypotension.
- Normalisation of ST segments.
- Absence of tachyarrhythmias.

6.12 September 2018 Laparotomy for ovarian malignancy

The third time this topic has been tested in the time period covered by this book, with virtually identical wording each time – but still only a 34.1% pass rate. The Chairs said, "The pass rate for this question was surprisingly low, since it has also been asked recently. Answers were very generic and lacked specificity for this condition and patients and may be a reflection of lack of experience. The practical aspects of anaesthesia for this patient were also lacking."

6.13 September 2020 Liver resection for hepatocellular carcinoma

a) State the five biochemical and clinical components of the Child Pugh Score. (5 marks)
b) State two features of liver anatomy and physiology that make it amenable to resection. (2 marks)
c) State five preoperative clinical features that increase the risk of post-hepatectomy liver failure after liver resection for hepatocellular carcinoma. (5 marks)
d) State four techniques that may be employed to minimise intraoperative venous blood loss during open surgery for liver resection. (4 marks)
e) State four elements of the Enhanced Recovery After Surgery recommendations for postoperative pain management following open liver surgery. (4 marks)

By September 2020, CRQ was the standard format for all questions. The College does not publish their CRQs, and so this CRQ is a "best guess" of the sorts of issues that would be likely to form the focus of a question on open surgery for liver resection. The Chairs' Report said that the pass rate was 49.6% and that "this question was judged to be one of the more difficult questions on the paper. The initial sections on liver anatomy and physiology were answered well, but the majority of candidates lost marks on parts (d) and (e) which required a more detailed knowledge of hepatic anaesthesia."

a) **State the five biochemical and clinical components of the Child Pugh Score. (5 marks)**

- Encephalopathy.
- Ascites.
- Raised bilirubin.
- Reduced albumin.
- Raised prothrombin time.

b) **State two features of liver anatomy and physiology that make it amenable to resection. (2 marks)**

- Segmental anatomy of liver permitting resection of some segments and leaving others.
- Hepatic regenerative capacity by hyperplasia of remaining hepatocytes *(the liver may reach its original size by six months after resection but may have functionally recovered by two to three weeks).*

c) **State five preoperative clinical features that increase the risk of post-hepatectomy liver failure after liver resection for hepatocellular carcinoma. (5 marks)**

- Diabetes *(due to alterations in liver metabolism, reduced immune function, and hepatic steatosis contributing to postoperative liver dysfunction).*
- Obesity.
- Metabolic syndrome.
- Malnutrition.
- Cholangitis.
- Age over 65 years.
- Higher ASA grade.
- Liver dysfunction: cirrhosis with elevated Child-Pugh or Model of End-Stage Liver Disease scores *(patients with hepatocellular carcinoma commonly have underlying liver cirrhosis with chronic liver dysfunction)*, steatohepatitis or chemotherapy-induced liver injury.
- Low future liver remnant volume *(as low as 20% is all that is required in an otherwise healthy liver but at least 50% is required in a patient with cirrhosis. CT and MRI can be used to estimate future liver remnant volume)* or extended liver resection, greater than 50%.

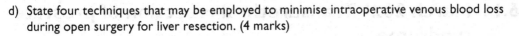

d) State four techniques that may be employed to minimise intraoperative venous blood loss during open surgery for liver resection. (4 marks)

Blood loss during resection while the afferent supply is occluded is mainly due to backflow from the valveless hepatic veins, and so efforts to maintain CVP < 5 cmH₂O help to reduce bleeding.

- Fluid restriction.
- Minimisation of PEEP.
- Reverse Trendelenburg positioning.
- Veno- and vasodilatory infusions such as GTN, remifentanil.
- Furosemide for its diuretic and venodilatory actions.

e) State four elements of the Enhanced Recovery After Surgery recommendations for postoperative pain management following open liver surgery. (4 marks)

- Thoracic epidural can provide excellent pain relief, but its use is limited by hypotension and impedance of early mobilisation.
- Multimodal analgesia is recommended.
- Inclusion of intrathecal opioids in multimodal analgesia is recommended.
- Continuous local anaesthetic wound infiltration catheters provide equivalent analgesia to thoracic epidural with lower complication rates.
- Local anaesthetic transversus abdominis plane blocks as part of multimodal analgesia improves pain control and reduces opioid use.

REFERENCES

Joliat G et al. Guidelines for perioperative care for liver surgery: Enhanced Recovery After Surgery (ERAS) Society recommendations 2022. *World J Surg.* 2023: 47: 11–34.

Patel J, Jones C, Amoako D. Perioperative management for hepatic resection surgery. *BJA Educ.* 2022: 22: 357–363.

Personal communication Dr Chris Jones, Consultant Anaesthetist, Royal Surrey County Hospital, Guildford, UK, 1st December 2022.

6.14 March 2021 Transurethral resection of prostate syndrome

a) State the level of spinal block required for surgery for transurethral resection of the prostate (TURP) and state why this level is required. (2 marks)
b) Explain why glycine is used as an irrigation fluid during TURP. (2 marks)
c) Give four intraoperative symptoms and signs of TURP syndrome. (4 marks)
d) Give five intraoperative risk factors for TURP syndrome apart from irrigation fluid choice. (5 marks)
e) State an equation for estimation of serum osmolality. (1 mark)
f) Give an advantage and a disadvantage of treatment of TURP syndrome with furosemide. (2 marks)
g) Give two complications of rapid correction of hyponatraemia. (2 marks)
h) Give two ECG features of hyponatraemia. (2 marks)

The pass rate for the CRQ on this subject was a fantastic 80%, and the Chairs' Report commented that it was a common topic in all parts of the exam and "reassuringly . . . answered well by most candidates." A CEACCP article from 2009 contains all the knowledge needed for this question. TURP syndrome is caused by excessive absorption of hypotonic irrigation fluid (glycine osmolarity 220 mmol/l, blood osmolality 275–295 mmol/kg) into the circulation. Volume changes cause cardiovascular complications. Hyponatraemia and hypo-osmolality cause neurological complications. Free water absorption into brain parenchyma causes raised intracranial pressure, water intoxication, and cerebral oedema resulting in burning sensations in the face and hands, headache, visual disturbance, confusion, restlessness, convulsions, and coma. Glycine (an inhibitory neurotransmitter) toxicity causes nausea, headache, transient blindness, and myocardial depression. It potentiates NMDA receptor activity causing encephalopathy and seizures. Magnesium stabilises NMDA receptors so is useful in managing seizures. Treatment would include supportive care, including use of furosemide, mannitol or hypertonic saline in selected cases with ongoing monitoring of electrolytes and serum osmolality, and seizure management.

a) **State the level of spinal block and required for surgery for transurethral resection of the prostate (TURP) and state why this level is required. (2 marks)**

- Height of spinal block required is T10.
- Pain innervation of bladder distension travels with sympathetic fibres that have their origin as high as T11.

b) **Explain why glycine is used as an irrigation fluid during TURP. (2 marks)**

Glycine was used commonly as an irrigation fluid when monopolar resection was standard management. Now, use of bipolar resectoscopes has obviated the need for a non-conductive fluid and so more isotonic fluids can be used. TURP syndrome is less common with the use of less hypotonic fluids. There is also a new range of methods of prostate ablation that do not involve diathermy.

- Non-conductive when using monopolar resectoscope.
- Good visibility, transparent.
- Non-haemolytic when absorbed.

c) **Give four intraoperative symptoms and signs of TURP syndrome. (4 marks)**

Take your pick – there is a wide range to choose from. I have grouped them according to body system to help you memorise them.

- Respiratory disturbance: tachypnoea, hypoxia, pulmonary oedema.
- Cardiovascular disturbance: initial hypertension due to fluid overload with reflex bradycardia, congestive heart failure, hypotension, cardiovascular collapse.

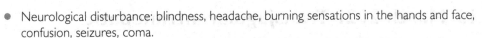

- Neurological disturbance: blindness, headache, burning sensations in the hands and face, confusion, seizures, coma.
- Gastrointestinal disturbance: nausea and vomiting.

d) Give five intraoperative risk factors for TURP syndrome apart from irrigation fluid choice. (5 marks)

- High intravesical pressure of irrigation fluid: failure to allow fluid to drain from bladder, excessive height (> 70 cm) above patient of irrigation fluid bag.
- Large quantities of irrigation fluid used.
- Low venous pressure (hypotensive or hypovolaemic patient).
- Prolonged surgery (more than an hour).
- Large blood loss (large numbers of open veins increases rate of absorption).
- Capsular or bladder perforation, allowing direct access of fluid into the peritoneum with rapid subsequent intravascular absorption.
- Large prostate.

e) State an equation for estimation of serum osmolality. (1 mark)

Osmolarity is the quantity of solute per litre of solvent and osmolality is per kilogram of solvent and therefore the equations for estimation relate to osmolarity, whereas osmolality is measured with an osmometer. However, the terms are often used interchangeably.

$$2\,(Na^+) + 2\,(K^+) + glucose + urea, \text{ in mmol/l}$$

$$OR \quad 2\,(Na^+) + glucose + urea, \text{ in mmol/l}$$

f) Give an advantage and a disadvantage of treatment of TURP syndrome with furosemide. (2 marks)

- Advantage: removal of free water in the event of pulmonary oedema.
- Disadvantage: worsening of the associated hyponatraemia.

g) Give two complications of rapid correction of hyponatraemia. (2 marks)

- Hypervolaemia.
- Cerebral oedema with risk of seizures.
- Central pontine myelinolysis.

h) Give two ECG features of hyponatraemia. (2 marks)

- Broadening QRS complexes.
- T wave inversion.

REFERENCE

O'Donnell A, Foo I. Anaesthesia for transurethral resection of the prostate. *Contin Educ Anaesth Crit Care Pain.* 2009; 9: 92–96.

6.15 March 2021 Transjugular intrahepatic portosystemic shunt

a) Give two respiratory and two cardiovascular consequences of chronic liver disease. (4 marks)
b) List four possible issues related to remote site working that should be considered when planning anaesthesia or sedation in the interventional radiology (IR) suite for a patient undergoing transjugular intrahepatic portosystemic shunt (TIPS). (4 marks)
c) Give four concerns regarding the use of sedation for a TIPS procedure. (4 marks)
d) Give two sedation scoring systems. (2 marks)
e) State two pharmacokinetic changes for midazolam in a patient with chronic liver failure. (2 marks)
f) Give two intraoperative and two postoperative complications of a TIPS procedure. (4 marks)

The pass rate for this question was an impressive 68.9%. The Chairs' Report said that "this question showed familiar failings in basic sciences. The effects of liver disease on cardiovascular/respiratory systems and pharmacokinetics were all poorly answered. Very few candidates demonstrated knowledge of sedation scores." There are some great BJA Education articles on chronic liver disease and one on TIPS that I have used for the basis of this question, and I have referenced them below. BJA Education articles should comprise a major part of your learning as the topics are planned by representatives of the College and are therefore highly relevant to the syllabus.

a) Give two respiratory and two cardiovascular consequences of chronic liver disease. (4 marks)

I have given a list below and in brackets I have offered a little bit of explanation about how some of these issues develop. You wouldn't need to include that level of detail in your exam answer, but I think that understanding something helps retention and is clinically more useful. Also, consider the other systemic effects of chronic liver disease:

- *Central nervous system: hepatic encephalopathy due to decreased metabolism of neurotoxins including ammonia and short-chain fatty acids.*
- *Endocrine: adrenal insufficiency and secondary hyperaldosteronism leading to water retention and hyponatraemia.*
- *Gastrointestinal: portal hypertension causing varices, ascites and splenomegaly.*
- *Haematological: coagulopathy due to reduced clotting factor synthesis (although procoagulant factor levels can also be affected), anaemia (multifactorial including gastrointestinal blood losses and hypersplenism), thrombocytopaenia (due to splenic sequestration and decreased production of hepatic thrombopoietin – however, function is usually preserved due to increased vWF production), hypofibrinogenaemia (initially an increase in fibrinogen may be seen as it is an acute phase protein).*
- *Renal: acute or chronic renal dysfunction as a result of progressively deteriorating renal perfusion resulting in pre-renal or intrinsic renal failure.*
- *Nutrition: malnutrition, sarcopenia, hypoglycaemia, hypoalbuminaemia, impaired wound healing.*

Respiratory:

- Mechanical lung compression from ascites and hepatomegaly resulting in hypoventilation, decreased FRC, atelectasis, and V/Q mismatch.
- Hepatic hydrothorax *(pleural effusion due to liver disease, not due to any coexisting cardiac or lung disease).*
- Hepatopulmonary syndrome *(dyspnoea and hypoxaemia due to intrapulmonary arteriovenous shunting).*

Cardiovascular:

- Hyperdynamic circulation with high cardiac output and low systemic vascular resistance *(initiated by portal hypertension and contributed to by collateral development, shear stress of vascular endothelial cells due to abnormal circulation resulting in release of vasodilatory mediators, and vasodilatory substances bypassing degradation in the liver).*
- Relative hypovolaemia secondary to systemic and splanchnic vasodilation.
- Cirrhotic cardiomyopathy *(diastolic dysfunction, prolonged Q-T interval, blunted contractile response to stress).*
- Portopulmonary hypertension *(intrapulmonary vasoconstriction and vascular remodelling in patients with portal hypertension in the absence of another cause).*

b) List four possible issues related to remote site working that should be considered when planning anaesthesia or sedation in the interventional radiology (IR) suite for a patient undergoing transjugular intrahepatic portosystemic shunt (TIPS). (4 marks)

I have taken these from the GPAS guidelines. They are applicable to all remote site work. You don't need to write so much detail in each of your answers, as the College repeatedly reminds us, only the first point will get a mark in each answer. However, I am mindful of the need for learning for the viva that comes after the written exam.

- Facilities: access to patient records, guidelines, clinical decision aids. Fully staffed recovery availability or other plan of post-procedure patient management should be made.
- Staffing: availability of skilled assistant with experience of working in IR, named consultant anaesthetist to supervise care, may be distant from main theatres and so availability of anaesthetic backup in case of complications.
- Equipment: need for usual equipment for safe provision of anaesthesia, including standard anaesthetic machine and monitoring for that Trust, piped oxygen and sufficient oxygen cylinder backup, tipping trolley (this function may not be feasible with the IR table), equipment to deal with possible massive haemorrhage, including rapid infuser and fluid warmers. Possibly prolonged procedure so patient warming necessary.
- Environment: consideration of how the procedure, IR equipment, and large numbers of staff will reduce access to the patient. Need to plan line insertion, length of airway circuit and fluid administration set to take this into consideration. May have low light levels in IR – ensure an alternative light source is available for drug checking and patient monitoring.
- Medications: ensure full access to the usual range of medications available in main theatres including emergency drugs, and drugs to deal with specific complications such as local anaesthetic toxicity and malignant hyperthermia.
- Processes: ensure patient labelling and pre-procedure checking is undertaken and that checking of the equipment and drugs stock is in line with that undertaken in main theatres.

c) Give four concerns regarding the use of sedation for a TIPS procedure. (4 marks)

- Risk of exacerbation or precipitation of hepatic encephalopathy may result in an uncooperative patient who may interfere with the safety of the ongoing procedure.
- Risk of reflux increased due to the presence of ascites and possibility of presence of blood in the stomach.
- Risk of impaired ventilatory capacity due to pre-existing lung complications of liver disease such as reduced FRC due to ascites or hepatopulmonary syndrome may result in significant desaturation with sedation in supine position for prolonged period.
- May be a very prolonged procedure resulting in discomfort due to prolonged period of lying supine on narrow, minimally padded table.
- Pain during balloon dilatation of the intrahepatic ducts may be severe and result in failure of the technique under sedation.

d) Give two sedation scoring systems. (2 marks)

- American Society of Anesthesiologists Continuum of Sedation.
- Modified Observer's Assessment of Alertness/Sedation Scale.
- Modified Ramsay Sedation Scale.

e) State two pharmacokinetic changes for midazolam in a patient with chronic liver failure. (2 marks)

- Greater proportion of unbound drug, and so greater effect, due to reduced synthesis of plasma proteins for binding of this usually highly protein bound drug.
- Reduced rate of hepatic metabolism and so prolongation of effect.

f) Give two intraoperative and two postoperative complications of a TIPS procedure. (4 marks)

Patients with cirrhosis develop raised portal pressure with effects that have been listed above. The consequences of raised portal pressure can be managed with treatments such as sodium restriction or diuretic use, banding of varices, draining of ascites and effusions, and treatment with lactulose and antibiotics for hepatic encephalopathy. Portal pressure can be lowered pharmacologically (beta blockade), by managing the liver disease (abstinence from alcohol, managing the viral hepatitis) or with TIPS. TIPS may be undertaken as an emergency where endoscopic control of variceal bleeding has failed, or in anticipation of future deterioration. A catheter is passed via the internal jugular vein to create a connection between a branch of the hepatic venous and portal venous circulation. It is balloon dilated and then stented to maintain patency. The complications are therefore based on the procedure itself and the effects of blood bypassing the liver and acutely increasing venous return.

Intraoperative:

- Complications of puncture of the internal jugular vein such as pneumothorax, haemothorax, brachial plexus injury, carotid puncture.
- Arrhythmia precipitation due to passage of the catheter in the right atrium.
- Massive haemorrhage due to portal venous rupture or inadvertent hepatic arterial puncture.

Postoperative:

- Precipitation of hepatic encephalopathy.
- Stent occlusion, thrombosis or dislodgement.
- Precipitation of heart failure.
- Sepsis.
- Contrast nephropathy and exacerbation of hepatorenal syndrome.

REFERENCES

Chana A, James M, Veale P. Anaesthesia for transjugular portosystemic shunt insertion. *BJA Educ.* 2016: 16: 405–409.

Gilbert-Kawai N, Hogan B, Milan Z. Perioperative management of patients with liver disease. *BJA Educ.* 2022: 22: 111–117.

Royal College of Anaesthetists. *Guidelines for the Provision of Anaesthesia Services (GPAS): chapter 7: guidelines for the provision of anaesthesia services in the non-theatre environment*, 2020.

Sheahan C, Mathews D. Monitoring and delivery of sedation. *BJA.* 2014: 113(suppl 2): ii37–ii47.

6.16 February 2023 Renal transplant

A patient with end-stage renal failure presents for a cadaveric kidney transplant.
a) State the most common cause of end-stage renal failure (ESRF) in the UK. (1 mark)
b) What is the most common comorbidity affecting patients with established ESRF in the UK? (1 mark)
c) List five issues relating to dialysis that should be ascertained prior to surgery for this patient. (5 marks)
d) State the perioperative threshold (g/l) for blood transfusion for this patient. (1 mark)
e) List three specific concerns for this patient regarding blood transfusion. (3 marks)
f) List two considerations regarding intraoperative fluid administration for this patient. (2 marks)
g) Give two considerations regarding arterial cannulation in this patient. (2 marks)
h) List three possible elements of a postoperative analgesic strategy following this patient's cadaveric renal transplant. (3 marks)
i) List two possible immediate side effects of rituximab infusion. (2 marks)

This is the third time that anaesthesia for renal transplantation has been examined in the Final FRCA written paper over the time period covered by this book. The Chairs found it "reassuringly well answered" with a pass rate of 67.9%. Alongside a focus on preoperative assessment and postoperative pain relief, which appeared in the September 2014 and March 2017 iterations, this CRQ has some more specific questioning regarding aspects of intraoperative care. Once again, the majority of detail is contained within a recent BJA Education article on the topic, which is referenced and well worth a read.

a) **State the most common cause of end-stage renal failure (ESRF) in the UK. (1 mark)**

- Diabetes mellitus.

b) **What is the most common comorbidity affecting patients with established ESRF in the UK? (1 mark)**

Patients are susceptible to accelerated development of ischaemic heart disease due to kidney failure and its impact on hypertension, diabetes and hypercholesterolaemia, as well as the inflammatory response that occurs due to dialysis, renal osteodystrophy and hyperhomocysteinaemia.

- Ischaemic heart disease.

c) **List five issues relating to dialysis that should be ascertained prior to surgery for this patient. (5 marks)**

- Method of dialysis and location of any lines or fistulae that warrant protection intraoperatively (positioning, location of intraoperative vascular access, site for blood pressure monitoring).
- Volume status (deplete and hypotensive following recent dialysis or overloaded and in need of dialysis before anaesthesia).
- Acid-base status.
- Electrolyte status.
- Necessary preoperative interval between dialysis sessions, ability to pass urine – will guide fluid administration perioperatively.
- Recent heparin use.

d) State the perioperative threshold (g/l) for blood transfusion for this patient. (I mark)

- < 70 g/l.

e) List three specific concerns for this patient regarding blood transfusion. (3 marks)

- Risk of alloimmunisation complicating future organ and blood compatibility.
- Risk of adverse outcome from e.g. cytomegalovirus due to immunosuppressed state (CMV-negative blood must be used if transfusion is necessary).
- Risk of hyperkalaemia.
- Risk of hyperviscosity affecting perfusion of newly grafted kidney.

f) List two considerations regarding intraoperative fluid administration for this patient. (2 marks)

- Need to maintain cardiac output to optimise renal perfusion (of both existing and transplanted kidney).
- Need to avoid hyperviscosity which may impair renal perfusion.
- Need to maintain adequate blood pressure for sake of new kidney and also for other organ perfusion, especially if patient is hypertensive or has any element of ischaemic heart or cerebrovascular disease.
- Need to avoid fluid overload in patient unable to regulate their own fluid status.
- Need to avoid excessive potassium administration.
- Balanced crystalloid is usually the optimum fluid for maintenance of acid-base and electrolyte status, with consideration for human albumin solution if indicated.

g) Give two considerations regarding arterial cannulation in this patient. (2 marks)

- Arterial cannulation may cause damage to artery that may otherwise be needed in future for fistula formation and must not be performed on the same limb as an existing fistula.
- Arterial cannulation gives ability to monitor mean arterial blood pressure on a beat-to-beat basis to help ensure it is continuously adequate for renal perfusion (> 90 mmHg or higher if patient is hypertensive).
- Arterial cannulation offers the ability to monitor cardiac output, which helps optimise fluid balance for renal perfusion.
- Arterial cannulation offers ability to closely monitor electrolytes and acid-base status, which may need manipulation.
- Arterial cannulation may be indicated in patients with cardiac comorbidities such as valvular or ischaemic heart disease.

h) List three possible elements of a postoperative analgesic strategy following this patient's cadaveric renal transplant. (3 marks)

- Regular paracetamol.
- Transversus abdominis plane blocks.
- Local anaesthesia wound catheters.
- Opioid PCA using an opioid that does not accumulate in renal failure e.g. fentanyl or oxycodone.
- Epidural analgesia *(risk of hypotension and therefore impact on new graft function limits use of epidural in postoperative pain relief such that these are rarely now used)*.

i) List two possible immediate side effects of rituximab infusion. (2 marks)

Rituximab is a monoclonal antibody active against CD20 protein on the surface of B-cells which results in cell death and so interferes with the immune response to implantation of a foreign tissue. It is one of the biological agents which may be given as part of the induction phase of immunosuppressant therapy of a patient receiving a renal transplant. Even if you have never read about this particular drug, you should know that biologics such as this are associated with immediate risk of allergic or anaphylactic responses and, in the longer term, are associated with a predisposition to severe and unusual infection.

- Anaphylaxis.
- Angioedema.
- Fever.
- Cytokine release syndrome *(a systemic inflammatory reaction characterised by bronchospasm, tachycardia and hypotension, which may last for several days).*
- Cardiac arrhythmias.

REFERENCE

Mayhew D, Ridgway D, Hunter J. Update on the intraoperative management of adult cadaveric renal transplantation. *BJA Educ.* 2016: 16: 53–57.

HEAD, NECK, MAXILLOFACIAL AND DENTAL SURGERY

7.1 September 2012 Maxillofacial trauma

A 23-year-old man is brought to the emergency department following an assault in a nightclub. He appears to have suffered significant mid-face fractures and is uncooperative with staff. You are asked to accompany him to the CT scanner.

a) Outline the immediate management plan for this patient. (5 marks)
b) List the options for securing the airway in this case and any advantage or disadvantage of the methods. (5 marks)
c) What problems should be anticipated before securing the airway? (10 marks)

This is the SAQ that appeared in September 2012. The Chair reported a pass rate of 51.3% and said that "Answers to this question were generally appropriate. It should be noted that 'securing the airway' using a laryngeal mask airway as a primary technique was not part of the model answer. Perhaps, a rapid sequence induction would be 'plan A' rather than an inhalational induction to achieve the definitive airway." A rapid sequence induction with cervical spine in-line manual immobilisation is likely to be top of the list for the airway plan, using video laryngoscopy and anticipating using a bougie or stylet to minimise the pressor response and possible neck movement that would be associated with obtaining the best possible view with direct laryngoscopy. Awake fibreoptic intubation is unlikely to be a good plan in an uncooperative patient with significant bleeding in the airway. A challenging airway should be anticipated, and so a second-generation supraglottic airway device may be required as a temporising measure to achieve oxygenation or to facilitate intubation in the event of intubation failure. It is unlikely to be safe to attempt to wake the patient up in the circumstances described, and so it would be important to be ready to secure the airway with surgical cricothyroidotomy having marked the cricothyroid membrane before starting the rapid sequence induction. With very severe facial trauma, it may be considered that intubation would not be possible, and consideration may have to be given to awake tracheostomy, but this is far from an ideal option in a confused and agitated patient who may have both a brain injury and a cervical spine injury. Even though the patient is at risk of exacerbating a brain or spinal injury due to their agitation, they currently appear to be maintaining an airway of sorts. An anaesthetist attending such a trauma call should resist the urge to anaesthetise the patient if they do not have a reasonable expectation that they will be able to achieve a secure airway; better to wait for support from anaesthetic, ENT or maxfax colleagues. Whatever the decision, the airway strategy should be discussed with the team, roles allocated, equipment checked, and a pre-RSI checklist used. The topic was revisited in a CRQ in September 2021, and you will see the answers there.

REFERENCE

McCullough A et al. Early management of the severely injured major trauma patient. *BJA*. 2014: 113: 234–241.

DOI: 10.1201/9781003388494-7

7.2 September 2014 Hemiglossectomy and free flap surgery

a) Give three benefits of a free flap reconstruction. (3 marks)
b) List the three main risk factors for oropharyngeal cancer. (3 marks)
c) List six likely comorbidities and preoperative issues that should be specifically sought and managed in a 54-year-old patient with base of tongue cancer presenting for a hemiglossectomy and radial forearm free flap reconstruction. (6 marks)
d) Give the equation that determines blood flow in blood vessels. (2 marks)
e) Four variables from the equation can be manipulated by anaesthetic technique in order to maximise blood flow – give a method of manipulation of each. (4 marks)
f) List two surgical causes of flap failure. (2 marks)

The pass rate for the SAQ on this topic was just 31.5%, and the Chair reported that "inexperience probably accounts for the poor pass rate for this question. Weak candidates suggested assessment of a potentially difficult airway as the important preoperative feature but ignored the comorbidities associated with causative factors such as smoking and alcohol consumption. The impacts of major physiological changes that are caused by such prolonged and invasive surgery were ignored. The role of the anaesthetist in influencing free-flap survival was particularly poorly answered." There is a lot of crossover with the content of the plastics syllabus in this question, and you'll find BJA Education articles that cover all of this required knowledge.

a) Give three benefits of a free flap reconstruction. (3 marks)

What are the benefits of a free flap reconstruction? Consider what the alternatives are, and it helps to organise your thoughts. An area of body that has had cancer removed could be covered by a graft (skin and subcutaneous tissues that are taken from elsewhere in the body and rely on development of vascular supply from the recipient site to survive) or a flap. The flap can be local (moving a chunk of tissue to cover a defect locally, taking its blood supply with it), pedicled (excising an area of tissue and moving it to some distant part of the body whilst retaining a pedicle through which the original blood supply still flows, for example a latissimus dorsi flap) and finally a free flap (where tissue is completely removed from the donor site and its blood vessels are anastomosed at the recipient site). You can visualise that a graft of skin and subcutaneous tissues alone will not give the functional or cosmetic result of a flap in this case, nor will it necessarily develop sufficient blood supply to survive, and there are no suitable nearby donor sites that could provide a local or pedicled flap.

- Better cosmetic outcome than a graft.
- Better functional outcome than a graft: e.g. bone can be used to reconstruct a functioning jaw into which dental implants can ultimately be inserted.
- Can be performed in an area where there is a lack of suitable local donor sites for local or pedicled flap.
- Better coverage than a graft for large and deep defects or of delicate underlying structures.
- Better healing and vascularisation than a graft.
- Possibility of retaining innervation as the whole neurovascular bundle can be anastomosed.

b) List the three main risk factors for oropharyngeal cancer. (3 marks)

- Tobacco smoking and chewing.
- High alcohol intake.
- Human papilloma virus infection.

c) List six likely comorbidities and preoperative issues that should be specifically sought and managed in a 54-year-old patient with base of tongue cancer presenting for a hemiglossectomy and radial forearm free flap reconstruction. (6 marks)

The question asks for comorbidities and preoperative issues that specifically relate to the patients who are likely to present for this sort of surgery – think about the patient, the condition that they have, and the operation that is going to be performed. I followed my usual alphabet approach. The stereotypical patient is a smoker, has high alcohol intake, is malnourished due to their high alcohol intake and presence of oral cancer, and may have had radiotherapy and chemotherapy already. Smoking and malnutrition are both risk factors for poor wound healing postoperatively and so flap failure. Finally, I have included diabetes and its control, not because this is a typical condition of the patients having this sort of surgery but because adequate control of diabetes, if present, is critical to postoperative wound healing in flap surgery.

- Difficult airway due to tumour and/or previous radiotherapy.
- Smoking-related lung disease.
- Ischaemic heart disease due to smoking.
- Pulmonary hypertension related to long-standing lung disease.
- Cardiomyopathy with heart failure and arrhythmias related to excessive alcohol intake.
- Chemotherapy-related heart disease.
- Risk of alcohol dependence which may result in withdrawal perioperatively.
- Ensure diabetes is adequately controlled, if present.
- Anaemia relating to alcoholism, poor nutritional status, chemotherapy.
- Malnutrition related to cancer cachexia, dysphagia, alcoholism, radiation mucositis, nausea and vomiting related to chemotherapy.

d) Give the equation that determines blood flow in blood vessels. (2 marks)

$$\text{Blood flow} = \frac{\Delta P\, \pi\, r^4}{8\eta l}$$

e) Four variables from the equation can be manipulated by anaesthetic technique in order to maximise blood flow – give a method of manipulation of each. (4 marks)

- Maintenance of arterial pressure:
  - Cardiac output directed fluid therapy to ensure appropriate filling.
  - Monitoring of anaesthesia depth to avoid excessive depth, which has a detrimental effect on blood pressure.
  - Consideration of withholding of on-the-day antihypertensive drugs such as ACE inhibitors and angiotensin-2 receptor blockers.
  - Use of vasopressors guided by cardiac output monitoring.
- Minimisation of venous pressure:
  - Ensuring adequately deep anaesthesia with no straining or lack of coordination with ventilator by using remifentanil infusion or muscle relaxant and monitoring depth of anaesthesia and/or train-of-four.
  - Use of cardiac output monitoring to avoid excessive fluid therapy, which will risk flap oedema and extramural pressure, which may impede venous outflow.
- Ensuring adequate blood vessel radius:
  - Using temperature monitoring to ensure that the surface to core body temperature difference (skin surface and core e.g. bladder, oesophageal) does not exceed 1.5°C to minimise risk of vasoconstriction, and use of forced air warmers, fluid warmers, and resistive heating mat.

— Ensuring that pain is adequately controlled to minimise risk of sympathetically mediated vasoconstriction.
— Use of cardiac output monitoring to avoid inappropriate vasopressor use.
— Monitoring of and responding to arterial blood gas to avoid alkalosis.
- Optimisation of blood viscosity:
  — Aim for haematocrit of 0.3–0.35 as this offers optimum balance between oxygen delivery and blood flow, using arterial blood gas monitoring, cardiac output monitoring to guide fluid management, and blood transfusion as required.
  — Maintenance of normothermia.

f) List two surgical causes of flap failure. (2 marks)

- Insufficient arterial supply:
  — Kinking at anastomosis site, anastomotic failure.
  — Thrombosis.
  — Vasospasm.
- Insufficient venous drainage:
  — Anastomotic kinking.
  — Compression due to haematoma.
  — Thrombosis.
  — Excessive flap handling causing oedema and impaired venous outflow.
- Reperfusion injury to flap tissue:
  — Excessive warm ischaemic time of flap tissue resulting in release of inflammatory mediators causing microvascular failure.
- Infection.

REFERENCES

Ahmed-Nusrath A. Anaesthesia for head and neck cancer surgery. *BJA Educ.* 2017: 17: 383–389.
Nimalan N, Branford O, Stocks G. Anaesthesia for free flap breast reconstruction. *BJA Educ.* 2016: 16: 162–166.

7.3 September 2015 Thyroidectomy

a) Which investigations are specifically indicated in the preoperative assessment of a patient presenting for thyroidectomy for treated thyrotoxicosis? (5 marks)
b) What particular issues must the anaesthetist consider during the induction, maintenance and extubation phases of anaesthesia for a euthyroid patient having a total thyroidectomy? (11 marks)
c) Describe the specific postoperative problems that may be associated with this operation. (4 marks)

The question above is the SAQ as it appeared in September 2015. As you can see, the SAQ format is very open-ended compared to CRQ and, in this case, essentially wanted a description of all key points relating to the management of a patient having a thyroidectomy from preoperative investigation through to the postoperative complications. The pass rate was only 31.9% with the Chairs reporting that "the first and last parts of this question on pre-operative tests and postoperative considerations were well answered. The majority of the marks were lost in the middle section on issues to be aware of during anaesthesia for elective thyroidectomy. Many . . . candidates concentrated on management of thyroid storm or difficult airway, both of which are relatively rare during such surgery. It is likely that some candidates failed to read the question correctly because it was clearly stated that the patient was euthyroid making thyroid storm very unlikely." The issues that would have been important to consider in the intraoperative phase would have included:

- *Shared airway surgery, patient's head distant to anaesthetist:*
  - *Padding of eyes (special care if exophthalmos associated with thyroid disease).*
  - *Secure taping of tube – not tying as may impair venous drainage.*
  - *Consideration of need for electromyography tube for recurrent laryngeal nerve protection – check electrodes and function before draping the patient.*
  - *Being alert to airway dislodgement/tube compression.*
  - *Head-up tilt to improve venous drainage but not so as to impair arterial supply.*
  - *Extensions on giving set.*
  - *Long circuit for anaesthetic machine.*
- *Drugs:*
  - *Maintenance via intravenous or inhalational route.*
  - *Remifentanil useful to minimise need for further muscle relaxant (especially if recurrent laryngeal nerve monitoring is used) and to achieve a degree of hypotension that will improve surgical field.*
  - *Vasopressor e.g. phenylephrine may be useful to achieve normotension towards the end of surgery to test haemostasis (may also check with a Valsalva manoeuvre).*
  - *High risk of nausea and vomiting, which may have deleterious effect on bleeding and haematoma formation postoperatively, give antiemetics – dexamethasone has added benefit of reducing airway oedema.*
  - *Plan for postoperative analgesia: important to ensure pain relief to limit sympathetic response which may increase the risk of postoperative bleeding. Intraoperative longer-acting opioid may be given intravenously followed by postoperative paracetamol, NSAIDs if not contraindicated, and oral morphine. Local anaesthetic with adrenaline infiltrated by the surgeon during surgery will contribute to postoperative pain management, and superficial cervical plexus blocks can be considered.*
- *DVT prophylaxis: intermittent pneumatic compression devices indicated due to surgery duration.*
- *Warming mattress/forced air warmer and warmed fluids indicated due to surgery duration.*
- *Recurrent laryngeal nerve monitoring intraoperatively – a neural integrity monitoring endotracheal tube with embedded electrodes may be used.*

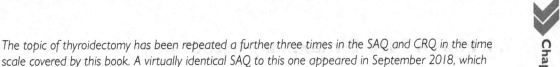

The topic of thyroidectomy has been repeated a further three times in the SAQ and CRQ in the time scale covered by this book. A virtually identical SAQ to this one appeared in September 2018, which I have converted into a CRQ with a few changes to make it more amenable to the CRQ format.

REFERENCE

Malhotra S, Sodhi V. Anaesthesia for thyroid and parathyroid surgery. *Contin Educ Anaesth Crit Care Pain*. 2007: 7: 55–58.

7.4 March 2018 Bimaxillary osteotomy

A 24-year-old woman is listed for a bimaxillary osteotomy.
a) Give three possible indications for bimaxillary osteotomy. (3 marks)
b) Give two approaches for management of the airway of this patient. (2 marks)
c) List three postoperative airway concerns for this patient. (3 marks)
d) List four ways in which intraoperative blood loss can be minimised. (4 marks)
e) List four possible clinical advantages in using remifentanil for this operation. (4 marks)
f) List four precautions that can reduce the risk of a retained throat pack post-surgery. (4 marks)

The pass rate for the SAQ on this topic was high, 71.1%. The Chairs reported that "despite the good pass rate the examiners felt that the candidates had little knowledge of the specifics of anaesthesia for this operation. Marks were scored in the section about the management of throat packs and in description of basic anaesthetic practice but there was a feeling that clinical experience was lacking, with some candidates not understanding the need for nasal intubation nor the reason for the operation."

a) Give three possible indications for bimaxillary osteotomy. (3 marks)

- Correction of dental malocclusion.
- Cosmesis.
- Correction of congenital head and neck conditions including secondary surgery after cleft palate repair.
- Severe obstructive sleep apnoea.

b) Give two approaches for management of the airway of this patient. (2 marks)

- Nasal intubation.
- Tracheostomy.
- Retromolar intubation.
- Submental intubation.

c) List three postoperative airway concerns for this patient. (3 marks)

- Risk of postoperative airway swelling or bleeding causing airway compromise.
- Intermaxillary fixation is sometimes applied at the end of surgery – a device to remove it must accompany the patient at all times in case of need for urgent removal.
- Risk of postoperative vomiting must be addressed as retching and vomiting will obstruct venous return, risking compromise of surgical haemostasis and may lead to airway bleeding.
- Risk of retention of throat pack.
- Risk of airway occlusion by blood clots that have not been adequately removed by suction at the end of surgery.

d) List four ways in which intraoperative blood loss can be minimised. (4 marks)

- Hypotensive anaesthesia (remifentanil as an adjunct to inhalational anaesthesia or as part of a total intravenous technique, deep volatile, clonidine, beta blockade, magnesium, dexmedetomidine, increased depth of propofol TCI if intravenous anaesthesia used).
- Head-up position to aid venous drainage.
- Use of adrenaline-containing local anaesthetic by surgeon.
- Avoidance of any restriction to venous drainage such as tube ties.
- Cessation of preoperative antiplatelet or anticoagulant drugs.
- Use of tranexamic acid.
- Mandibular and maxillary nerve blocks undertaken by the surgeon may help to minimise the peaks of blood pressure and hence blood loss associated with stimulating parts of the surgery.

e) List four possible clinical advantages in using remifentanil for this operation. (4 marks)

- Induced hypotension to reduce intraoperative bleeding risk.
- Readily titratable in response to the highly stimulating parts of surgery.
- Facilitates smooth wake-up and extubation, which is important to ensure integrity of the surgery.
- Reduced risk of postoperative nausea and vomiting if used as part of a total intravenous anaesthesia compared to inhalational use – vomiting may compromise surgical integrity and necessitate removal of maxillary fixation.

f) List four precautions that can reduce the risk of a retained throat pack post-surgery. (4 marks)

- Agreement at pre-list briefing as to who will insert and remove the pack.
- Throat packs should not be stored in the anaesthetic room.
- Throat packs should be allocated by the scrub-nurse and will be included in the swab count.
- The throat pack sticker should be applied directly to the tube.
- Removal of the pack must be confirmed in recovery handover.

REFERENCES

Beck J, Johnston K. Anaesthesia for cosmetic and functional maxillofacial surgery. *Contin Educ Anaesth Crit Care Pain*. 2014: 14: 38–42.

Jozefowicz E et al. The effect of tranexamic acid on blood loss in orthognathic surgery: a randomized, placebo-controlled, equivalence study. *Int J Oral Maxillofac Surg*. 2022: 51: 637–642.

National Patient Safety Agency. *Safer practice notice: reducing the risk of retained throat packs after surgery*, 2009.

Safe Anaesthesia Liaison Group, RCoA. *Patient safety*, update January to March 2016.

7.5 September 2018 Thyroidectomy

a) List four preoperative investigations that may be specifically indicated in the preoperative assessment of a patient with treated thyrotoxicosis presenting for thyroidectomy for a large goitre that extends retrosternally, giving the reason for each investigation listed. (4 marks)

b) Complete the following table, giving three possible airway issues that may be encountered during intubation for this patient (3 marks), and a possible strategy to manage each of these risks. (3 marks)

c) List three complications of surgery that may result in difficulties at extubation. (3 marks)

d) Give two symptoms and/or signs of hypocalcaemia as a consequence of parathyroid gland damage during thyroid surgery. (2 marks)

e) List three signs suggestive of airway compromise due to acute haematoma development following thyroidectomy. (3 marks)

f) Give two drugs that may be considered as part of the management of a patient with suspected haematoma following thyroidectomy. (2 marks)

The Chairs' Report for the SAQ on this topic (identical bar a few words compared to the September 2015 version) stated a pass rate of 46.6%. They said that "candidates answered this question in very general terms and answers lacked specific details. Answers demonstrated lack of experience in this field. There was also a degree of failing to read the question which asked why they would do tests, candidates just gave a list." The difficulty in being specific enough in answers has hopefully improved with changing to the CRQ format; however, the need to read the questions and to learn from past topics persists.

a) List four preoperative investigations that may be specifically indicated in the preoperative assessment of a patient with treated thyrotoxicosis presenting for thyroidectomy for a large goitre that extends retrosternally, giving the reason for each investigation listed. (4 marks)

- Thyroid function tests – to confirm the patient is euthyroid.
- Full blood count – carbimazole and propylthiouracil can cause agranulocytosis, and surgical blood loss may be significant.
- Serum calcium – assess baseline levels as may drop postoperatively.
- ECG – should show normal rate if euthyroid, may be bradycardic if ongoing beta blockade.
- Fibreoptic nasendoscopy – to assess likely ease of visualisation of larynx at laryngoscopy and to assess for pre-existing vocal cord palsies associated.
- CT scan – to assess for tracheal compression or deviation.

b) Complete the following table, giving three possible airway issues that may be encountered during intubation for this patient (3 marks), and a possible strategy to manage each of these risks. (3 marks)

Airway issue	Management strategy
Possible deterioration in tracheal compression on lying down in the presence of a large goitre.	Check what happens to patient's airway on lying down before induction, and consider head-up tilt for induction or awake intubation technique.
Possible tracheal narrowing due to compression.	Smaller size endotracheal tube may be required.
In a "can't intubate, can't oxygenate" situation, the obstruction to the airway may be distal to the level of the cricothyroid membrane.	Rigid bronchoscopy by surgeon may be a more appropriate rescue technique than front-of-neck access.
Desaturation during management of difficult airway.	Consider use of HFNO.
Tracheal deviation.	Consideration of awake fibreoptic intubation.

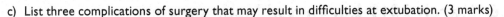

c) List three complications of surgery that may result in difficulties at extubation. (3 marks)

- Tracheomalacia consequent to a large and long-standing retrosternal goitre.
- Recurrent laryngeal nerve damage resulting in stridor.
- Laryngeal oedema resulting in stridor.
- Failure of haemostasis causing bleeding and compression of airway.

d) Give two symptoms and/or signs of hypocalcaemia as a consequence of parathyroid gland damage during thyroid surgery. (2 marks)

- Perioral tingling.
- Tingling of fingers.
- Tetany.
- Twitching.

e) List three signs suggestive of airway compromise due to acute haematoma development following thyroidectomy. (3 marks)

The final two subsections are based on the DAS management of haematoma after thyroid surgery guidelines that were issued in 2021. I have put in bold the letter that contributes to the overall acronym DESATS.

- **D**ifficulty swallowing/discomfort.
- N**E**WS score suggestive of bleeding.
- **S**welling of neck.
- Patient appears **a**nxious.
- **T**achypnoea/difficulty breathing.
- **S**tridor
- Desaturation.

f) Give two drugs that may be considered as part of the management of a patient with suspected haematoma following thyroidectomy. (2 marks)

- Tranexamic acid.
- Dexamethasone.

REFERENCES

Ahmed-Nusrath A. Anaesthesia for head and neck cancer surgery. *BJA Educ.* 2017: 17: 383–389.

Iliff H et al. Management of haematoma after thyroid surgery: systematic review and multidisciplinary consensus guidelines from the Difficult Airway Society, the British Association of Endocrine and Thyroid Surgeons and the British Association of Otorhinolaryngology, Head and Neck Surgery. *Anaesthesia.* 2021: 77: 82–95.

Malhotra S, Sodhi V. Anaesthesia for thyroid and parathyroid surgery. *Contin Educ Anaesth Crit Care Pain.* 2007: 7: 55–58.

7.6 March 2019 Laryngeal laser surgery

A 77-year-old man is scheduled for laser surgery to a laryngeal tumour.
a) State what is meant by the acronym LASER. (1 mark)
b) List three types of lasing media that are used in medical treatments and give an example of each. (3 marks)
c) List five measures that should be taken to protect staff when lasers are in use. (5 marks)
d) List four ways in which the risk of an airway fire can be minimised when using laser in the airway. (4 marks)
e) An airway fire develops during laser laryngeal surgery. A member of the theatre team has activated the fire alarm, dialled the emergency hospital number to report the location and nature of the fire and has left to bring a carbon dioxide fire extinguisher into theatre. List four steps that should be undertaken to extinguish the airway fire. (4 marks)
f) List three options for patient oxygenation during tubeless laryngeal surgery. (3 marks)

The Chairs reported a good pass rate of 67% when this question appeared as an SAQ but commented that "it would appear from some answers . . . that many candidates had minimal experience of laryngeal surgery and were unclear as to methods used to ventilate/oxygenate patients during this type of surgery." There is a great BJA Education article referenced below which describes the techniques in detail. I have added a subsection to my CRQ about the management of airway fire – it is one of the emergencies covered in the Association of Anaesthetists' Quick Reference Handbook and so there are "definitive" answers that can easily be made the basis of a question.

a) **State what is meant by the acronym LASER. (1 mark)**

- Light amplification by the stimulated emission of radiation.

b) **List three types of lasing media that are used in medical treatments and give an example of each. (3 marks)**

- Solid e.g. ruby, neodynium yttrium aluminium garnet (Nd-YAG).
- Semiconductor e.g. gallium arsenide.
- Liquid e.g. rhodamine 6G in methanol.
- Gas e.g. carbon dioxide, argon.

c) **List five measures that should be taken to protect staff when lasers are in use. (5 marks)**

- Use restricted to a list of authorised users.
- All staff must have been educated in laser hazards – authorised users, those assisting the user, and those who will be present in the controlled area.
- Carbon dioxide fire extinguisher availability wherever laser is used.
- Eye protection for all staff in the laser-controlled area suitable for the specific laser.
- Doors locked and windows covered with signage to indicate laser being used in the theatre.
- Use of equipment with matt surfaces that will dissipate the laser beam rather than reflect it as a narrow beam.
- Laser protection supervisor for every clinical area where laser is used to ensure safe use.

d) **List four ways in which the risk of an airway fire can be minimised when using laser in the airway. (4 marks)**

- Use of air rather than nitrous oxide.
- Use of lowest possible fraction of inspired oxygen – ideally below 25%.
- Stopping oxygen supply before laser is activated when using tubeless technique.

- Non-flammable, non-reflective endotracheal tube if used.
- Use of saline instead of air in endotracheal tube cuffs (*has a higher specific heat capacity and reduces risk of ignition of the cuff*).
- Use of water-based gel to cover facial hair.
- Gauze and pledgets that are used in the airway to be soaked in saline.
- Ensuring that any alcoholic skin prep used e.g. on the patient's face, has fully dried before application of any drapes and that drapes are applied in such a way that they cannot trap oxygen-rich anaesthetic gases.
- Removal of any non-essential equipment or gauze from the airway when laser is in use.
- Use of non-reflective surgical instruments.

e) **An airway fire develops during laser laryngeal surgery. A member of the theatre team has activated the fire alarm, dialled the emergency hospital number to report the location and nature of the fire and has left to bring a carbon dioxide fire extinguisher into theatre. List four steps that should be undertaken to extinguish the airway fire. (4 marks)**

- Stop laser.
- Discontinue ventilation AND fresh gas flow.
- Remove tracheal tube if on fire.
- Remove flammable material from airway.
- Flood airway with 0.9% saline.

f) **List three options for patient oxygenation during tubeless laryngeal surgery. (3 marks)**

- High pressure source ventilation either with an automated high frequency jet ventilation device (*e.g. Monsoon with which a pressure limit and frequency rate can be set, has the facility for end-tidal carbon dioxide measurement, and which has a function to reduce the fraction of inspired oxygen to .21 when laser is to be used*) or with a manual low frequency device (*e.g. Sanders jet ventilator or Manujet*) via a transtracheal, transglottic or supraglottic attachment or catheter. (*Ventilation via supraglottic catheter will make vocal cords move, and etCO$_2$ cannot be measured but gives the surgeon an unobstructed view. Use of a transglottic catheter or transtracheal cannula enables etCO$_2$ monitoring and the cords move less, but there is a risk of barotrauma. A transglottic catheter will slightly obscure the view.*)
- High-flow nasal oxygenation. (*Provides oxygenation, humidification and PEEP. Need to maintain upper airway patency to facilitate oxygen movement from nasal passages to glottis. Prolonged use may result in absorption atelectasis, and there is no mechanism for CO$_2$ removal or monitoring.*)
- Spontaneous ventilation with oxygen delivered via low-flow nasal cannulae or a narrow transglottic catheter. (*Useful if surgeon wants to visually assess airway function.*)
- Apnoeic oxygenation with low-flow nasal cannulae. (*Would rarely be used now as HFNO offers significant advantages.*)

REFERENCES

Association of Anaesthetists of Great Britain and Ireland. *Quick reference handbook 3–7 patient fire v1*, 2018.

Kitching A, Edge C. Lasers and surgery. *BJA CEPD Rev.* 2003: 8: 143–146.

Medicines and Healthcare Products Regulatory Agency. *Lasers, intense light source systems and LEDs – guidance for safe use in medical, surgical, dental and aesthetic practices*, 2015.

Pearson K, McGuire B. Anaesthesia for laryngo-tracheal surgery, including tubeless field techniques. *BJA Educ.* 2017: 17: 242–248.

7.7 March 2020 Thyroidectomy

Blood test	Result	Normal range
Thyroid-stimulating hormone (TSH)	0.14 mU/L	0.4–4.0 mU/L
Free T4	35.6 pmol/L	9.0–25.0 pmol/L
Free T3	14.1 pmol/L	3.5–7.8 pmol/L

a) Give three possible underlying diagnoses consistent with the blood tests in the table. (3 marks)
b) List three signs of hyperthyroidism. (3 marks)
c) List three oral medications used in the management of hyperthyroidism (3 marks) along with their mechanisms of action. (3 marks)
d) A euthyroid patient who had a large goitre extending retrosternally is in PACU following a thyroidectomy. Give three possible reasons for postoperative hoarseness. (3 marks)
e) The patient then develops neck swelling, respiratory distress and stridor with oxygen saturations dropping to 85% which is unresponsive to sitting up and administration of high flow oxygen. After calling for the adult cardiac arrest team and help from a senior surgeon, detail the five next steps that you would take. (5 marks)

The pass rate for the CRQ on this topic was 90.6%, and the Chairs said that it had "the highest overall pass rate for this paper." The CRQ that appears here is not that set by the College but is based on similar themes. I have also avoided repeating the content from the previous questions about thyroidectomy. Despite the great pass rate, the Chairs highlighted this particular question as one where the candidates failed to read the question, listing symptoms instead of signs of hyperthyroidism and, when asked about what investigations would be needed preoperatively, some candidates wrote that they wanted a CT scan despite this being shown in the introduction to the question.

a) **Give three possible underlying diagnoses consistent with the blood tests in the table. (3 marks)**

Note that the free T4 and T3 are high, with a low TSH level. The issue is therefore not a problem with the pituitary, as it has appropriately downregulated its TSH production in response to the high T4 and T3. I have given a very full list, but this is an anaesthetic exam, so stick to the common ones towards the top of the list.

- Graves' disease (the commonest cause, an autoimmune disease, will have raised thyroid-stimulating hormone receptor antibodies).
- Toxic multinodular goitre.
- Solitary hypersecreting adenoma.
- Early stages of thyroiditis (e.g. postpartum or subacute) causing temporary hyperthyroidism followed by return to eu- or hypothyroidism.
- Ectopic thyroid hormone production by a cancer.
- Trophoblastic tumour.
- Amiodarone use.
- Excessive iodine intake.

b) **List three signs of hyperthyroidism. (3 marks)**

- Tachypnoea.
- Tachycardia or tachyarrhythmia.
- Systolic hypertension.
- Tremor.
- Pelvic girdle and shoulder myopathy.

- Weight loss.
- Exophthalmos with conjunctival injection and chemosis.

c) **List three oral medications used in the management of hyperthyroidism (3 marks) along with their mechanisms of action. (3 marks)**

Drug	Mechanism of action
Beta antagonist	Antagonism of the potentiation of adrenergic signalling by T4 and T3, therefore reducing the symptoms and signs of thyrotoxicosis.
Carbimazole	Inhibition of thyroid peroxidase in the thyroid gland to inhibit T4 and T3 production.
Propylthiouracil	Inhibition of thyroid peroxidase in the thyroid gland to inhibit T4 and T3 production. Inhibits peripheral deiodinase to decrease peripheral conversion of T4 to T3.
Radioactive iodine	Uptake by the cells of the thyroid gland leading to their destruction.

d) **A euthyroid patient who had a large goitre extending retrosternally is in PACU following a thyroidectomy. Give three possible reasons for postoperative hoarseness. (3 marks)**

- Laryngeal oedema or other laryngeal injury due to airway manipulation.
- Unilateral recurrent laryngeal nerve injury.
- Tracheomalacia.

e) **The patient then develops neck swelling, respiratory distress and stridor with oxygen saturations dropping to 85% which is unresponsive to sitting up and administration of high flow oxygen. After calling for the adult cardiac arrest team and help from a senior surgeon, detail the five next steps that you would take. (5 marks)**

This final section is based on the new guidelines developed by DAS in association with groups representing endocrine, ENT, and head and neck surgeons. Like other guidelines by well-recognised national organisations, it can be used as a definitive marking scheme. I have put in bold the letters that constitute the acronym SCOOP.

- **S**kin exposure.
- **C**ut subcuticular sutures.
- **O**pen skin wound.
- **O**pen strap muscles to expose the trachea.
- **P**ack – use a pack to cover the wound.

REFERENCES

De Leo S, Lee S, Braverman L. Hyperthyroidism. *Lancet.* 2016: 388(10047): 906–918.

Iliff H et al. Management of haematoma after thyroid surgery: systematic review and multidisciplinary consensus guidelines from the Difficult Airway Society, the British Association of Endocrine and Thyroid Surgeons and the British Association of Otorhinolaryngology, Head and Neck Surgery. *Anaesthesia.* 2021: 77: 82–95.

Malhotra S, Sodhi V. Anaesthesia for thyroid and parathyroid surgery. *Contin Educ Anaesth Crit Care Pain.* 2007: 7: 55–58.

National Institute for Health and Care Excellence. *Thyroid disease: assessment and management: NG145*, November 2019.

7.8 September 2020 Middle ear surgery

a) Explain the indication for facial nerve monitoring in middle ear surgery. (1 mark)
b) Explain two methods of facial nerve monitoring during middle ear surgery. (2 marks)
c) Give three anaesthetic approaches to facilitate the use of intraoperative facial nerve monitoring during middle ear surgery and a disadvantage of each. (3 marks)
d) Give three possible benefits of the use of remifentanil during middle ear surgery. (3 marks)
e) Apart from pharmacological manipulation of blood pressure, give three techniques, with their underlying physiological principles, that may improve the surgical field during mastoidectomy. (6 marks)
f) Give three reasons why patients having middle ear surgery are prone to postoperative nausea and vomiting (PONV). (3 marks)
g) Give two reasons why the use of nitrous oxide as part of the anaesthetic technique should be avoided in middle ear surgery. (2 marks)

The CRQ on this topic appeared to be heavily based on a BJA Education article from 2019, referenced below. The Chairs reported a pass rate of 65% and said, "This is an area of the syllabus that candidates would be expected to know. The question was deemed by the examiners to be one of the easier questions on the paper and this was reflected in the good pass rate for this question."

a) **Explain the indication for facial nerve monitoring in middle ear surgery. (1 mark)**

- The facial nerve runs through the tympanic cavity where it is at risk of injury during middle ear surgery. *(It is enclosed within the bony facial canal, but this is sometimes lacking in areas, increasing the risk of injury.)*

b) **Explain two methods of facial nerve monitoring during middle ear surgery. (2 marks)**

- EMG monitoring of facial nerve – two electrodes are placed in a muscle of facial expression (often orbicularis oris or orbicularis oculi), and a potential difference confirmed which indicates facial nerve activity. High potential differences later in surgery indicate stimulation of the facial nerve which may indicate that it is at risk of damage. An audible alarm can be set to trigger above a certain potential difference.
- Use of a monopolar stimulator probe to confirm the location (and also function) of the facial nerve during surgery.
- Drill burrs may have the nerve stimulator function built in so that there is an audible alarm if they come too close to the facial nerve.

c) **Give three anaesthetic approaches to facilitate the use of intraoperative facial nerve monitoring during middle ear surgery and a disadvantage of each. (3 marks)**

- Use of a single dose of intermediate or short-acting muscle relaxant at start of surgery to facilitate intubation and then no further doses given – effects may not have fully worn off by the time the surgeon has started operating in the at-risk area.
- Intubation under deep anaesthesia with no muscle relaxants given – may result in suboptimal intubating conditions or cardiovascular compromise in attaining the depth of anaesthesia necessary for intubation.
- Use of a supraglottic airway device thus obviating the need for muscle relaxation – not all patients are suitable for supraglottic airway use e.g. in cases of morbid obesity or reflux disease, and it may be more difficult to control ventilation adequately for the duration of the surgery.

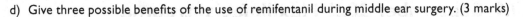

d) **Give three possible benefits of the use of remifentanil during middle ear surgery. (3 marks)**

- May be used to provide a degree of hypotension to improve the surgical field (if this is appropriate for the patient).
- May be used to reduce response to surgical stimulation in a patient who is not having ongoing neuromuscular blocking agent administration.
- Can facilitate a smooth extubation – important for maintaining integrity of surgical outcome as coughing and retching will increase middle ear pressure.
- Can be used in combination with propofol for a total intravenous technique that may reduce postoperative nausea and vomiting in what is typically very emetogenic surgery.

e) **Apart from pharmacological manipulation of blood pressure, give three techniques, with their underlying physiological principles, that may improve the surgical field during mastoidectomy. (6 marks)**

- 10-degree reverse Trendelenburg to improve venous drainage.
- Using minimum PEEP in ventilated patients to reduce intrathoracic pressure and so improve venous drainage.
- Avoid tracheal tube ties or extreme lateral rotation of the head to avoid impeding venous drainage.
- Optimising ventilation to avoid hypercapnia, which causes acidosis and therefore vasodilation, and also sympathetic activation and therefore increase in blood pressure.

f) **Give three reasons why patients having middle ear surgery are prone to postoperative nausea and vomiting (PONV). (3 marks)**

- Prolonged surgery.
- Direct stimulation of the vestibular system by drilling adjacent to inner ear.
- Suction-irrigation acting as a caloric vestibular stimulant.
- Age demographic of patient – children and younger adults at greater risk of PONV than older adults.

g) **Give two reasons why the use of nitrous oxide as part of the anaesthetic technique should be avoided in middle ear surgery. (2 marks)**

- Nitrous oxide will diffuse back out of the middle ear after surgery faster than nitrogen can diffuse in, resulting in a subatmospheric middle ear pressure, which may compromise the outcome of delicate surgery.
- Nitrous oxide use will increase risk of postoperative nausea and vomiting.

REFERENCE

Pairaudeau C, Mendonca C. Anaesthesia for major middle ear surgery. *BJA Educ.* 2019: 19: 136–143.

7.9 September 2021 Maxillofacial trauma

A patient is brought in by ambulance to the emergency department with maxillofacial trauma following a fall of 3 metres.

a) Give four possible indications for intubation in this case. (4 marks)
b) List four issues that may make intubation challenging for this patient. (4 marks)
c) Define what is meant by a Le Fort III fracture. (1 mark)
d) Apart from the difficulties in intubation associated with the fracture itself, list three perioperative airway concerns for a patient having surgery for an isolated Le Fort III fracture. (3 marks)
e) List two factors that may make a planned extubation "at risk." (2 marks)
f) List three strategies that could be considered in the management of an "at risk" extubation. (3 marks)
g) List the three pieces of equipment required for emergency front-of-neck access in the event of a "can't intubate, can't oxygenate" situation. (3 marks)

Many of the issues raised in the September 2012 SAQ about maxillofacial trauma were addressed more specifically in this question. The September 2021 CRQ paper was discounted, and the candidates scored on the MCQ component only as there were problems with text entry with the online exam format. As a consequence, no Chairs' Report was issued. The subsections in this question are assessing whether you would make sensible decisions if faced with such an emergency in ED and whether you are familiar with DAS guidelines. From the College's point of view, such guidelines make a fantastic basis for a question as the answers are definitive.

a) **Give four possible indications for intubation in this case. (4 marks)**

- Actual or impending airway compromise due to the maxillofacial injuries.
- Actual or impending airway compromise due to altered or reducing level of consciousness.
- Suspected brain injury – to control physiological parameters to reduce risk of secondary brain injury.
- To facilitate management or surgery for other urgent, painful, and significant injuries such as thoracic or abdominal trauma.
- Respiratory failure due to associated thoracic trauma.
- To facilitate management, transfer, or imaging of agitated or confused patient who may cause themselves further injury due to inability to cooperate.
- Associated traumatic cardiac arrest.

b) **List four issues that may make intubation challenging for this patient. (4 marks)**

- Foreign bodies in airway e.g. teeth, vomit, blood.
- Soft tissue and laryngotracheal oedema due to trauma may render the airway narrower.
- Posterior displacement of fractured facial bones may make face mask preoxygenation painful, a face mask seal difficult to achieve, and laryngoscopy challenging.
- Confusion or agitation may make it difficult to effectively preoxygenate and position the patient for intubation.
- The need for manual in-line stabilisation of the neck will limit ability to obtain a good laryngoscopy view.
- Ability to communicate with the patient prior to induction may be limited – they may have other comorbidities that might lead to an increased risk of difficulty at intubation.

c) Define what is meant by a Le Fort III fracture. (1 mark)

- Craniofacial dissociation caused by fracture extending from frontonasal and frontomaxillary sutures along medial orbital wall, orbital floor then lateral orbital wall to zygomatic arch bilaterally.

d) Apart from the difficulties in intubation associated with the fracture itself, list three perioperative airway concerns for a patient having surgery for an isolated Le Fort III fracture. (3 marks)

- Route of intubation; consideration of nasal or submental intubation or tracheostomy as surgery will involve ensuring dental occlusion and postoperative intermaxillary fixation.
- Risk of damage or obstruction of airway device due to surgery itself.
- Consideration of need for postoperative ventilation due to further airway swelling.
- Risk of postoperative bleeding and airway compromise requiring urgent removal of intermaxillary fixation and possible reintubation.

e) List two factors that may make a planned extubation "at risk." (2 marks)

- Uncertain ability to oxygenate.
- Reintubation is potentially difficult.
- Presence of general risk factors such as cardiovascular, respiratory, metabolic or neuromuscular comorbidities.

f) List three strategies that could be considered in the management of an "at risk" extubation. (3 marks)

- Use of advanced techniques such as laryngeal mask exchange, remifentanil for extubation or airway exchange catheter.
- Postponement of extubation until conditions can be optimised.
- Tracheostomy.

g) List the three pieces of equipment required for emergency front-of-neck access in the event of a "can't intubate, can't oxygenate" situation. (3 marks)

- Scalpel, number 10 blade.
- Bougie.
- Cuffed 6.0 ID endotracheal tube.

REFERENCES

Frerk C et al. Difficult Airway Society guidelines 2015 for management of unanticipated difficult intubation in adults. *BJA*. 2015: 115: 827–848.

McCullough A et al. Early management of the severely injured major trauma patient. *BJA*. 2014: 113: 234–241.

Morosan M, Parbhoo A, Curry N. Anaesthesia and common oral and maxillo-facial emergencies. *Contin Educ Anaesth Crit Care Pain*. 2012: 12: 257–262.

Popat M et al. Difficult Airway Society guidelines for the management of tracheal extubation. *Anaesthesia*. 2012: 67: 318–340.

7.10 September 2022 Thyroidectomy

This question addressed similar aspects of management of patients for thyroidectomy as the other questions on the same topic. The pass rate was 68.2%, and the Chairs commented that the "question was considered by examiners to be one of the harder questions on the paper, but reassuringly it was answered well. The first section, on the mechanism of action of drugs, was poorly answered. The more clinical aspects of this question . . . was where weaker candidates also dropped marks."

MANAGEMENT OF RESPIRATORY AND CARDIAC ARREST

8.1 September 2011 Temperature control

a) Define hypothermia. (1 mark)
b) State the approach to temperature management that should be adopted in a comatose patient who has suffered a cardiac arrest and has now achieved return of spontaneous circulation (ROSC). (2 marks)
c) List four methods that may be used to achieve the desired temperature for a patient whose body temperature has exceeded the desired range. (4 marks)
d) List three putative cerebral physiological benefits of prevention of pyrexia following ROSC. (3 marks)
e) List seven adverse systemic effects of hypothermia. (7 marks)
f) List three changes to the standard Advanced Life Support algorithms that are made when treating a patient who is hypothermic when in cardiac arrest. (3 marks)

NICE guidance from 2011 advised cooling to 32–34°C for comatose patients who had achieved return of spontaneous circulation after cardiac arrest. Later that year, an SAQ featured in the Final exam on active cooling of such patients and the related complications. However, subsequent research resulted in a change to targeted temperature management of 32–36°C as no extra benefit was found from extreme cooling, but some significant harms were. This is the current approach to patient management in the UK.

Moving on to 2022, research has found no benefit in cooling cardiac arrest patients to below normal temperature at all but instead focuses on "temperature control," the monitoring and active treatment of pyrexia, should it occur. The European Resuscitation Council and European Society of Intensive Care Medicine guidelines have adopted this change, but my answer reflects current UK practice. UK practice may change, and NICE are undertaking a review of their 2011 guidance this year. The CRQ that follows is therefore only loosely based on the original SAQ and has provided the opportunity to look at other aspects of hypo- and hyperthermia. This is also a reminder that guidelines change, and it is important to keep up with them for your clinical practice and also your exam revision.

a) **Define hypothermia. (1 mark)**

- Core body temperature < 35°C.

b) **State the approach to temperature management that should be adopted in a comatose patient who has suffered a cardiac arrest and has now achieved return of spontaneous circulation (ROSC). (2 marks)**

- Targeted temperature management to a range of 32–36°C for 24 hours followed by gradual rewarming with control of pyrexia for at least a further 48 hours.

DOI: 10.1201/9781003388494-8

c) List four methods that may be used to achieve the desired temperature for a patient whose body temperature has exceeded the desired range. (4 marks)

- Exposing the patient.
- Use of antipyretic drugs.
- Reduction of ambient temperature.
- Use of wet towels and ice packs.
- Active intravascular cooling device using cooled intravenous fluid.
- Surface cooling device with electronic feedback system for targeted temperature management.

d) List three putative cerebral physiological benefits of prevention of pyrexia following ROSC. (3 marks)

The rationale for active cooling that was previously undertaken for neuroprotection following cardiac arrest is the same rationale as for the avoidance of pyrexia. However, there is an acknowledged gap in the evidence now as no studies have yet compared outcomes between patients in whom normothermia is targeted and patients in whom pyrexia is left untreated.

- Reduced cerebral metabolic rate for oxygen ($CMRO_2$), resulting in reduced oxygen and glucose demand.
- Suppression of release of oxygen free radicals during reperfusion after cardiac arrest.
- Suppression of destructive neuroexcitotoxic cascade (glutamate release, receptor activation, leading to intracellular calcium overload and cell death).
- Reduction of expression of pro-apoptotic signals.
- Reduction of cerebral oedema associated with reperfusion.

e) List seven adverse systemic effects of hypothermia. (7 marks)

This is no longer relevant to management of post-cardiac arrest patients but is relevant to the effects of cardiopulmonary bypass, to the adverse consequences of exposure and immersion, and to failure to adequately maintain body temperature perioperatively. It was the focus of an SAQ question in 2010. Also consider the pharmacological effects: hypothermia increases the tissue solubility of volatile anaesthetics resulting in delayed recovery, reduces hepatic metabolism, and slows the rate of Hoffman degradation.

Respiratory:

- Increased risk of pneumonia.
- Risk of respiratory failure due to inability to manage the increased carbon dioxide release from shivering.

Cardiovascular:

- Increased catecholamine release, increased systemic vascular resistance, increased myocardial workload and so increased oxygen demand, with risk of ischaemia.
- Arrhythmias.
- Shivering increases oxygen demand.
- Cardiac arrest < 30°C.

Neurological:

- Decline in cognitive function, confusion.
- Slurred speech, loss of motor coordination.

Endocrine:

- Reduced insulin release with increased insulin resistance resulting in elevated blood glucose.

Gastrointestinal:

- Reduced motility compromising enteral nutrition.
- Rarely, pancreatitis.

Haematological:

- Reduced platelet number (sequestered in spleen and liver) and function results in prolonged bleeding time.
- Decreased clotting factor function.

Immune, infection:

- Impaired immune function, overall increased risk of sepsis, surgical site infection.

Renal:

- Diuresis and loss of electrolytes resulting in risk of hypovolaemia and effects of electrolyte imbalance such as arrhythmia.

Hepatic:

- Slowed metabolism rate.

Metabolic:

- Lactic acidosis.
- Impaired enzyme function in all enzymatic pathways.

f) **List three changes to the standard Advanced Life Support algorithms that are made when treating a patient who is hypothermic when in cardiac arrest. (3 marks)**

- If ventricular fibrillation persists after three shocks, delay further shocks until core temperature > 30°C.
- Withhold adrenaline if core temperature is < 30°C.
- Increase administration intervals for adrenaline to 6–10 minutes if core temperature is 30–34°C.
- Rewarm, ideally with extracorporeal life support.

REFERENCES

National Institute for Health and Care Excellence. *Therapeutic hypothermia following cardiac arrest: interventional procedures guidance: IPG386*, March 2011.

Resuscitation Council UK. *Post-resuscitation care*, May 2021. www.resus.org.uk/library/2021-resuscitation-guidelines/post-resuscitation-care-guidelines. Accessed 28th April 2023.

Resuscitation Council UK. *Special circumstances guidelines*, May 2021. www.resus.org.uk/library/2021-resuscitation-guidelines/special-circumstances-guidelines. Accessed 6th March 2023.

Riley C andrzejowski J. Inadvertent perioperative hypothermia. *BJA Educ.* 2018: 18: 227–233.

Sandroni C et al. ERC-ESICM guidelines on temperature control after cardiac arrest in adults. *Intensive Care Med.* 2022: 48: 261–269.

The TTM Trial Investigators. Targeted temperature management at 33°C versus 36°C after cardiac arrest. *N Engl J Med.* 2013: 369: 2197–2206.

8.2 March 2022 Adult tachyarrhythmia

A 60-year-old patient with a history of atrial fibrillation (AF) presents for elective knee arthroplasty.

a) List three elements of your preoperative examination of the patient that relate to assessment of their AF. (3 marks)

b) List three non-cardiac causes of AF. (3 marks)

c) State the mechanism of action of apixaban. (1 mark)

d) The patient has normal renal function – for how long should apixaban be stopped preoperatively if a neuraxial technique is planned? (1 mark)

e) List three patient risk factors for the development of vertebral canal haematoma. (3 marks)

f) Twenty minutes into the operation under spinal anaesthesia, the patient's heart rate rises to 150 bpm – state four reversible causes of this. (4 marks)

g) You have treated all reversible causes, but the patient's heart rate remains at 150 bpm and the ECG now shows myocardial ischaemia. State three things you would do now. (3 marks)

h) The patient is stable, but the ECG monitor now shows a regular broad complex tachycardia. Give two further pharmacological options for treating this rhythm. (2 marks)

The Chairs' Report of the original CRQ commented that this was 'the worst performing question on the paper', with a pass rate of 43.2%. "The latter sections relating to the management of atrial fibrillation were answered poorly. Knowledge of the Resuscitation Council UK guidelines on the management of adult tachycardia would have benefited candidates in answering this question."

a) **List three elements of your preoperative examination of the patient that relate to assessment of their AF. (3 marks)**

* Assess whether currently in AF; presence of an irregularly irregular pulse.
* Assess whether currently adequately rate controlled: 60–80 bpm at rest.
* Assessment for possible underlying cause e.g.:
    — Evidence of Graves' disease (goitre, exophthalmos, pretibial myxoedema).
    — Evidence of previous cardiac surgery (sternotomy, venous harvest scar, mechanical valve on auscultation).
    — Evidence of congenital heart disease or valvular heart disease: abnormal heart sounds.
* Assess for evidence of heart failure associated with AF; dyspnoea, paroxysmal nocturnal dyspnoea, pulmonary oedema, pitting oedema, raised JVP, low BP.
* Absent a wave on JVP.

b) **List three non-cardiac causes of AF. (3 marks)**

Cardiac causes of AF may be related to previous myocardial infarction, valvular (often mitral) heart disease, hypertension (especially if there is consequent left ventricular hypertrophy), congenital heart disease, and sick sinus syndrome.

* Pulmonary embolism.
* Pulmonary hypertension.
* Sepsis.
* Thyrotoxicosis or thyroid storm.
* Stress.
* Excessive caffeine.
* Excessive alcohol.
* High vagal tone causing nocturnal episodes.

c) **State the mechanism of action of apixaban. (I mark)**

The clue is in the name – apiXAban.

- Factor 10a inhibitor.

d) **The patient has normal renal function – for how long should apixaban be stopped preoperatively if a neuraxial technique is planned? (I mark)**

The patient is likely to be on high dose apixaban (5 mg twice a day) for stroke prevention in AF. They have normal renal function and are under 80 years of age. The advice from the most up-to-date consensus, the joint ESAIC/ESRA guidelines, is used for this answer. The Association of Anaesthetists' guideline of 2013 states that apixaban "prophylaxis" should be stopped 24–48 hours before spinal anaesthesia but does not offer advice on treatment dose, unlike its approach to some other DOACs. Finally, this is for elective surgery; the advice would be different if it was urgent.

- 72 hours.

e) **List three patient risk factors for the development of vertebral canal haematoma. (3 marks)**

- Coagulopathy:
  - Inherited or acquired disorders of platelets or coagulation.
  - Liver failure.
  - Uraemia.
  - Sepsis.
  - Major trauma.
- Increased risk of traumatic neuraxial access or multiple attempts:
  - Obesity.
  - Increased age (this may also relate to slower metabolism of antiplatelet or anticoagulant drugs that have been stopped preoperatively).
  - Spinal deformity e.g. scoliosis.

f) **Twenty minutes into the operation under spinal anaesthesia, the patient's heart rate rises to 150 bpm – state four reversible causes of this. (4 marks)**

- Failure of spinal anaesthesia resulting in pain (*this is unlikely twenty minutes into the operation*).
- Patient anxiety (if awake or minimally sedated).
- Sympathetic response to vasodilation, hypovolaemia (including blood loss), hypoxia, or hypercapnea.
- Fast AF due to e.g. electrolyte abnormalities, including hypokalaemia and hypomagnesaemia, myocardial ischaemia, hypovolaemia.
- Critical incident e.g. anaphylaxis, tension pneumothorax, local anaesthetic toxicity, fat or air embolus, malignant hyperthermia, thyroid storm.
- Iatrogenic e.g. administration of ephedrine or atropine.

g) **You have treated all reversible causes, but the patient's heart rate remains at 150 bpm and the ECG now shows myocardial ischaemia. State three things you would do now. (3 marks)**

This is a critical incident. In a viva situation, do not forget the general points of calling for help, applying oxygen if you have not already done so, and asking the surgeons to stop operating whilst you stabilise the patient. According to the adult tachycardia guidelines of the Resuscitation Council UK, reversible causes have been addressed, a "life threatening feature," myocardial ischaemia, is present and so:

- Ensure adequate sedation or anaesthesia.
- Synchronised DC cardioversion at maximum defibrillator output (for AF) up to 3 attempts.

- If unsuccessful, give 300 mg amiodarone iv over 15–20 minutes.
- Consider a further synchronised DC shock.

h) **The patient is stable, but the ECG monitor now shows a regular broad complex tachycardia. Give two further pharmacological options for treating this rhythm. (2 marks)**

- Magnesium 2 g over 10 minutes.
- Amiodarone 900 mg over 24 hours.

REFERENCES

Abhay B, Edward R. Atrial fibrillation. *BJA Educ.* 2006: 6: 219–224.

Ashken T, West S. Regional anaesthesia in patients at risk of bleeding. *BJA Educ.* 2021: 21: 84–94.

Association of Anaesthetists of Great Britain and Ireland, Obstetric Anaesthetists' Association and Regional Anaesthesia UK: regional anaesthesia and patients with abnormalities of coagulation. *Anaesthesia.* 2013: 68: 966–972.

Cook T, Counsell D, Wildsmith J. Major complications of central neuraxial block: report on the third National Audit Project of the Royal College of Anaesthetists. *BJA.* 2009: 102: 179–190.

Kietaibl S et al. Regional anaesthesia in patients on antithrombotic drugs: Joint European Society of Anaesthesiology and Intensive Care and European Society of Regional Anaesthesia guidelines. *Eur J Anaesthesiol.* 2022: 39: 100–132.

Resuscitation Council UK. *Adult tachycardia guideline*, May 2021. www.resus.org.uk/sites/default/files/2021-04/Tachycardia%20Algorithm%202021.pdf. Last accessed 6th March 2023.

NON-THEATRE

9.1 September 2013 Cardioversion

You are asked to anaesthetise a 75-year-old man for an urgent DC cardioversion on the coronary care unit (CCU). He has a broad complex tachycardia of 150 beats/minute but is maintaining a systolic blood pressure of 70 mmHg and has a Glasgow Coma Score of 13/15.

a) List three advantages and three disadvantages of providing anaesthesia in the CCU. (6 marks)
b) List four patient factors that must be taken into consideration when choosing an anaesthetic technique for cardioversion. (4 marks)
c) State three anaesthetic complications that may occur as a consequence of the procedure. (3 marks)
d) State three non-anaesthetic complications that may occur as a consequence of the procedure. (3 marks)
e) The patient returns three months later for a cardiac ablation under anaesthesia. Describe four issues relevant to anaesthesia for ablation procedures that must be considered when planning care, beyond those that needed consideration for cardioversion. (4 marks)

The Chair's Report for the SAQ on this topic gave good insight to the issues considered important by the College. They said that the pass rate was 45.7% and that the "question proved difficult for many candidates . . . The advantages of providing anaesthesia in a coronary care unit for a maximum of 3 marks included the following: avoiding the transfer of an unstable patient to theatre; cardiology department skills readily available; specialist equipment and drugs are immediately accessible; allows earlier treatment. The most important disadvantage was anaesthetising a patient in a remote and unfamiliar environment. This statement needed to be expanded to include the potential lack of monitoring (capnography), anaesthetic drugs, recovery, and skilled assistance. Few candidates mentioned the difficulty in complying with the filling in of a WHO checklist. . . . Some of the factors that should have been considered before commencing anaesthesia included valid consent, recent investigations, starvation status and a potential need for intra- or inter-hospital transfer."

a) List three advantages and three disadvantages of providing anaesthesia in the CCU. (6 marks)

My list of disadvantages of providing anaesthesia on CCU is taken from the issues discussed in the RCoA GPAS "Guidelines for the Provision of Anaesthesia Services in the Non-theatre Environment 2020." It is important to keep these sorts of issues in your mind as they feature in other questions concerning non-theatre duties and also in questions on other topics, for example vascular, where anaesthesia may be undertaken in the radiology suite.

Advantages:

- Don't need to transfer unstable patient.
- Minimises delays to treatment.
- Close availability of cardiology specialist equipment, drugs, and staff.
- Don't need an operating theatre so not delayed by e.g. capacity on emergency list.

Disadvantages:

- Remote, unfamiliar environment; must ensure adequate size for anaesthesia equipment and provision as well as access for a resuscitation team if necessary, and room must be readily accessible to the rest of the hospital building for transfer of patient or equipment if needed.
- Possible lack of availability of standard anaesthesia monitoring, especially capnography.
- May have limited availability of anaesthetic drugs, oxygen (piped or sufficient cylinder supply), suction, difficult airway equipment.
- Availability of appropriate investigations, including coagulation, electrolytes, ECG, and possibly echocardiogram.
- Availability of skilled assistant.
- Compliance with team briefing, WHO checklist, venous thromboembolism assessment.
- Availability of adequate recovery care and facilities.
- Adequacy of trainee competencies; should have had induction in the area and have completed the relevant higher units of training.
- Availability of named consultant supervision.
- Availability of timely anaesthetic support if problems encountered.
- Must have access to the usual anaesthetic guidelines and patient record-keeping systems.

b) **List four patient factors that must be taken into consideration when choosing an anaesthetic technique for cardioversion. (4 marks)**

- Period of starvation.
- Reflux.
- Anticipated difficult airway.
- Any other investigation results – time for these may be limited by patient condition and potential for further deterioration.
- Other medical history. May have limited history as patient has a GCS score of 13.
- Likelihood of whether this is an isolated broad complex tachycardia or the presenting feature of an ischaemic myocardial event.
- Post-cardioversion plans, need for transfer elsewhere for further management e.g. cardiac catheter laboratory.
- Consent.

c) **State three anaesthetic complications that may occur as a consequence of the procedure. (3 marks)**

There are risks associated with all anaesthetics. However, the issues specific to this situation are as follows:

- Aspiration secondary to full stomach.
- Deterioration in cardiovascular stability due to anaesthetic agents and arrhythmia or asystole associated with cardioversion.
- Failure to gain important anaesthetic history information from patient due to reduced GCS and urgency of situation.
- Risk of awareness.

d) **State three non-anaesthetic complications that may occur as a consequence of the procedure. (3 marks)**

- Arterial embolism causing stroke, cardiac ischaemia.
- Asystole, pulseless ventricular tachycardia, ventricular fibrillation.
- Burns.
- Electrical injury to staff.
- Pulmonary oedema.

e) The patient returns three months later for a cardiac ablation under anaesthesia. Describe four issues relevant to anaesthesia for ablation procedures that must be considered when planning care, beyond those that needed consideration for cardioversion. (4 marks)

This part of the question did not feature in the original SAQ, but I have added it as anaesthesia in the cardiac catheterisation laboratory is a growing field and a potential focus for future questions relevant to remote site anaesthesia.

- Likely fixed non-tipping table – safer to induce anaesthesia on tipping trolley before transfer to table.
- Lengthy procedure – care for pressure points, temperature monitoring, sedation may not be tolerated.
- Use of radiography – protection of staff is necessary, access to patient due to presence of C-arm may be restricted.
- Low light levels – possible difficulties with drug management or patient monitoring.
- Choice of anaesthetic technique guided by patient and procedural factors.
- Invasive arterial and/or central venous access may be required.
- Special considerations – requirement of trans-oesophageal echocardiography during the procedure would necessitate intubation, some procedures require heparinisation and ACT monitoring, movement by the patient may preclude effective treatment so neuromuscular blocking drug or remifentanil infusion required.

REFERENCES

Ashley E. Anaesthesia for electrophysiology procedures in the cardiac catheter laboratory. *Contin Educ Anaes Crit Care Pain.* 2012: 12: 230–236.

Knowles P, Press C. Anaesthesia for cardioversion. *BJA Educ.* 2017: 17: 166–171.

Royal College of Anaesthetists. *Guidelines for the provision of anaesthesia services: chapter 7: guidelines for the provision of anaesthesia services in the non-theatre environment 2020.* www.rcoa.ac.uk/sites/default/files/documents/2020-02/GPAS-2020-07-ANTE.pdf. Accessed 10th March 2023.

9.2 March 2015 Electro-convulsive therapy

A 55-year-old patient is due to have electro-convulsive therapy (ECT) for severe depression. They take lithium and fluoxetine.
a) List five patient-specific preoperative considerations for ECT. (5 marks)
b) List three cardiovascular effects of ECT. (3 marks)
c) State four other physiological consequences of ECT. (4 marks)
d) List three types of physical injuries that may occur during ECT. (3 marks)
e) List three anaesthetic implications of lithium treatment. (3 marks)
f) List two anaesthetic implications of fluoxetine treatment. (2 marks)

The Chair reported a 13.3% pass rate with 54.4% of candidates receiving a poor fail for the SAQ on this topic. "Performance on this question was highly variable as reflected by the pass and poor fail rates, and the item was strongly discriminatory. Examiners felt that trainees did not have adequate experience of supervised working in non-theatre locations. Few seem to be attending ECT sessions; for example, many candidates did not realise suxamethonium would be given and did not appreciate that myalgia is a common side effect. Many thought that ECT could not be conducted safely in an isolated environment. Consent and mental health issues, problems with patient communication and the likelihood of comorbidity did not feature in many scripts. Of concern was failure to understand the significance of lithium or fluoxetine therapy, as patients appearing on routine theatre lists may be taking these drugs; few candidates made mention of the potentiation of relaxants or volatile anaesthetic agents by lithium."

ECT:

- *Used for severe, medication-resistant depression (especially with associated psychomotor retardation) and also mania, catatonia, psychosis, and schizophrenia including in pregnant women.*
- *Tonic-clonic seizure of specific duration (15–120 seconds) is induced.*
- *Both electrodes on the nondominant hemisphere minimises cognitive side effects.*
- *Electrode positioned on each side if speed of recovery is the most important factor.*
- *Repeat twice a week for up to 12 treatments until no further improvement.*

a) List five patient-specific preoperative considerations for ECT. (5 marks)

- Capacity for consent; patient may be under section.
- Psychiatric illness may make it difficult to obtain full medical history from the patient, may affect compliance with treatment for comorbidities, may affect recent oral intake (consider dehydration and electrolyte disturbance).
- Anaesthetic assessment; check for significant reflux (commonly do not use airway adjuncts in ECT), dentition (bite block will be used).
- Assess for comorbidities that specifically affect suitability for ECT; significant ischaemic heart disease, cardiac failure (ventricular dysfunction noted in normal hearts for up to six hours afterwards), significant valvular disease, raised intracranial or intraocular pressure, untreated cerebral aneurysm, recent cerebrovascular accident, unstable fracture or cervical spine.
- Check for implantable cardioverter defibrillator (ICD) (which should be deactivated) or permanent pacemaker (which may be set into a fixed mode, depending on underlying pathology). Liaise with cardiac physiologist.
- ECT tends to happen in sites remote from main theatres: ensure full staffing, monitoring, equipment, recovery facilities – if patient has significant comorbidities, consider need for relocation to more central, supported site.

b) **List three cardiovascular effects of ECT. (3 marks)**

- Brief (15 seconds) parasympathetic response with bradycardia and risk of asystole.
- Then, prominent sympathetic response with increased heart rate and blood pressure, therefore increased myocardial oxygen consumption and risk of ischaemia or infarction.
- Risk of post-procedure myocardial stunning with reduced ejection fraction – risk of heart failure.

c) **State four other physiological consequences of ECT. (4 marks)**

- Airway; risk of laryngospasm, increased salivation secondary to parasympathetic phase.
- Respiratory; risk of aspiration.
- Neurological; increased cerebral oxygen consumption and intracranial pressure. Risk of intracranial haemorrhage, transient ischaemic defects, status epilepticus. More commonly, disorientation and memory loss.
- Gastrointestinal; increased gastric pressure risking reflux.
- Cutaneomusculoskeletal; seizure increases peripheral oxygen consumption and results in raised lactate, raised temperature, and myalgia.

d) **List three types of physical injuries that may occur during ECT. (3 marks)**

- Dental damage due to seizure plus bite block.
- Intraoral damage due to biting.
- Musculoskeletal damage and fractures are rare since use of muscle relaxant.
- Myalgia due to seizure and use of suxamethonium.

e) **List three anaesthetic implications of lithium treatment. (3 marks)**

- Potentiation of effect of neuromuscular blocking drugs.
- Possible reduction in anaesthetic dose requirement due to reduction in brainstem catecholamine release.
- Renally excreted. Nonsteroidal anti-inflammatory drugs reduce lithium excretion and can result in toxic levels.
- Nephrogenic diabetes insipidus – consider patient fluid status.
- Narrow therapeutic index – ensure recent level check.
- Risk of serotonin syndrome if co-administration with serotonin reuptake inhibitors e.g. fentanyl, tramadol, meperidine or $5HT_3$ receptor antagonists e.g. ondansetron.
- Reduced seizure threshold.
- Cardiac arrhythmias are a side effect, worse if toxic.
- Omit for 24 hours prior to anaesthesia for major surgery.

f) **List two anaesthetic implications of fluoxetine treatment. (2 marks)**

- Risk of serotonin syndrome if co-administration with serotonin reuptake inhibitors e.g. fentanyl, tramadol, meperidine or $5HT_3$ receptor antagonists e.g. ondansetron.
- Inhibits CYP2D6, thus preventing metabolism from codeine to morphine, and tramadol to its active form, so no analgesic effect would be obtained.
- Co-administration with NSAIDs increases bleeding risk due to both drugs having separate impact on reducing platelet activity.

REFERENCES

The Handbook of Perioperative Medicines UKCPA. *UK Clinical Pharmacy Association: lithium.* www.ukcpa-periophandbook.co.uk/medicine-monographs/lithium. Accessed 10th March 2023.

Royal College of Psychiatrists. *Statement on electroconvulsive therapy (ECT): position statement CERT01/17*, February 2017. www.rcpsych.ac.uk/docs/default-source/about-us/who-we-are/electroconvulsive-therapy-ect-ctee-statement-feb17.pdf?sfvrsn=2f4a94f9_2. Accessed 10th March 2023.

Uppal V, Dourish J, Macfarlane A. Anaesthesia for electroconvulsive therapy. *Contin Educ Anaesth Crit Care Pain.* 2010: 10: 192–196.

9.3 September 2016 Magnetic resonance imaging

You are asked to transfer an intubated intensive care patient for a magnetic resonance imaging (MRI) scan.

a) What is meant by the terms magnetic resonance (MR) safe and MR conditional in relation to equipment used in the MRI scanner room? (2 marks)
b) State the SI unit of magnetic flux density. (1 mark)
c) State the field contour within which the "MR environment" is defined. (1 mark)
d) State five precautions that should be taken to prevent burns caused by monitoring equipment used in an MRI scanner. (5 marks)
e) List six other precautions you would take to minimise the risks associated with MRI. (6 marks)
f) List five possible contraindications to an MRI scan. (5 marks)

The Chairs' Report stated a pass rate of 45.8% pass and said, "Despite the fact that many candidates will have accompanied patients to the MRI scanner, knowledge of the specific precautions needed to prevent harm during such a procedure was poor. Points were lost by concentrating on the difficulties of anaesthesia in a remote location, which, whilst important, were not what was asked for." I have added the subsections about magnetic field strength to the original SAQ to add some Primary-specific knowledge that may be tested in a CRQ.

a) **What is meant by the terms magnetic resonance (MR) safe and MR conditional in relation to equipment used in the MRI scanner room? (2 marks)**

- MR Safe: these devices pose no MR-related hazards to patients or staff when used according to instructions and can therefore be used in any MR setting.
- MR Conditional: this equipment poses no MR-related hazard in a specified MR environment under specific conditions of use e.g. static field strength, rate of change of magnetic field.

b) **State the SI unit of magnetic flux density. (1 mark)**

- Tesla.

c) **State the field contour within which the "MR environment" is defined. (1 mark)**

Within this area there is risk of projectile damage from ferromagnetic objects, risk of heating from radiofrequency coils, and risk associated with implanted devices. This is also called the "5 Gauss line," Gauss being another unit of magnetic flux density (1 Tesla = 10,000 Gauss).

- 5 Gauss, or 0.5 milliTesla (mT).

d) **State five precautions that should be taken to prevent burns caused by monitoring equipment used in an MRI scanner. (5 marks)**

- Use only MR safe monitoring equipment or MR conditional equipment that has been deemed appropriate to use in that scanner.
- Check all equipment prior to use, that it is intact, that there is no breach in any insulating surfaces that might risk metal touching skin.
- Fibreoptic cables for ECG and pulse oximeter eliminate use of electrical current, which may result in induction currents and burns to underlying skin.
- Telemetric monitor to eliminate the risk of induction currents in connecting leads.
- ECG leads should be high impedance, braided and short to minimise risk of induction currents. ECG electrodes must be MR safe.

- Do not allow any cables to coil or cross each other as induction of current can result from capacitance coupling.
- Ensure leads are positioned to exit the scanner down the centre rather than at the side of the patient to keep them away from the radiofrequency (RF) coils.
- Separate leads from patient's skin with e.g. foam insulating padding.

e) List six other precautions you would take to minimise the risks associated with MRI. (6 marks)

The superconductor coil windings of the MRI magnets are kept at 4K by liquid helium. If the coils rise in temperature, the helium will escape as a gas and bring the oxygen content of the room down to a dangerous level, necessitating urgent evacuation.

- Equipment check; ensure all equipment to be used is MR safe or MR conditional and has been checked as safe to use on that scanner.
- Checklist; all staff and patients to complete checklist to ensure no contraindications to entering MRI scanner (see *answer to (f) for more detail*).
- Ferromagnetic objects: staff and patient to remove all ferromagnetic objects from clothes/ pockets to avoid the possibility of them becoming projectiles; ensure all equipment e.g. trolley, is non-ferromagnetic, remove oxygen cylinders etc.; some clothes e.g. sportswear, contain silver fibres – cotton hospital gown to be worn; drug delivery patches may contain metal – remove due to risk of burns.
- Padding over RF coils; ensure padding is intact to prevent direct contact between patient and coils.
- Ear protection; for all patients, anaesthetised or not, due to high noise levels in scanner.
- Monitoring equipment and breathing circuit; check that there is sufficient length by checking planned range of movement of MRI table before leaving the scanning room.
- Inaccessibility of airway; meticulous securing of airway to ensure it does not become dislodged with movement as difficult to access once in scanner.
- Monitoring; telemetric monitoring to facilitate the presence of monitoring screen in control room, reduces risk of failing to notice abnormalities.
- Remote site anaesthesia; ensure senior support available, ensure orientation with equipment/location/emergency kit prior to commencement, especially as some equipment will be unfamiliar as it is MR safe and therefore different to that used elsewhere. Ensure identical monitoring standards to those used elsewhere can be achieved; awareness of low light levels often used in radiology.
- Risks of gadolinium-based contrast agents:
  - Avoid contrast if eGFR is less than 30 ml/min.
  - Risk of nephrogenic sclerosing fibrosis if patient is in ESRF.
  - Do not repeat contrast within seven days.
  - Avoid in pregnancy unless absolutely necessary.
  - Drugs to manage anaphylaxis to be readily available.
- Awareness of quench evacuation procedures and evacuation in case of need to treat patient for cardiac arrest.

f) List five possible contraindications to an MRI scan. (5 marks)

There are few absolute contraindications – most situations need further evaluation and are dependent on the specifications of the scanner and the implanted medical device. Devices may not be compatible with the scanner because of their ferromagnetic content and thus propensity to move within the magnetic field and also depending on whether they can be exposed to the specific frequency of radiofrequency pulses generated by the scanner. MRI scanners in clinical use are mostly 1.5–3 Tesla, and

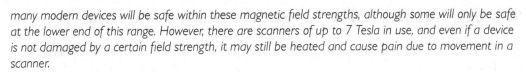

many modern devices will be safe within these magnetic field strengths, although some will only be safe at the lower end of this range. However, there are scanners of up to 7 Tesla in use, and even if a device is not damaged by a certain field strength, it may still be heated and cause pain due to movement in a scanner.

- Recent surgery involving ferromagnetic clips or implants (including neurosurgical clips and cochlear implants).
- Ferromagnetic material (or shrapnel) in eye.
- Intra-aortic balloon pumps, ventricular assist devices, some aortic stent grafts.
- Neurostimulators.
- Programmable shunts for hydrocephalus.
- Implantable cardiac devices, valves and stents.
- Passive implanted devices e.g. breast implants, vascular access ports, orthopaedic implants.
- Neurostimulators.

REFERENCES

British Institute of Radiology. MR safety. www.bir.org.uk/media/376620/day_2_field_strength_finalr. pdf. Accessed 10th March 2023.

Reddy U, White M, Wilson S. Anaesthesia for magnetic resonance imaging. Contin Educ Anaesth Crit Care Pain. 2012: 12: 140–144.

Wilson S et al. Association of Anaesthetists and the Neuro Anaesthesia and Critical Care Society of Great Britain and Ireland: guidelines for the safe provision of anaesthesia in magnetic resonance units 2019. Anaesthesia. 2019: 74: 638–650.

9.4 September 2018 Magnetic resonance imaging

You are asked to transfer an intubated intensive care patient for a magnetic resonance imaging (MRI) scan.

a) What is meant by the term "magnetic resonance conditional" in relation to equipment used in the MRI scanner room? (1 mark)

b) What precautions should be taken to prevent burns caused by monitoring equipment used in an MRI scanner? (6 marks)

c) Describe other precautions you should take while this patient is having an MRI scan. (8 marks)

d) What are the relative/absolute contraindications to an MRI scan for any patient? (5 marks)

Reproduced here in its original format, this SAQ was an almost exact repeat of that asked in September 2016. This reiterates the value of going over poorly answered questions and topics when preparing for the Final FRCA. It seemed like most people had not taken this opportunity as the pass rate was lower than the previous time at 38.1%. The Chairs said, "This question was poorly answered, although again showed good correlation with overall performance. Most candidates did not concentrate on anaesthesia for MRI but instead discussed remote location only. The lack of understanding of the risks inherent in looking after a patient during an MRI scan is worrying as this is a frequent task for anaesthetists and intensive care doctors at this level." Remote location is just one small aspect of the risks of managing an anaesthetised patient in the MRI scanner.

ORTHOPAEDIC SURGERY

10.1 March 2015 Revision hip surgery and bone cement implantation syndrome

An 80-year-old patient is to undergo second stage revision of a total hip arthroplasty for treated deep joint infection.
a) List five specific preoperative considerations relevant to this patient. (5 marks)
b) Give seven important features of the intraoperative anaesthetic management of this case. (7 marks)
c) List four patient risk factors for bone cement implantation syndrome (BCIS). (4 marks)
d) List four measures that can be taken to prevent or minimise the effect of BCIS. (4 marks)

The Chair's Report for the SAQ on this topic (which has been minimally altered to create a CRQ) said that "examiners felt that this question should have proved relatively easy, so the pass [46.8%] and poor fail [17.7%] rates are surprising. Inexperience probably accounts for these results. Strong candidates considered issues such as anticipated blood loss and analgesia. Weak candidates focused on infection control issues and ignored the information that the patient had been treated. This question had a very strong correlation with overall candidate scores." Answering the first two parts of the question will have been mostly dependent on having had relevant clinical experience, reinforcing the importance of learning from every case you are involved in. I know it says that weaker candidates focused on infection control issues, but I would never anaesthetise a patient for this surgery without assuring myself that treatment had been effective. The last two parts were based on the BCIS guideline that was published in the same year, again highlighting the importance of keeping up to date with current issues and guidance.

a) List five specific preoperative considerations relevant to this patient. (5 marks)

- Ensure adequate treatment of infection by assessment of symptoms and signs, and by white cell count and CRP level. Plan for perioperative antibiotics with microbiology input.
- Anaemia more common in elderly and after chronic infection – ensure it is adequately managed before this elective surgery to reduce the risk of perioperative blood transfusion.
- Reduced mobility may have resulted in deconditioning. Early physiotherapy input should be planned.
- Dietician input for nutritional assessment and management if weight loss has occurred or appetite compromised as a consequence of chronic infection.
- Advanced age of patient therefore increased risk of comorbidities that will require assessment and management, especially respiratory disease, ischaemic heart disease, valvular heart disease, which will influence choice of anaesthesia.
- Plan for location of postoperative care, which will be dependent on discussion with surgeon regarding complexity of surgery, likelihood of blood loss, presence of comorbidities.

DOI: 10.1201/9781003388494-10

b) **Give seven important features of the intraoperative anaesthetic management of this case. (7 marks)**

In attempting to come up with a suitable list of important features, I have followed the alphabet again. It helped organise my thoughts in the absence of a more obvious way of addressing this question. I have put the point about BCIS down the bottom to minimise repeating answers in the various subsections.

- Increased risk of postoperative delirium due to patient's age: avoidance of long-acting sedative drugs, minimisation of opioids through inclusion of regional or neuraxial techniques, depth of anaesthesia monitoring if GA.
- Significant risk of blood loss with this type of surgery: cell salvage, ensure adequate starting haemoglobin, prepare cross-matched blood, include neuraxial technique, use of tranexamic acid, consider invasive monitoring.
- Further risk of joint infection; antibiotic prophylaxis as discussed with microbiologist in line with previous sensitivities, maintenance of normothermia.
- High deep vein thrombosis risk due to elderly patient, major lower limb orthopaedic surgery, prolonged surgery: mechanical prophylaxis intraoperatively, plan for mechanical and pharmacological postoperatively, maintain hydration.
- Risks of renal dysfunction due to advanced age, hypotension associated with blood loss, and neuraxial technique: consider invasive monitoring, ensure adequate hydration, use of vasopressor, avoidance of nephrotoxic agents.
- Patient positioned laterally for prolonged period; elderly patient at risk of pressure sores so ensure adequate protection, and inability to tolerate position may impact on anaesthetic choices.
- Choice of anaesthetic technique: spinal anaesthesia unlikely to offer adequate duration, sedation may need to be deep to tolerate prolonged lateral positioning with CSE, epidural or spinal catheter, neuraxial and regional techniques may offer an anaesthesia-sparing approach if GA used.
- High risk of bone cement implantation syndrome due to age and gender; take steps to mitigate risk.

c) **List four patient risk factors for bone cement implantation syndrome (BCIS). (4 marks)**

- Increasing age.
- Significant cardiopulmonary disease.
- Diuretic treatment.
- Male sex.

d) **List four measures that can be taken to prevent or minimise the effect of BCIS. (4 marks)**

- Avoid use of cement where surgically appropriate or where patient's physiological status dictates.
- Communication; preoperative assignation of roles in the event of BCIS, surgeon to inform anaesthetist before applying cement, anaesthetist to acknowledge.
- Surgical management:
  — Wash and dry femoral canal.
  — Apply cement in retrograde fashion using cement gun with a suction catheter and intramedullary plug in the femoral shaft.
  — Avoid vigorous pressurisation of cement in at risk patients.

- Anaesthetic management:
  - Ensure adequate resuscitation pre- and intraoperatively – aim for blood pressure within 20% of pre-induction value.
  - Monitor for cardiorespiratory compromise; blood pressure (invasive if high-risk patient) and $etCO_2$ (if general anaesthesia).
  - Prepare vasopressors in case of cardiovascular collapse.

REFERENCES

Association of Anaesthetists of Great Britain and Ireland. Safety guideline: reducing the risk from cemented hemiarthroplasty for hip fracture 2015. *Anaesthesia*. 2015: 70: 623–626.

Robinson H, Medlock G, Cranfield K. Anaesthesia for revision hip surgery. *ATOTW*. 2017: 363. https://resources.wfsahq.org/atotw/anaesthesia-for-revision-hip-surgery/. Accessed 20th January 2023.

10.2 September 2019 Revision hip surgery and blood loss

A 76-year-old patient presents for revision hip surgery following periprosthetic infection. The patient weighs 50 kg. Preoperative haemoglobin is 85 g/l and MCV is 90 fL.

a) List three possible causes of anaemia in this patient. (3 marks)

b) List four perioperative risks that are increased in patients with anaemia. (4 marks)

c) At what level of predicted intraoperative blood loss should cell salvage be considered? (1 mark)

d) List four acute physiological intraoperative implications of one litre blood loss for this patient. (4 marks)

e) List three nonsurgical intraoperative strategies that can help to reduce blood loss for this patient. (3 marks)

f) At what level of haemoglobin (g/l) does NICE recommend perioperative blood transfusion? (1 mark)

g) List four risks associated with intraoperative allogeneic blood transfusion. (4 marks)

The Chairs' Report said that the original CRQ question was "very relevant to anaesthetic practice and yet [candidates] performed surprisingly poorly. In general the answers given were not specific to the scenario. Candidates failed to comment on the significance of one litre of blood loss as compared to a patient's total blood volume. Instead, candidates gave vague statements on the effects of blood loss, which did not answer the question." I don't know what was asked in the original CRQ but have created a CRQ here which I hope provides learning surrounding acute intraoperative blood loss.

a) List three possible causes of anaemia in this patient. (3 marks)

The question describes a normocytic (MCV 80–95 fL) anaemia, which has several causes.

- Functional iron deficiency (anaemia of chronic disease): may relate to chronic periprosthetic infection or an underlying systemic joint disease e.g. rheumatoid arthritis, or an unrelated comorbidity e.g. chronic kidney disease or malignancy.
- Bone marrow disorders e.g. aplastic anaemia.
- Sickle cell anaemia.
- Vitamin B deficiencies.
- Haemolysis (due to haemoglobinopathies or autoimmune haemolytic anaemia).

b) List four perioperative risks that are increased in patients with anaemia. (4 marks)

Almost every organ function can be disturbed by anaemia because of reduced oxygen-carrying capacity and oxygen delivery by the blood, together with the increased perioperative oxygen demand as a result of the surgical stress response.

- Cardiovascular events, including myocardial infarction and stroke.
- Infections including respiratory, urinary, and surgical site.
- Venous thromboembolism.
- Acute kidney injury.
- Unplanned ICU admission, longer hospital stay.
- Thirty-day mortality.
- Blood transfusion requirement with its associated risks.

c) **At what level of predicted intraoperative blood loss should cell salvage be considered? (1 mark)**

This is recommended in the two Association of Anaesthetists' guidelines referenced below. The guideline on cell salvage advises specific consent for patients with active infection, but there is no clear evidence of contraindication.

- Predicted blood loss > 500 ml or > 10% blood volume.

d) **List four acute physiological intraoperative implications of one litre blood loss for this patient. (4 marks)**

The circulating blood volume in an adult is roughly 70 ml/kg, so 3.5 litres in this patient. Therefore, one litre blood loss accounts for just under 30% of the circulating volume and may be poorly tolerated. This is on the border between class II and class III haemorrhagic shock. Tachypnoea and altered mentation would be seen in a non-anaesthetised patient.

- Development of haemorrhagic shock type II due to loss of just under 30% of total blood volume with resulting hypoperfusion and dysfunction of organs.
- Hypoperfusion causing anaerobic metabolism and lactic acidosis.
- Sympathetic response to volume loss with tachycardia, peripheral vasoconstriction and risk of cardiac ischaemia.
- Activation of the renin-angiotensin-aldosterone system with reduction in urine output and vasoconstriction.
- Development of coagulopathy and exacerbation of further bleeding.
- Systemic inflammatory response causing release of vasodilatory and myocardial depressant mediators which will have a negative effect on the initial compensatory mechanisms.

e) **List three nonsurgical intraoperative strategies that can help to reduce blood loss for this patient. (3 marks)**

Read the question – it specifically asks for intraoperative strategies, and therefore preoperative measures (or surgical measures) would not get you the marks here:

- Regional or neuraxial anaesthesia.
- Avoidance of hypothermia, aiming for core body temperature > 35°C.
- Avoidance of acidosis, aiming for pH > 7.2.
- Avoidance of hypocalcaemia, aiming for ionised calcium > 1 mmol/l.
- Use of antifibrinolytic drugs i.e. tranexamic acid.
- (Hypotensive anaesthesia or acceptance of low intraoperative blood pressure is a useful technique to reduce blood loss for other surgeries but unlikely to be useful in hip revision surgery in an elderly patient.)

f) **At what level of haemoglobin (g/l) does NICE recommend perioperative blood transfusion? (1 mark)**

NICE recommendations are in line with Association of Anaesthetists' guidelines.

- > 70 g/l (or 80 g/l in patients with underlying cardiac disease).

g) List four risks associated with intraoperative allogeneic blood transfusion. (4 marks)

- Transfusion errors resulting in incompatible blood transfusion and haemolytic reaction.
- Development of atypical antibodies making future blood cross-matching more challenging.
- Administration of cold blood with low 2,3 DPG and no clotting factor content causing a negative impact on blood clotting.
- Immunomodulation.
- Transfusion-associated circulatory overload.
- Non-haemolytic transfusion reactions.
- Infection.
- Transfusion-associated graft-versus-host disease.
- Increased morbidity and mortality – evidence suggests this risk is independent of the risks associated with the cause of need for transfusion.

REFERENCES

Hans G, Jones N. Preoperative anaemia. *CEACCP*. 2013: 13: 71–74.

Klein A et al. AAGBI guidelines: the use of blood components and their alternatives 2016. *Anaesthesia*. 2016: 71: 829–842.

Klein A et al. Association of Anaesthetists' guidelines: cell salvage for peri-operative blood conservation 2018. *Anaesthesia*. 2018: 73: 1141–1150.

Robinson H, Medlock G, Cranfield K. Anaesthesia for hip revision surgery. *ATOTW*. 2017: 363. https://resources.wfsahq.org/wp-content/uploads/363_english.pdf. Accessed 20th January 2023.

Thakrar S, Clevenger B, Mallett S. Patient blood management and perioperative anaemia. *BJA Educ*. 2017: 17: 28–34.

10.3 March 2020 Ankylosing spondylitis

A 42-year-old patient with a history of ankylosing spondylitis presents for cervical spine surgery.

a) Which Human Leukocyte Antigen (HLA) allele is associated with the development of ankylosing spondylitis? (1 mark)

b) List three articular features of ankylosing spondylitis which may predispose to difficult airway management. (3 marks)

c) List three approaches to minimising cervical extension during airway management in a patient with ankylosing spondylitis. (3 marks)

d) Give two respiratory complications of ankylosing spondylitis of relevance to the anaesthetist. (2 marks)

e) Give two cardiovascular complications that may affect patients with ankylosing spondylitis. (2 marks)

f) List three neurological complications that may affect patients with ankylosing spondylitis. (3 marks)

g) List three types of drugs used in the treatment of ankylosing spondylitis apart from analgesics and NSAIDs. (3 marks)

h) List three possible causes of postoperative airway obstruction relevant to this case. (3 marks)

The Chairs' Report of the original CRQ said "examiners were surprised at the lack of knowledge on this topic. The condition is important and frequently seen therefore candidates should have known it in more detail than was demonstrated. The pass rate [of 24.4%] for this question was the lowest overall."

a) Which Human Leukocyte Antigen (HLA) allele is associated with the development of ankylosing spondylitis? (1 mark)

- HLA B27.

b) List three articular features of ankylosing spondylitis which may predispose to difficult airway management. (3 marks)

- Temporomandibular joint involvement resulting in restricted mouth opening.
- Cervical spine involvement with instability, fusion, and fragility resulting in restricted movement.
- Kyphosis resulting in difficulty positioning.
- Cricoarytenoid joint involvement (rare) which may lead to hoarseness and dyspnoea which may be exacerbated by airway instrumentation.

c) List three approaches to minimising cervical extension during airway management in a patient with ankylosing spondylitis. (3 marks)

Ankylosing spondylitis is an autoimmune condition which causes ossification of inflamed vertebral ligaments resulting in reduced movement between vertebrae and impingement on nerve roots. Eventually, the spine can become rigid and fixed in flexion. There is a predisposition to osteoporosis which results in risk of fracture with minimal movement due to the rigidity of the spine.

- Manual in-line stabilisation or rigid collar use during laryngoscopy (however, this is associated with increased difficulty of laryngoscopy and risk of failed airway management).
- Use of video laryngoscope with stylet or bougie.
- Laryngeal mask use or intubating laryngeal mask if intubation is required.
- Awake or asleep fibreoptic intubation.
- Awake surgical tracheostomy (although this may not be feasible in the presence of a significant fixed flexion deformity).

d) **Give two respiratory complications of ankylosing spondylitis of relevance to the anaesthetist. (2 marks)**

- Kyphosis causing restrictive lung defect.
- Costovertebral joint involvement resulting in restrictive lung defect.
- Upper lobe pulmonary fibrosis.

e) **Give two cardiovascular complications that may affect patients with ankylosing spondylitis. (2 marks)**

- Valve disease (aortic or mitral regurgitation).
- Conduction disorders.
- Increased risk of ischaemic heart disease.

f) **List three neurological complications that may affect patients with ankylosing spondylitis. (3 marks)**

- Peripheral nerve impingement by bony overgrowth.
- Cauda equina syndrome.
- Spinal cord damage due to compression, subluxation, fractures due to fragility.
- Vertebrobasilar insufficiency (due to cervical spine disease).
- Focal epilepsy.

g) **List three types of drugs used in the treatment of ankylosing spondylitis apart from analgesics and NSAIDs. (3 marks)**

- Disease-modifying anti-rheumatic drugs e.g. sulfasalazine, methotrexate.
- Anti-TNF drugs e.g. infliximab, adalimumab.
- Other monoclonal antibody drugs active against interleukins e.g. secukinumab.
- JAK inhibitors e.g. upadacitinib.
- Corticosteroids.

h) **List three possible causes of postoperative airway obstruction relevant to this case. (3 marks)**

- Haematoma compressing airway.
- Laryngopharyngeal oedema due to both prolonged surgery and prone positioning.
- Migration or displacement of any implant used.
- Intraoperative damage to the recurrent laryngeal nerve associated with anterior cervical surgery.
- Cricoarytenoid joint disease causing fixed vocal cords and so minimal oedema related to e.g. intubation may cause airway obstruction.

REFERENCES

Hunninger A, Calder I. Cervical spine surgery. *Contin Educ Anaes Crit Care Pain.* 2007: 7: 81–84.
Wiles M. Airway management in patients with suspected or confirmed traumatic spinal cord injury: a narrative review of current evidence. *Anaesthesia.* 2022: 77: 1120–1128.
Woodward L, Kam P. Ankylosing spondylitis: recent developments and anaesthetic implications. *Anaesthesia.* 2009: 64: 540–548.

PERIOPERATIVE MEDICINE

11.1 September 2011 Chronic liver disease

a) List the commonest causes of chronic liver disease in adults. (3 marks)
b) Outline the effects of chronic liver disease on organ systems. (12 marks)
c) What elements constitute the Child-Pugh scoring system? (5 marks)

This is the SAQ that appeared in September 2011 for which there is no Chair's Report. A virtually identical SAQ appeared in March 2015, and so I have addressed most of the content there. For 5 marks, part (c) asks for the "elements that constitute the Child-Pugh scoring system," and the answer is:

- *Ascites.*
- *Bilirubin.*
- *Prothrombin time.*

- *Albumin.*
- *Encephalopathy.*

If more detail is required, each of these variables is quantified and given a score from 1, least severe, to 3, most severe. The numbers are added up and the patient assigned to Child's category A, B or C. Based on population studies, an individual's Child's category can be used to predict their overall survival and also their likely mortality associated with surgery.

	1	2	3
Bilirubin (micromol/l)	< 34	34–50	> 50
Albumin (g/l)	> 35	28–35	< 28
Prothrombin time (s > control)	< 4	4–6	> 6
Encephalopathy	None	Mild (Grades I–II)	Marked (Grades III–IV)
Ascites	None	Mild	Marked

Used as a risk prediction tool for patients undergoing abdominal surgery:

< 7 = Child's A, < 5% mortality
7–9 = Child's B, 25% mortality
> 9 = Child's C, 50% mortality

Or just for assessing overall mortality risk:

One-year survival

A: 100%
B: 80%
C: 45%

REFERENCE

Vaja R, McNicol L, Sisley I. Anaesthesia for patients with liver disease. *Contin Educ Anaesth Crit Care Pain.* 2010: 10: 15–19.

11.2 March 2012 Chronic kidney disease

You are asked to anaesthetise a patient with chronic kidney disease (CKD stage ≥ 4).
a) List two possible respiratory issues that should be considered preoperatively. (2 marks)
b) List three possible cardiovascular issues that should be considered preoperatively. (3 marks)
c) List three possible endocrine issues that should be considered preoperatively. (3 marks)
d) List five pharmacokinetic issues that should be considered. (5 marks)
e) List four factors that should be considered when planning overall perioperative fluid requirements. (4 marks)
f) List three issues that should be considered when planning postoperative analgesia for this patient. (3 marks)

The Chair reported a 59% pass rate for the SAQ on this topic. The question asks about patients with CKD ≥ 4, which would therefore include patients established on dialysis as well as those who are currently being managed without. The original SAQ asked, "(b) Outline the pharmacological factors that must be considered." This clearly led to a variety of approaches of response as the Chair's Report stated that "many candidates listed specific drugs that they would or would not use in patients with CKD but failed to comment on general issues such as alterations of protein binding, volume of distribution, excretion of drugs, antihypertensive medication and accumulation of active metabolites." I have reworded that subsection with, I hope, a little more specificity.

a) List two possible respiratory issues that should be considered preoperatively. (2 marks)

- Assessment of fluid status; fluid overload can result in pulmonary oedema and pleural effusion, which reduces FRC and results in V/Q mismatch.
- If using CAPD, need to drain fluid as it will result in diaphragmatic splinting and reduction of FRC.
- If patient has had a previous transplant, patient may be immunosuppressed – need to assess for possibility of respiratory infection.

b) List three possible cardiovascular issues that should be considered preoperatively. (3 marks)

- Hypertension.
- Risk of ischaemic heart disease – process is accelerated in patients with CKD.
- Risk of left ventricular hypertrophy with subsequent decompensation and failure.
- Calcified and poorly functioning heart valves.
- Arrhythmias related to electrolyte disturbance, left ventricular hypertrophy and myocardial fibrosis.
- Presence of arteriovenous fistula or other vascular access device which will have an impact on site of perioperative line placement.

c) List three possible endocrine issues that should be considered preoperatively. (3 marks)

- Diabetes; a common cause of CKD, and CKD itself leads to increased insulin resistance. Also, long-term steroid treatment for the underlying disease that may have caused the CKD and immunosuppressants used in the management of renal transplant may lead to insulin resistance that requires treatment.
- Glucocorticoid supplementation; if taking steroids for a previous transplant or for an autoimmune cause of kidney failure, supplementation will be required perioperatively.
- Secondary hyperparathyroidism that can result in bone fragility and electrolyte imbalance.

d) List five pharmacokinetic issues that should be considered. (5 marks)

Remember; absorption, distribution, metabolism, excretion.

- Absorption of oral drugs may be slowed by gastroparesis, increased gastric pH, and small bowel oedema due to fluid overload.
- Hypoalbuminaemia, competition for binding to albumin by organic acids, and altered binding site conformation due to acidic environment all increase free and therefore active acidic drug availability.
- Increased concentration of alpha-1-glycoprotein increases binding of and therefore reduces effect of basic drugs.
- Hydrophilic drugs show an increased volume of distribution due to increased extracellular water, and so the serum concentration may decrease, especially with a loading dose.
- Altered metabolism due to impact of multiple drugs on cytochrome P450 with some enzymes induced and some inhibited.
- Reduced excretion of renally excreted drugs and their metabolites.

e) List four factors that should be considered when planning overall perioperative fluid requirements. (4 marks)

- Patient's dry weight.
- Patient's current weight.
- Patient's current dialysis mode, if applicable, and when dialysis last took place.
- Patient's ability to produce urine.
- Likely blood and fluid losses intraoperatively.
- Any period of restricted intake pre- and postoperatively.

f) List three issues that should be considered when planning postoperative analgesia for this patient. (3 marks)

- Contraindication to NSAIDs due to direct nephrotoxic effect, reduction in renal blood flow, increased bleeding risk, and reduction in potassium excretion.
- Reduced rate of renal excretion of active morphine metabolite, morphine-6-glucuronide, risking sedation and respiratory depression – need to reduce repeat doses or avoid use. Similar risk with codeine and dihydrocodeine.
- Tramadol is 30% excreted unchanged by kidney so risk of sedation and respiratory depression with its use. Also epileptogenic as seizure threshold reduced by uraemia.
- Hypotension associated with neuraxial techniques will lead to kidney hypoperfusion, which risks further impairment of function but cannot be treated with liberal fluid use due to risk of fluid overload.

REFERENCES

Chowdhury S, McLure H. Chronic kidney disease and anaesthesia. *BJA Educ.* 2022: 22: 321–328.
Mayhew D, Ridgway D, Hunter J. Update on the intraoperative management of adult cadaveric renal transplantation. *BJA Educ.* 2016: 16: 53–57.

11.3 March 2012 Patient blood management

A 57-year-old patient is scheduled for resection of a colonic carcinoma in three weeks' time. The haemoglobin is 100 g/l at time of referral to the pre-assessment clinic.

a) List two preoperative approaches that may reduce the risk of intraoperative allogeneic blood use. (2 marks)

b) List six intraoperative anaesthetic and surgical approaches that may reduce the risk of intraoperative allogeneic blood and blood component use. (6 marks)

c) List three aspects of the bedside check of a blood unit prior to transfusion. (3 marks)

d) List five signs that may indicate an acute transfusion reaction in this patient intraoperatively. (5 marks)

e) Give four additional pre- and intraoperative measures that should be taken or considered if the patient refuses blood transfusion. (4 marks)

The Chair's Report gave a 45.2% pass rate on the SAQ on this topic. They found the lack of knowledge of blood checking procedure "particularly disappointing." I have used updated sources to validate my answers to this CRQ as a decade has passed since 2012.

a) List two preoperative approaches that may reduce the risk of intraoperative allogeneic blood use. (2 marks)

If this surgery was fully elective, then surgery should be delayed in order to properly optimise the patient's haemoglobin.

- Antiplatelet and anticoagulant medications should be reviewed and stopping for appropriate duration preoperatively considered.
- Haemoglobin level should be optimised according to haematinics – it is likely to be an iron deficiency anaemia related to colonic carcinoma but may only be partially responsive to an iron infusion due to the presence of active cancer.

b) List six intraoperative anaesthetic and surgical approaches that may reduce the risk of intraoperative allogeneic blood and blood component use. (6 marks)

Depending on the nature of surgery, don't forget to ensure that positioning minimises the risk of obstructing venous drainage.

- Patient warming to maintain temperature > 36°C.
- Consideration of cell salvage use if blood loss greater than 500 ml anticipated.
- Consideration of tranexamic acid use if blood loss greater than 500 ml anticipated.
- Application of a restrictive transfusion threshold (Hb 70 g/l) if appropriate for the patient.
- Use of laparoscopic technique.
- Consideration of use of topical haemostatic agents.
- Application of single unit blood transfusion policy with reassessment of need between units.
- Use of point-of-care haemoglobin and coagulation testing.

c) List three aspects of the bedside check of a blood unit prior to transfusion. (3 marks)

- Perform check in close proximity to patient using their wristband, which should have four core identifiers: first name, last name, date of birth, a patient identification number.
- Check four core identifiers match those on blood unit.
- Check the compatibility label attached to the blood unit has the same 14-digit number as the sticker on the blood unit bag.
- Check blood unit expiry date and time.
- Visually check bag for leakage, discolouration, clots or clumps.

d) List five signs that may indicate an acute transfusion reaction in this patient intraoperatively. (5 marks)

- Fever.
- Rash.
- Angioedema.
- Hypoxia.
- Wheeze.
- Hypotension, cardiovascular collapse.
- Bleeding diathesis with acute onset.

e) Give four additional pre- and intraoperative measures that should be taken or considered if the patient refuses blood transfusion. (4 marks)

- Preoperative discussion about acceptability of all blood components, risks of refusing blood component administration, ascertainment of lack of any coercion or undue influence on decision-making, and advance decision paperwork completed accordingly.
- Discussion of process of cell salvage and acute normovolaemic haemodilution and their acceptability to the patient.
- Discussion of location for surgery e.g. if current hospital does not have capacity for cell salvage.
- Consideration (in conjunction with haematologist) of erythropoietin use alongside haematinics preoperatively.
- Discussion of status regarding blood product acceptability alongside the WHO checklist.
- Use of paediatric sampling bottles.
- Controlled hypotension if suitable for the individual patient.
- Consideration of desmopressin use in the event of bleeding.

REFERENCES

Association of Anaesthetists of Great Britain and Ireland. AAGBI guidelines: the use of blood components and their alternatives 2016. *Anaesthesia.* 2016: 71: 829–842.

Klein A et al. Association of Anaesthetists: anaesthesia and peri-operative care for Jehovah's witnesses and patients who refuse blood. *Anaesthesia.* 2018a: 74: 74–82.

Klein A et al. Association of Anaesthetists' guidelines: cell salvage for perioperative blood conservation 2018. *Anaesthesia.* 2018b: 73: 1141–1150.

Tinegate H et al. Guideline on the investigation and management of acute transfusion reactions prepared by the BCSH blood transfusion task force. *Br J Haem.* 2012: 159: 143–153.

11.4 September 2013 Enhanced recovery after surgery

A 74-year-old patient is scheduled for a primary total hip replacement.
a) List four potential benefits of an enhanced recovery programme for this type of surgery. (4 marks)
b) List five preoperative elements of an enhanced recovery protocol that should be implemented in the weeks leading up to admission. (5 marks)
c) List two preoperative elements of an enhanced recovery protocol that should be implemented in the 24 hours leading up to the time of surgery. (2 marks)
d) List five elements of intraoperative anaesthetic patient management for enhanced recovery. (5 marks)
e) List four elements of early postoperative pain management. (4 marks)

Since this topic was tested as an SAQ, the ERAS Society has issued recommendations for enhanced recovery after joint replacement and GIRFT has created a good practice guideline for the same. My answers are therefore based on these two sources. There has been criticism of the ERAS guideline in that the literature reviewed was from over five decades and therefore didn't necessarily reflect studies involving the sorts of approaches and techniques that may be viewed as current standard practice, and that much of the guidance was extrapolated from other sources and not from procedure-specific data. The Chair's Report from 2013 gave a list of factors that formed part of the model answer, and much of it is the same as the list I have given here in 2022 with just a few notable changes. Nonetheless, you don't need to remember it all to pass the question – the Chair said that it had been deemed an easy question, meaning that 14 marks out of 20 were necessary for a pass. There are more things to write down than points available, so this should be achievable. Despite this, the pass rate was only 49.9%.

a) **List four potential benefits of an enhanced recovery programme for this type of surgery. (4 marks)**

- Reduction of physiological stress.
- Maintenance and support of homeostasis and physiological function.
- Reduced length of stay.
- Reduction in complications.
- Reduction in healthcare costs per procedure.
- Maximisation of case numbers/reduction of waiting list times.
- Reduction of on the day cancellation.
- Reduction in surgical site infection.
- Improved patient experience/reduction in patient anxiety.

b) **List five preoperative elements of an enhanced recovery protocol that should be implemented in the weeks leading up to admission. (5 marks)**

- Preoperative education and counselling ("joint school" – to include input from physiotherapy, occupational therapy, nurse specialists, pain management team and may include dietetic input, weight management, and exercise advice).
- Smoking cessation for four weeks or more before surgery.
- Alcohol cessation programme attendance for patients who misuse alcohol.
- Identification, investigation and treatment of anaemia.
- Optimisation of diabetic control.
- Pharmacological optimisation of chronic diseases such as hypertension, heart disease, COPD.

- Optimisation of preoperative pain management and reduction in opioid use where feasible.
- MRSA and MSSA screening and treatment.
- Medication checking to ensure correct advice given regarding perioperative medication management (e.g. antiplatelets, ACE inhibitors).

c) **List two preoperative elements of an enhanced recovery protocol that should be implemented in the 24 hours leading up to the time of surgery. (2 marks)**

- Clear fluid to be taken until two hours or less preoperatively and solids up to six hours preoperatively.
- Consideration of use of high-energy drinks preoperatively.
- Staggered admission on day of surgery to minimise fasting and reduce anxiety.
- Patient prewarming.
- Oral opioid premedication.
- Showering with antimicrobial body wash preoperatively.

d) **List five elements of intraoperative anaesthetic patient management for enhanced recovery. (5 marks)**

- Single-shot spinal anaesthetic with light sedation as standard.
- General anaesthesia with fast-acting, rapid offset agents if neuraxial technique contraindicated (+/– nerve blocks).
- Avoidance of intrathecal opioid to minimise need for urinary catheterisation.
- Multimodal, opioid-sparing analgesia to be initiated intraoperatively, including intravenous paracetamol and local anaesthetic infiltration to incision site.
- Ketamine at induction for patients with chronic pain issues.
- Prophylactic antiemetics to be initiated intraoperatively.
- Intravenous and deep tissue topical administration of tranexamic acid.
- Antibiotic prophylaxis as per local policy 30 minutes prior to skin incision.
- Maintenance of normothermia.

e) **List four elements of early postoperative pain management. (4 marks)**

- Use of ice therapy.
- Assessment of pain at rest and on movement.
- Regular oral paracetamol.
- Regular ibuprofen if eGFR > 60, not on aspirin, and no other contraindications.
- Oral opioids for a maximum of 48 hours.
- Use of music for anxiolysis and improvement of patient satisfaction.

REFERENCES

Getting It Right First Time. *Hip and knee pathway guidance*, November 2020. https://gettingitrightfirsttime.co.uk/wp-content/uploads/2022/05/Hip-and-Knee-Pathway-Supporting-Guidance-2020-v7.1.pdf. Last accessed 8th December 2022.

Kehlet H, Memtsoudis S. ERAS guidelines for hip and knee replacement – need for reanalysis of evidence and recommendations? *Acta Orthop.* 2020: 91: 243–245.

Wainwright T et al. Consensus statement for perioperative care in total hip replacement and total knee replacement surgery: Enhanced Recovery After Surgery (ERAS) society recommendations. *Acta Orthop.* 2020: 91: 3–19.

11.5 September 2014 Rheumatoid arthritis

A 72-year-old patient with long-standing severe rheumatoid arthritis (RhA) presents for total knee replacement.
a) In the table below, list four joints that may be affected by RhA and indicate why their involvement has implications for anaesthesia. (8 marks)
b) Give two respiratory complications of RhA. (2 marks)
c) Give three cardiovascular complications of RhA. (3 marks)
d) Give three neurological complications of RhA. (3 marks)
e) Give two contributing causes for anaemia in patients with RhA. (2 marks)
f) List two possible hepatic complications of RhA. (2 marks)

The Chair said that the SAQ on this topic was one of the easiest on the paper but that the overall pass rate seemed very low at 41.9%, "given that patients with rheumatoid arthritis are regularly encountered in daily practice, particularly for arthroplasty procedures. The answers given by most candidates reveal a poor understanding of important factors in the preoperative assessment of these patients. Many scripts demonstrated a 'medical student' level of appreciation of the topic e.g. writing 'the neck' in response to the first question on joints affected by the disease."

a) In the table below, list four joints that may be affected by RhA and indicate why their involvement has implications for anaesthesia. (8 marks)

Rheumatoid arthritis is characterised by a chronic, destructive, symmetrical polyarthritis of mainly peripheral joints (fingers, elbows, ankles) but also more proximal joints (shoulders, neck, knees, hips). Any of these may be relevant as they will impact on positioning for regional and general anaesthesia as well as surgery itself, but they may also be the focus of the operation the patient is having.

Joint problem	Implications for anaesthesia
Temporomandibular joint swelling, degeneration.	Impact on mouth opening – restriction may necessitate fibreoptic nasal intubation.
Cricoarytenoid joint fixation.	May cause preoperative hoarseness – just a small degree of postoperative oedema could result in airway compromise.
Atlantoaxial subluxation.	Excessive movement may cause cord compression – may necessitate fibreoptic intubation.
Cervical ankylosis.	Limits neck extension – may cause difficult airway.
Costovertebral and costotransverse joint ankylosis.	Restrictive lung defect.
Interphalangeal joints and metacarpophalangeal joints inflammation, swelling, pain.	Inability to manage a PCA.

b) Give two respiratory complications of RhA. (2 marks)

- Fibrosing alveolitis causing restrictive defect.
- Pleurisy with effusion.
- Nodules.
- Costochondral disease causing reduced chest wall compliance.

c) Give three cardiovascular complications of RhA. (3 marks)

- Inflammatory pericarditis and pericardial effusion leading gradually to a restrictive pericarditis requiring pericardectomy. Rarely leads to tamponade.
- Rheumatoid nodules in any layer of the heart damaging valve function, causing conduction defects, and rarely congestive cardiac failure.
- Accelerated atherosclerosis and coronary artery disease due to chronic inflammatory state.

d) Give three neurological complications of RhA. (3 marks)

- Peripheral nerve entrapment (e.g. common peroneal, ulnar, median).
- Mononeuritis multiplex due to associated vasculitis.
- Glove-and-stocking peripheral neuropathy.
- Autonomic dysfunction.
- Compression of nerve roots, especially cervical spine.

e) Give two contributing causes for anaemia in patients with RhA. (2 marks)

- Normochromic, normocytic anaemia of chronic disease.
- Iron deficiency anaemia due to chronic gastrointestinal losses with NSAID or prednisolone treatment.
- Bone marrow depression due to disease-modifying anti-rheumatic drugs (e.g. methotrexate, hydroxychloroquine).

f) List two possible hepatic complications of RhA. (2 marks)

- Steatosis.
- Fibrosis.
- Cirrhosis — may relate to disease process or e.g. methotrexate.
- Intrahepatic small vessel arteritis.
- Amyloidosis — rare.
- Asymptomatic elevation of transaminases and cholestatic enzymes.

REFERENCE

Fombon F, Thompson J. Anaesthesia for the adult patient with rheumatoid arthritis. *Contin Educ Anaesth Crit Care Pain*. 2006: 6: 235–239.

11.6 September 2014 Myotonic dystrophy

A 35-year-old man presents for a laparoscopic cholecystectomy. He was diagnosed with myotonic dystrophy 10 years ago.
a) What is myotonic dystrophy, and how is it inherited? (2 marks)
b) What are the problems of myotonic dystrophy relevant to anaesthesia? (10 marks)
c) Outline the important aspects of preoperative assessment and intraoperative management that are specific to myotonic dystrophy. (8 marks)

This is the SAQ that featured in the September 2014 exam. The pass rate was just 6.5%. The Chair's Report said that "the prevalence of myotonic dystrophy is comparatively high, and anaesthetists are much more likely to encounter a patient with this condition than one with malignant hyperthermia risk. Poorly applied general anaesthesia causes significant morbidity and mortality in myotonic patients, and the disease is rightly considered an 'old chestnut,' which all clinicians should be able to manage appropriately. Most candidates had very poor knowledge of this subject, confusing myotonia with forms of muscular dystrophy whose prevalence is rarer. However, strong candidates scored significantly in excess of the pass mark, which suggests that their preparation for the Final FRCA examination was better. Most weak individuals thought incorrectly that suxamethonium was contraindicated due to a risk of hyperkalaemia and failed to mention the importance of preoperative echocardiography in detecting any associated cardiomyopathy. This question was a poor discriminator as so many candidates scored very poorly, and remedial reading on the topic is recommended for the majority of this cohort." Despite it being considered an "old chestnut," I have struggled to find comprehensive, up-to-date journal articles on the anaesthetic management of myotonic dystrophy.

For this particular SAQ, I also struggled with how you could answer parts (b) and (c) without repetition of content. Hopefully, the move to CRQ format will alleviate this issue. Meantime, here is a systems-based summary of myotonic dystrophy.

Airway:

- *Delayed gastric emptying and pharyngeal muscle wasting increases risk of aspiration – consider need for rapid sequence induction but avoiding use of suxamethonium.*

Respiratory:

- *Bulbar weakness leads to weak cough, risk of aspiration and increased likelihood of respiratory tract infection.*
- *Bulbar weakness can lead to obstructive sleep apnoea – may need NIV.*
- *Respiratory muscle weakness can lead to respiratory failure (may be using NIV long term), especially in the postoperative period.*
- *Centrally driven respiratory depression which can lead to central sleep apnoea and an exaggerated respiratory depressant response to opioids, sedative agents and intravenous anaesthetic agents.*
- *Restrictive lung defect due to progressive spinal deformity.*

Cardiovascular:

- *Progressive risk of conduction defects and arrhythmia – may result in sudden death – need regular ECG checks and may have pacemaker +/- ICD.*
- *Cardiomyopathy: progressive left ventricular failure leading to heart failure – need regular checks with echocardiography or CMR.*
- *Pulmonary hypertension secondary to chronic hypoventilation.*
- *Risk of embolic stroke due to predisposition to arrhythmia.*

Neurological:

- *Can result in reduced intelligence, may occasionally lead to problems with capacity and consent.*
- *Early cataracts affect vision.*

Endocrine:

- *Increased risk of insulin resistance or type 2 diabetes mellitus.*
- *Increased risk of hypothyroidism.*
- *Hypogonadism.*

Pharmacological:

- *Suxamethonium and neostigmine may trigger myotonia.*
- *Non-depolarising neuromuscular blocking agents may have prolonged action in the presence of muscle wasting. Consider using a smaller dose of short-acting agents e.g. atracurium, cis-atracurium. Sugammadex has been used without adverse incident – it is important that muscle relaxation is adequately reversed given the pre-existing risk of hypoventilation and respiratory failure.*
- *Anaesthetic agents have a more profound effect on respiratory function, vasodilation, and depressed cardiac function.*

Gastrointestinal:

- *Delayed gastric emptying, risk of reflux.*
- *Tendency to constipation due to reduced intestinal motility.*
- *Increased risk of gallstones due to impaired smooth muscle activity.*

Cutaneomusculoskeletal:

- *Muscle wasting. Careful padding of pressure points required. Care to avoid precipitating myotonia due to pain, or percussive or electrical stimulation.*

Metabolic:

- *At risk of myotonia due to hypothermia or shivering. Intraoperative warming essential with monitoring of effect.*

Obstetric:

- *Dysfunctional labour due to smooth muscle effects of the disease.*

REFERENCES

Ferschl M et al. *Practical suggestions for the anesthetic management of a myotonic dystrophy patient.* Myotonic Dystrophy Foundation. www.myotonic.org/sites/default/files/pages/files/MDF_PracticalSuggestionsDM1_AAnesthesi2_17_21.pdf. Accessed 9th December 2022.

Marsh S, Ross N, Pittard A. Neuromuscular disorders and anaesthesia: part 1: generic anaesthetic management. *Contin Educ Anaesth Crit Care Pain.* 2011: 11: 115–118.

Marsh S, Pittard A. Neuromuscular disorders and anaesthesia: part 2: specific neuromuscular disorders. *Contin Educ Anaesth Crit Care Pain.* 2011: 11: 119–123.

McNally E. Clinical care recommendations for cardiologists treating adults with myotonic dystrophy. *J Am Heart Assoc.* 2020: 9: 1–7.

Trip J et al. Drug treatment for myotonia (review). *Cochrane Database Syst Rev.* 2006: (1): Article No. CD004762.

11.7 March 2015 Chronic liver disease

a) List three common causes of chronic liver disease in adults. (3 marks)
b) Give two risk classification scoring systems that can be used to help predict perioperative risk in patients with chronic liver disease. (2 marks)
c) Give five pharmacokinetic issues that should be considered in the perioperative care of a patient with severe chronic liver disease. (5 marks)
d) Explain three respiratory issues associated with chronic liver disease that are of relevance to safe provision of anaesthesia. (3 marks)
e) Explain three cardiovascular issues associated with chronic liver disease that are of relevance to safe provision of anaesthesia. (3 marks)
f) List four possible perioperative precipitants of hepatic encephalopathy. (4 marks)

The SAQ on this topic in March 2015 was virtually identical to that from September 2011 but only had a 54.0% pass rate with 35.8% of candidates receiving a poor fail. The Chair said that the "question proved the most discriminatory question of the paper. Many candidates showed poor general knowledge of liver disease. Weak candidates were unable to associate the effects of chronic liver disease with the consequences for anaesthesia, which raises concerns for safe practice." The SAQ again asked candidates to "outline the Child-Pugh scoring system" but this time also asked for an explanation of "how this may be used to stratify mortality risk." I have addressed this back with the September 2011 SAQ. The SAQ also asked "which systemic effects of chronic liver disease are of importance to the anaesthetist and why," which would require the candidate to address all body systems. Only the respiratory, cardiovascular and neurological systems are included in my CRQ below, so here is a brief summary of some of the impact of chronic liver disease on some of the other body systems.

Airway:

- *Risk of reflux due to raised intra-abdominal pressure due to ascites. Rapid sequence induction and premedication with proton pump inhibitor required.*

Gastrointestinal:

- *Risk of varices and gastric erosions with consequent blood loss – stomach may therefore be full of blood necessitating rapid sequence induction. Oesophageal Doppler contraindicated in the presence of varices.*
- *Risk of spontaneous bacterial peritonitis.*

Haematological:

- *Anaemia due to chronic blood loss from gastrointestinal tract, hypersplenism-induced haemolysis, chronic illness, and malnutrition.*
- *Coagulopathy due to failure to synthesise most clotting factors, but prothrombotic tendency due to associated failure to synthesise factors such as protein C, protein S, and antithrombin alongside an increased production of von Willebrand's factor and factor VIII.*
- *Thrombocytopaenia due to splenic sequestration and impaired production, as well as platelet dysfunction.*
- *Normal or high fibrinogen (an acute phase protein) levels in early stages of disease followed by reduced production in later stages of disease as well as hyperfibrinolysis.*
- *Overall, coagulation is dysregulated, and viscoelastic testing e.g. ROTEM or TEG will allow a global assessment of coagulation that the traditional approach of monitoring prothrombin time or INR does not.*

Immune, infection:

- *Reduced immune function, infection prone.*

Renal:

- *Hepatorenal syndrome (renal dysfunction occurring because of chronic poor perfusion due to the disproportionately low SVR in relation to circulating volume. Renal arteries vasoconstrict in response to the activation of the renin-angiotensin-aldosterone system and sympathetic nervous system, but renal perfusion remains inadequate nonetheless).*
- *Secondary hyperaldosteronism contributes to ascites, effusions, and peripheral oedema.*

Metabolic:

- *Depletion of hepatic and muscle glycogen stores increases risk of hypoglycaemia.*
- *Electrolyte disturbance due to hormonal responses to widespread vasodilation.*

a) **List three common causes of chronic liver disease in adults. (3 marks)**

- Alcoholic liver disease.
- Non-alcoholic fatty liver disease (caused by obesity, diabetes).
- Viral hepatitis, B and C.
- Autoimmune causes: primary biliary cholangitis, sclerosing cholangitis.
- Metabolic disease: Wilson's, haemochromatosis, alpha-1-antitrypsin deficiency.
- Toxins, drugs.
- Right heart failure.

b) **Give two risk classification scoring systems that can be used to help predict perioperative risk in patients with chronic liver disease. (2 marks)**

The first two listed are most commonly used.

- Child-Pugh score/Child-Turcotte-Pugh score.
- Model for End-Stage Liver Disease (MELD).
- American Society of Anesthesiologists (ASA) Physical Status.
- Mayo Clinic postoperative mortality risk in patients with cirrhosis calculator.
- VOCAL-Penn model.

c) **Give five pharmacokinetic issues that should be considered in the perioperative care of a patient with severe chronic liver disease. (5 marks)**

Remember; absorption, distribution, metabolism, excretion.

- Increased bioavailability of oral medications due to portosystemic shunting or reduced first pass metabolism.
- Increased volume of distribution of water-soluble drugs as increased total body water causes a reduction in concentration (e.g. NMBD).
- Increased free fraction of highly protein bound drugs due to reduction in liver manufacture of plasma proteins, resulting in increased drug activity and side effects (e.g. thiopentone and propofol).
- Reduction in rate of metabolism of hepatically metabolised drugs thus prolonging pharmacological action (e.g. opioids, NMBD).
- Reduction in rate of metabolism of prodrugs into their active form (e.g. codeine), thus reducing their effectiveness.

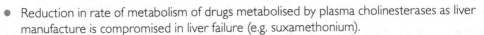

- Reduction in rate of metabolism of drugs metabolised by plasma cholinesterases as liver manufacture is compromised in liver failure (e.g. suxamethonium).
- Reduced rate of excretion of renally excreted drugs in the presence of hepatorenal syndrome.

d) **Explain three respiratory issues associated with chronic liver disease that are of relevance to safe provision of anaesthesia. (3 marks)**

- Diaphragmatic splinting due to ascites, resulting in basal atelectasis, V/Q mismatch, reduced functional residual capacity. May require diuresis, paracentesis with albumin replacement, and sodium and water restriction preoperatively in order to improve ventilatory mechanics.
- Pleural effusions and hepatic hydrothorax *(ascites fluid entering the thorax)* can impact on lung expansion, impairing gas exchange. May need to be drained preoperatively.
- Hepatopulmonary syndrome: failure of clearance of vasodilatory mediators causes pulmonary vasodilation, V/Q mismatch, and thus hypoxia that cannot be corrected by administration of oxygen. *Causes platypnoea (shortness of breath relieved by lying down) and orthodeoxia (decreased oxygen saturations on sitting up).*

e) **Explain three cardiovascular issues associated with chronic liver disease that are of relevance to safe provision of anaesthesia. (3 marks)**

- Reduction in clearance and/or increased production of vasodilatory mediators and increased intestinal bacterial translocation, resulting in an inflammatory response which results in vasodilation with consequential sodium and water retention resulting in increased heart rate and cardiac output. Hypovolaemia will be poorly tolerated under anaesthesia but excessive fluid administration will lead to further increases in venous return with risk of pulmonary oedema and hepatic congestion.
- Cirrhotic cardiomyopathy; systolic and diastolic dysfunction thought to be related to changes in ion conductance in heart muscle, fibrosis and oedema, altered autonomic input, and increased exposure to cardiodepressant mediators. Perioperative stress may result in decompensation and congestive cardiac failure.
- Portopulmonary hypertension and right ventricular dysfunction – pulmonary hypertension due to increased venous return due to portosystemic shunting and increased overall blood volume. Intraoperative hypoxia, hypercapnia, or positive pressure ventilation may lead to right heart failure.
- Heart disease associated with the underlying cause of chronic liver disease e.g. dilated cardiomyopathy associated with excessive alcohol intake, or ventricular hypertrophy associated with haemochromatosis. Perioperative stress may lead to decompensation.
- Pericardial effusion may result in inability to cope with either increases or decreases in circulating volume.

f) List four possible perioperative precipitants of hepatic encephalopathy. (4 marks)

Hepatic encephalopathy is incompletely understood. It is associated with an increase in ammonia, which then bypasses liver metabolism due to portosystemic shunting, thus increasing delivery to the brain, where it is converted to glutamine in astrocytes. Excessive glutamine from increased ammonia delivery results in cell oedema and ultimately whole brain oedema resulting in a range of presentations from mild confusion through to coma with brain herniation. Lactulose acidifies the gut to decrease ammonia absorption and oral antibiotics such as rifaximin or vancomycin will reduce the population of ammonia-producing gut bacteria.

- Gastrointestinal bleed.
- Infection.
- Sedative drugs.
- Hypoglycaemia.
- Hypotension.
- Hypoxia.
- Electrolyte disturbance.

REFERENCES

Gilbert-Kawai N, Hogan B, Milan Z. Perioperative management of patients with liver disease. *BJA Educ.* 2022: 22: 111–117.

Kiamanesh D et al. Monitoring and managing hepatic disease in anaesthesia. *BJA.* 2013: 111(suppl 1): i50–i61.

Moller S, Henriksen J. Cirrhotic cardiomyopathy: a pathophysiological review of circulatory dysfunction in liver disease. *Heart.* 2002: 87: 9–15.

Vaja R, McNicol L, Sisley I. Anaesthesia for patients with liver disease. *Contin Educ Anaesth Crit Care Pain.* 2010: 10: 15–19.

11.8 September 2016 Enhanced recovery after surgery

A 74-year-old patient is scheduled for a primary total hip replacement.

a) What are the potential benefits of an enhanced recovery ("fast-track") programme for this type of surgery? (4 marks)

b) List the preoperative (6 marks), intraoperative (7 marks) and postoperative (3 marks) measures that should be included in the enhanced recovery programme for this patient.

This is the SAQ that appeared in September 2016. The Chairs stated a pass rate of 59.4% and said that "this was predicted to be an easy question, and whilst most candidates answered it well, some did not appear to know the reasons for having an enhanced recovery program nor what the elements of it would be. This is surprising given that most hospitals now run such programs for their patients in various surgical areas." It is even more surprising that this was not well answered when you consider that a virtually identical question (with the Chairs' Report offering a really detailed list of what was required to pass) appeared just a few years earlier. It is worth looking at the enhanced recovery principles of other types of surgery as this is an important area of perioperative medicine.

11.9 March 2017 Anaemia

A patient scheduled for primary elective total knee replacement is found to be anaemic, with a haemoglobin level of 90 g/L.

a) List five perioperative consequences that may be associated with preoperative anaemia. (5 marks)

b) List four physiological adaptations that offset the effects of anaemia. (4 marks)

c) Give five perioperative events that may worsen the effects of anaemia. (5 marks)

d) List two blood test findings that would specifically support a diagnosis of iron deficiency as the cause of microcytic hypochromic anaemia. (2 marks)

e) Give the blood test finding that would support a diagnosis of functional iron deficiency in the presence of a microcytic hypochromic anaemia. (1 mark)

f) Give three blood test findings that would be supportive of a diagnosis of haemolytic anaemia. (3 marks)

The SAQ on this topic had a pass rate of just 29.5%. The Chairs said that "detailed knowledge of the consequences of anaemia and the physiological adaptations accompanying it was lacking. In particular, candidates scored poorly [when] asked about blood tests used to help classify anaemia." The wording of this part of the question in the SAQ was "What further blood tests may help in the classification of this anaemia? (5 marks)." I think that this could have led to a very long list of possible blood tests. I hope that the candidate may be a little more directed in a CRQ-style question, and I have altered the wording in my CRQ that follows to ask much more specific questions.

a) **List five perioperative consequences that may be associated with preoperative anaemia. (5 marks)**

- Cancellation and, therefore, delayed treatment.
- Increased length of hospital stay, increased length of ICU stay, increased all-cause morbidity and mortality.
- Increased risk of cardiac events, including myocardial infarction.
- Increased risk of respiratory, urinary, and wound infections.
- Increased risk of thromboembolic events.
- Delayed wound healing.
- Increased need for allogeneic blood transfusion and its risks.

b) **List four physiological adaptations that offset the effects of anaemia. (4 marks)**

- Increased oxygen extraction by tissues thus reducing SvO_2. Brain and heart already have high extraction ratios and so are unable to compensate further.
- Increased cardiac output: as a response to reduced systemic vascular resistance due to decreased blood viscosity, and also sympathetic response to hypoxia causing tachycardia.
- Redistribution of cardiac output to areas of high demand such as brain and heart.
- Rightward shift of oxygen dissociation curve due to increased 2,3 DPG, thus reducing the affinity of haemoglobin for oxygen, favouring oxygen offloading at tissues.

c) **Give five perioperative events that may worsen the effects of anaemia. (5 marks)**

- Increased oxygen requirement due to shivering, pain, stress response, fever.
- Hypoxaemia due to inadequate oxygen therapy, failure to adequately manage the airway, hypoventilation due to drug effects – results in overall reduced oxygen delivery.
- Blood loss due to surgery.
- Hypothermia causing leftward shift of oxygen dissociation curve.

- Reduced erythropoiesis due to inflammatory response.
- Reduced cardiac output due to anaesthetic agents.

d) List two blood test findings that would specifically support a diagnosis of iron deficiency as the cause of microcytic hypochromic anaemia. (2 marks)

Ferritin is the form in which iron is stored with protein in cells (especially macrophages and hepatocytes) and transferrin, as the name suggests, is the protein that moves iron around the blood stream to the point of use, the bone marrow, where it is incorporated into new red blood cells. The overall lack of iron in iron deficiency anaemia would mean that a lower proportion of transferrin is bound with iron, resulting in a low transferrin saturation. However, there is upregulation of the amount of transferrin in response to this situation, causing a high total iron binding capacity due to increased transferrin levels. Iron deficiency anaemia is a hypochromic, microcytic anaemia, but there are other causes of this – the following tests are the ones that would lead you to the diagnosis of iron deficiency.

- Low ferritin < 30 mcg/ml.
- Low transferrin saturation OR high total iron binding capacity/high transferrin.
- Low reticulocyte iron content.

e) Give the blood test finding that would support a diagnosis of functional iron deficiency in the presence of a microcytic hypochromic anaemia. (1 mark)

Acute phase mediators upregulate hepcidin, which binds to and degenerates ferroportin, the "doorway" that iron uses to get out of storage in macrophages and hepatocytes and into the body via the duodenal enterocytes. This results in ferritin levels remaining normal, but iron being unavailable for transport to the bone marrow to be incorporated into new red blood cells. It is thought to be an adaptive response to deprive any invading pathogen from benefiting from the body's iron stores. Markers of inflammation such as CRP or ESR or white cell count may be elevated in functional iron deficiency (anaemia of chronic disease) but may also be present in anaemias due to all sorts of other reasons.

- Normal or high ferritin.

f) Give three blood test findings that would be supportive of a diagnosis of haemolytic anaemia. (3 marks)

Physiological attempts to compensate for this type of anaemia will result in increased bone marrow production and so a high reticulocyte count. Lactate dehydrogenase is released from the breakdown of red blood cells, and haptoglobin is responsible for binding to free plasma haemoglobin to facilitate its removal from the blood stream by the liver.

- High reticulocyte count.
- Elevated lactate dehydrogenase.
- High serum iron.
- High free plasma haemoglobin.
- Low plasma haptoglobin.

REFERENCES

Clevenger B, Richards T. Pre-operative anaemia. *Anaesthesia.* 2015: 70(suppl 1): 20–28.

Guideline for Management of Anaemia in the Perioperative Pathway. London: Centre for Perioperative Care, 2022.

Hans G, Jones M. Preoperative anaemia. *Contin Educ Anaesth Crit Care Pain.* 2013: 13: 71–74.

11.10 September 2017 Cardiopulmonary exercise testing

The SAQ on this topic had a very poor pass rate of 24.3% with the Chairs commenting that it "was not well answered, which is surprising given the widespread use of cardiopulmonary exercise testing. The inclusion of perioperative medicine in the curriculum will hopefully lead to more exposure to this and other preoperative testing methods and to a greater understanding of risk assessment in general." The same aspects of knowledge about cardiopulmonary exercise testing were addressed in March 2022, and so I have addressed the topic there.

11.11 September 2017 Obstructive sleep apnoea

a) List four of the elements of the STOP-BANG assessment for a patient with suspected obstructive sleep apnoea (OSA). (4 marks)
b) State how the STOP-BANG assessment is used to quantify risk of OSA. (3 marks)
c) List three possible underlying causes for OSA. (3 marks)
d) List four cardiovascular comorbidities associated with OSA. (4 marks)
e) List three lifestyle issues that should be addressed in a patient with a recent diagnosis of OSA. (3 marks)
f) List three elements of intraoperative management of a patient with OSA. (3 marks)

The Chairs' Report for this question when it appeared as an SAQ revealed a 43.3% pass rate. The Chairs said that the "pass rate for this question was surprisingly low. Most candidates knew the elements of the STOP-BANG assessment but few knew how to use the score to quantify risk . . . those who remembered the importance of such things as the use of perioperative CPAP, short-acting anaesthetic agents, neuromuscular monitoring and of ensuring full reversal of muscle relaxation scored well here and tended to do well overall."

a) List four of the elements of the STOP-BANG assessment for a patient with suspected obstructive sleep apnoea (OSA). (4 marks)

S – loud snoring.
T – daytime tiredness.
O – observed cessation in breathing.
P – high blood pressure, treated or untreated.
B – BMI greater than 35 kg/m^2.
A – age greater than 50 years.
N – neck circumference greater than 40 cm.
G – male gender.

b) State how the STOP-BANG assessment is used to quantify risk of OSA. (3 marks)

- Score of 2 or less virtually excludes sleep apnoea.
- Score of 3–4 indicates intermediate risk of sleep apnoea.
- Score of 5–8 indicates high risk of sleep apnoea.

c) List three possible underlying causes for OSA. (3 marks)

OSA is most commonly associated with obesity and conditions associated with obesity. However, OSA happens because of a reduction in pharyngeal tone during sleep compromising an already altered airway, resulting in periods of partial or complete obstruction. There are a number of underlying conditions that can cause such an altered airway.

- Obesity.
- Congenital conditions associated with craniofacial abnormalities such as Down's syndrome, or Treacher Collins.
- Neuromuscular disorders such as myotonic dystrophy.
- History of mid-face fracture.
- ENT disorders such as adenotonsillar hypertrophy, deviated nasal septum, nasal polyps.
- Endocrine disorders such as hypothyroidism and acromegaly.

d) List four cardiovascular comorbidities associated with OSA. (4 marks)

Recurrent arousal from sleep results in disrupted sleep and adreno-cortical activation resulting in increased heart rate and blood pressure. OSA is a pro-inflammatory state which causes endothelial dysfunction and enhanced platelet activation. Recurrent episodes of hypoxia associated with apnoea or hypopnoea lead to hypoxic pulmonary vasoconstriction resulting in increased afterload to the right heart with consequent hypertrophy and, ultimately, failure.

- Arrhythmias.
- Hypertension.
- Diastolic and systolic ventricular dysfunction OR biventricular failure OR congestive heart failure.
- Pulmonary hypertension.
- Myocardial infarction.
- Stroke and TIA.

e) List three lifestyle issues that should be addressed in a patient with a recent diagnosis of OSA. (3 marks)

- Weight loss/prevention of further weight gain.
- Smoking cessation.
- Reduction of alcohol intake.
- Sleep hygiene.

f) List three elements of intraoperative management of a patient with OSA. (3 marks)

- Anticipation and planning for difficult airway.
- Avoidance of general anaesthesia if feasible with the use of neuraxial, regional, or local anaesthetic techniques.
- Use of short-acting agents such as desflurane, propofol, and remifentanil.
- Use of neuromuscular monitoring, full reversal using sugammadex if necessary, awake extubation.
- Use of multimodal analgesia to reduce/avoid need for long-acting opioid.

REFERENCES

American Society of Anesthesiologists. Practice guidelines for the perioperative management of patients with obstructive sleep apnea: an updated report by the American Society of Anesthesiologists task force on perioperative management of patients with obstructive sleep apnea. *Anesthesiology.* 2014: 120(2): 268–286.

Hall A. Sleep physiology and the perioperative care of patients with sleep disorders. *BJA Educ.* 2014: 15: 167–172.

Martinez G, Faber P. Obstructive sleep apnoea. *Contin Educ Anaesth Crit Care Pain.* 2011: 11: 5–8.

National Institute for Health and Care Excellence. *Obstructive sleep apnoea/hypopnoea syndrome and obesity hypoventilation syndrome in over 16s: NG202,* August 2021.

Society for Obesity and Bariatric Anaesthesia UK. *Recommendations for screening and management of sleep disordered breathing (SDB) in patients undergoing bariatric surgery: SOBA-UK consensus document,* 2016. www.dropbox.com/s/7njcdrrjfqgcyp1/SOBA%20OSA%20Guideline%202016.pdf?dl=0. Last accessed 16th December 2022.

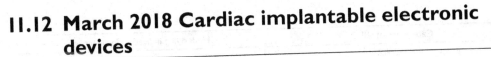

11.12 March 2018 Cardiac implantable electronic devices

a) List four categories of cardiac implantable electronic device (CIED) and an underlying indication for each. (8 marks)
b) List three aspects of function of a CIED for which reprogramming should be considered preoperatively. (3 marks)
c) State the reason for possible failure of arrhythmia management by a pacemaker in a patient having surgery that involves diathermy. (1 mark)
d) List four approaches to maximise the safety of intraoperative diathermy use in a patient who has a pacemaker for management of sinus bradycardia. (4 marks)
e) List two non-pharmacological steps in the management of severe intraoperative bradycardia in a patient with circulatory compromise and no pacemaker response. (2 marks)
f) List two pharmacological approaches to the management of severe intraoperative bradycardia in a patient with circulatory compromise and no pacemaker response. (2 marks)

When this topic appeared in an SAQ, the pass rate was 44.6%. The Chairs commented that it was "not a well answered question. Section (a) [List the possible indications for the insertion of cardiac implantable electronic devices. (5 marks)], in particular, was poorly answered reflecting a lack of basic medical knowledge. The section on management in the perioperative phase was well answered which is reassuring as it is important for patient safety."

a) List four categories of cardiac implantable electronic device (CIED) and an underlying indication for each. (8 marks)

Categories of CIED	Underlying indication for insertion
Permanent pacemaker.	• Symptomatic sinus node disease. • Third-degree heart block. • Second-degree type 2 heart block. • Infranodal second-degree heart block type 1. • Alternating bundle branch block. • Unexplained syncope and bifascicular block. • Severe, unpredictable, recurrent syncope with documented pauses.
Cardiac resynchronisation therapy device (may be a pacemaker or may have associated defibrillation capacity).	• Symptomatic heart failure with LVEF ≤ 35% despite optimal medical therapy with left bundle branch block QRS ≥ 130 ms. • Symptomatic heart failure with LVEF ≤ 35% despite optimal medical therapy with QRS ≤ 150 ms. • Heart failure NYHA class III or IV with LVEF ≤ 35% despite optimal medical therapy in atrial fibrillation with QRS ≥ 130 ms. • Symptomatic atrial fibrillation with uncontrolled heart rate in patient who is a candidate for atrioventricular junction ablation.

(Continued)

(Continued)

Categories of CIED	Underlying indication for insertion
Implantable cardioverter defibrillator.	• Primary prevention of serious arrhythmia in at risk patients e.g. due to familial condition increasing risk of sudden death in conjunction with poor prognostic indicators such as systolic dysfunction, NYHA II–III, gene abnormalities, history of VF or VT (long QT, Brugada, HOCM, arrhythmogenic right ventricular dysplasia) or following surgical repair of congenital heart disease. • Secondary prevention for people who have survived cardiac arrest due to a ventricular arrhythmia; have sustained, symptomatic VT; or have asymptomatic VT in association with heart failure with LVEF ≤ 35% and NYHA classification of ≤ III.
Implantable loop recorder.	• For investigation of symptoms possibly attributable to cardiac arrhythmia not detected on standard ECG, 24 hours or 72 hours cardiac monitoring.

b) **List three aspects of function of a CIED for which reprogramming should be considered preoperatively. (3 marks)**

The indication for changing to an asynchronous mode i.e. 0 at the third letter of the pacemaker function description, is generally when a patient is highly reliant on their pacemaker for achieving cardiac output. This may be seen on an ordinary 12-lead ECG if a pacing spike precedes most complexes, or on a pacemaker testing report. If diathermy is interpreted as cardiac electrical activity, then the pacemaker wouldn't trigger, and there is a risk of asystole. A default pacing rate is therefore chosen for these patients.

- Response mode changed to asynchronous pacing when there is significant pacemaker dependency.
- Advanced CIED functions may cause unhelpful rate changes perioperatively e.g. rate response function using minute ventilation to regulate pacing, sleep/rest mode especially if surgery late in the day.
- Defibrillator function should be switched off to eliminate risk of firing in response to electromagnetic interference if diathermy is used.

c) **State the reason for possible failure of arrhythmia management by a pacemaker in a patient having surgery that involves diathermy. (1 mark)**

- Interpretation by the pacemaker of diathermy current as cardiac electrical current and therefore failure of appropriate rate response.

d) **List four approaches to maximise the safety of intraoperative diathermy use in a patient who has a pacemaker for management of sinus bradycardia. (4 marks)**

- Consideration of use of asynchronous mode if surgical site is above the umbilicus.
- Use of bipolar rather than monopolar diathermy where feasible.
- Application of diathermy plate to direct current path away from pacemaker.
- Short rather than long bursts of diathermy.
- Visual assessment of impact of diathermy use on ECG monitoring confirmed with pulse palpation/invasive blood pressure monitoring of electrical capture if in doubt.

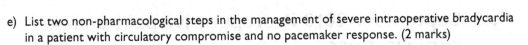

e) List two non-pharmacological steps in the management of severe intraoperative bradycardia in a patient with circulatory compromise and no pacemaker response. (2 marks)

- Correction of any abnormality of PaO_2, $PaCO_2$, acid-base balance or electrolyte level.
- Transcutaneous pacing.

f) List two pharmacological approaches to the management of severe intraoperative bradycardia in a patient with circulatory compromise and no pacemaker response. (2 marks)

- Atropine 500 mcg repeated to a maximum of 3 mg.
- Glycopyrrolate 200 mcg iv.
- Isoprenaline 5 mcg/min ivi.
- Adrenaline 2–10 mcg/min ivi.

Aminophylline, dopamine and glucagon in the case of a beta-blocker of calcium channel blocker overdose can be considered, but these are not first line.

REFERENCES

British Heart Rhythm Society. *British Heart Rhythm Society guidelines for the management of patients with cardiac implantable electrical devices (CIEDs) around the time of surgery*, January 2016, revised February 2019. https://bhrs.com/wp-content/uploads/2019/05/Revised-guideline-CIED-and-surgery-Feb-19.pdf. Last accessed 24th January 2023.

Bryant H et al. Perioperative management of patients with cardiac implantable electronic devices. *BJA Educ.* 2016: 16: 388–396.

National Institute for Health and Care Excellence. *Implantable cardioverter defibrillators and cardiac resynchronisation therapy for arrhythmias and heart failure: TA314*, June 2014. www.nice.org.uk/guidance/ta314/chapter/1-Guidance. Last accessed 24th January 2023.

Resuscitation Council UK. *Adult Advanced Life Support guidelines: adult bradycardia guideline*, 2021. www.resus.org.uk/sites/default/files/2021-04/Bradycardia%20Algorithm%202021.pdf. Last accessed 24th January 2023.

Task Force on Cardiac Pacing and Cardiac Resynchronization Therapy of the European Society of Cardiology (ESC). 2021 ESC guidelines on cardiac pacing and cardiac resynchronization therapy. *Eur Heart J.* 2021: 00: 1–94.

Zeppenfeld K et al. 2022 ESC guidelines for the management of patients with ventricular arrhythmias and the prevention of sudden cardiac death: developed by the task force for the management of patients with ventricular arrhythmias and the prevention of sudden cardiac death of the European Society of Cardiology (ESC) endorsed by the Association for European Paediatric and Congenital Cardiology (AEPC). *Eur Heart J.* 2022: 40: 3997–4126.

11.13 September 2018 Postoperative pulmonary complications

a) List four postoperative pulmonary complications that may occur following non-cardiothoracic surgery. (4 marks)

b) List four patient-related (4 marks) and two surgery-related (2 marks) risk factors for postoperative pulmonary complications following non-cardiothoracic surgery.

c) List four aspects of general anaesthesia that may contribute to postoperative pulmonary complications. (4 marks)

d) List two preoperative strategies that may be considered to reduce the risk of postoperative pulmonary complications in the weeks leading up to surgery. (2 marks)

e) List two intraoperative strategies that may be considered to reduce the risk of postoperative pulmonary complications. (2 marks)

f) List two postoperative strategies that may be considered to reduce the risk of postoperative pulmonary complications. (2 marks)

The pass rate for this question when it appeared as an SAQ was 63.2%. I have changed it very little to turn it into a CRQ, mainly just dividing the final part into pre-, intra-, and postoperative strategies. The Chairs said, "This is a question on a topic of great relevance to everyday practice and was reassuringly answered relatively well. The pass rate was good and the candidates generally exhibited good knowledge. However, there were still common errors in particular the last section gave lists of complications rather than strategies to avoid them. This may be an example of not reading the question properly." Just a year before this question appeared, there was a BJA Education article titled "Postoperative pulmonary complications following non-cardiothoracic surgery" – I know I am repeating myself, but please use BJA Education articles in your revision. There was also a BJA article in the same year on the same topic.

a) List four postoperative pulmonary complications that may occur following non-cardiothoracic surgery. (4 marks)

You should be able to reach a suitable list based on your own clinical experience – this list is straight out of a table in the BJA Education article I mentioned.

- Atelectasis.
- Pneumonia.
- Respiratory failure.
- Pleural effusion.
- Pneumothorax.
- Bronchospasm.
- Aspiration pneumonitis.

b) List four patient-related (4 marks) and two surgery-related (2 marks) risk factors for postoperative pulmonary complications following non-cardiothoracic surgery.

This list comes from the BJA Education article and also the BJA article referenced. I have ordered the patient risk factors such that those with more evidence to support their identification as a significant risk factor are towards the top of the list. A lack of evidence does not, of course, mean that they are not risk factors, but the evidence to support a risk factor can only be found if a well-planned study has been designed to find it. Cardiac and thoracic surgery are also associated with increased risk, but the question specifically asks about non-cardiothoracic surgery.

Patient:

- Age > 60 years.
- ASA ≥ 2.
- Functional dependency or frailty.
- Congestive heart failure.
- Chronic obstructive pulmonary disease, lung disease associated with chest X-ray abnormality, preoperative oxygen saturations < 96%.
- Chronic liver disease, hypoalbuminaemia, ascites.
- Smoking.
- Anaemia with haemoglobin < 10 g/l.
- Recent upper respiratory tract infection.
- Obstructive sleep apnoea.
- Male sex.
- Pulmonary hypertension.
- Diabetes mellitus.
- Impaired cognition or delirium.
- Excessive alcohol use.
- Weight loss > 10% within 6 months, or BMI < 18.5 kg/m^2.
- Disseminated cancer.
- BMI > 40 kg/m^2.
- Long-term steroid use.
- Preoperative sepsis or shock.

Surgery:

- Emergency surgery.
- Prolonged surgery, > 3 hours.
- Surgery type: abdominal, head and neck, major vascular and neurosurgery.

c) **List four aspects of general anaesthesia that may contribute to postoperative pulmonary complications. (4 marks)**

- Anaesthetic agents and opioids impair response to hypoxia and hypercapnia, impair hypoxic pulmonary vasoconstriction, reduce cough, and impair mucociliary function.
- Dry anaesthetic gases cause mucus plugging, atelectasis, V/Q mismatch.
- Residual neuromuscular block reduces ventilatory efficiency, impairs cough and swallow, resulting in increased atelectasis, hypoxia, aspiration, and increased risk of negative pressure pulmonary oedema.
- Absorption atelectasis following prolonged periods of 100% oxygen.
- Failure to manage pain, especially in abdominal surgery, may cause reduced mobilisation, failure to cough, failure to deep breathe, mucus plugging, V/Q mismatch, and hypoxia.
- In a spontaneously ventilating patient who is supine under general anaesthesia, the closing capacity approaches FRC resulting in collapse of small airways, atelectasis, and V/Q mismatch.

d) List two preoperative strategies that may be considered to reduce the risk of postoperative pulmonary complications in the weeks leading up to surgery. (2 marks)

The answers to the final three questions are again taken from the BJA Education article but have been updated based on newer publications, as referenced.

- Optimisation of existing cardiorespiratory disease.
- Early smoking cessation.
- Prehabilitation exercise programmes.

e) List two intraoperative anaesthetic strategies that may be considered to reduce the risk of postoperative pulmonary complications. (2 marks)

- Lung protective ventilatory strategy.
- Short-acting NMBD with quantitative monitoring.
- Goal-directed fluid therapy.

f) List two postoperative strategies that may be considered to reduce the risk of postoperative pulmonary complications. (2 marks)

- Adequate analgesia.
- Early mobilisation.
- Lung expansion techniques, respiratory physiotherapy.

REFERENCES

Assouline B et al. Preoperative exercise training to prevent postoperative pulmonary complications in adults undergoing major surgery: a systematic review and meta-analysis with trial sequential analysis. *Ann Am Thorac Soc.* 2021: 18: 678–688.

Davies O et al. Postoperative pulmonary complications following non-cardiothoracic surgery. *BJA Educ.* 2017: 17: 295–300.

Jessen M et al. Goal-directed haemodynamic therapy during general anaesthesia for noncardiac surgery: a systematic review and meta-analysis. *BJA.* 2021: 128: 416–433.

Miskovic A, Lumb A. Postoperative pulmonary complications. *BJA.* 2017: 118: 317–334.

11.14 March 2019 End-stage renal failure

a) List three of the commonest causes of end-stage renal failure (ESRF) in the United Kingdom. (3 marks)
b) List two respiratory complications of ESRF of importance to the anaesthetist. (2 marks)
c) List three cardiovascular complications of ESRF of importance to the anaesthetist. (3 marks)
d) List three possible causes of anaemia in ESRF. (3 marks)
e) List three acute physiological or metabolic disturbances that may be seen in a patient who has just had haemodialysis. (3 marks)
f) List six key practical considerations when providing general anaesthesia for a patient with ESRF on haemodialysis. (6 marks)

Renal failure features commonly in the Final written exam and so it should; it is a commonly encountered comorbidity. The Chairs reported a pass rate for the SAQ of 70.7% and said it was an "important topic that was generally well answered. Poorer candidates tended to struggle in [the complications of ESRF of importance to the anaesthetist, and the key practical considerations when providing anaesthesia for a patient with ESRF on haemodialysis] and this may be a reflection of a lack of clinical experience. . . . In the last section, candidates who scored poorly tended to give generic answers with little explanation of the practical considerations in this group of patients."

a) **List three of the commonest causes of end-stage renal failure (ESRF) in the United Kingdom. (3 marks)**

I have listed these in order of incidence.

- Diabetes mellitus.
- Glomerulonephritis.
- Polycystic kidney disease.
- Hypertension.
- Pyelonephritis.
- Renal vascular disease.

b) **List two respiratory complications of ESRF of importance to the anaesthetist. (2 marks)**

- Fluid overload causing pulmonary oedema and impaired gas exchange.
- Pleural effusion.
- Fibrinous pleuritis.
- Pulmonary calcification and restrictive lung defect.
- Predisposition to pneumonia due to oedema and immunosuppressed state of ESRF.
- Obstructive sleep apnoea.

c) **List three cardiovascular complications of ESRF of importance to the anaesthetist. (3 marks)**

- Accelerated coronary artery disease.
- Hypertension (*results from ESRF due to factors such as activation of the renin-angiotensin-aldosterone system, increased arterial stiffness, endothelial dysfunction, activation of the sympathetic nervous system, and sodium and water retention. It is also a cause of ESRF, and may be a side effect of immunosuppressive drugs*).
- Arrhythmia due to calcification of conduction pathways and electrolyte imbalance.
- Valvular dysfunction due to calcification.
- Pericardial effusion.

d) **List three possible causes of anaemia in ESRF. (3 marks)**

- Lack of erythropoietin production.
- Anaemia of chronic disease.
- Iron deficiency anaemia due to altered appetite or absorption with illness, frequent blood sampling, loss with dialysis, and gastrointestinal losses due to uraemic-induced gastritis.

e) **List three acute physiological or metabolic disturbances that may be seen in a patient who has just had haemodialysis. (3 marks)**

- Hypotension and tachycardia due to intravascular fluid depletion.
- Electrolyte changes, including hypokalaemia, risking arrhythmia.
- Dialysis disequilibrium syndrome – cerebral oedema with associated symptoms.
- Hypoglycaemia.
- Acute blood loss due to needling complications and associated heparin use.

f) **List six key practical considerations when providing general anaesthesia for a patient with ESRF on haemodialysis. (6 marks)**

- Protection of fistula (no cannulation or taking of blood pressure on that limb, protection when positioning)/line (avoid use, strict asepsis if becomes necessary).
- Protection of veins and arteries for future fistula formation (avoid use of subclavian line for central line as it risks stenosis and loss of use of that arm for future fistula formation, use arterial monitoring only when necessary and as distal as possible).
- Consider need for reversal of heparin if dialysed recently and surgery is urgent.
- Recent heparin administration may render neuraxial approaches inappropriate.
- Consider need for preoperative dialysis if approaching usual timing of dialysis or risk starting surgery fluid overloaded, hyperkalaemic, and uraemic if this is not done.
- Consider haemodynamic status of the patient if they have had recent dialysis – may require cautious volume loading to facilitate stable induction.
- Consider how haemodialysis will be delivered postoperatively if the surgery necessitates inpatient stay – patient may need to be relocated to a hospital that offers on-site haemodialysis.
- Consideration of appropriate drugs for use in patients with ESRF – avoid drugs that accumulate e.g. morphine, nephrotoxins e.g. NSAIDs if the patient still passes urine, and suxamethonium if there is hyperkalaemia/high-normal potassium level.
- Plan for management of the patient's regular medications, which may include: immunosuppressants that shouldn't be stopped perioperatively; steroids, which may require the patient to receive supplementation; diabetes management, which may need adjustment during perioperative starvation; and ACE inhibitors, which may need to be paused preoperatively to avoid haemodynamic instability.

REFERENCES

Bradley T et al. Anaesthetic management of patients requiring vascular access surgery for renal dialysis. *BJA Educ.* 2017: 17: 269–274.

Mayhew D et al. Update on the intraoperative management of adult cadaveric renal transplantation. *BJA Educ.* 2016: 16: 53–57.

11.15 March 2019 Prehabilitation

a) What is prehabilitation in perioperative medicine? (1 mark)
b) List three outcome benefits of a prehabilitation programme. (3 marks)
c) List six specific issues that are addressed as part of medical optimisation in a prehabilitation programme. (6 marks)
d) Give three ways in which a prehabilitation exercise programme may improve a patient's cardiorespiratory physiology. (3 marks)
e) Give two benefits of carbohydrate preloading. (2 marks)
f) Give three possible benefits of nutritional optimisation preoperatively. (3 marks)
g) List two psychologically supportive interventions that may be used in prehabilitation. (2 marks)

The pass rate for the SAQ on this topic was 71.4%. The Chairs said, "Prehabilitation is topical and relevant to clinical practice, covering both perioperative medicine and basic sciences. This was a new question and was anticipated to be difficult for the candidates. Reassuringly this was well answered by the majority of candidates and had a good pass rate." Difficult SAQs required 10–11/20 in order to pass. They also said that the "basic sciences component of the question [regarding impact of prehabilitation on cardiovascular physiology] along with the benefits of carbohydrate preloading . . . were both poorly answered." In 2017 an article titled "Prehabilitation" appeared in the BJA Education; its text reads like a marking scheme for this question, and I have relied on it entirely for my answers here.

a) What is prehabilitation in perioperative medicine? (1 mark)

- The process of enhancing an individual's functional capacity to enable them to withstand a forthcoming stressor such as major surgery.

b) List three outcome benefits of a prehabilitation programme. (3 marks)

- Reduced length of stay.
- Less postoperative pain.
- Fewer postoperative complications.
- Reduced cost per case to the health service/ability to provide care to more patients.

c) List six specific issues that are addressed as part of medical optimisation in a prehabilitation programme. (6 marks)

- Smoking cessation.
- Alcohol reduction.
- Weight optimisation.
- Anaemia management.
- Blood glucose control.
- Pharmacological optimisation of chronic diseases such as hypertension, heart disease, COPD.

d) Give three ways in which a prehabilitation exercise programme may improve a patient's cardiorespiratory physiology. (3 marks)

Raising fitness above a patient's previous baseline means that the inevitable postoperative dip (due to the catabolic effects of the physiological challenge that is surgery) might not bring them below the critical level required for day-to-day functioning, or will bring them below that level for a shorter time period.

- Increased stroke volume (physiological ventricular hypertrophy in response to longer-term exercise) and hence cardiac output.
- Increased skeletal and respiratory muscle mitochondrial numbers increases the capacity for peripheral oxygen utilisation, increasing VO_2 max.
- Increased blood flow to the lungs for gas exchange due to pulmonary vasodilation.
- Improved respiratory muscle strength resulting in an ability to sustain ventilation at a higher rate and larger tidal volume.
- Development of greater numbers of capillaries in skeletal muscle reducing the afterload to the heart.

e) Give two benefits of carbohydrate preloading. (2 marks)

- Reduces insulin resistance.
- Promotes anabolism.
- Reduces protein (muscle) catabolism.
- Maintains muscle and liver glycogen stores during a period of starvation.

f) Give three possible benefits of nutritional optimisation preoperatively. (3 marks)

- Improved immune function/reduction in perioperative infection risk.
- Improved wound healing.
- Reduction in risk of organ dysfunction.
- Improved functional recovery.
- Improved muscle bulk/reduction in loss of muscle bulk.

g) List two psychologically supportive interventions that may be used in prehabilitation. (2 marks)

- Procedural instruction.
- Relaxation techniques.
- Cognitive interventions.
- Support groups with similar patients.

REFERENCES

Banugo P, Amoako D. Prehabilitation. *BJA Educ.* 2017: 17: 401–405.
Gillis C, Wischmeyer P. Pre-operative nutrition and the elective surgical patient: why, how and what? *Anaesthesia.* 2019: 74: 27–35.

11.16 September 2019 Aortic stenosis

a) List two underlying causes of aortic stenosis. (2 marks)
b) Give values for the peak aortic flow velocity (m/s), mean transaortic pressure gradient (mmHg), and valve area (cm²) that would indicate severe aortic stenosis. (3 marks)
c) List three cardiac investigations that may be used in assessment of the severity of aortic stenosis. (3 marks)
d) List three classical presenting features of aortic stenosis. (3 marks)
e) Describe the changes that occur to the left ventricle with worsening aortic stenosis, initially compensating for its effect and latterly resulting in decompensation and display of the presenting features described. (5 marks)
f) List four haemodynamic goals during surgery for a patient with severe aortic stenosis. (4 marks)

Aortic stenosis features in the exam on two other occasions in the time period covered by this book, and these questions can be found in the cardiothoracic chapter as they relate to interventions for aortic stenosis, whereas this CRQ is relevant to the perioperative management of a patient with aortic stenosis undergoing any type of surgery. The Chairs said that the pass rate for the CRQ on this topic was 66.7% and that "aortic stenosis is a common condition, and its pathophysiology and management should be known to candidates sitting this exam. Candidates continue to underestimate the importance of basic sciences and how they underpin anaesthesia. . . . Candidates were unable to discuss in any detail the changes that occur in the left ventricle in patients with aortic stenosis." I don't know exactly what was asked in the CRQ in the exam, but clearly the College wanted the candidates to know about the progressive changes to the left ventricle with worsening aortic stenosis, and so I have included a section on this with more detail than is likely to be needed to aid understanding.

a) List two underlying causes of aortic stenosis. (2 marks)

- Bicuspid aortic valve or other congenital valve abnormality.
- Rheumatic fever.
- Calcification of the aortic valve.

b) Give values for the peak aortic flow velocity (m/s), mean transaortic pressure gradient (mmHg), and valve area (cm²) that would indicate severe aortic stenosis. (3 marks)

It is now recognised that aortic stenosis may occur in the absence of elevated flow velocity or mean pressure gradient – it is the valve area that is the unifying diagnostic criterion.

- Peak aortic jet velocity > 4 m/s.
- Mean transaortic pressure gradient > 40 mmHg.
- Valve area < 1.0 cm² (equal to an indexed valve area of < 0.6 cm/m² BSA).

c) List three cardiac investigations that may be used in assessment of the severity of aortic stenosis. (3 marks)

ECG and BNP do not give diagnostic input into the severity of aortic stenosis.

- Transthoracic or trans-oesophageal echocardiogram (to assess valve area, peak flow velocity, mean pressure gradient, assess for regurgitation, and to assess for consequences of aortic stenosis such as left ventricular hypertrophy, presence of mitral regurgitation, pulmonary artery pressure, post-stenotic ascending artery dilatation).
- Left heart catheter invasive haemodynamic measurements.

- Low-dose dobutamine stress testing in conjunction with echo or invasive haemodynamic measurements.
- Cardiac CT to measure aortic valve calcium score.
- Cardiac MRI.
- Exercise testing *(to confirm absence of symptoms)*.

d) List three classical presenting features of aortic stenosis. (3 marks)

- Presyncope, syncope.
- Dyspnoea, heart failure.
- Angina.
- Sudden death.

e) Describe the changes that occur to the left ventricle with worsening aortic stenosis, initially compensating for its effect and latterly resulting in decompensation and display of the presenting features described. (5 marks)

Remember that coronary perfusion pressure is the difference between aortic diastolic pressure and left ventricular end diastolic pressure. As blood passes through the narrowed valve, it accelerates, gaining kinetic energy. By the law of conservation of energy, it loses pressure, resulting in reduced perfusion pressure to the coronary arteries.

- Increased left ventricular systolic pressure results in compensatory left ventricular hypertrophy, thus preserving systolic function.
- Left ventricular hypertrophy increases oxygen demand but also decreases oxygen supply.
- Bulkier ventricle relaxes less effectively in diastole leading to diastolic dysfunction.
- Progression of diastolic dysfunction and ventricular hypertrophy lead to subendocardial ischaemia.
- Progression of diastolic dysfunction leads to pulmonary congestion and shortness of breath.
- Ejection fraction deteriorates in the face of progressive outflow restriction, reduced end diastolic volume due to worsening diastolic dysfunction, left ventricular dilatation, and myocardial dysfunction due to an imbalance between oxygen demand and supply.

f) List four haemodynamic goals during surgery for a patient with severe aortic stenosis. (4 marks)

I have included some detail about how these goals could be achieved in case you are asked about the conduct of anaesthesia necessary to achieve the desired haemodynamic goals for a patient with aortic stenosis.

- Maintenance of preload *(cardiac output dependent on adequate diastolic filling which is compromised by the increased bulk of the left ventricle)*.
- Maintenance of sinus rhythm *(contribution of atrial contraction to left ventricular filling increasingly important – maintain normal acid-base status, gas exchange, and electrolyte levels, and ensure continuation of medications for arrhythmias)*.
- Maintenance of normal heart rate *(tachycardia results in shortened diastolic time which will further impair filling and coronary perfusion – bradycardia is also problematic as a very hypertrophic heart is unable to compensate for reduction in cardiac output due to bradycardia with increased stroke volume)*.
- Maintenance of cardiac contractility *(this is impaired with the development of hypertrophy – avoidance of excessive anaesthetic agents, ensuring normal gas exchange and acid-base status, use of inotropic support as guided by invasive monitoring)*.

- Maintenance of afterload/blood pressure *(to preserve coronary perfusion – avoidance of excessive anaesthetic depth, caution with use of neuraxial techniques, use of vasopressors as guided by invasive monitoring).*

REFERENCES

Chacko M, Weinberg L. Aortic valve stenosis: perioperative anaesthetic implications of surgical replacement and minimally invasive interventions. *Contin Educ Anaesth Crit Care Pain.* 2012: 12: 302–306.

National Institute for Health and Care Excellence. *Heart valve disease presenting in adults: investigation and management: NG208,* November 2021.

Nishimura R et al. 2014 AHA/ACC guideline for the management of patients with valvular heart disease: executive summary. *Circulation.* 2014: 129: 2440–2492.

11.17 September 2019 Myasthenia gravis

a) List three clinical features of myasthenia gravis. (3 marks)
b) State the most common underlying cause of muscle weakness in myasthenia gravis. (1 mark)
c) List three comorbidities that patients with myasthenia gravis are at elevated risk of developing. (3 marks)
d) List four possible triggers, of relevance to the anaesthetist, of a myasthenic crisis. (4 marks)
e) List three management strategies for the treatment of myasthenia gravis. (3 marks)
f) State three elements of management of neuromuscular blockade with a non-depolarising agent for a patient with myasthenia gravis. (3 marks)
g) State the altered response to suxamethonium in patients with myasthenia gravis. (1 mark)
h) List two drugs that may be used in the management of a cholinergic crisis. (2 marks)

The Chairs said that the pass rate for the CRQ on this topic was 54.9%. "The knowledge component of this question was answered well. However, the more clinical aspects of this question . . . were answered poorly."

a) List three clinical features of myasthenia gravis. (3 marks)

- Ocular muscle weakness, ptosis, diplopia.
- Generalised muscle weakness, limbs and trunk, symmetrical, more marked proximally.
- Respiratory and bulbar muscle weakness, including respiratory failure.
- Fatiguability – symptoms least severe in the morning, worse with exercise/muscle use, improve with rest.

b) State the most common underlying cause of muscle weakness in myasthenia gravis. (1 mark)

Some patients are seronegative, and some have antibodies against MuSK or LRP4, which are involved in inducing acetylcholine receptor clustering and therefore function at the neuromuscular junction.

- B-cell autoantibody production against acetylcholine receptors resulting in their conformational change and degradation and thus failure of nerve transmission at the neuromuscular junction.

c) List three comorbidities that patients with myasthenia gravis are at elevated risk of developing. (3 marks)

Thymoma is a more common association in patients with early onset of disease. Myasthenia gravis is also associated with a range of other autoimmune conditions.

- Thymoma.
- Autoimmune thyroid disease.
- Systemic lupus erythematosus.
- Rheumatoid arthritis.
- Dermatopolymyositis.
- Addison's disease.
- Cardiac involvement: ECG changes, myocarditis, conduction disorders, ventricular tachycardia, sudden death.

d) List four possible triggers, of relevance to the anaesthetist, of a myasthenic crisis. (4 marks)

A myasthenic crisis is when there is insufficient nerve transmission at the neuromuscular junction to facilitate normal muscle function, resulting in severe respiratory and bulbar muscle weakness necessitating invasive ventilation. It can be the mode of presentation of myasthenia gravis.

- Infection.
- Surgery.
- Residual neuromuscular block after anaesthesia.
- Pain.
- Hypo- or hyperthermia.
- Alteration to myasthenia gravis treatment.
- Pregnancy.
- Stress.
- Sleep deprivation.
- Drugs e.g. aminoglycosides, beta-blockers, corticosteroids, macrolide antibiotics, calcium channel blockers, magnesium, phenytoin.

e) List three management strategies for the treatment of myasthenia gravis. (3 marks)

Thymectomy may be required to remove a thymoma and also to remove the source of autoantibodies.

- Symptomatic treatment with acetylcholinesterase inhibitors (e.g. pyridostigmine with oral antimuscarinic drug to reduce muscarinic adverse effects).
- Long-term immunosuppression (options include corticosteroids, azathioprine, mycophenolate mofetil, methotrexate, ciclosporin, rituximab).
- Acute immunomodulation with intravenous immunoglobulin or plasma exchange in the event of acute deterioration or significant bulbar and respiratory symptoms.
- Thymectomy for patients with thymoma and younger patients with positive anti-AChR antibodies.

f) State three elements of management of neuromuscular blockade with a non-depolarising agent for a patient with myasthenia gravis. (3 marks)

Myasthenia gravis leads to a lack of functional acetylcholine receptors – only a small dose of a non-depolarising agent is therefore required to produce an effect equivalent to that in a patient not affected by myasthenia gravis.

- Use of 1/10th usual dose required for intubation and titrated incrementally if required.
- Use of train-of-four monitoring, ideally quantitative.
- Reversal with sugammadex.
- Avoidance, if possible, of neostigmine which may trigger cholinergic crisis. If use is necessary, use small dose initially and titrate upwards to effect.

g) State the altered response to suxamethonium in patients with myasthenia gravis. (1 mark)

The reverse is the case with a depolarising agent – there aren't many receptors, and so more drug is required. Due to the possible complications associated with its use, consideration should be given as to whether neuromuscular blockade is absolutely necessary in patients with myasthenia gravis or whether intubation can be achieved with deep inhalational anaesthesia or a TIVA technique. Positive pressure ventilation, however, will help to reduce respiratory muscle fatigue and reduce the risk of postoperative respiratory failure.

- Resistance to effect/need increased dose/dose must be increased by approximately 2.5 times/risk of phase II neuromuscular block.

h) List two drugs that may be used in the management of a cholinergic crisis. (2 marks)

A cholinergic crisis has the opposite cause to a myasthenic crisis – it occurs when too much acetylcholine is present in the neuromuscular junction due to excessive anticholinergic drug treatment. The symptoms are those of muscarinic receptor stimulation (like organophosphate poisoning).

- Atropine.
- Glycopyrrolate.

REFERENCE

Daum P et al. Perioperative management of myasthenia gravis. *BJA Educ.* 2021: 21: 414–419.

11.18 March 2020 Parkinson's disease

a) List three classical motor symptoms used in the clinical diagnosis of Parkinson's disease. (3 marks)
b) List four airway and respiratory issues that patients with Parkinson's disease are at increased risk of and their possible perioperative consequences. (4 marks)
c) List three drug classes that are used in the routine management of Parkinson's disease, giving an explanation for the function of each. (3 marks)
d) List two drug options, with their routes of administration, that can be considered for perioperative management of Parkinson's disease when drug administration via the enteral route is not feasible. (2 marks)
e) Give three complications that may be encountered in the event of interruptions to the administration of anti-Parkinson's therapy, giving features for each. (6 marks)
f) Give two classes of antiemetic drug, and an example for each, that should be avoided in the perioperative management of nausea and vomiting in patients with Parkinson's disease due to their antidopaminergic activity. (2 marks)

The Chairs reported that the pass rate for the CRQ on this topic was high at 70.9% despite it being deemed "one of the more difficult questions on the paper." There was a great BJA Education article on Parkinson's disease in 2017 which contained all the information you would have needed to pass or, indeed, all the information you would need as a safe starting point for managing patients with Parkinson's disease in your day-to-day practice. The Chairs commented that "the pharmacological components of this question were where the candidates tended to drop marks. Weaker candidates were unable to describe the features of withdrawal of medication in these patients."

a) **List three classical motor symptoms used in the clinical diagnosis of Parkinson's disease. (3 marks)**

Parkinson's disease occurs as a consequence of loss of dopaminergic neurones in the pars compacta of the substantia nigra. It may be seen in association with other conditions (so-called Parkinson's-plus conditions), such as progressive supranuclear palsy, and may be associated with neuropsychiatric conditions, dementia and autonomic dysfunction. The diagnosis is a clinical one based on the presence of typical features, the exclusion of other conditions, and response to treatment.

- Bradykinesia.
- Muscular rigidity/stiffness of movement.
- Resting tremor (usually asymmetrical, 4–6 Hz).
- Postural instability (not caused by visual, vestibular, cerebellar, or proprioceptive dysfunction).

b) **List four airway and respiratory issues that patients with Parkinson's disease are at increased risk of and their possible perioperative consequences. (4 marks)**

Patients with Parkinson's disease are at an increased risk of perioperative morbidity and mortality due to airway and respiratory issues as well as the increased risk of falls, delirium, postoperative ileus, and deep vein thrombosis. Many of the airway and respiratory issues listed below are interlinked, but however you phrase your answers, just make sure you aren't repeating the same points.

- Upper airway dysfunction resulting in increased risk of failure to clear secretions, atelectasis, aspiration with consequent pneumonia, laryngospasm after extubation.
- Increased risk of obstructive sleep apnoea in Parkinson's disease with increased risk of apnoea and hypoxia following anaesthesia.

- Restrictive pulmonary defect due to rigidity, bradykinesia, or dyskinesia of respiratory muscles affecting gas exchange and ventilation perioperatively.
- Respiratory muscle dyskinesis and bradykinesia increases the risk of respiratory failure postoperatively.
- Fixed flexion deformity of cervical spine may lead to difficulties with intubation.

c) **List three drug classes that are used in the routine management of Parkinson's disease, giving an explanation for the function of each. (3 marks)**

- Dopamine precursor – converted to dopamine after crossing blood-brain barrier, to replace the role of endogenous dopamine *(i.e. levodopa)*.
- Peripherally acting dopamine decarboxylase inhibitor – reduce the non-CNS effects of dopamine *(e.g. carbidopa)*.
- Dopamine agonists – to mimic the effect of endogenous dopamine in the CNS *(e.g. pramipexole, rotigotine, apomorphine, bromocriptine)*.
- Monoamine oxidase B inhibitors (MAOBIs) – reduce the breakdown of dopamine by MAOB *(e.g. selegiline)*.
- Catechol-O-methyl transferase inhibitors (COMTIs) – reduce breakdown of dopamine by COMT *(e.g. entacapone)*.
- Amantadine, from the class adamantines – reduces dopamine reuptake, stimulates dopamine release.
- Acetylcholinesterase inhibitors – to re-establish balance between dopaminergic and acetylcholine mediated pathways in the basal ganglia *(e.g. rivastigmine)*.

d) **List two drug options, with their routes of administration, that can be considered for perioperative management of Parkinson's disease when drug administration via the enteral route is not feasible. (2 marks)**

These are both dopamine agonists.

- Rotigotine – transdermal patch.
- Apomorphine – subcutaneous infusion.

e) **Give three complications that may be encountered in the event of interruptions to the administration of anti-Parkinson's therapy, giving features for each. (6 marks)**

- "Off" period: increasing rigidity, tremor and bradykinesia leading up to the time that the next dopaminergic drug is due or in the early stages of a delayed dose.
- Antidopaminergic syndrome/Parkinsonism-hyperpyrexia syndrome/neuroleptic malignant syndrome/neuroleptic malignant-like syndrome following withdrawal of levodopa: muscle rigidity, fever, cardiovascular instability, agitation, delirium, coma.
- Dopaminergic agonist withdrawal syndrome: anxiety, depression, nausea, sweating, pain, dizziness, dysphoria, sleep disturbance.

f) **Give two classes of antiemetic drug, and an example for each, that should be avoided in the perioperative management of nausea and vomiting in patients with Parkinson's disease due to their antidopaminergic activity. (2 marks)**

- Phenothiazines e.g. prochlorperazine.
- Butyrophenones e.g. droperidol (but very little domperidone crosses the blood brain barrier and so can be used).
- Benzamide derivative i.e. metoclopramide.

REFERENCES

Chambers D et al. Parkinson's disease. *BJA Educ.* 2017: 17: 145–149.

National Institute for Health and Care Excellence. *Parkinson's disease in adults: NG71*, July 2017.

Sveberg Dietrichs E, Dietrichs E. Time to replace the term neuroleptic malignant syndrome with antidopaminergic syndrome? *Lancet Psychiat.* 2022: 9: 348.

UK Parkinson's Disease Society. *UK Parkinson's Society brain bank clinical diagnostic criteria.* www.ncbi.nlm.nih.gov/projects/gap/cgi-bin/GetPdf.cgi?id=phd000042. Last accessed 30th January 2023.

11.19 March 2020 Drug-eluting stents

a) List three issues that must be evaluated when considering the optimal timing of elective surgery in a patient receiving dual antiplatelet therapy (DAPT) with aspirin and clopidogrel following percutaneous coronary intervention (PCI) involving a drug-eluting stent (DES). (3 marks)

b) State the minimum time period of DAPT following PCI with DES before consideration should be given to proceeding with urgent non-cardiac surgery on aspirin as a sole antiplatelet. (1 mark)

c) Give a strategy for perioperative management of a patient who urgently requires surgery that requires discontinuation of DAPT in advance of the planned timing of cessation. (1 mark)

d) State the recommended duration of DAPT in a patient who has had PCI with DES as management of an acute coronary syndrome. (1 mark)

e) List four patient factors, evaluated at the time of coronary stenting, that have been found to increase the risk of bleeding during DAPT. (4 marks)

f) List four patient characteristics that may increase the risk of stent thrombosis following PCI with DES. (4 marks)

g) List three types of surgery where the risk of continuation of aspirin as a sole antiplatelet agent may outweigh the benefit to a patient who had PCI with DES four years previously. (3 marks)

h) List three types of antiplatelet agents used in the management of patients with DES, PCI and acute coronary syndromes and give their mechanisms of action. (3 marks)

A CRQ in March 2020 focussed on drug-eluting stents. The Chairs quoted a pass rate of 74.7% and said that the "question correlated very well with overall performance. It was [a] well answered question, with candidates giving comprehensive answers. The management of patients with drug-eluting stents has become a common clinical problem and this was reflected in a good pass rate." The approach to management of DAPT in patients with stents has changed in recent years with a much more individualised approach now being taken, and so it is difficult to know what questions could be asked that would have a really definitive answer. The College has shown through its questioning in all of the sections of the exam that they want us to have a good understanding of the mechanisms of action of antiplatelet agents.

a) List three issues that must be evaluated when considering the optimal timing of elective surgery in a patient receiving dual antiplatelet therapy (DAPT) with aspirin and clopidogrel following percutaneous coronary intervention (PCI) involving a drug-eluting stent (DES). (3 marks)

- Risk of delay to elective surgery.
- Risk of bleeding and its consequences if surgery performed whilst taking one or both antiplatelet agents.
- Risk of stent thrombosis especially if one or both antiplatelet agents is stopped perioperatively.
- Implications of antiplatelet agents on mode of anaesthesia.

b) State the minimum time period of DAPT following PCI with DES before consideration should be given to proceeding with urgent non-cardiac surgery on aspirin as a sole antiplatelet. (1 mark)

If a patient is at high risk for stent thrombosis, then the risk-benefit assessment may indicate waiting for six months of DAPT to elapse before surgery. Where DAPT has been interrupted early to facilitate

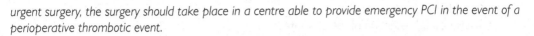

urgent surgery, the surgery should take place in a centre able to provide emergency PCI in the event of a perioperative thrombotic event.

- One month.

c) **Give a strategy for perioperative management of a patient who urgently requires surgery that requires discontinuation of DAPT in advance of the planned timing of cessation. (1 mark)**

- Intravenous bridging with an antiplatelet agent (e.g. eptifibatide or tirofiban, both glycoprotein IIb/IIIa inhibitors which are reversible, or cangrelor, an intravenous reversible P2Y$_{12}$ ADP receptor inhibitor).

d) **State the recommended duration of DAPT in a patient who has had PCI with DES as management of an acute coronary syndrome. (1 mark)**

If the patient has had their DES in the context of stable coronary artery disease, then the recommended duration of DAPT is six months, unless the patient has an excessive bleeding risk, and must be considered on a case-by-case basis in patients having stents that have bioresorbable scaffolds which have been associated with an increased risk of stent thrombosis.

- Twelve months unless the patient has an excessive bleeding risk.

e) **List four patient factors, evaluated at the time of coronary stenting, that have been found to increase the risk of bleeding during DAPT. (4 marks)**

These risk factors contribute to the PRECISE-DAPT score that can be used to guide the duration of a patient's DAPT. Up-to-date European Society of Cardiology guidance has a focus on aiming to individualise DAPT duration depending on a patient's bleeding and thrombosis risk.

- Low haemoglobin/anaemia.
- Leucocytosis.
- Increasing age.
- Reduced creatinine clearance.
- Previous episode of spontaneous bleeding.

f) **List four patient characteristics that may increase the risk of stent thrombosis following PCI with DES. (4 marks)**

- Cigarette smoking.
- Diabetes mellitus.
- Congestive heart failure/LVEF < 30%.
- Previous PCI.
- Previous MI.
- MI as the indication for PCI and DES.

g) **List three types of surgery where the risk of continuation of aspirin as a sole antiplatelet agent may outweigh the benefit to a patient who had PCI with a DES four years previously. (3 marks)**

- Spinal surgery.
- Intracranial surgery.
- Intraocular surgery.
- Transbronchial operations.
- Vascular reconstructions.

- Complex visceral surgery.
- Transurethral resection of the prostate.

h) **List three types of antiplatelet agents used in the management of patients with DES, PCI and acute coronary syndromes and give their mechanisms of action. (3 marks)**

Examples of P2Y$_{12}$ADP receptor blockers include clopidogrel, prasugrel, ticagrelor and cangrelor. The first three are taken orally, whereas cangrelor is administered intravenously. The first two are thienopyridines and irreversibly antagonise the P2Y$_{12}$ ADP receptor, whereas ticagrelor and cangrelor are reversible in their action on the receptor. Cangrelor is rapidly deactivated in the circulation by dephosphorylation resulting in a negligibly active metabolite whereas the others are metabolised in the liver. Ticagrelor can be reversed rapidly with bentracimab. Clopidogrel is a prodrug which is activated by the CYP2C19 enzyme and is subject to inter-individual variation in effectiveness due to genetic polymorphism, and interactions with drugs metabolised by the same pathways. The glycoprotein IIb/IIIa inhibitors are administered intravenously, and examples include abciximab, eptifibatide and tirofiban.

- Aspirin, a nonsteroidal anti-inflammatory drug: irreversible inhibition of cyclo-oxygenase therefore reducing production of thromboxane A2 which is responsible for platelet activation and aggregation.
- P2Y$_{12}$ receptor inhibitors: inhibition of the binding of ADP to the P2Y$_{12}$ ADP receptor thus preventing activation of the glycoprotein IIb/IIIa receptors.
- Glycoprotein IIb/IIIa receptor blockers: prevent cross-linking of fibrinogen to glycoprotein IIb/IIIa receptors on platelets.

REFERENCES

Ganesh R et al. Platelets for anaesthetists: part 2: pharmacology. *BJA Educ.* 2016: 16: 140–145.
Reed-Poysden C, Gupta K. Acute coronary syndromes. *BJA Educ.* 2015: 15: 286–293.
Valgimigli M et al. 2017 ESC focused update on dual antiplatelet therapy in coronary artery disease developed in collaboration with EACTS: the task force for dual antiplatelet therapy in coronary artery disease of the European Society of Cardiology (ESC) and the European Association for Cardiothoracic Surgery (EACTS). *Eur Heart J.* 2018: 39: 213–260.

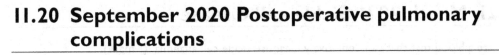

11.20 September 2020 Postoperative pulmonary complications

I have covered this topic already earlier in this chapter. The Chairs said the pass rate was 63.5% for the CRQ on this topic and that the "question correlated very well with overall performance. It was [a] well answered question, with candidates giving very comprehensive answers. It was only the last stem, on the pathophysiology of atelectasis, that candidates struggled with."

11.21 March 2021 Sickle cell disease

a) State a blood test that can definitively diagnose sickle cell anaemia. (1 mark)
b) State the inheritance of sickle cell anaemia. (1 mark)
c) Give the two major pathological consequences of sickling. (2 marks)
d) What are reticulocytes and what does a raised blood reticulocyte count represent? (2 marks)
e) Give three airway or respiratory complications of sickle cell anaemia. (3 marks)
f) Give two cardiovascular complications of sickle cell anaemia. (2 marks)
g) Give two indications for splenectomy in sickle cell anaemia. (2 marks)
h) Explain the role of hydroxycarbamide in the management of sickle cell disease. (1 mark)
i) Give the target haemoglobin and HbS% for a 15-year-old boy with sickle cell disease undergoing a splenectomy. (2 marks)
j) Give four perioperative factors that may increase the risk of sickling in this patient. (4 marks)

The Chairs reported a pass rate of 65.2% for the CRQ on this topic and said that the "knowledge components of this question were poorly answered. Very few candidates were aware of the systemic effects of sickle cell disease. The anaesthetic-related questions were better answered, though surprisingly only one third of candidates got full marks for naming the peri-operative factors that may precipitate sickling." Actual clinical experience in managing patients with sickle cell disease will vary considerably depending on where in the world or in the UK you have worked, but there was a comprehensive guideline on patient management produced by the Association of Anaesthetists in 2021.

a) State a blood test that can definitively diagnose sickle cell anaemia. (1 mark)

The Sickledex test, or rapid sickle solubility test, cannot definitively diagnose sickle cell anaemia. It is a test that lyses red blood cells and then checks how much the resulting haemoglobin is dissolved in a solvent – HbS is less soluble than normal haemoglobin. However, the test may give a false negative in neonates or if the patient has been recently transfused and won't differentiate between sickle cell disease and trait. It also won't reveal whether the patent has a combination of haemoglobinopathies, for example, thalassaemia alongside sickle cell disease. Haemoglobinopathy screening is now part of the standard newborn blood spot testing.

- Haemoglobinopathy screen using electrophoresis, chromatography or mass spectrometry.

b) State the inheritance of sickle cell anaemia. (1 mark)

A genetic mutation of chromosome 11 causes a change from a glutamic acid to a valine in the beta globin gene. This renders the resulting haemoglobin liable to polymerisation especially when it has a low oxygen saturation, resulting in deformation of the red blood cell into a sickle shape. Homozygosity, SS, is associated with sickling within the physiological range of oxygen saturations, whereas heterozygosity, AS, will only tend to result in sickling at oxygen saturations well below that encountered in venous blood. The latter is therefore sickle cell trait.

- Autosomal recessive.

c) Give the two major pathological consequences of sickling. (2 marks)

There are lots of different names of the range of consequences of sickle cell anaemia, but they are all as a result of one or other of these two processes.

- Small vessel obstruction by sickled cells and consequent endothelial inflammation resulting in acute and chronic organ damage and pain.
- Shorter lifespan of sickled cells resulting in haemolytic anaemia.

d) **What are reticulocytes, and what does a raised blood reticulocyte count represent? (2 marks)**

- Reticulocytes are immature red blood cells.
- A raised count indicates that the bone marrow has increased the production process of new red blood cells in response to the increased loss due to haemolysis.

e) **Give three airway or respiratory complications of sickle cell anaemia. (3 marks)**

Adenotonsillar hyperplasia may be due to the haemopoietic function of adenotonsillar tissue in the face of chronic haemolytic anaemia, the higher frequency of respiratory tract infections, or a compensatory mechanism in response to reduced splenic function. Acute chest syndrome results from an area of hypoventilation in the lungs due to, for example, infection or postoperative atelectasis resulting in low oxygen saturations of associated capillaries causing sickling and haemolysis of the red blood cells which, alongside an inflammatory response from the endothelium, will result in vaso-occlusion and therefore a downward vicious circle with areas of lung infarction. The consequences are pain, fever, respiratory failure, and infiltrates on chest radiograph.

- Obstructive sleep apnoea or adenotonsillar hypertrophy.
- Acute chest syndrome.
- Chronic restrictive lung disease.
- Increased susceptibility to pneumonia due to chronic lung damage and hyposplenism.

f) **Give two cardiovascular complications of sickle cell anaemia. (2 marks)**

- Pulmonary hypertension. *This is due to lung damage and infarction of pulmonary vessels.*
- Ischaemic stroke. *Vaso-occlusion in the cerebral vasculature results in stroke in up to 10% of children. Transcranial Doppler can identify those most at risk, who can be managed with blood transfusion to reduce the percentage of sickle haemoglobin.*
- Congestive heart failure. *Consequent to pulmonary hypertension, direct damage to cardiac blood supply, and chronic fluid overload in patients with frequent transfusion.*

g) **Give two indications for splenectomy in sickle cell anaemia. (2 marks)**

- Acute large splenic infarction.
- Hypersplenism. *Recurrent episodes of vaso-occlusion result in enlargement of the spleen causing increased retention and destruction of red blood cells, thus exacerbating anaemia.*
- Acute splenic sequestration crisis. Mostly affects very young children, occurs due to vaso-occlusion resulting in rapid enlargement and sequestration resulting in hypovolaemic shock and pancytopenia.

h) **Explain the role of hydroxycarbamide in the management of sickle cell disease. (1 mark)**

At birth, haemoglobin is mostly in the form of haemoglobin F, $\alpha_2\gamma_2$. This fetal haemoglobin has a higher oxygen affinity compared to adult forms. This is necessary to allow loading of oxygen onto fetal haemoglobin at a partial pressure of oxygen in the placenta that encourages offloading from the maternal haemoglobin. Most haemoglobin in an adult is haemoglobin A, $\alpha_2\beta_2$, with a small percentage of both haemoglobin A_2, $\alpha_2\delta_2$, and fetal haemoglobin. As it does not contain beta chains, fetal haemoglobin is not affected by sickle cell disease. Another name for hydroxycarbamide is hydroxyurea.

- Hydroxycarbamide increases the production of fetal haemoglobin, which interferes with the polymerisation of HbS and so reduces the tendency to sickle.

i) Give the target haemoglobin and HbS% for a 15-year-old boy with sickle cell disease undergoing a splenectomy. (2 marks)

- Target haemoglobin: 100 g/l.
- Target HbS%: < 30%.

j) Give four perioperative factors that may increase the risk of sickling in this patient. (4 marks)

- Dehydration: excessive starvation times, bleeding, intraoperative fluid losses, failure to keep up with urine output *(recurrent vaso-occlusion in the kidneys results in progressive failure to concentrate urine and, ultimately, renal failure)*.
- Hypotension: due to general anaesthetic drugs or regional or neuraxial techniques may result in hypoperfusion, stasis and consequent hypoxia and sickling.
- Hypoxia: failure to adequately manage the airway or ventilation of an anaesthetised patient, hypoventilatory effects of anaesthetic, opioid analgesic and sedative drugs, postoperative atelectasis.
- Infection as a consequence of surgery.
- Hypothermia leading to shivering, blood stasis and consequent hypoxia.
- Hypercapnia and its consequent acidosis result in pulmonary vasoconstriction and consequent poor gas exchange with risk of hypoxia.
- Acidosis associated with complications from surgery will result in pulmonary vasoconstriction and consequent poor gas exchange with risk of hypoxia.

REFERENCES

Akrimi S, Simiyu V. Anaesthetic management of children with sickle cell disease. *BJA Educ.* 2018: 18: 331–336.

Morven W et al. Haemoglobinopathy and sickle cell disease. *Contin Educ Anaesth Crit Care Pain.* 2010: 10: 24–28.

Walker I et al. Guideline on the peri-operative management of patients with sickle cell disease. *Anaesthesia.* 2021: 76: 805–817.

11.22 September 2021 Delayed recovery after general anaesthesia

a) List six comorbidities associated with a delayed return to consciousness after general anaesthesia. (6 marks)
b) Give three reasons why elderly patients are at increased risk of delayed return to consciousness after general anaesthesia. (3 marks)
c) List three possible reasons for delayed return of consciousness after general anaesthesia after cardiac surgery. (3 marks)
d) Explain two mechanisms by which opioids may contribute to a delayed return of consciousness after general anaesthesia. (2 marks)
e) A patient is breathing spontaneously via an endotracheal tube 60 minutes after the cessation of anaesthesia, remains on full monitoring, and is haemodynamically stable but has not opened their eyes. List six steps you would consider to establish and manage the cause. (6 marks)

It was the online September 2021 sitting of the CRQ that was beset with technical issues resulting in the CRQ being removed from contributing to the overall exam grade. There was therefore no Chairs' comment on the CRQ on this topic. Just one year before the CRQ on this topic appeared, it was the focus of a BJA Education article. It included a suggested pathway for approaching the management and diagnosis of underlying cause of a patient with delayed return to consciousness after general anaesthesia, and I have relied on this for my answers.

a) **List six comorbidities associated with a delayed return to consciousness after general anaesthesia. (6 marks)**

I don't think you need to give such full answers as these to get the six marks, but I think it is worth you giving as wide a variety of responses as possible, not just listing six different pulmonary pathologies that may result in delayed return to consciousness. Also, the question didn't ask why they may cause delayed return of consciousness, but I have added the detail here for clarity.

- Comorbidities causing reduced central respiratory drive e.g. OSA, obesity hypoventilation syndrome, intracranial pathology, pre-existing lung disease associated with chronic carbon dioxide retention.
- Neuromuscular disorders e.g. myasthesia gravis, motor neurone disease, muscular dystrophies, Gullain-Barré syndrome.
- Pulmonary pathology causing V/Q mismatch e.g. COPD, interstitial lung disease.
- Acute and chronic hepatic disease *(impact on drug metabolism and reduction in plasma protein production will result in increased free fraction of highly protein bound drugs).*
- Acute and chronic renal failure *(failure to excrete drugs or their active metabolites, increased protein excretion has an impact on free fraction of highly protein bound drugs).*
- Endocrine diseases e.g. hypothyroidism (decreased minute ventilation, impaired hepatic drug metabolism, reduced plasma volume and hyponatraemia), diabetes (ketonaemia, hypoglycaemia).
- Cardiac failure (reduced cardiac output and pleural effusion reduces respiratory drug washout, renal and hepatic function compromise may occur due to heart failure).
- Pre-existing neurocognitive decline that may increase susceptibility to sedating effects of anaesthetic and sedative agents as well as agents that disturb cholinergic balance.

b) Give three reasons why elderly patients are at increased risk of delayed return to consciousness after general anaesthesia. (3 marks)

- Decline in CNS function leading to increased sensitivity to sedative effects of anaesthetic agents, sedative drugs, and opioid analgesics.
- Proportionally increased adipose component to overall body mass such that lipophilic drugs have a larger volume of distribution causing a prolonged effect.
- Reduced water component to overall body mass resulting in higher peak concentration of hydrophilic drugs.
- Impairment of liver or kidney function with age results in reduced clearance of drugs and their active metabolites.

c) List three possible reasons for delayed return of consciousness after general anaesthesia after cardiac surgery with cardiopulmonary bypass. (3 marks)

- Hypothermia and rapid rewarming.
- Haemorrhagic stroke associated with anticoagulation.
- Embolic stroke (air from bypass circuit, thrombi from vessel manipulation, and failure to adequately anticoagulate).
- Ischaemic stroke due to failure to maintain adequate MAP for adequate cerebral perfusion during bypass.
- Electrolyte or acid-base disturbance.

d) Explain two mechanisms by which opioids may contribute to a delayed return of consciousness after general anaesthesia. (2 marks)

- Direct sedation via opioid receptors.
- Respiratory depression causing hypercarbia.

e) A patient is breathing spontaneously via an endotracheal tube 60 minutes after the cessation of anaesthesia, remains on full monitoring and is haemodynamically stable but has not opened their eyes. List six steps you would consider to establish and manage the cause. (6 marks)

- Neurological assessment: check GCS, check pupillary response, check return of neuromuscular function.
- Check core temperature.
- Check arterial blood gas for oxygenation, carbon dioxide, electrolytes, acid-base status and blood glucose.
- Review anaesthetic chart and notes for possible risk factors: pre-existing patient risk factors, surgical risk factors, drug risk factors.
- Consider use of reversal and antidote drugs depending on neurological assessment and knowledge of drugs given e.g. sugammadex or neostigmine/glycopyrrolate, flumazenil, naloxone.
- Brain imaging e.g. CT head.

REFERENCES

Tan A, Amoako D. Postoperative cognitive dysfunction after cardiac surgery. *Contin Educ Anaesth Crit Care Pain*. 2013: 13: 218–223.

Thomas E et al. Delayed recovery of consciousness after general anaesthesia. *BJA Educ*. 2020: 20: 173–179.

11.23 September 2021 Myotonic dystrophy

A 35-year-old man presents for a laparoscopic cholecystectomy. He was diagnosed with myotonic dystrophy ten years ago.

a) What is myotonic dystrophy? (1 mark)
b) State the mode of inheritance of myotonic dystrophy. (1 mark)
c) List three possible respiratory complications of myotonic dystrophy that are of relevance to anaesthesia. (3 marks)
d) List three possible cardiac complications of myotonic dystrophy that are of relevance to anaesthesia. (3 marks)
e) List two cardiovascular responses to hypercarbia. (2 marks)
f) List three possible causes of hypercarbia in an anaesthetised patient. (3 marks)
g) List two drugs that can precipitate myotonia in susceptible patients. (2 marks)
h) Give three non-drug triggers of myotonia in the perioperative period. (3 marks)
i) Give two strategies in the management of a myotonic crisis. (2 marks)

Again, there was no Chairs' Report for this exam.

a) **What is myotonic dystrophy? (1 mark)**

- An inherited disorder of chloride or sodium channel, altering conductance, affecting skeletal, smooth, and cardiac muscle resulting in myotonia (delayed relaxation of muscle contraction) with associated multisystem effects.

b) **State the mode of inheritance of myotonic dystrophy. (1 mark)**

Anticipation is the worsening of the disease with successive generations.

- Autosomal dominance and may demonstrate anticipation.

c) **List three possible respiratory complications of myotonic dystrophy that are of relevance to anaesthesia. (3 marks)**

Patients may be on NIV to manage obstructive sleep apnoea or progressive respiratory failure. Lung function tests and blood gas analysis may be indicated preoperatively. Patients who are not already established on NIV should be considered for the need for postoperative NIV or invasive ventilation, especially after body cavity surgery.

- Bulbar weakness leads to weak cough, risk of aspiration, and increased likelihood of respiratory tract infection.
- Bulbar weakness can lead to obstructive sleep apnoea.
- Respiratory muscle weakness can lead to respiratory failure, especially in the postoperative period.
- Centrally driven respiratory depression which can lead to central sleep apnoea and an exaggerated respiratory depressant response to opioids, sedative agents, and intravenous anaesthetic agents.
- Restrictive lung defect due to progressive spinal deformity.

d) **List three possible cardiac complications of myotonic dystrophy that are of relevance to anaesthesia. (3 marks)**

Arrhythmia or heart failure may be the presenting feature of myotonic dystrophy, and cardiac complications are the second most common cause of death after respiratory failure. These patients require regular ECG checks and monitoring for cardiomyopathy with echocardiogram or CMR. They may have a pacemaker +/– ICD.

- Progressive risk of conduction defects and arrhythmia – may result in sudden death.
- Cardiomyopathy; progressive left ventricular failure leading to heart failure.
- Pulmonary hypertension secondary to chronic hypoventilation.
- Risk of embolic stroke due to predisposition to arrhythmia.

e) List two cardiovascular responses to hypercarbia. (2 marks)

- Hypertension.
- Vasodilation.
- Tachycardia.
- Raised pulmonary artery pressure.

f) List three possible causes of hypercarbia in an anaesthetised patient. (3 marks)

Patients with myotonic dystrophy are not thought to have an increased risk of malignant hyperthermia compared to the general population.

- Hypoventilation.
- Rebreathing due to faulty breathing circuit (increasing dead space) or exhausted soda lime.
- Increased carbon dioxide due to hypermetabolic state such as fever, malignant hyperthermia, thyroid storm.
- Increased absorption in laparoscopic surgery.

g) List two drugs that can precipitate myotonia in susceptible patients. (2 marks)

The pain of propofol injection has been reported to trigger myotonia and therefore it has been suggested that lidocaine be added to reduce this risk. However, it is not the propofol itself causing the myotonia. It is imperative that patients with myotonic dystrophy who have had neuromuscular blocking agents as part of their anaesthetic technique should be adequately reversed before extubation. Sugammadex has been used without issue.

- Suxamethonium.
- Neostigmine.

h) Give three non-drug triggers of myotonia in the perioperative period. (3 marks)

- Hypothermia.
- Electrical nerve stimulation e.g. during nerve block, when checking train-of-four, with diathermy.
- Shivering in response to neuraxial block.
- Pain.
- Percussive stimulation of the muscle.

i) Give two strategies in the management of a myotonic crisis. (2 marks)

- Removal or cessation or management of trigger.
- Class I antiarrhythmics, sodium channel blockers e.g. lidocaine, phenytoin.

REFERENCES

Ferschl M et al. *Practical suggestions for the anesthetic management of a myotonic dystrophy patient.* Myotonic Dystrophy Foundation. www.myotonic.org/sites/default/files/pages/files/MDF_PracticalSuggestionsDM1_AAnesthesi2_17_21.pdf. Accessed 9th December 2022.

Marsh S, Ross N, Pittard A. Neuromuscular disorders and anaesthesia: part 1: generic anaesthetic management. *Contin Educ Anaesth Crit Care Pain.* 2011: 11: 115–118.

Marsh S, Pittard A. Neuromuscular disorders and anaesthesia: part 2: specific neuromuscular disorders. *Contin Educ Anaesth Crit Care Pain.* 2011: 11: 119–123.

McNally E. Clinical care recommendations for cardiologists treating adults with myotonic dystrophy. *J Am Heart Assoc.* 2020: 9: 1–7.

Trip J et al. Drug treatment for myotonia (review). *Cochrane Database Syst Rev.* 2006: (1): Article No. CD004762.

11.24 March 2022 Patient blood management

The Chairs' Report for the CRQ on this topic gave a pass rate of 59.7% and said it "was a well answered question, with candidates giving comprehensive answers. Candidates only struggled to answer the question on the factors that aid clot formation." A BJA Education article about perioperative blood management is a useful read in addition to the Association of Anaesthetists' guidelines that I referenced after the question on the same topic in March 2012. It states that pH > 7.2, core body temperature > 35°C (a degree less than the advised lower limit in the Association guidelines for minimising perioperative blood loss), and ionised calcium > 1 mmol/l are necessary for optimal clot formation.

REFERENCE

Thakrar S et al. Patient blood management and perioperative anaemia. *BJA Educ.* 2017: 17: 28–34.

11.25 March 2022 Cardiopulmonary exercise testing

a) List three components of the equipment used in cardiopulmonary exercise testing (CPET). (3 marks)
b) Give four reasons for stopping CPET before maximal effort has been achieved. (4 marks)
c) Define anaerobic threshold and give the units by which it is measured. (2 marks)
d) Give two ways in which anaerobic threshold (AT) can be determined from the results of CPET. (2 marks)
e) List two core measures of exercise capacity (apart from AT) that can be determined from CPET. (2 marks)
f) Give three circumstances where CPET using a bicycle may not be practical for use as a preoperative assessment tool. (3 marks)
g) Name four scoring systems that may be used to help predict perioperative risk before major elective non-cardiac surgery. (4 marks)

The pass rate for the original CRQ on this topic was 59.7%, much better than the pass rate for the SAQ on CPET in 2017. The Chairs commented that "pre-operative assessment and the use of CPET in the stratification of risk is an area of the syllabus that candidates should know. Candidates should be able to interpret the results produced by CPET testing. The sections relating to the CPET variables were the sections where candidates dropped the majority of their marks." The BJA Education article on CPET referenced below really is a beginner's guide to the nine-panel plot – follow it up with a bit more detail from the POETTS article.

a) List three components of the equipment used in cardiopulmonary exercise testing. (3 marks)

- Electromagnetically braked cycle ergometer (or hand crank).
- Rapid gas analyser.
- Pressure differential pneumotachograph.
- Noninvasive blood pressure, ECG, and oxygen saturation monitoring.

b) Give four reasons for stopping CPET before maximal effort has been achieved. (4 marks)

- Hypotension.
- Arrhythmia.
- Claudication.
- ECG changes consistent with ischaemia.
- Ischaemic chest pain.
- Musculoskeletal pain.
- Dyspnoea or significant oxygen desaturation.
- Severe hypertension.
- Reduced consciousness or confusion.

c) Define anaerobic threshold and give the units by which it is measured. (2 marks)

- Anaerobic threshold is the point at which oxygen demand of the body exceeds the capacity of the cardiopulmonary system to supply it, triggering a change to ATP generation through anaerobic metabolism resulting in lactate production.
- ml O_2/kg/min.

d) Give two ways in which anaerobic threshold (AT) can be determined from the results of a CPET. (2 marks)

VCO_2 increases proportionally with VO_2 until capacity for oxygen delivery is exceeded and anaerobic metabolism starts resulting in a greater proportion of carbon dioxide being produced compared to oxygen delivered. Below is an abbreviated approach to the determination of AT.

- V-slope method: change in the linear graph of VCO_2 plotted against VO_2 such that the increase in VCO_2 causes the line to start to follow a new, steeper gradient; AT is the VO_2 at that inflection point.
- The nadir of the VE/VO_2 curve: this demonstrates hyperventilation relative to VO_2, that ventilation is now being driven by the anaerobic production of carbon dioxide.

e) **List two core measures of exercise capacity (apart from AT) that can be determined from CPET. (2 marks)**

There are a multitude of measurements of a patient's physiology that can be determined from CPET, but these, along with AT, are ones that relate to exercise capacity.

- Peak oxygen consumption, VO_2 peak, in ml/kg/min.
- Peak work rate, WRpeak, in Watts.

f) **Give three circumstances where CPET using a bicycle may not be practical for use as a preoperative assessment tool. (3 marks)**

This is not the same as contraindications, which can be found in the references below. Many of these issues can be overcome and so only "may" make CPET impractical.

- Exercise-limiting peripheral vascular disease.
- Lower limb amputation that has compromised ability to cycle.
- Severe arthritis.
- Learning difficulties or dementia sufficient to impair ability to follow instructions, or other communication difficulties such as profound deafness.
- Balance or coordination problems.
- Inability to tolerate mouthpiece/face mask due to e.g. claustrophobia.
- Lack of motivation.

g) **Name four scoring systems that may be used to help predict perioperative risk before major elective non-cardiac surgery. (4 marks)**

- American Society of Anesthesiologists (ASA) Physical Status classification.
- Physiological and Operative Severity Score for the enUmeration of Mortality and Morbidity (POSSUM).
- Surgical Outcome Risk Tool (SORT).
- American College of Surgeons Surgical Risk Calculator (ACS NSQIP).
- Charlson Age Comorbidity Index (CACI).
- Revised Cardiac Risk Index (RCRI).

REFERENCES

Barnett S, Moonesinghe S. Clinical risk scores to guide perioperative management. *Postgrad Med J.* 2011: 87: 535–541.

Chambers D, Wisely N. Cardiopulmonary exercise testing – a beginner's guide to the nine-panel plot. *BJA Educ.* 2019: 19: 158–164.

Levett D et al. Perioperative Exercise Testing and Training Society (POETTS): perioperative cardiopulmonary exercise testing (CPET): consensus clinical guidelines on indications, organisation, conduct and physiological interpretation. *BJA.* 2018: 120: 484–500.

Minto G, Biccard B. Assessment of the high-risk perioperative patient. *Contin Educ Anaesth Crit Care Pain.* 2014: 14: 12–17.

11.26 September 2022 Robotic surgery

a) Give two reasons why carbon dioxide is the gas used for creating the pneumoperitoneum used in robotic laparoscopic surgery. (2 marks)
b) List three possible complications that may occur in the process of accessing the peritoneal cavity for creation of a pneumoperitoneum. (3 marks)
c) List two airway complications associated with robotic laparoscopic cystectomy. (2 marks)
d) List two respiratory complications associated with robotic laparoscopic cystectomy. (2 marks)
e) List five surgical and anaesthetic factors that contribute to the risk of development of compartment syndrome of the lower limbs during robotic laparoscopic cystectomy. (5 marks)
f) List three neurological complications related to positioning for robotic laparoscopic cystectomy. (3 marks)
g) List three other possible complications of positioning for robotic laparoscopic cystectomy. (3 marks)

The Chairs reported a 48.4% pass rate for the CRQ on this topic, "one of the lower pass rates" of the paper. They said that it "appeared that many candidates had minimal experience of robotic surgery" and that answers to some sections "seemed to indicate that many candidates were unclear as to the practicalities of positioning patients during this type of surgery." The CRQ also asked about the components of enhanced recovery in the context of surgery, but as this has been covered elsewhere in this book, I have not addressed it here.

a) **Give two reasons why carbon dioxide is the gas used for creating the pneumoperitoneum used in robotic laparoscopic surgery. (2 marks)**

- High blood solubility and so less likely to cause significant gas embolism in the event of intravascular insufflation.
- Will not support combustion when diathermy is used.

b) **List three possible complications that may occur in the process of accessing the peritoneal cavity for creation of a pneumoperitoneum. (3 marks)**

- Damage to organ or blood vessel resulting in major haemorrhage.
- Insufflation of vessel causing gas embolism.
- Subcutaneous or mediastinal emphysema.
- Pneumothorax.

c) **List two airway complications associated with robotic laparoscopic cystectomy. (2 marks)**

- Accidental extubation/bronchial intubation with movement into Trendelenburg positioning.
- Airway oedema resulting in postoperative stridor and respiratory distress due to prolonged surgery in head-down position.

d) **List two respiratory complications associated with robotic laparoscopic cystectomy. (2 marks)**

- Atelectasis due to pneumoperitoneum and steep Trendelenburg positioning.
- Baro- and volutrauma as increased airway pressures and tidal volumes are used to counteract effects of diaphragmatic splinting and raised partial pressures of carbon dioxide associated with pneumoperitoneum.
- Risk of pulmonary aspiration due to passive regurgitation of gastric contents.

e) **List five surgical and anaesthetic factors that contribute to the risk of development of compartment syndrome of the lower limbs during robotic laparoscopic cystectomy. (5 marks)**

- Steep Trendelenburg positioning.
- Lithotomy positioning using leg supports.
- Often very long duration of surgery.
- Use of antiembolism stockings or intermittent pneumatic compression devices.
- Hypotension associated with anaesthetic technique such as neuraxial block or deep general anaesthesia.
- Use of vasoactive medication.
- Limited intravenous fluid use.

f) **List three neurological complications related to positioning for robotic laparoscopic cystectomy. (3 marks)**

- Brachial plexus injuries related to use of e.g. shoulder bolsters or beanbags.
- Common peroneal nerve injury due to pressure caused by lithotomy leg supports.
- Sciatic, femoral or lateral cutaneous nerve injury due to excessive flexion associated with lithotomy positioning.
- Cerebral oedema resulting in delayed return to consciousness postoperatively.

g) **List three other possible complications of positioning for robotic laparoscopic cystectomy. (3 marks)**

- Patient sliding resulting in fall from table, loss of monitoring or intravascular access, or injury from surgical instruments that have been fixed in place.
- Pressure sores affecting areas in contact with restraint devices.
- Conjunctival oedema.
- Gastric content reflux causing conjunctival burns or oral ulceration.
- Deep vein thrombosis.

REFERENCE

Carey B et al. Anaesthesia for minimally invasive abdominal and pelvic surgery. *BJA Educ.* 2019: 19: 254–260.

11.27 September 2022 Liver disease

The Chairs' Report of the original CRQ said that the pass rate was 76.7%, commenting that "this was a well answered question, with candidates giving very comprehensive answers. Candidates only really struggled with the pharmacological component of the question." The content included that which has been addressed earlier in this chapter, but they also wanted candidates to appreciate the distinction between acute and chronic liver disease. Interestingly, this was covered in the BJA Education article on liver disease that appeared earlier in the year.

Acute liver disease:

- *New onset liver failure as evidenced by jaundice, coagulopathy and encephalopathy in a patient without pre-existing cirrhosis.*
- *Hyperacute if onset is less than 7 days, acute if less than 4 weeks, sub-acute if less than 12 weeks.*

Chronic liver disease:

- *Progressive deterioration in hepatic function over 28 weeks or more.*

REFERENCE

Gilbert-Kawai N, Hogan B, Milan Z. Perioperative management of patients with liver disease. *BJA Educ.* 2022: 22: 111–117.

12.1 September 2012 Transversus abdominis plane block

a) Between which muscles do the nerves that supply cutaneous innervation for the anterior abdominal wall lie? (2 marks)
b) State the nerves that are responsible for the sensory innervation of the anterior abdominal wall. (3 marks)
c) List three types of surgery in which a transversus abdominis plane (TAP) block could be used. (3 marks)
d) List three potential benefits of performing a TAP block for abdominal surgery. (3 marks)
e) Give two limitations of TAP block as part of an analgesic approach for abdominal surgery. (2 marks)
f) State the boundaries of the triangle of Petit. (3 marks)
g) List two approaches to ultrasound-guided TAP block. (2 marks)
h) List two specific complications of TAP blocks. (2 marks)

The Chair's Report of the original SAQ said there was a 67.4% pass rate, commenting that "the question was relevant and topical. Many candidates had poor knowledge of the innervation of the anterior abdominal wall. Overall was answered well." Regional nerve blocks have peaks of popularity and interest – make sure you know about the current hot favourites.

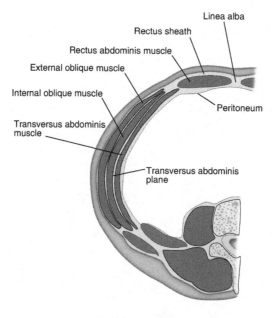

Abdominal wall.

DOI: 10.1201/9781003388494-12

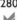

a) **Between which muscles do the nerves that supply cutaneous innervation for the anterior abdominal wall lie? (2 marks)**

- Internal oblique.
- Transversus abdominis.

b) **State the nerves that are responsible for the sensory innervation of the anterior abdominal wall. (3 marks)**

- Branches of anterior rami of T7–12/T7–12 thoracoabdominal nerves. (*The anterior rami of the thoracic spinal nerves each send a branch to give sensory innervation to the anterior abdominal wall, both the skin and the underlying muscle. T6–9 supplies above the umbilicus, T10 supplies umbilical level, and T11–12 supply below the umbilicus.*)
- Iliohypogastric nerve (*cutaneous innervation includes the suprapubic region*).
- Ilioinguinal nerve (*cutaneous innervation includes the inguinal region, as well as medial thigh and external genitalia*).

c) **List three types of surgery in which a transversus abdominis plane (TAP) block could be used. (3 marks)**

TAP block provides parietal pain relief to the anterior abdominal wall (not effective for visceral pain) from T7 to L1 level. Spread above the umbilicus level is unreliable, so it is useful for any surgery involving anterior abdominal wall where the incision is below the level of the umbilicus:

- Gynaecological e.g. abdominal hysterectomy.
- Obstetric e.g. caesarean section.
- Urological e.g. retropubic prostatectomy.
- General surgical e.g. appendicectomy, lower abdominal open colorectal surgery.

d) **List three potential benefits of performing a TAP block for abdominal surgery. (3 marks)**

- Reduced opioid requirement, useful in patients for whom opioids may be undesirable e.g. those with respiratory or renal disease.
- Alternative analgesic option for patients in whom neuraxial technique is contraindicated e.g. patients with coagulopathy (*however, unlikely to be as effective as neuraxial technique*).
- Offers pain relief after emergency caesarean, where urgency has not permitted neuraxial technique.
- No associated motor block or urinary retention compared to neuraxial technique and so earlier return to mobilisation and no need for urinary catheter – may be useful as part of an enhanced recovery approach.

e) **Give two limitations of TAP block as part of an analgesic approach for abdominal surgery. (2 marks)**

- TAP blocks only block parietal nerves and so no visceral pain relief is provided.
- Short duration of analgesia.
- Variable spread of local anaesthetic in the fascial plane and anatomical variety result in variable outcome.
- Bilateral blocks required, large doses of local anaesthetic may be indicated, may be limited by maximum permitted doses.

f) State the boundaries of the triangle of Petit. (3 marks)

The triangle of Petit was used in guiding needle placement in a landmark-guided TAP block, although ultrasound guidance for TAP blocks is now the gold standard.

- Iliac crest inferiorly.
- Anterior border of latissimus dorsi posteriorly.
- Posterior border of external oblique anteriorly.

g) List two approaches to ultrasound-guided TAP block. (2 marks)

- "Classical"/lateral approach (*ultrasound probe placed transversely in the mid-axillary line, in between the twelfth rib and iliac crest, needling anterior-to-posterior*).
- Subcostal approach (*ultrasound probe placed obliquely parallel to the costal margin, needling medial-to-lateral – more useful when aiming to anaesthetise T6–T9, whose cutaneous branches enter the TAP plane medial to the anterior axillary line and may be missed by a classical/lateral TAP block*).
- Posterior approach (*evolved from the initial landmark TAP block, the ultrasound is placed transversely in the mid-axillary line and moved posteriorly until the posterior end of the TAP is reached, needling anterior-to-posterior, may provide better analgesia to the lateral abdominal wall*).

h) List two specific complications of TAP blocks. (2 marks)

Don't just write "nerve damage, bleeding, failure" – explain the specific issues associated with this particular block.

- Failure: there is significant variation in degree of local anaesthetic spread with TAP block.
- Local anaesthetic toxicity: large volumes of local anaesthetic are used, especially if bilateral block, and the plane is vascular.
- Risks of incorrect site of injection is reduced with the use of ultrasound but include intraperitoneal injection, intrahepatic injection, bowel perforation or haematoma.
- Transient femoral nerve block.

REFERENCES

Onwochei A, Børglum J, Pawa A. Abdominal wall blocks for intrabdominal surgery. *BJA Educ.* 2018: 18: 317–332.

Townsley P, French J. Transversus abdominis plane block. *ATOTW.* 2011: 239.

Yarwood J, Berrill A. Nerve blocks of the anterior abdominal wall. *Contin Educ Anaesth Crit Care Pain.* 2010: 10: 182–186.

12.2 March 2013 Regional anaesthesia for shoulder surgery

a) List six specific nerves that must be blocked to achieve effective local anaesthesia for shoulder surgery. (6 marks)
b) List six possible neurological complications of an interscalene block. (6 marks)
c) State five anaesthetic measures that can help to reduce all types of neurological damage during shoulder surgery. (5 marks)
d) Give one surgical measure that can help to reduce all types of neurological damage during shoulder surgery. (1 mark)
e) Give two possible advantages of carrying out shoulder surgery in conscious patients using regional anaesthesia. (2 marks)

The Chair's Report of the original SAQ found that the question was answered well with a 69.2% pass rate. They said that "if an open question is asked on the possible neurological complications of a block, then this will include damage to both the peripheral and central nervous system. Some candidates focused on the peripheral nerves only." Parts (c) and (d) in my CRQ were merged into one in the original SAQ, and the Chair said, "The answer . . . required an account of both anaesthetic and surgical factors that would reduce neurological damage. This included 'avoiding interscalene block' in the first place. The question was a very good discriminator."

a) **List six specific nerves that must be blocked to achieve effective local anaesthesia for shoulder surgery. (6 marks)**

To get the six points, you need only list the nerves. I have included more detail as it is useful information for the sake of the viva.

Nerve	Area supplied
Supraclavicular nerve *(C3,4)*	*Skin above clavicle, shoulder tip and first two intercostal spaces anteriorly. For awake surgery, would either need to perform superficial cervical plexus block OR infiltrate around posterior port site.*
Suprascapular nerve, *branch of the upper trunk (C4–6).*	*Acromioclavicular joint, capsule, glenohumeral joint.*
Axillary nerve *(C5, 6).*	*Inferior aspect of capsule and glenohumeral joint.*
Upper lateral cutaneous nerve of arm, branch of axillary nerve *(C5, 6).*	*Skin over deltoid.*
Musculocutaneous nerve *(C5–7).*	*Very variable input.*
Medial cutaneous nerve of arm, medial cord of brachial plexus *(C8, T1).*	*Skin of medial arm and axilla.*

b) **List six possible neurological complications of an interscalene block. (6 marks)**

- Phrenic nerve block or damage leading to breathing difficulties in susceptible patients.
- Stellate ganglion block or damage leading to transient Horner's syndrome.
- Recurrent laryngeal nerve palsy leading to hoarse voice.
- Inadvertent spinal anaesthesia.
- Inadvertent epidural anaesthesia.
- Direct nerve damage of any of the nerves intended to be blocked, causing temporary or permanent neuropraxia.
- Syrinx or cavity formation as a consequence of injection into the cervical cord resulting in paraplegia.
- Seizures due to local anaesthesia toxicity or injection into the vertebral artery.

c) State five anaesthetic measures that can help to reduce all types of neurological damage during shoulder surgery. (5 marks)

Nerve damage is a risk during any operation and may occur in relation to nerve blocks, general anaesthesia, surgery and positioning. Be really careful when reading the questions to establish exactly what they are asking. Each of the points below are a separate measure, but they are grouped for ease of learning.

Nerve block:

- Full asepsis, use of 0.5% chlorhexidine spray, air dried, to minimise risk of infection and neurotoxicity.
- Adequate training, use of ultrasound, awake patient, appropriate needle length, low pressure injection, to minimise risk of neuropraxia.
- Avoid nerve blocks altogether to eliminate risk of nerve damage from regional anaesthesia.

General anaesthesia:

- Ensuring adequate filling, appropriate use of vasopressors and leg elevation, and avoidance of excessive depth of anaesthesia to minimise risk of cerebral hypoperfusion in the beach chair position.
- Ensuring adequate padding to protect eyes from pressure damage that may cause optic neuropathy.

Positioning:

- Care with positioning on table (to avoid excessive stretch on brachial plexus in beach chair or lateral positioning) and use of padding (especially at ulnar and common peroneal nerves in lateral position) to minimise risk of neuropraxias.

d) Give one surgical measure that can help to reduce all types of neurological damage during shoulder surgery. (1 mark)

- Appropriate training and careful technique to minimise risk of contusion or traction (rarely laceration) of nerves (axillary nerve close to inferior shoulder capsule is particularly vulnerable) during surgery.
- Minimisation of arm abduction to reduce risk of brachial plexus stretch injury.

e) Give two possible advantages of carrying out shoulder surgery in conscious patients using regional anaesthesia. (2 marks)

- Reduction of risk of hypotension and adverse effect on cerebral perfusion in the beach chair position.
- Avoidance of general anaesthesia and large opioid doses therefore reduction in postoperative nausea and vomiting, more rapid return to normal diet, facilitation of case as day surgery.
- Increased patient engagement in their own care and pathology.
- More efficient theatre utilisation if block room model followed.

REFERENCES

Beecroft C, Coventry D. Anaesthesia for shoulder surgery. *Contin Educ Anaesth Crit Care Pain.* 2008: 8: 193–198.

Hewson D, Oldman M, Bedforth N. Regional anaesthesia for shoulder surgery. *BJA Educ.* 2019: 19: 98–104.

12.3 September 2014 Ankle blocks

a) List five nerves that can be blocked at ankle level for foot surgery. (5 marks)
b) For each of these nerves, describe their sensory distribution within the foot. (5 marks)
c) Give the anatomical landmarks for an ankle block which aid correct placement of local anaesthesia for each nerve. (5 marks)
d) Give five advantages and disadvantages of an ankle block. (5 marks)

The CRQ above is virtually unchanged from its SAQ format. The pass rate for the question was 65.9%, and the Chairs commented that "common clinical subjects tend to score well in the SAQ paper and discriminate between strong and weak candidates as was the case for this question. Weak candidates had poor anatomical knowledge or failed to list the advantages of this specific block, giving instead the features common to any local anaesthetic technique. Poor candidates tended to describe features of blocks at the popliteal level, perhaps due to failing to read the question thoroughly as ankle level was highlighted. The importance of candidates retaining knowledge of the basic sciences has been highlighted before."

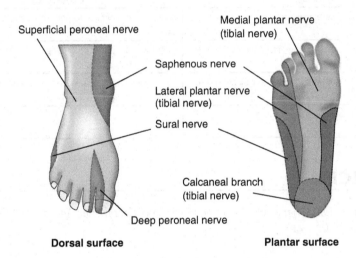

Cutaneous innervation of the foot.

a) List five nerves that can be blocked at ankle level for foot surgery. (5 marks)
b) For each of these nerves, describe their sensory distribution within the foot. (5 marks)
c) Give the anatomical landmarks for an ankle block which aid correct placement of local anaesthesia for each nerve. (5 marks)

I have grouped the answers into a table for ease of learning.

Nerve	Sensory distribution	Anatomical landmarks
Tibial:	Heel and plantar aspect of the foot.	Midway between medial malleolus and tip of calcaneum, inject posteriorly to the posterior tibial artery.
Deep peroneal:	1st/2nd toe web space.	2–3 cm distal to the intermalleolar line, palpate extensor hallucis longus. Lateral to this is the dorsalis pedis artery: inject either side.

(Continued)

(Continued)

Nerve	Sensory distribution	Anatomical landmarks
Superficial peroneal:	Dorsum of the foot excluding 1st/2nd toe web space.	Find tibial ridge, insert needle and direct towards lateral malleolus raising a subcutaneous wheal.
Sural:	Plantar aspect 4th/5th web space and 5th toe, and lateral aspect of the foot.	Infiltrate subcutaneously between lateral malleolus and Achilles tendon.
Saphenous:	Medial aspect of the foot and ankle.	Find saphenous vein anterior to medial malleolus: inject subcutaneously from here posteriorly as far as the Achilles tendon.

d) Give five advantages and disadvantages of an ankle block. (5 marks)

Advantages	Disadvantages
Provides good postoperative analgesia.	Can be uncomfortable to perform in awake or unsedated patients.
May avoid general anaesthesia in high-risk patients.	Risk of vascular puncture causing haematoma. Saphenous vein particularly at risk.
Relatively simple technique with low risk of local anaesthetic toxicity.	If a tourniquet is to be used, does not alleviate tourniquet pain.
Minimal motor block; can therefore be used for bilateral procedures.	

REFERENCE

Kopka A, Serpell M. Distal nerve blocks of the lower limb. *Contin Educ Anaesth Crit Care Pain.* 2005: 5: 166–170.

12.4 September 2015 Regional anaesthesia for shoulder surgery

a) Which specific nerves must be blocked to achieve effective local anaesthesia for shoulder surgery? (6 marks)
b) What are the possible neurological complications of an interscalene block? (6 marks)
c) Outline the measures available to reduce all types of neurological damage during shoulder surgery. (8 marks)

I have reproduced the original SAQ here – it was identical to that from March 2013 and yet the pass rate was only 48.3%. Topics recur with regularity; if you do no other preparation for this exam, at least look at the past papers. The Chairs' Report said, "This question also correlated well with overall performance. The anatomy was not well known to a lot of the candidates, so quite a few marks were lost here. This is a recurring theme in the Final exam – remember that anatomy relevant to clinical practice is likely to be included. Failure to read the question again caused some candidates to lose marks. Part (b) asked specifically for possible neurological complications of an interscalene block and quite a few candidates wrote about non-neurological complications."

12.5 March 2017 Fascia iliaca compartment block

An 80-year-old woman is admitted to your hospital having sustained a proximal femoral (neck of femur) fracture in a fall.

a) List three pharmacological best practice elements of this patient's pain management while awaiting surgery. (3 marks)

b) You decide to perform a fascia iliaca compartment block as part of her multimodal analgesia. Give the borders of the fascia iliaca compartment. (4 marks)

c) List the three nerves that you are attempting to block. (3 marks)

d) List two benefits of inclusion of a fascia iliaca compartment block in the pain management strategy for this patient. (2 marks)

e) State why a fascia iliaca block alone is insufficient for provision of anaesthesia for fractured neck of femur surgery. (1 mark)

f) Give two anatomical approaches to performing ultrasound-guided fascia iliaca compartment block. (2 marks)

g) State two specific complications of fascia iliaca block. (2 marks)

h) Give three alternative peripheral nerve blocks that may be used in the management of patients having proximal femoral fracture surgery. (3 marks)

The original SAQ on this topic had a pass rate of only 22.2%! Beware a reappearance. The SAQ was quite different to my CRQ below as a large proportion of the marks were available for writing about the technique of performing an ultrasound-guided fascia iliaca compartment block. As this is not really the style of a CRQ, I wonder if this sort of detail is more likely to be questioned in the viva. However, you can still be asked detailed questions about anatomy, and as the Chairs' Report said, "There was general lack of knowledge of anatomy."

a) **List three pharmacological best practice elements of this patient's pain management while awaiting surgery. (3 marks)**

- Regular paracetamol unless contraindicated.
- Opioids if required but aim to limit opioid intake, especially long-acting opioids.
- NSAIDs not recommended.

b) **You decide to perform a fascia iliaca compartment block as part of her multimodal analgesia. Give the borders of the fascia iliaca compartment. (4 marks)**

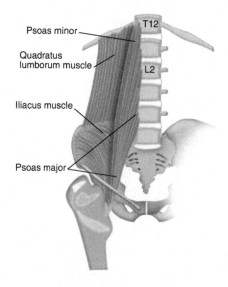

Posterior border of fascia iliaca.

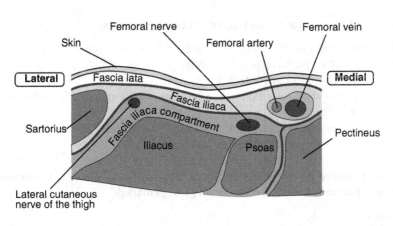

Fascia iliaca compartment.

- Anteriorly: posterior surface of fascia iliaca.
- Posteriorly: anterior surface of iliacus and psoas major muscles.
- Medially: origin of psoas major and vertebral column from which it originates.
- Laterally: origin of iliacus muscle along the inner aspect of the iliac crest.

c) List the three nerves that you are attempting to block. (3 marks)

- Femoral.
- Lateral cutaneous nerve of the thigh.
- Obturator.

d) List two benefits of inclusion of a fascia iliaca compartment block in the pain management strategy for this patient. (2 marks)

- Avoidance of longer-acting opioids which may contribute to the risk of delirium and respiratory depression especially in the context of renal dysfunction.
- May reduce the need for sedative or analgesic drugs for positioning for spinal anaesthesia, thus reducing the risk of delirium.
- Contribute to better overall pain experience.
- Are associated with a reduced time to remobilisation.
- May facilitate examination and radiological assessment on first presentation.
- Are not contraindicated in anticoagulated patients in whom a spinal anaesthetic would be contraindicated.

e) State why a fascia iliaca block alone is insufficient for provision of anaesthesia for fractured neck of femur surgery. (1 mark)

- Innervation of posterior aspect of hip capsule and ischiocapsular ligaments is from the sciatic plexus.

f) Give two anatomical approaches to performing ultrasound-guided fascia iliaca compartment block. (2 marks)

- Suprainguinal.
- Infrainguinal.

g) State two specific complications of fascia iliaca block. (2 marks)

- Femoral nerve block causing quadriceps weakness, or femoral nerve damage.
- Peritoneal puncture (suprainguinal technique).
- Bladder puncture (suprainguinal technique).
- Compartment block so reliant on large quantities of local anaesthetic, with risk of local anaesthetic toxicity.
- Femoral artery and/or vein puncture with risk of vascular injection with local anaesthetic toxicity, pseudoaneurysm formation, or haematoma.

h) Give three alternative peripheral nerve blocks that may be used in the management of patients having proximal femoral fracture surgery. (3 marks)

- Femoral nerve block.
- 3-in-1 block.
- Pericapsular nerve group block.
- Lumbar plexus block.
- Quadratus lumborum block.
- Erector spinae block.

REFERENCES

Griffiths R et al. Guideline by the Association of Anaesthetists: guideline for the management of hip fractures 2020. *Anaesthesia*. 2021: 76: 225–237.

National Institute for Health and Care Excellence. *Management of hip fractures in adults CG124*, June 2011, updated January 2023.

New York School of Regional Anaesthesia. *Ultrasound-guided fascia iliaca block*. www.nysora.com/ultrasound-guided-fascia-iliaca-block. Accessed 12th January 2018.

O-Reilly N, Desmet M, Kearns R. Fascia Iliaca compartment block. *BJA Educ*. 2019: 19: 191–197.

Shelton C, White S. Anaesthesia for hip fracture repair. *BJA Educ*. 2020: 20: 142–149.

12.6 September 2022 Brachial plexus

a) From which spinal nerve roots does the brachial plexus originate? (1 mark)
b) List the dermatomes that a successful interscalene block will reliably anaesthetise. (3 marks)
c) List four peripheral nerves that would need to be blocked to facilitate awake shoulder surgery. (4 marks)
d) List four patient factors that increase the likelihood of development of nerve injury after peripheral nerve block. (4 marks)
e) List three mechanisms of injury that may cause nerve damage during peripheral nerve block. (3 marks)
f) State what is meant by "triple monitoring" in the context of performing peripheral nerve blockade. (3 marks)
g) Assuming appropriate patient selection, preparation, antisepsis and use of "Stop Before You Block," list two other strategies that may help reduce the risk of nerve injury during peripheral nerve blockade. (2 marks)

The Chairs' Report of the original CRQ stated that brachial plexus blocks "is a common question in all parts of the exam and an area of the curriculum that candidates would be expected to know. Though well answered, the sections on anatomy were poorly answered. A lack of knowledge of basic sciences is a recurring theme in the Final exam." Nonetheless, the pass rate was a fantastic 79%.

a) From which spinal nerve roots does the brachial plexus originate? (1 mark)

- Anterior rami of spinal nerve roots C5-T1. *(There is variable input from C4 and T2).*

b) List the dermatomes that a successful interscalene block will reliably anaesthetise. (3 marks)

C8 and T1 are not reliably blocked leading to preserved sensation in the ulnar nerve distribution and/or the medial cutaneous nerve of the arm. An interscalene block is therefore not usually suitable as a sole technique for procedures on the distal forearm, wrist or hand.

- C5 – posterolateral aspect of upper arm.
- C6 – upper arm, posterolateral aspect of forearm.
- C7 – posterior forearm, lateral aspect of hand.

c) List four peripheral nerves that would need to be blocked to facilitate awake shoulder surgery. (4 marks)

This is the same question as was asked in the March 2013 question.

d) List four patient factors that increase the likelihood of development of nerve injury after peripheral nerve block. (4 marks)

- Pre-existing peripheral neuropathy.
- Electrolyte abnormalities.
- Cigarette smoking.
- Obesity.
- Diabetes mellitus.
- Hypertension.
- Anatomical abnormalities causing pre-existing nerve stretch or pressure e.g. at thoracic outlet, or joint instability due to e.g. rheumatoid arthritis.

e) List three mechanisms of injury that may cause nerve damage during peripheral nerve block. (3 marks)

- Direct trauma.
- Compression.
- Local anaesthesia neurotoxicity.
- Stretch.

f) State what is meant by "triple monitoring" in the context of performing peripheral nerve blockade. (3 marks)

- Use of ultrasound.
- Use of peripheral nerve stimulator to ensure absence of motor response at 0.2 mA.
- In-line pressure monitoring to avoid injection pressure > 25 psi.

g) Assuming appropriate patient selection, preparation, antisepsis and use of "Stop Before You Block," list two other strategies that may help reduce the risk of nerve injury during peripheral nerve blockade. (2 marks)

- Awake patient.
- Echogenic needle.
- Short-bevelled needle.
- Tangential approach to the nerve.
- Needle repositioning if paraesthesia encountered.
- Avoidance of intraneural injections.
- Local anaesthetic concentration as low as possible.
- Avoidance of adrenaline use around poorly vascularised nerves.

REFERENCES

Betteridge N, Taylor A, Hartley R. Clinical anatomy of the nerve supply to the upper limb. *BJA Educ.* 2021: 21: 462–471.

Hewson D, Oldman M, Bedforth N. Regional anaesthesia for shoulder surgery. *BJA Educ.* 2019: 19: 98–104.

Raju P, Coventry D. Ultrasound-guided brachial plexus blocks. *Contin Educ Anaes Crit Care Pain.* 2014: 14: 185–191.

Topor B, Oldman M, Nicholls B. Best practices for safety and quality in peripheral regional anaesthesia. *BJA Educ.* 2020: 20: 341–347.

13 SEDATION

13.1 September 2015 Sedation for dental procedures

You are asked to sedate a frightened adult patient for insertion of dental implants in an outpatient dental chair.

a) Complete the table to show the four levels of sedation in the American Society of Anaesthesiologists' (ASA) continuum of sedation (top row) (4 marks) and the relevant clinical features seen at each level (rows below). (4 marks)

b) Give two pharmacodynamic or pharmacokinetic attributes of remimazolam that are advantageous for the purposes of conscious sedation in the dentist chair when compared to other benzodiazepines. (2 marks)

c) Give two pharmacodynamic or pharmacokinetic attributes of ketamine that are advantageous for the purposes of conscious sedation in the dentist chair when compared to other sedative options. (2 marks)

d) Give two advantages in the use of nitrous oxide for the purposes of conscious sedation in the dentist chair when compared to other sedative options. (2 marks)

e) List three other drugs that may be used (3 marks) and their methods of administration (3 marks), when providing sedation for this patient.

The "Standards for Conscious Sedation in the Provision of Dental Care" was published in April 2015. In the following exam, there was a question based on sedation for outpatient dental care. The Chairs' Report on the original SAQ gave a 62.1% pass rate and said, "This is an important topic and was generally well answered despite some confusion caused by the inclusion of a table that required completion. It had the highest pass rate of all the questions." The guideline has since been updated in 2020, with a new statement about the use of remimazolam this year.

a) Complete the table to show the four levels of sedation in the American Society of Anesthesiologists' (ASA) continuum of sedation (top row) (4 marks) and the relevant clinical features seen at each level (rows below). (4 marks)

The clinical features follow the alphabet, A, B, C, D. Then remembering what goes into each box is straightforward.

DOI: 10.1201/9781003388494-13   293

Level of sedation / Clinical features	Minimal sedation – anxiolysis	Moderate sedation – conscious sedation	Deep sedation	General anaesthesia
A Airway:	Unaffected.	No intervention required.	Intervention may be required.	Intervention often required.
B Spontaneous ventilation:	Unaffected.	Adequate.	May be inadequate.	Frequently inadequate.
C Cardiovascular function:	Unaffected.	Usually maintained.	Usually maintained.	May be impaired.
D Responsiveness:	Normal response to verbal stimulation.	Purposeful response to verbal or light tactile stimulation.	Purposeful response to repeated or painful stimulation.	No response.

b) **Give two pharmacodynamic or pharmacokinetic attributes of remimazolam that are advantageous for the purposes of conscious sedation in the dentist chair when compared to other benzodiazepines. (2 marks)**

- Faster onset of action.
- Rapid metabolism by plasma esterases and return to pre-sedated state.
- Negligibly active metabolites.

c) **Give two pharmacodynamic or pharmacokinetic attributes of ketamine that are advantageous for the purposes of conscious sedation in the dentist chair when compared to other sedative options. (2 marks)**

- Cardiovascular stability.
- Inherent analgesic effect.
- Preservation of protective airway reflexes.

d) **Give two advantages in the use of nitrous oxide for the purposes of conscious sedation in the dentist chair when compared to other sedative options. (2 marks)**

- Inherent analgesic effect.
- No cannulation required.
- Rapid offset of effect.
- Patient able to drive themselves home after 30 minutes, no escort required.

e) **List three other drugs that may be used (3 marks) and their methods of administration (3 marks), when providing sedation for this patient.**

This is the rest of the full list given in the "Standards for Conscious Sedation in the Provision of Dental Care" document.

- Temazepam – oral.
- Midazolam – intravenous, oral or intranasal route.
- Fentanyl – intravenous route (single small dose, wait until peak effect, followed by cautious intravenous midazolam titration).
- Propofol – intravenous as patient- or target-controlled sedation – can give a titrated dose of midazolam first.
- Sevoflurane in oxygen or with nitrous oxide – inhalation.

REFERENCES

American Society of Anaesthesiologists. *Continuum of depth of sedation: definition of general anesthesia and levels of sedation/analgesia*, Last amended October 2019. www.asahq.org/standards-and-guidelines/continuum-of-depth-of-sedation-definition-of-general-anesthesia-and-levels-of-sedationanalgesia. Accessed 13th March 2023.

Intercollegiate Advisory Committee for Sedation in Dentistry. *Standards for conscious sedation in the provision of dental care (v1.1)*. The Dental Faculties of the Royal Colleges of Surgeons and the Royal College of Anaesthetists, 2020.

Intercollegiate Advisory Committee for Sedation in Dentistry. *Remimazolam for intravenous conscious sedation for dental procedures*, 9th January 2023. www.rcseng.ac.uk/dental-faculties/fds/publications-guidelines/standards-for-conscious-sedation-in-the-provision-of-dental-care-and-accreditation/. Accessed 13th March 2023.

Sneyd J. Developments in procedural sedation for adults. *BJA Educ.* 2022: 22: 258–264.

14 TRAUMA AND STABILISATION

14.1 March 2012 Fractured neck of femur

A 90-year-old woman sustains a fractured neck of femur following a fall. She is scheduled for surgery.
a) What aspects of this patient's care will have the greatest impact on outcome? (9 marks)
b) Outline the recommendations made by The National Institute for Health and Clinical Excellence (2011) for the management of acute pain in this patient. (6 marks)
c) What causes of a fall in this patient might impact on the anaesthetic management? (5 marks)

This SAQ, reproduced above in its original form, focussed on the 2011 NICE guidance on hip fracture care which was updated in 2023. The Chair said that the pass rate was 52.9% but that "a significant number of candidates gave a generic answer without relating to the current NICE guidelines. A significant number of candidates in section (b) failed to concentrate on the management of pain and digressed to general aspects of care." The question reappeared in March 2014 – the only wording change was that it asked for "best practice for the management of pain in this patient." The Chair's Report then said that the pass rate was 53.1% and that it was "straightforward for candidates who had read one of the recent guidelines published by NICE or the AAGBI, and a number of individuals gained maximum marks. The question proved highly discriminatory between generally strong and generally weak candidates." This shows just how clear the link is between guideline publication and exam topics in the Final FRCA, and how you will pick up points for being aware of topical clinical issues. I have made a CRQ in place of the March 2014 SAQ, which addresses the issues surrounding hip fracture care with answers based on contemporaneous guidelines and statements.

DOI: 10.1201/9781003388494-14

14.2 March 2014 Fractured neck of femur

A 90-year-old woman sustains a fractured neck of femur following a fall. She is scheduled for surgery.

a) Apart from selection of the appropriate surgical technique, give five factors that contribute to best patient care in the context of hip fracture. (5 marks)

b) List three pharmacological best practice elements of the patient's pain management while awaiting surgery. (3 marks)

c) List two regional anaesthetic techniques that can be used as part of the patient's pain management strategy. (2 marks)

d) List two benefits of inclusion of regional anaesthetic techniques in the pain management strategy for this patient. (2 marks)

e) State the perioperative transfusion thresholds for hip fracture patients. (2 marks)

f) List six causes of the fall in this patient that might impact on the anaesthetic management. (6 marks)

There is a great BJA Education article, referenced below, that draws together the key current guidelines that are relevant to hip fracture care.

a) **Apart from selection of the appropriate surgical technique, give five factors that contribute to best patient care in the context of hip fracture. (5 marks)**

These best practice points are from NICE guidance, NHS England Best Practice Tariffs, Association of Anaesthetists' guidance, and the National Hip Fracture Database report. There are slight variations in wording (especially with regard to timing of surgery) between the sources but the overall message emphasises rapid surgery and multidisciplinary input on recovery and prevention of future fractures, with the aim of returning the patient to their original residence.

- Surgery within 36 hours of (or on the day of or the day after) admission (or from the time of the fracture, if it occurred in hospital) on a planned trauma list with consultant or other senior staff supervision.
- Geriatrician assessment within 72 hours of admission.
- Mobilisation with physiotherapist to commence no later than the day after surgery.
- Preoperative cognitive assessment using abbreviated mental test score.
- Fracture prevention assessment to include specialist falls and bone health assessment.
- Nutritional assessment.
- Postoperative delirium assessment using the 4 "As" Test (4AT).

b) **List three pharmacological best practice elements of the patient's pain management while awaiting surgery. (3 marks)**

- Regular paracetamol unless contraindicated.
- Opioids if required but aim to limit opioid intake, especially long-acting opioids.
- NSAIDs not recommended.

c) **List two regional anaesthetic techniques that can be used as part of the patient's pain management strategy. (2 marks)**

The use of fascia iliaca block as an easily teachable technique with low risk profile has had a lot of focus. It can readily be performed in the emergency department with the potential of transforming the patient's pain experience from admission onwards. The first three listed feature in the guidelines, but there are a number of blocks that may be utilised.

- Fascia iliaca block.
- Femoral nerve block.
- 3-in-1 block.
- Pericapsular nerve group block.
- Lumbar plexus block.
- Quadratus lumborum block.
- Erector spinae block.

d) **List two benefits of inclusion of regional anaesthetic techniques in the pain management strategy for this patient. (2 marks)**

- Avoidance of longer-acting opioids which may contribute to the risk of delirium and respiratory depression especially in the context of renal dysfunction.
- May reduce the need for sedative or analgesic drugs for positioning for spinal anaesthesia, thus reducing the risk of delirium.
- Contribute to better overall pain experience.
- Are associated with a reduced time to remobilisation.
- May facilitate examination and radiological assessment on first presentation.
- Are not contraindicated in anticoagulated patients in whom a spinal anaesthetic would be contraindicated.

e) **State the perioperative transfusion thresholds for hip fracture patients. (2 marks)**

- > 90 g/l for frail patients with fractured neck of femur.
- > 100 g/l for patients with a history of ischaemic heart disease or who fail to remobilise on the first postoperative day due to dizziness or fatigue.

f) **List six causes of the fall in this patient that might impact on the anaesthetic management. (6 marks)**

Take your pick of six from the list below – I have grouped them as I used the alphabet to think of all possible causes of a fall that might impact on the safe provision of anaesthesia (I want you to see that this is a useful approach), but you wouldn't need to do that in the exam.

- Respiratory; exacerbation of chronic obstructive pulmonary disease, pneumonia. Regional anaesthesia may be preferable to avoid interference with lung mechanics.
- Cardiovascular; brady- or tachyarrhythmias, myocardial infarction, valvular heart disease (e.g. aortic stenosis), structural abnormalities (e.g. hypertrophic obstructive cardiomyopathy). Higher levels of monitoring such as invasive blood pressure and cardiac output monitoring may be employed in the presence of significant comorbidities. Neuraxial techniques relatively contraindicated by left ventricular outflow-limiting disease.
- Neurological; stroke, peripheral neuropathy, dementia, Parkinson's. Confusion or other difficulty with positioning may cause problems with complying with neuraxial approach. Pre-existing neuropathy should be documented prior to any form of anaesthesia.
- Endocrine; diabetes mellitus causing hypoglycaemia or diabetic ketoacidosis. Awake surgery would permit ongoing neurological monitoring (once fit for surgery).

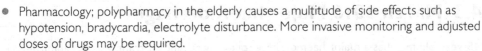

- Pharmacology; polypharmacy in the elderly causes a multitude of side effects such as hypotension, bradycardia, electrolyte disturbance. More invasive monitoring and adjusted doses of drugs may be required.
- Infection, immune; sepsis causing confusion, hypoxia. Sepsis may contraindicate neuraxial technique.
- Cutaneoumusculoskeletal; arthritic conditions causing pain and deformity. May cause difficulty with positioning for regional or neuraxial techniques.

REFERENCES

Griffiths R et al. Guideline by the Association of Anaesthetists: guideline for the management of hip fractures 2020. *Anaesthesia.* 2021: 76: 225–237.

National Institute for Health and Care Excellence. *Management of hip fractures in adults: CG124,* June 2011, updated January 2023.

National Institute for Health and Care Excellence. *Hip fracture in adults quality standard: QS16.* NHS England, March 2012, updated January 2023.

NHS England. *Consultation on 2021/2022 national tariff payment system: annex DtC: guidance on best practice tariffs,* March 2021. www.england.nhs.uk/wp-content/uploads/2021/03/21-22NT_Annex-DtC-Best-practice-tariffs.pdf. Accessed 21st March 2023.

Royal College of Physicians. *National hip fracture database annual report 2019.* London: Royal College of Physicians, 2019.

Shelton C, White S. Anaesthesia for hip fracture repair. *BJA Educ.* 2020: 20: 142–149.

14.3 March 2016 Major haemorrhage

A 45-year-old man has a major haemorrhage following significant trauma and is admitted to your emergency department. He does not have a head injury.
a) Give one definition of major haemorrhage. (1 mark)
b) Define massive transfusion. (1 mark)
c) List five signs of major haemorrhage. (5 marks)
d) List three elements of damage control resuscitation. (3 marks)
e) Give two laboratory target values for infusion of blood products other than packed red cells during major haemorrhage. (2 marks)
f) List four immune complications of a massive blood transfusion. (4 marks)
g) List four non-immune complications of a massive blood transfusion. (4 marks)

The Chairs' Report following the original SAQ reported an 85.3% pass rate stating, "It is reassuring that candidates have sound knowledge of the management of major haemorrhage and of the complications of massive transfusion." The AAGBI guideline "The Use of Blood Components and Their Alternatives," brings together three previous AAGBI guidelines concerning blood management. It is clinically useful to read and contains plenty of material that could be the basis of future questions.

a) Give one definition of major haemorrhage. (1 mark)

There are lots of definitions referred to in the guideline. Pick your favourite.

- Loss of more than one blood volume within 24 hours (70 ml/kg or 5 litres for a 70 kg adult).
- 50% of total blood volume loss in < 3 hours.
- Bleeding > 150 ml/min.
- Bleeding that results in systolic blood pressure < 90 mmHg or heart rate > 110 bpm.

b) Define massive transfusion. (1 mark)

As per the ATLS guidelines:

- Transfusion of more than ten units of blood in 24 hours OR
- More than four units of blood in one hour.

c) List five signs of major haemorrhage. (5 marks)

The ATLS manual gives a table of the changes in these signs that are associated with class I-IV haemorrhagic shock, with values for the accompanying worsening base deficit.

- Increased heart rate.
- Decreased blood pressure.
- Decreased pulse pressure.
- Increased respiratory rate.
- Decreased urine output.
- Decreased GCS.

d) List three elements of damage control resuscitation. (3 marks)

- Early haemorrhage control; pressure, tourniquets, surgery, interventional radiology techniques.
- Permissive hypotension; allowing a lower-than-normal blood pressure whilst maintaining, with volume alone (i.e. not vasopressors), an adequate preload and blood pressure for cerebration and other essential organ perfusion.

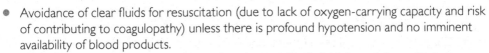

- Avoidance of clear fluids for resuscitation (due to lack of oxygen-carrying capacity and risk of contributing to coagulopathy) unless there is profound hypotension and no imminent availability of blood products.
- Management of trauma-induced coagulopathy, empirically initially and then with use of laboratory or point-of-care results. Initial management is 1 g tranexamic acid and administration of red blood cells and FFP in 1:1 ratio, with two five-unit pools of cryoprecipitate, and a pack of platelets.

e) Give two laboratory target values for infusion of blood products other than packed red cells during major haemorrhage. (2 marks)

The target fibrinogen in obstetric haemorrhage is 2 g/l.

- Fresh frozen plasma if INR greater than 1.5.
- Cryoprecipitate if fibrinogen less than 1.5 g/l.
- Platelets if platelet count less than 75×10^9/l.

f) List four immune complications of a massive blood transfusion. (4 marks)

I have put in a few details of the mechanisms of some of these reactions because I find it easier to remember something when I understand it, but this is not actually asked for. The first four of these listed are early reactions, and the rest occur at a variable time after transfusion.

- Immediate haemolytic reaction due to ABO incompatibility due to human error.
- Febrile non-haemolytic transfusion reactions: reaction to donor leucocyte antigens, risk lower now that units are leucodepleted.
- Allergic or anaphylactic reaction: recipient immunoglobulin E versus donor proteins present especially in plasma-rich components e.g. FFP but also in packed red cells.
- Transfusion-related acute lung injury (TRALI): donor leucocyte antibodies reacting with human leucocyte antigens (HLA) and human neutrophil antigens (HNA) in the recipient.
- Delayed haemolytic transfusion reaction due to re-exposure after sensitisation (from e.g. pregnancy or previous blood transfusion) to a more minor grouping such as Kidd or rhesus.
- Immune sensitisation causing issues with cross match for future blood transfusions.
- Transfusion-associated graft-versus-host disease: viable donor lymphocytes engraft in immunosuppressed recipient and mount immune response to recipient cells.
- Post-transfusion purpura: previous sensitisation to a platelet antigen e.g. during pregnancy and then re-exposure to that antigen after transfusion results in indiscriminate platelet destruction. Rare since blood leucodepletion.

g) List four non-immune complications of a massive blood transfusion. (4 marks)

Iron overload is another non-immunological risk of blood transfusion, but this takes place after a series of blood transfusions e.g. with transfusion-dependent anaemias, rather than a single massive transfusion.

- Overwhelming infection due to bacterial contamination. Rare, occurs more commonly with platelets which are stored at 22°C.
- Transfusion-associated circulatory overload (TACO).
- Hyperkalaemia: potassium content in stored blood rises with time due to loss of activity of red blood cell Na/K ATPase pump.
- Citrate toxicity: large amounts of citrate in fresh frozen plasma and platelets, binds calcium resulting in hypocalcaemia, impacts on cardiac conduction and coagulation.
- Acid-base disturbance: citric acid from anticoagulant and lactic acid from stored cells may cause acidosis in critically unwell patients, but their metabolism leads to alkalosis.
- Hypothermia.

- Air embolism.
- Thrombophlebitis.
- Coagulation abnormalities if other blood components not given appropriately.
- Viral infection such as hepatitis A, B or C, HIV, CMV.
- Parasitic infection e.g. malaria, toxoplasma.
- vCJD: risk reduced since universal leucodepletion of donated blood, exclusion of donors who have received blood transfusions in UK, sourcing of plasma for fractionation from abroad.

REFERENCES

American College of Surgeons. *Advanced trauma life support: student course manual*, 10th edition. Chicago: American College of Surgeons, 2018.

Association of Anaesthetists of Great Britain and Ireland. AAGBI guidelines: the use of blood components and their alternatives 2016. *Anaesthesia.* 2016: 71: 829–842.

Joint United Kingdom (UK) Blood Transfusion and Tissue Transplantation Services Professional Advisory Committee. *Handbook of transfusion medicine.* www.transfusionguidelines.org/transfusion-handbook/publication-information. Accessed 21st March 2023.

National Institute for Health and Care Excellence. *Blood transfusion: NG24*, November 2015.

14.4 March 2016 Nonfatal drowning

A 20-year-old man is brought to the emergency department having been pulled from a river where he got into difficulties whilst swimming.
a) List four key aspects of the history for a patient who has suffered nonfatal drowning. (4 marks)
b) List four specific investigations relevant to the assessment of a patient who has suffered nonfatal drowning, giving one reason for the relevance of each. (8 marks)
c) List four possible respiratory complications in a patient presenting after nonfatal drowning. (4 marks)
d) List four causes of hypotension in a patient extracted after submersion in a river. (4 marks)

The Chairs' Report of the original SAQ found a pass rate of 57.9%. Drowning is the process of respiratory impairment following immersion or submersion in a liquid. It is fatal or nonfatal – older terminologies such as dry-drowning, wet-drowning or near-drowning are no longer used.

a) **List four key aspects of the history for a patient who has suffered nonfatal drowning. (4 marks)**

- Medical history; seek possible medical cause for nonfatal drowning such as epilepsy, arrhythmia, cardiac history, uncontrolled diabetes.
- Toxins; drugs, alcohol ingestion.
- Trauma; may have associated injuries e.g. from a boat, diving, debris in water, foul play.
- Scene; timings, duration of submersion, contaminants in water, type of water (*this question says river*), ambient and water temperature ("cold water" is less than 20°C, "warm water" is above). Witnesses useful.

b) **List four specific investigations relevant to the assessment of a patient who has suffered nonfatal drowning, giving one reason for the relevance of each. (8 marks)**

- Core body temperature:
  - Impact on algorithm management of cardiac arrest.
  - Guides re-warming if patient does not require intubation.
- Capillary blood glucose:
  - Poor control of diabetes may be cause of events.
  - Target normal blood glucose to maximise neurological outcome.
- Arterial blood gases:
  - Likely hypoxic, hypercapnic, with lactic acidosis.
- Venous blood:
  - Urea, creatinine, creatine kinase. Acute kidney injury may develop from myoglobinuria, hypoxaemia, hypoperfusion, haemolysis.
  - Electrolytes. Occasionally, electrolyte changes from fluid shifts.
  - Full blood count and coagulation. Disseminated intravascular coagulation may occur.
  - Toxicological assays for drugs and alcohol which may have precipitated the event.
- 12-lead ECG:
  - Risk of arrhythmias due to hypothermia, hypoxia, acid-base disturbance.
  - May identify underlying cardiac event.
- Chest X-ray:
  - Identification of ARDS.
- Transthoracic echo:
  - May help optimise cardiovascular management in the presence of instability.
- Trauma imaging:
  - Cervical spine imaging, CT of the head, as indicated by history and examination.

- Microbiology:
  - Sputum or tracheal aspirates once intubated. May help with antimicrobial management in the presence of developing sepsis.

c) **List four possible respiratory complications in a patient presenting after nonfatal drowning. (4 marks)**

- Fluid aspiration washes out surfactant leading to alveolar collapse and atelectasis.
- Acute pulmonary oedema follows the aspiration of hypotonic fluid.
- Bronchospasm follows introduction of fluid or other foreign material into the airways.
- Attempted ventilation against reflex laryngospasm can cause alveolar rupture and acute emphysema.
- Inhaled toxins e.g. pollutants, chlorine, particulate material can directly cause pulmonary dysfunction.
- Aspiration of stomach contents due to reduced consciousness level.
- Development of ARDS.
- Acute pneumonia. *Pseudomonas* and *Aeromonas* are common in water and can cause pneumonia within hours.

d) **List four causes of hypotension in a patient extracted after submersion in a river. (4 marks)**

- Decrease in afterload due to loss of hydrostatic effect of water.
- Acute heart failure due to profound hypoxia, and hypothermia induced, sympathetically mediated, vasoconstriction.
- Arrhythmias, myocardial depression (and, eventually, cardiac arrest) due to acid-base disturbance, hypoxia, hypercapnia, electrolyte disturbance, hypothermia, and high catecholamine levels.
- Intravascular depletion due to pulmonary and systemic extravasation.
- Cardio-depressant and vasodilatory effect of proinflammatory mediators due to SIRS response to nonfatal drowning.
- Hypotensive effect of any associated injuries e.g. due to haemorrhage, spinal shock.

REFERENCES

Carter E, Sinclair R. Drowning. *Contin Educ Anaesth Crit Care Pain*. 2011: 11: 210–213.
RCEM Learning. Wen Tao Kark W. *Drowning: Royal College of Emergency Medicine*, Published 29th February 2020. www.rcemlearning.co.uk/reference/drowning/#1568890491084-3a97dd39-a049. Accessed 21st March 2023.

14.5 March 2018 Nonfatal drowning

A 20-year-old man is brought to the emergency department having been pulled from a river following a near drowning.
  a) What relevant features in the history are important? (5 marks)
  b) What investigations are required? (8 marks)
  c) He has a Glasgow Coma Score of 13 but is found to have an arterial oxygen partial pressure of 6 kPa (45 mmHg) breathing 4 l/min of oxygen via a variable performance mask. Outline your management of this patient. (7 marks)

This is the original SAQ from March 2018, which was the same as that from March 2016. The pass rate this time was 62.4%, and the Chairs deemed it an "easy" question. However, as in 2016, the Chairs commented that the answers to the management section were poor with candidates concentrating solely on intubation and ventilation and demonstrating little knowledge of any other management. For the sake of a possible viva, I have therefore answered section (c) below.

  c) He has a Glasgow Coma Score of 13 but is found to have an arterial oxygen partial pressure of 6 kPa (45 mmHg) breathing 4 l/min of oxygen via a variable performance mask. Outline your management of this patient. (7 marks)

I would call for help and adopt an ABCDE trauma team management approach to this patient, assessing and treating him simultaneously as issues are revealed.

A:

  - Open airway, administer 15 l oxygen via non-rebreathe mask, prepare for rapid sequence induction (RSI) if patient unable to maintain own airway or does not respond rapidly to measures to improve breathing adequacy.
  - Cervical spine control with all airway manoeuvres if there is any possibility of injury.
  - If PaO_2 and GCS not rapidly improving with higher inhaled oxygen concentration, proceed with RSI (stomach likely full of water), intubate.

B:

  - Consider orogastric or nasogastric (if no associated head injury) tube to empty stomach of water and facilitate ventilation.
  - Lung protective ventilation: 6 ml/kg, high PEEP, 100% oxygen initially.
  - CXR may demonstrate ARDS, foreign body aspiration (e.g. sand — consider bronchoalveolar lavage).

C:

  - Large-bore intravenous access.
  - Intravascular depletion occurs due to pulmonary and systemic extravasation.
  - Warmed intravenous fluids with cardiac output monitoring guidance.
  - Arterial cannulation to monitor blood pressure and blood gases. Aim MAP greater than 80–90 mmHg for neuroprotection if concerns about neurological injury.
  - Inotropes or vasopressors may be required.
  - Monitor for and manage arrhythmias caused by hypothermia, acid-base or electrolyte disturbance.
  - Catheterise. Monitor urine output as an indicator of end-organ perfusion.

D:

If concerns about neurological injury, manage secondary brain injury risks:

- Maintain $PaCO_2$ between 4.5 and 5.0 kPa (permissive hypercapnia in line with lung protection would otherwise be the aim).
- Adequate sedation (and analgesia) to reduce $CMRO_2$.
- Muscle paralysis if needed to facilitate ventilation to desired PaO_2 and $PaCO_2$ and if patient not synchronising with ventilator.
- Facilitate venous drainage by 30-degree head-up tilt, avoidance of tight tube ties.
- Maintain normoglycaemia.
- Warm to 34°C only; warmed fluids, forced air warming, electrical warming pads for 24 hours (fully rewarm if patient doesn't require intubation).

E:

- Manage coexisting injuries or precipitating causes.

REFERENCES

Carter E, Sinclair R. Drowning. *Contin Educ Anaesth Crit Care Pain.* 2011: 11: 210–213.

RCEM Learning. Wen Tao Kark W. *Drowning: Royal College of Emergency Medicine*, Published 29th February 2020. www.rcemlearning.co.uk/reference/drowning/#1568890491084-3a97dd39-a049. Accessed 21st March 2023.

14.6 February 2023 Fractured neck of femur

a) State the time frame within which patients presenting with fractured neck of femur should have their surgery. (1 mark)
b) List five reasons for which it may be acceptable to delay surgical fixation in a patient presenting with a fractured neck of femur. (5 marks)
c) List four patient factors that increase the 30-day mortality risk in patients admitted with hip fracture. (4 marks)
d) State the mechanism of action of apixaban and, assuming normal renal function, state the interval after which it is acceptable to perform a spinal anaesthetic following the last dose. (2 marks)
e) List five aspects of the conduct of anaesthesia for fractured neck of femur that support best patient outcomes. (5 marks)
f) List three possible barriers to next-day mobility after fractured neck of femur surgery. (3 marks)

This is the third time fractured neck of femur surgery has been the focus of a Final question in the time frame of this book, and there are a number of areas of factual recall tested relating to the best practice guidelines published by the Association of Anaesthetists in 2020. In the same year, there was a BJA article reviewing anaesthesia for hip fracture surgery so it should have come as no surprise that this common topic was re-examined shortly after. The Chairs reported a pass rate of 66.8% and commented that the topic was one that "most candidates will have experience of in their day to day practice."

a) **State the time frame within which patients presenting with fractured neck of femur should have their surgery. (1 mark)**

Delayed surgery is associated with increased 30-day mortality. There is slight variety in recommendations but the following is an appropriate answer:

- Surgery within 36 hours of (or on the day of or the day after) admission (or from the time of the fracture, if it occurred in hospital).

b) **List five reasons for which it may be acceptable to delay surgical fixation in a patient presenting with a fractured neck of femur. (5 marks)**

Historically, patients presenting with fractured neck of femur have been subjected to delayed surgery due to a range of reasons. Current recommendations identify eight "acceptable" reasons for delay, if the benefit from correcting the issue is deemed to outweigh the risk of delay. However, it is also emphasised that 36 hours should be enough time to sufficiently address the reversible nature of most of these issues. NICE guidance also refers to volume depletion as being a reason for delay, but this should be very rapidly correctable.

- Hb < 80 g/l (aim instead for 90 g/l in all patients and > 100 g/l in those with cardiovascular disease).
- Sodium < 120 or > 150 mmol/l.
- Potassium < 2.8 or > 6 mmol/l.
- Uncontrolled diabetes.
- Acute heart failure.
- Correctable tachyarrhythmia with ventricular rate > 120 bpm.
- Chest infection with sepsis.
- Reversible coagulopathy.

c) **List four patient factors that increase the 30-day mortality risk in patients admitted with hip fracture. (4 marks)**

The following points are those which contribute to the Nottingham Hip Fracture Score. In addition to the use of this scoring system, Association of Anaesthetists' guidance advises the use of a frailty score to help predict discharge destination, scoring to detect postoperative delirium with the use of the 4 "As" Test (4AT), and assessment of risk of acute kidney injury with, for example, Nottingham Hip Fracture Risk Score for Kidney Injury.

- Advanced age.
- Male sex.
- Reduced cognitive function (reduced abbreviated mental test score).
- Anaemia.
- Institutional living prior to admission.
- Two or more active comorbidities.
- Active malignancy (apart from squamous or basal cell malignancy) within the past 20 years.

d) **State the mechanism of action of apixaban and, assuming normal renal function, state the interval after which it is acceptable to perform a spinal anaesthetic for hip fracture surgery following the last dose. (2 marks)**

The acceptable time interval for spinal anaesthesia specifically for hip fracture surgery is different to that quoted in other guidance on the basis that the risk-benefit assessment pushes in favour of early fixation of hip fracture using whichever anaesthesia modality is deemed the most appropriate for the individual patient.

- Factor Xa inhibitor.
- Acceptable time to neuraxial technique is 24 hours.

e) **List five aspects of conduct of anaesthesia for fractured neck of femur that support best patient outcomes. (5 marks)**

Current evidence does not support either general or neuraxial anaesthesia as supportive of better outcomes, rather the focus should be on the manner in which either is delivered.

- General principles:
  - Intraoperative regional anaesthesia (alongside spinal or general anaesthesia) as part of a multimodal analgesia approach to reduce the need for long-acting psychoactive agents.
  - Avoidance of hypotension (*systematic reviews show an increase in mortality if MAP < 80 mmHg for > 10 mins*).
  - Minimisation of risk of postoperative delirium by avoiding use of long-acting sedatives, long-acting opioids, antipsychotics, centrally acting anticholinergics, and antihistamines.
- Conduct of spinal anaesthesia:
  - Limitation of spinal bupivacaine dose to < 10 mg.
  - Avoidance of intrathecal opioids (using fentanyl only if opioid deemed necessary).
- Conduct of general anaesthesia:
  - Avoidance of excessive depth of anaesthesia by using EEG-based assessment of anaesthetic depth and age-adjusted minimum alveolar concentration monitoring.
  - Maintenance of spontaneous respiration to minimise atelectasis, barotrauma, and hypotension associated with positive pressure ventilation.

f) List three possible barriers to next-day mobility after fractured neck of femur surgery. (3 marks)

The following list is not exhaustive, but these factors are identified in the Association of Anaesthetists' guidance as those which can be influenced by anaesthetic management.

- Ongoing pain.
- Hypotension.
- Constipation or diarrhoea.
- Nausea and vomiting.
- Urinary retention.
- Postoperative delirium.
- Anaemia.

REFERENCES

Griffiths R et al. Guideline by the Association of Anaesthetists: guideline for the management of hip fractures 2020. *Anaesthesia.* 2021: 76: 225–237.

Maxwell M, Moran C, Moppett I. Development and validation of a preoperative scoring system to predict 30 day mortality in patients undergoing hip fracture surgery. *BJA.* 2008: 101: 511–517.

National Institute for Health and Care Excellence. *Management of hip fractures in adults: CG124,* June 2011, updated January 2023.

National Institute for Health and Care Excellence. *Hip fracture in adults quality standard: QS16,* March 2012, updated January 2023.

NHS England. *Consultation on 2021/2022 national tariff payment system: annex DtC: guidance on best practice tariffs,* March 2021. www.england.nhs.uk/wp-content/uploads/2021/03/21-22NT_ Annex-DtC-Best-practice-tariffs.pdf. Accessed 21st March 2023.

Royal College of Physicians. *National hip fracture database annual report 2019.* London: Royal College of Physicians, 2019.

Shelton C, White S. Anaesthesia for hip fracture repair. *BJA Educ.* 2020: 20: 142–149.

INTENSIVE CARE
MEDICINE

15.1 September 2011 Acute respiratory distress syndrome

An almost identical question appeared in the March 2017 paper, and so I will address this question there. The precise definition of ARDS changed between 2012 and 2017, and so it was an obvious choice for appearing in the exam again. The topic of ARDS featured again in March 2022 with extra questions about proning, making it very topical.

DOI: 10.1201/9781003388494-15

15.2 March 2012 Diabetic ketoacidosis

a) Give the three diagnostic criteria for diabetic ketoacidosis (DKA). (3 marks)
b) Give the two components of initial insulin management of a known diabetic adult patient admitted with DKA. (2 marks)
c) State the immediate fluid management of an adult patient admitted with DKA with systolic blood pressure < 90 mmHg. (1 mark)
d) State the equation for calculation of anion gap. (1 mark)
e) List three biochemical findings of severe DKA in an adult that may warrant High Dependency Unit (HDU) referral. (3 marks)
f) List three clinical findings of severe DKA in an adult that may warrant HDU referral. (3 marks)
g) Give three patient groups or patient comorbidities that may indicate need for HDU referral of an adult patient with DKA. (3 marks)
h) Give four common complications of DKA management. (4 marks)

"The Management of Diabetic Ketoacidosis in Adults" was published in 2010, DKA featured in the exam in 2012, and then the guidance was updated in 2021, making this topic a likely focus for an exam question in the near future. The authors of the guideline comment on the wide variation in hospital guidelines for the management of DKA and the variation in adherence to them. It is therefore worth making yourself familiar with their single-page summary guideline for the sake of your clinical practice as well as the exam. The question had a 57.2% pass rate when it appeared as an SAQ in March 2012.

a) **Give the three diagnostic criteria for diabetic ketoacidosis (DKA). (3 marks)**

- Blood glucose concentration > 11 mmol/l OR known to be diabetic.
- Blood or capillary ketone concentration > 3 mmol/l OR ketonuria 2+ on urine dip.
- Bicarbonate concentration of < 15 mmol/l AND/OR pH < 7.3.

b) **Give the two components of initial insulin management of a known diabetic adult patient admitted with DKA. (2 marks)**

- Commence a fixed rate intravenous insulin infusion at 0.1 unit/kg/h.
- Continue whatever long-acting insulin the patient takes at the usual dose and time.

c) **State the immediate fluid management of an adult patient admitted with DKA with systolic blood pressure < 90 mmHg. (1 mark)**

- 500 ml 0.9% sodium chloride over 10–15 minutes.

d) **State the equation for calculation of anion gap. (1 mark)**

- $(Na^+ + K^+) - (Cl^- + HCO_3^-)$

e) **List three biochemical findings of severe DKA in an adult that may warrant High Dependency Unit (HDU) referral. (3 marks)**

- Blood ketones > 6 mmol/l.
- Venous bicarbonate < 5 mmol/l.
- Venous pH < 7.1.
- Hypokalaemia on admission < 3.5 mmol/l.
- Anion gap > 16.

f) List three clinical findings of severe DKA in an adult that may warrant HDU referral. (3 marks)

- GCS <12.
- Oxygen saturation < 92% on air.
- Systolic blood pressure < 90 mmHg.
- Pulse > 100 bpm or < 60 bpm.

g) Give three patient groups or patient comorbidities that may indicate need for HDU referral of an adult patient with DKA. (3 marks)

- Young adults aged 18–25 years.
- Elderly.
- Pregnant.
- Significant comorbidity including heart or kidney failure.

h) Give four common complications of DKA management. (4 marks)

- Hypo or hyperkalaemia with/without cardiac arrhythmia.
- Hypoglycaemia *(risking brain injury or death)*.
- Cerebral oedema *(more likely in young adults and children, due to excessive fluid administration and fluid shifts associated with DKA treatment)*.
- Transient acute kidney injury.
- Venous thromboembolism *(may occur in association with a central venous catheter)*.

REFERENCE

Joint British Diabetes Societies for Inpatient Care. *The management of diabetic ketoacidosis in adults*, Revised June 2021.

15.3 March 2012 Venous thromboembolism

a) List two respiratory symptoms of pulmonary thrombo-embolism. (2 marks)
b) List three respiratory signs of pulmonary thrombo-embolism. (3 marks)
c) List two neurological features of pulmonary thrombo-embolism. (2 marks)
d) Give three ECG changes that may be associated with pulmonary thrombo-embolism. (3 marks)
e) List two clinical presentations which indicate a diagnosis of "high-risk" pulmonary thrombo-embolism. (2 marks)
f) Give two tests that may be used to confirm the diagnosis in a patient suspected of having high-risk pulmonary thrombo-embolism. (2 marks)
g) List two absolute contraindications for pharmacological thrombolytic treatment for patients with high-risk pulmonary thrombo-embolism. (2 marks)
h) Give two interventional or surgical management options for the treatment of high-risk pulmonary thrombo-embolism. (2 marks)
i) Give two specific risks to a patient with high-risk pulmonary thrombo-embolism if initiation of invasive ventilation is required as part of their management. (2 marks)

The question had a 77.5% pass rate when it appeared as an SAQ.

a) List two respiratory symptoms of pulmonary thrombo-embolism. (2 marks)

- Dyspnoea.
- Pleuritic chest pain *(pleural irritation due to distal emboli causing pulmonary infarction)*.
- Haemoptysis.

b) List three respiratory signs of pulmonary thrombo-embolism. (3 marks)

- Cyanosis/low oxygen saturations.
- Pleural rub.
- Tachypnoea/increased work of breathing.
- Wheeze.

c) List two neurological features of pulmonary thrombo-embolism. (2 marks)

- Syncope/pre-syncope.
- Anxiety/apprehension.

d) Give three ECG changes that may be associated with pulmonary thrombo-embolism. (3 marks)

- Tachycardia.
- Atrial arrhythmia, especially atrial fibrillation.
- Signs of right ventricular strain: S1Q3T3 or T wave inversion in V1-V4 or QR pattern in V1.
- Pulseless electrical activity.

e) List two clinical presentations which indicate a diagnosis of "high-risk" pulmonary thrombo-embolism. (2 marks)

- Cardiac arrest.
- Obstructive shock; hypotension in association with end-organ hypoperfusion.
- Persistent hypotension.

f) Give two tests that may be used to confirm the diagnosis in a patient suspected of having high-risk pulmonary thrombo-embolism. (2 marks)

- Echocardiography.
- CTPA.

g) List two absolute contraindications for pharmacological thrombolytic treatment for patients with high-risk pulmonary thrombo-embolism. (2 marks)

- History of haemorrhagic stroke or stroke of unknown cause.
- Ischaemic stroke within the past six months.
- Central nervous system neoplasm.
- Major trauma, surgery, or head injury in the previous three weeks.
- Bleeding diathesis.
- Active bleeding.

h) Give two interventional or surgical management options for the treatment of high-risk pulmonary thrombo-embolism. (2 marks)

The answer does not include caval filter – indications for this would be recurrent venous thrombo-embolism when already on anticoagulation or venous thrombo-embolism and a contraindication to anticoagulation.

- Percutaneous catheter-directed therapy *(femoral artery access for catheter, mechanical or ultrasound fragmentation, thrombus aspiration, may be combined with in situ reduced dose thrombolysis)*.
- Surgical embolectomy.

i) Give two specific risks to a patient with high-risk pulmonary thrombo-embolism if initiation of invasive ventilation is required as part of their management. (2 marks)

- Hypotensive and negatively inotropic effects of anaesthetic induction agents on an already haemodynamically compromised patient.
- Deterioration of venous return and hence right heart cardiac output due to positive pressure ventilation.

REFERENCE

Konstantinides S et al. 2019 ESC guidelines for the diagnosis and management of acute pulmonary embolism developed in collaboration with the European Respiratory Society (ERS). *Eur Respir J.* 2019: 54: 1901647.

15.4 March 2013 Tricyclic antidepressant overdose

a) State the mechanism of action for therapeutic effect of tricyclic antidepressants (TCA). (1 mark)
b) Complete the following table to list three further receptor actions of TCAs giving an effect of that receptor action for each. (6 marks)
c) Give two therapeutic interventions that can be considered in the management of TCA overdose if within one hour of ingestion. (2 marks)
d) List three possible indications for intubation and invasive ventilation for patients following a TCA overdose. (3 marks)
e) List four treatments that can be used in the management of hypotension and arrhythmia in the presence of TCA overdose. (4 marks)
f) Apart from sinus tachycardia, give two ECG changes that can result from TCA overdose. (2 marks)
g) Give one drug that should be avoided for management of seizures in TCA overdose. (1 mark)
h) Give the drug class of choice for management of seizures in TCA overdose. (1 mark)

The Chair's Report quoted a pass rate of 65% for the SAQ on this topic. Mixed acidosis from TCA overdose will cause reduction in plasma protein binding of the drug making more of it available for competition at sodium and alpha receptors. Correction of acidosis through controlled ventilation and with sodium bicarbonate, which also increases the presence of sodium at sodium receptors to compete with the action of TCA, are important approaches to improving cardiovascular stability.

a) State the mechanism of action for therapeutic effect of tricyclic antidepressants (TCA). (1 mark)

- Inhibition of reuptake of serotonin and noradrenaline into the presynaptic terminals thus raising their concentration for postsynaptic receptor activation.

b) Complete the following table to list three further receptor actions of TCAs giving an effect of that receptor action for each. (6 marks)

Receptor action	Clinical effect
Sodium channel antagonism.	Cardiac depression, decrease in cardiac output, hypotension. Arrhythmias, seizures.
Alpha adrenergic direct antagonism.	Hypotension.
Anticholinergic effects.	Mydriasis, tachycardia, hypotension, ileus, irritability, confusion, seizures, coma, urinary retention, pyrexia.

c) Give two therapeutic interventions that can be considered in the management of TCA overdose if within one hour of ingestion. (2 marks)

- Activated charcoal administration.
- Gastric lavage (*if airway is protected either by patient being fully awake or intubated*).

d) List three possible indications for intubation and invasive ventilation for patients following a TCA overdose. (3 marks)

- Fluctuation in consciousness/GCS < 8/reduction of GCS that compromises airway protection.
- Hypoventilation contributing to acidosis.
- Refractory seizures.

e) List four treatments that can be used in the management of hypotension and arrhythmia in the presence of TCA overdose. (4 marks)

- Fluid resuscitation.
- 8.4% sodium bicarbonate (correction of acidosis and increased competition at sodium receptors).
- Alpha agonist e.g. adrenaline infusion.
- Magnesium sulphate for treatment of dysrhythmia.
- Intravenous glucagon.

f) Apart from sinus tachycardia, give two ECG changes that can result from TCA overdose. (2 marks)

- QRS prolongation.
- QTc prolongation.
- R/S ratio > 0.7 in aVR.
- Nodal or ventricular arrhythmia.

g) Give one drug that should be avoided for management of seizures in TCA overdose. (1 mark)

- Phenytoin. *Phenytoin given in the presence of an overdose of TCA can raise phenytoin levels risking toxicity and ventricular arrhythmias.*

h) Give the drug class of choice for management of seizures in TCA overdose. (1 mark)

- Benzodiazepines.

REFERENCES

Body R. *Guideline for the management of tricyclic antidepressant overdose.* The College of Emergency Medicine, 2009.

Kerr G, McGuiffie A, Wilkie S. Tricyclic antidepressant overdose: a review. *Emerg Med J.* 2001: 18: 236–234.

15.5 September 2013 Acute kidney injury and renal replacement therapy on intensive care

a) List five perioperative risk factors for development of acute kidney injury. (5 marks)
b) List four patient risk factors for development of acute kidney injury perioperatively. (4 marks)
c) List four indications for renal replacement therapy (RRT) in the intensive care setting. (4 marks)
d) List three types of RRT available on intensive care. (3 marks)
e) Give two possible complications associated with the use of heparin for systemic anticoagulation for maintenance of the extracorporeal circuit during RRT on intensive care. (2 marks)
f) Give two possible complications associated with the use of citrate for regional anticoagulation for maintenance of the extracorporeal circuit during RRT on intensive care. (2 marks)

The SAQ on this topic had a 59.1% pass rate. The question concerned RRT and its indications only, not the risk factors for development of acute kidney injury that I have added here. The original question asked the candidates to "outline the . . . mechanisms of solute and water removal by RRT" for 6 of the 20 marks. It is difficult to see how this could be phrased for a CRQ, but this is important knowledge nonetheless, and so I have reproduced the answer here.

Haemofiltration for removal of water:

- *Blood pumped through extracorporeal circuit that incorporates a semipermeable membrane.*
- *Hydrostatic pressure drives plasma water across the membrane – this is ultrafiltration.*
- *Small molecules (less than 50 kDa) are dragged across the membrane with the water by convection.*
- *Ultrafiltrate is discarded, and replacement fluid added according to desired fluid balance.*

Haemodialysis for removal of solutes:

- *Blood pumped through an extracorporeal circuit that incorporates a dialyser (semipermeable membrane separating blood from crystalloid solution, the dialysate).*
- *Solutes move from high concentration to low according to Fick's law of diffusion.*
- *To maintain concentration gradients, the dialysate flows countercurrent to the flow of the blood.*
- *Solutes of small size, low volume of distribution and low levels of plasma protein binding are most readily dialysed.*

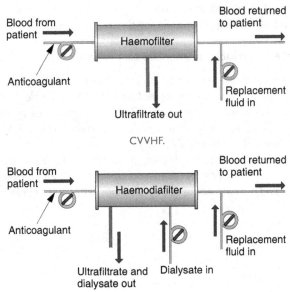

CVVHF.

CVVHDF.

a) List five perioperative risk factors for development of acute kidney injury. (5 marks)

- Poor renal perfusion due to e.g. hypovolaemia, dehydration, bleeding.
- Hypotension due to e.g. heart failure, dehydration, iatrogenic causes.
- Locally impaired renal circulation due to e.g. medication (NSAIDs, ACE inhibitors, angiotensin-2 receptor blockers), abdominal compartment syndrome, vascular cross-clamping.
- Systemic inflammation causing acute tubular injury due to e.g. systemic sepsis, major surgery, cardiopulmonary bypass.
- Exogenous nephrotoxins e.g. aminoglycosides, contrast.
- Rhabdomyolysis due to e.g. trauma necessitating surgery, prolonged or major surgery, vascular cross-clamp.
- Post-renal obstruction e.g. following surgery for kidney stone disease (misplaced stent or residual stone), urinary retention (due to bladder clots after bladder or prostate surgery).

b) List four patient risk factors for development of acute kidney injury perioperatively. (4 marks)

- Increasing age.
- Male sex.
- Chronic kidney disease.
- Chronic liver disease.
- Congestive cardiac failure/poor cardiorespiratory reserve.
- Hypertension.
- Diabetes mellitus.

c) List four indications for renal replacement therapy (RRT) in the intensive care setting. (4 marks)

Although it is a rise in creatinine or a reduction in urine output that would indicate a diagnosis of AKI, these are not indications for initiation of RRT. Early initiation of RRT before development of the complications of AKI listed below has not been shown to improve outcomes.

- Fluid overload/pulmonary oedema due to AKI not controlled with medical management.
- Hyperkalaemia due to AKI not controlled with medical management.
- Metabolic acidosis.
- Symptomatic uraemia (encephalopathy, pericarditis, bleeding, nausea) due to AKI.
- Overdose with a dialysable drug or toxin.
- Management of pre-existing chronic kidney disease.

d) List three types of RRT available on intensive care. (3 marks)

- Intermittent haemodialysis (*cheaper, efficient, but more rapid fluid shifts may not be tolerated in haemodynamically unstable or head injured patients. Not available in all ICUs*).
- Continuous renal replacement therapies (CRRTs) i.e. continuous venovenous haemofiltration (CVVHF), continuous venovenous haemodialysis (CVVHD), continuous venovenous haemodiafiltration (CVVHDF).
- Peritoneal dialysis of a patient already using this form of RRT. *Peritoneal dialysis is feasible in ICU but does not have the efficiency of haemodialysis, may cause problems with diaphragmatic splinting in ventilated patients, and is not appropriate in patients with intra-abdominal pathology.*

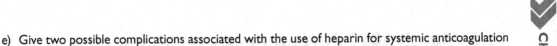
e) Give two possible complications associated with the use of heparin for systemic anticoagulation for maintenance of the extracorporeal circuit during RRT on intensive care. (2 marks)

- Heparin-induced thrombocytopenia (immune or non-immune mediated).
- Increased risk of haemorrhage.
- Heparin resistance associated with reduced antithrombin III production in critically ill patients.

f) Give two possible complications associated with the use of citrate for regional anticoagulation for maintenance of the extracorporeal circuit during RRT on intensive care. (2 marks)

- Alkalosis *(due to conversion of citrate to bicarbonate)*.
- Acidosis *(due to accumulation of citrate)*.
- Hypocalcaemia *(due to binding with citrate and removal with effluent)*.
- Hypomagnesemia *(due to binding with the citrate-calcium complex and removal with effluent)*.

REFERENCES

Gemmell L et al. Renal replacement therapy in critical care. *BJA Educ.* 2017: 17: 88–93.

Gross J, Prowle J. Perioperative acute kidney injury. *BJA Educ.* 2014: 15: 213–218.

The STARRT-AKI Investigators for the Canadian Critical Care Trials Group, the Australian and New Zealand Intensive Care Society Clinical Trials Group, the United Kingdom Critical Care Research Group, the Canadian Nephrology Trials Network and the Irish Critical Care Trials Group. *N Engl J Med.* 2020: 383: 240–251.

15.6 March 2014 Percutaneous tracheostomy

The SAQ on this topic addressed the indications for, contraindications to, and complications of percutaneous tracheostomy all of which were addressed in a CRQ from September 2019 which can be found in the airway chapter. The pass rate for this SAQ in 2014 was high at 79.4%. The Chair said, "This question is highly relevant to modern critical care practice, and the involvement of trainees in PCT procedures is reflected by the very high pass rate. Most marks were lost in the section on complications but in general this question was well answered. It was obvious which candidates had observed or performed significant numbers of PCTs and which had not."

15.7 September 2014 Propofol infusion syndrome

a) List six clinical features of propofol infusion syndrome. (6 marks)
b) List five possible risk factors for the development of propofol infusion syndrome in adult intensive care patients. (5 marks)
c) List three laboratory findings that might be expected in a case of propofol infusion syndrome. (3 marks)
d) Give two approaches to minimising the risk of development of propofol infusion syndrome. (2 marks)
e) List four aspects of management of propofol infusion syndrome. (4 marks)

Propofol infusion syndrome – previously known as propofol-related infusion syndrome – is a rare but potentially fatal metabolic syndrome to which children are more at risk, resulting in the cessation of use of long-term propofol infusions in children. There are a range of presenting features with no single feature being present universally. The pathophysiology is not fully established but is thought to relate to a disruptive effect of propofol on the respiratory chain leading to reduced ATP production and consequent cell hypoxia and death (hence an impact on organ function) and development of acidosis. The increased risk of development of the syndrome in children may relate to a smaller glycogen store in children compared to adults, thus increasing the risk of lack of glucose as a substrate for respiratory chain function. The Chair stated a pass rate of 35.8% for the SAQ on this topic and said, "This question was felt to be hard to answer and was assigned a low pass mark after the Angoff process. It proved to be another very strong discriminator between candidates and was answered poorly in the main. Weak candidates had no real knowledge of the subject and did not appreciate that the cardiovascular consequences of the syndrome predominate. Many referred incorrectly to the precipitation of liver failure. Trainees undertaking a block of intensive care medicine will use propofol sedation for some patients so it is important that they understand any potential complications." "Hard questions," for the SAQ, had a pass mark of 10–11/20. A CEACCP article (the forerunner of the BJA Education journal) on this topic was published in 2013, a year before this question appeared. Recent BJA Education articles should be a major focus of your revision.

a) **List six clinical features of propofol infusion syndrome. (6 marks)**

- Metabolic acidosis.
- ECG changes.
- Rhabdomyolysis.
- Acute kidney injury.
- Hyperkalaemia.
- Lipidaemia.
- Cardiac failure.
- Pyrexia.
- Elevated liver enzymes, hepatomegaly.
- Elevated lactate.

b) **List five possible risk factors for the development of propofol infusion syndrome in adult intensive care patients. (5 marks)**

The risk factors for propofol infusion syndrome have not been fully established, but this was the question asked in the 2014 SAQ. There are many confounding factors making establishment of a clear list of risks challenging, especially as the source material is mainly case report based. Many of the risks may therefore be just associations. Traumatic brain injury may be associated with a higher cumulative dose of propofol in an effort to control intracranial pressure, thus increasing risk. Alternatively, it may be that an exaggerated stress response in traumatic brain injury, and other severe critical illnesses, leads to high catecholamine and glucocorticoid secretion. Glucocorticoids may impact on mitochondrial function and trigger myofilament derangement and hence muscle damage. Catecholamines will result in increased cardiac output and subsequent clearance from the blood of propofol, possibly leading to increased doses to maintain the same sedative effect. High exogenous catecholamine administration may be a marker of critical illness disease severity, or result from treatment of the developing haemodynamic compromise of propofol infusion syndrome. Alternatively, both catecholamines and glucocorticoids lead to a switch of energy substrate from carbohydrate-based metabolism to lipolysis, resulting in an increased free fatty acid concentration.

- Cumulative propofol dose/prolonged infusion/high infusion rates.
- Traumatic brain injury.
- Increased severity of critical illness, sepsis.
- High exogenous or endogenous catecholamines.
- High exogenous or endogenous glucocorticoids.
- Low carbohydrate intake.
- Genetic mitochondrial defects.
- Younger age.

c) **List three laboratory findings that might be expected in a case of propofol infusion syndrome. (3 marks)**

- Raised creatine kinase.
- Raised lactate OR low pH.
- Elevated potassium.
- Elevated creatinine OR reduction in eGFR.
- Elevated transaminases.
- Raised triglycerides.

d) **Give two approaches to minimising the risk of development of propofol infusion syndrome. (2 marks)**

- Multimodal sedation/lowest dose of propofol for shortest duration.
- Consideration of alternative sedative drug for use in patients with high vasopressor requirements or who are receiving exogenous steroids.
- Maintenance of adequate carbohydrate supply (glucose infusion, parenteral nutrition, or enteral nutrition).
- Monitoring of markers of onset of syndrome: creatine kinase, pH, lactate.
- Avoidance of propofol use in patients with known or suspected mitochondrial disorders.

e) **List four aspects of management of propofol infusion syndrome. (4 marks)**

- Immediate cessation of propofol infusion and initiation of alternative sedative agent.
- Administration of a glucose source, i.e. dextrose infusion, while monitoring blood glucose and treating with insulin if indicated.
- Medical management of hyperkalaemia.
- Fluid treatment for hypotension and acidosis/raised lactate.
- Ventilatory management to compensate for metabolic acidosis.
- Standard management of arrhythmias.
- Renal replacement therapy for treatment of acidosis and hyperkalaemia in association with acute kidney injury – may also help clear the water-soluble metabolites of propofol that will accumulate due to acute kidney injury although will not increase the rate of excretion of the lipophilic propofol itself.
- Consideration of ECMO for patients unresponsive to more conservative treatments.

REFERENCES

Hemphill S. Propofol infusion syndrome: a structured literature review and analysis of published case reports. *BJA*. 2019: 122: 448–459.

Will Loh N, Nair P. Propofol infusion syndrome. *Contin Educ Anaesth Crit Care Pain*. 2013: 13: 200–202.

15.8 March 2015 Intensive care unit-acquired weakness

a) Define intensive care unit-acquired weakness (ICU-AW). (1 mark)
b) List three types of ICU-AW that may occur. (3 marks)
c) List six risk factors for the development of ICU-AW. (6 marks)
d) List two pre-existing patient characteristics that are associated with an increased risk of ICU-AW. (2 marks)
e) List four features that contribute to the clinical diagnosis of ICU-AW. (4 marks)
f) List two neurophysiological tests that may be used to determine the type of ICU-AW. (2 marks)
g) List two aspects of ICU care that may reduce the development of ICU-AW. (2 marks)

The SAQ in March 2015 called this condition critical illness weakness, but it seems that the term intensive care unit-acquired weakness is more commonly in use. The pass rate was only 30.4% with a poor fail rate of 46.6%. The Chair said, "This question was anticipated to be difficult for the candidates, and the pass and poor fail rates reflect this expectation. The subject matter is topical and an important consideration in the management of critically ill patients. Many candidates had no idea that the definition excluded pre-existing pathology, and that the weakness was symmetrical with cranial nerve sparing. Few candidates had knowledge of the use of nerve conduction studies, and even fewer mentioned the MRC scale of scoring muscle power. The importance of preparing detailed notes on mandatory units of training when revising for the Final FRCA is exemplified by this question."

I think it is difficult to revise for topics that are poorly understood. There are many theories about the cause of ICU-AW, but little that has been proven. It is likely to be multifactorial. The multiorgan failure that has resulted in ICU admission will cause a systemic inflammatory process with circulation of inflammatory mediators, net catabolic effect, and high blood glucose which may all cause direct damage to nerves and muscles. Mitochondria may also be damaged – energy release necessary for cell function will be compromised and cell death may result. Hypotension and vasoconstriction caused by cardiovascular compromise and use of vasopressors respectively will result in poor blood supply to nerves and muscles. Denervation due to neuromuscular blocking agent use and the process of ICU-AW on the nerves, alongside immobility, will lead to muscle atrophy. Corticosteroids may cause direct damage to myocytes. There may be involvement of autoantibodies against sodium channels which will interfere with nerve transmission and muscle action potential generation. There was a CEACCP article on this topic in 2012 – BJA Education and CEACCP articles are really important in your revision. Remember that as a "difficult" question, you would only have needed 10–11/20 to pass.

a) **Define intensive care unit–acquired weakness (ICU-AW). (1 mark)**

- Clinically detected weakness in critically ill patients in whom there is no plausible aetiology other than critical illness OR clinically detectable, symmetrical, peripheral (not involving cranial nerves, thus facial sparing) weakness in critically ill patient that is not pre-existing.

b) **List three types of ICU-AW that may occur. (3 marks)**

It can affect nerves, muscles, or both.

- Critical illness polyneuropathy.
- Critical illness myopathy.
- Critical illness polyneuropathy and myopathy/critical illness neuromyopathy.

c) List six risk factors for the development of ICU-AW. (6 marks)

- Multiorgan failure due to any underlying cause – risk increased with increased duration.
- Prolonged mechanical ventilation/immobility.
- Hyperglycaemia.
- Severe sepsis, severe SIRS.
- Glucocorticoids.
- Neuromuscular blocking agents.
- Electrolyte imbalance.
- Hyperosmotic pressure.
- High lactate.
- Parenteral nutrition.
- Inappropriate vasoactive drug use.
- Abnormal calcium concentration.

d) List two pre-existing patient characteristics that are associated with an increased risk of ICU-AW. (2 marks)

- Female sex.
- Increasing age.

e) List four features that contribute to the clinical diagnosis of ICU-AW. (4 marks)

- Development of weakness after onset of critical illness.
- Generalised, symmetrical, flaccid weakness, usually sparing cranial nerves (*facial grimacing but no peripheral movement in response to painful stimulus*).
- There may be associated sensory loss, but not autonomic involvement.
- Other causes excluded.
- Dependence on mechanical ventilation.
- Low muscle strength (as assessed by Medical Research Council standardised assessment).

f) List two neurophysiological tests that may be used to determine the type of ICU-AW. (2 marks)

Ever keen to ensure that you understand and don't just list (or maybe it's me that needs the explanation), here is a little more detail about the why. Nerve conduction studies will measure the speed of an electrical impulse from one point to another on a sensory nerve and the evoked amplitude (sensory nerve action potential, SNAP). It will also measure the speed of an electrical impulse along a motor nerve and the compound motor action potential (CMAP) that results. A reduced amplitude would indicate an issue with the axon of the nerves, as is the case in ICU-AW, and a slowing of the conduction would indicate myelin loss which is not associated with ICU-AW. An electromyograph (EMG) requires a cooperative patient to keep a specific muscle still and then use that muscle voluntarily, and the resulting action potentials (motor unit action potential, MUAP) are measured with a needle electrode. Muscle motor action potentials in the absence of voluntary muscle use may indicate a denervated muscle having spontaneous activity, and a weak muscle will have a smaller amplitude of MUAP on voluntary contraction. Normal nerve conduction with abnormal EMG may indicate a muscle problem. Only the action potentials from muscle fibres very close to the needle tip will be measured. As many patients on intensive care are unable to cooperate with a test that involves spontaneous muscle movement, another test comparing direct muscle stimulated CMAP (dmCMAP) to nerve stimulated CMAP (neCMAP) can elucidate the variable contributions of nerve and muscle to the patient's weakness. However, this test is not in widespread clinical use.

- Nerve conduction studies.
- Electromyographic studies.
- Electrophysiological study comparing nerve-stimulated and direct muscle-stimulated muscle action potentials.

g) **List two aspects of ICU care that may reduce the development of ICU-AW. (2 marks)**

- Early physiotherapy/early mobilisation.
- Reduction in ventilator dependent days using approaches to facilitate weaning.
- Optimisation of nutrition to include sufficient amino acids such as glutamine and antioxidants.
- Close management of blood glucose.

REFERENCES

Appleton R, Kinsella J. Intensive care unit-acquired weakness. *Contin Educ Anaesth Crit Care Pain.* 2012: 12: 62–66.

Bromberg M. An electrodiagnostic approach to the evaluation of peripheral neuropathies. *Phys Med Rehabil Clin N Am.* 2013: 24: 153–168.

Intiso D. ICU-acquired weakness: should medical sovereignty belong to any specialist? *Crit Care.* 2018: 22: 1.

15.9 September 2015 Ventilator-associated pneumonia

a) Define the term ventilator-associated pneumonia (VAP). (1 mark)
b) List five clinical and investigational findings that may indicate the presence of VAP. (5 marks)
c) List eight factors that may increase the risk of VAP development. (8 marks)
d) List two elements of endotracheal tube design that may help reduce the risk of VAP development. (2 marks)
e) List two aspects of ventilator circuit management that may help reduce the risk of VAP development. (2 marks)
f) List two other measures that may reduce the risk of VAP development. (2 marks)

The Chairs said that the SAQ on this topic had a 44.3% pass rate. "This is a common condition that candidates should have seen, so it was surprising that it was quite poorly answered. Very few candidates were able to give a definition of VAP or to give details of the care bundles used in its prevention and treatment. Merely stating 'a care bundle would be used' suggests inadequate depth of knowledge." However, there are a range of definitions of VAP which has contributed to the difficulty in comparing rates between units, studies and countries, including the duration of ventilation necessary for the pneumonia to be classified as ventilator-associated. This question was substantially repeated in September 2018 and again as a CRQ in February 2023, with some rewording of the last section to focus on the term "care bundle," which is also a common viva topic.

a) Define the term ventilator-associated pneumonia (VAP). (1 mark)

- Nosocomial lung infection occurring more than 48 hours after commencement of ventilation via tracheal intubation *(whether that is an endotracheal tube or a tracheostomy).*

b) List five clinical and investigational findings that may indicate the presence of VAP. (5 marks)

There are a range of different scoring systems to aid diagnosis that include clinical, microbiological and radiological factors. However, studies have shown that there is a big element of inter-individual variation, and the scoring systems lack sensitivity and specificity.

- Leucocytosis.
- Fever.
- Purulent secretions.
- Infiltrates on chest radiograph or other radiological imaging e.g. ultrasound, CT.
- Reduction in patient oxygenation/need for increase in FiO_2.
- Culture or positive gram stain or PCR testing of pathogenic bacteria on tracheal aspirate sample.

c) List eight factors that may increase the risk of VAP development. (8 marks)

The presence of an endotracheal tube is included in the definition of VAP and therefore would not be a correct answer here. They increase the risk of development of pneumonia by causing loss of the cough reflex, biofilm development on the inner surface of the tube, pooling of secretions on top of the cuff that then gain access via channels caused by folds in the cuff.

- Nasogastric tube *(colonisation, predisposition to sinusitis and, therefore, a pool of infected secretions on cuff of tube).*
- Nasal intubation *(predisposition to sinusitis and therefore a pool of infected secretions).*
- Positive pressure ventilation *(forces bacteria to distal airways).*
- Long duration of mechanical ventilation.

- Dysfunction in immune response associated with critical illness (*e.g. reduced level of salivary fibronectin, which normally protects against oropharyngeal colonisation with aerobic gram negative bacilli and Staphylococci, impaired phagocytosis*).
- Severe burns.
- Supine position increasing risk of gastro-oesophageal reflux.
- Low GCS/excessive sedation.
- Enteral feeding (*due to risk of aspiration, but for the purposes of overall morbidity and mortality, enteral feeding is still preferable overall to no/parenteral feeding*).
- Previous surgery.

d) List two elements of endotracheal tube design that may help reduce the risk of VAP development. (2 marks)

- Subglottic suction port (*this allows suction of the secretions that are below the vocal cords but above the cuff*).
- Tapered cuff of ultra-thin polyurethane to avoid channelling.
- Antimicrobial coating to discourage biofilm development.

e) List two aspects of ventilator circuit management that may help reduce the risk of VAP development. (2 marks)

- Avoidance of routine ventilator circuit changes (*excessive manipulation of ventilator circuits being thought to contribute to VAP due to draining of contaminated humidification condensate into endotracheal tube*).
- Minimisation of circuit disconnections e.g. by using closed circuit suctioning.
- Hand hygiene and glove wearing during necessary interruptions to the circuit.

f) List two other measures that may reduce the risk of VAP development. (2 marks)

These are elements of a ventilator care bundle. A care bundle is a group of evidence-based interventions that relate to a particular aspect of patient care. The strength of evidence supporting the individual components varies; some elements may just be accepted as good practice. Nonetheless, the aim of care bundle use is that the implementation of all of the components together should result in better patient outcomes. Care bundles are readily auditable. Think about the care bundles for sepsis management or reduction of surgical infection (part of the WHO checklist). Oral decontamination with chlorhexidine is no longer recommended and is actually associated with an increased mortality risk. General oral hygiene is still supported as a way of minimising dental complications and for maintenance of normal intraoral flora. Gastric ulcer prophylaxis with a PPI raises gastric pH and may therefore increase colonisation with pathogenic organisms.

- Patient to be positioned 30–45 degrees head up to reduce risk of passive reflux and aspiration.
- Cuff pressure checking (20–30 cm H_2O or 2 cm H_2O above peak inflation pressure to minimise risk of secretion movement below cuff).
- Daily sedation interruption to help reduce length of ventilator dependency.
- Daily spontaneous breathing assessment to check for readiness for extubation.

REFERENCES

American Thoracic Society, Infectious Diseases Society of America. Management of adults with hospital-acquired and ventilator-associated pneumonia: 2016 clinical practice guidelines by the Infectious Diseases Society of America and the American Thoracic Society. *Clin Infect Dis.* 2016: 63: e61–e111.

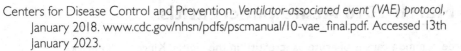

Centers for Disease Control and Prevention. *Ventilator-associated event (VAE) protocol,* January 2018. www.cdc.gov/nhsn/pdfs/pscmanual/10-vae_final.pdf. Accessed 13th January 2023.

Gunasekera P, Gratrix A. Ventilator-associated pneumonia. *BJA Educ.* 2016: 16: 198–202.

Hellyer T et al. The Intensive Care Society recommended bundle of interventions for the prevention of ventilator-associated pneumonia. *JICS.* 2016: 17: 238–243.

Kalanuria A, Zai W, Mirski M. Ventilator-associated pneumonia in the ICU. *Crit Care.* 2014: 18: 208.

15.10 March 2016 Acute pancreatitis

a) List three common causes of acute pancreatitis in the United Kingdom. (3 marks)
b) Give the two subtypes of acute pancreatitis. (2 marks)
c) Give three diagnostic criteria for acute pancreatitis. (3 marks)
d) State the classification of severity of acute pancreatitis. (3 marks)
e) List three local complications of acute pancreatitis. (3 marks)
f) Give two targets for fluid resuscitation in the initial phase of acute pancreatitis. (2 marks)
g) List two approaches to reduce the risk of pulmonary complications of acute pancreatitis. (2 marks)
h) List two possible long-term sequelae of acute pancreatitis. (2 marks)

There was a 53.6% pass rate for the SAQ on this topic. The Chair said, "This is a condition seen commonly in intensive care. Many candidates did not mention alcohol as a cause in part (a). Few candidates could describe the classification of severity of acute pancreatitis. . . . Also, some candidates tended to give a generic answer to part (d), describing the management of sepsis, rather than the specific management of acute pancreatitis as asked. This resulted in them losing marks in this section." Part (d) had asked, "What are the specific principles of managing severe acute pancreatitis in a critical care environment? (11 marks)." It is these long, open-ended questions that the change to CRQ format has removed. Instead you are likely to get questions targeted at specific aspects of the overall management, in the way I have attempted to mimic in my CRQ here. Meantime, the BJA Education article referenced below gives a great summary that would have been a perfect answer to the old SAQ part (d).

a) **List three common causes of acute pancreatitis in the United Kingdom. (3 marks)**

- Gallstones.
- Excessive alcohol intake.
- Neoplasm resulting in obstruction *(head of pancreas or periampullary primary, or metastasis from breast, renal, gastric, ovarian, lung).*

Other common causes include autoimmune diseases such as sclerosing cholangitis, viral infections such as CMV and the hepatitides, trauma following surgery or ERCP, cystic fibrosis, hypercalcaemia, hypertriglyceridaemia, and idiopathic, but not scorpion bites.

b) **Give the two subtypes of acute pancreatitis. (2 marks)**

- Interstitial oedematous pancreatitis.
- Necrotising pancreatitis.

c) **Give three diagnostic criteria for acute pancreatitis. (3 marks)**

These are the revised Atlanta criteria, with two out of three being necessary to make a diagnosis.

- Abdominal pain consistent with acute pancreatitis (acute, persistent, severe, epigastric pain, often radiating to the back).
- Serum lipase or amylase at least three times greater than the upper limit of normal.
- Characteristic radiological findings, usually contrast-enhanced CT.

d) **State the classification of severity of acute pancreatitis. (3 marks)**

- Mild acute pancreatitis: no organ failure, no local or systemic complications.
- Moderately severe acute pancreatitis: organ failure that resolves within 48 hours and/or local or systemic complications.
- Severe acute pancreatitis: organ failure persisting more than 48 hours.

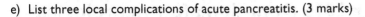

e) List three local complications of acute pancreatitis. (3 marks)

- Acute peripancreatic fluid collection.
- Acute necrotic collection.
- Walled-off necrosis.
- Pancreatic pseudocyst.
- Splenic, superior mesenteric or portal vein thrombosis.
- Pseudoaneurysm formation of splenic or gastroduodenal artery with risk of intra-abdominal haemorrhage.
- Pancreatic fistulae.
- Abdominal compartment syndrome.
- Paralytic ileus.

f) Give two targets for fluid resuscitation in the initial phase of acute pancreatitis. (2 marks)

- Normalisation of lactate.
- Urine output > 0.5 ml/kg/h.

g) List two approaches to reduce the risk of pulmonary complications of acute pancreatitis. (2 marks)

- Avoidance of excessive intravenous fluids especially after the initial resuscitation phase.
- Early, effective analgesia to reduce the risk of hypoventilation.
- Supplementary oxygen including as high-flow nasal oxygen to reduce the need for invasive ventilation and its associated complications.

h) List two possible long-term sequelae of acute pancreatitis. (2 marks)

- Chronic pancreatitis.
- Exocrine insufficiency.
- Endocrine insufficiency.
- Pseudocyst formation.
- Gastric outlet obstruction.
- Long-term consequences of critical illness – cognitive and psychiatric consequences, physical consequences e.g. failure to return to pre-morbid functioning, ongoing renal insufficiency, intensive care unit–acquired weakness.

REFERENCES

Banks P et al. Classification of acute pancreatitis – 2012: revision of the Atlanta classification and definitions by international consensus. *Gut.* 2013: 62: 102–111.
MacGoey P et al. Management of patients with acute pancreatitis. *BJA Educ.* 2019: 19: 240–245.

15.11 September 2016 Donation after neurological death

a) List the two essential preconditions that must be met prior to testing an adult patient for neurological death. (2 marks)
b) State the values that should be seen on arterial blood gas analysis in a previously well patient prior to commencement of apnoea testing. (2 marks)
c) State the value that should be seen on arterial blood gas analysis at the end of apnoea testing that (alongside allowing a period of five minutes to elapse) would indicate completion of the test. (1 mark)
d) State which nerves are tested by vestibulo-ocular reflex testing. (3 marks)
e) State the method for vestibulo-ocular reflex testing. (3 marks)
f) Give two causes of hypotension following neurological death. (2 marks)
g) List two biochemical changes of diabetes insipidus. (2 marks)
h) List three drugs, with their indications, that may be initiated after confirmation of neurological death to maximise organ function. (3 marks)
i) List two measures undertaken to optimise donor lung condition for the purposes of transplantation. (2 marks)

The SAQ on this topic had a 68.8% pass rate. The Chairs said that the "examiners anticipated that candidates would find this question difficult but gratifyingly most achieved enough marks to pass and demonstrated good knowledge of this important topic." The Organ Donation and Transplantation website has a lot of information about the physiology behind neurological death and the subsequent deterioration as well as the practicalities of identifying donors and optimising their organ function prior to donation. There is a link to their extended care bundle which gives clear targets for treatment for optimisation.

a) List the two essential preconditions that must be met prior to testing an adult patient for neurological death. (2 marks)

- Evidence of irreversible brain damage of known aetiology.
- Patient must have GCS 3 and be on mechanical ventilation with apnoea. Haemodynamic instability, medications (sedation and NMBD), hypothermia, abnormal glucose level and electrolyte imbalance must be ruled out as causes of the patient's condition.

b) State the values that should be seen on arterial blood gas analysis in a previously well patient prior to commencement of apnoea testing. (2 marks)

- $PaCO_2 \geq 6.0$ kPa.
- pH < 7.4 OR $[H^+]$ > 40 nmol/l.

c) State the value that should be seen on arterial blood gas analysis at the end of apnoea testing that (alongside allowing a period of five minutes to elapse) would indicate completion of the test. (1 mark)

- $PaCO_2$ rise > 0.5 kPa.

d) State which nerves are tested by vestibulo-ocular reflex testing. (3 marks)

- Cranial nerve III/oculomotor.
- Cranial nerve VI/abducens.
- Cranial nerve VIII/vestibulocochlear.

e) State the method for vestibulo-ocular reflex testing. (3 marks)

- Ensure visualisation of tympanic membranes.
- Head flexed at 30 degrees.

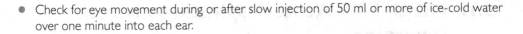

- Check for eye movement during or after slow injection of 50 ml or more of ice-cold water over one minute into each ear.

f) Give two causes of hypotension following neurological death. (2 marks)

- Dehydration following the onset of diabetes insipidus and neurogenic pulmonary oedema.
- Left ventricular impairment with reduced cardiac output following sympathetic storm.
- Refractory vasodilation due to loss of sympathetic tone and adrenoceptor desensitisation.

g) List two biochemical changes of diabetes insipidus. (2 marks)

- Increased serum osmolality (and reduced urine osmolality).
- Hypokalaemia.
- Hypernatremia.

h) List three drugs, with their indications, that may be initiated after confirmation of neurological death to maximise organ function. (3 marks)

A range of drugs may be necessary to optimise donor organ function, but I have restricted my answer to those listed in the Donor Optimisation Extended Care Bundle. Desmopressin is a synthetic analogue of vasopressin with high antidiuretic effects but minimal vasopressor effects.

- Methylprednisolone (given to all donors) to attenuate the systemic inflammation of neurological death.
- Vasopressin if vasopressor is required, to facilitate cessation of adrenaline or noradrenaline – will also treat diabetes insipidus.
- Insulin infusion to maintain blood glucose 4–10 mmol/l.
- Dobutamine or dopamine for inotropic support.
- Desmopressin may be required to treat diabetes insipidus.
- Low molecular weight heparin to minimise risk of thromboembolic disease.

i) List two measures undertaken to optimise donor lung condition for the purposes of transplantation. (2 marks)

- Lung recruitment manoeuvres after apnoea testing.
- Lung protective ventilation strategy – tidal volumes 4–8 ml/kg, PEEP 5–10 cmH$_2$O.
- Chest physiotherapy, suctioning, repositioning.
- 30–45° head-up positioning.
- Maintenance of endotracheal tube cuff inflation.
- Bronchoscopy and bronchial lavage.

REFERENCES

Faculty of Intensive Care Medicine. *Form for the diagnosis of death using neurological criteria {long version}.* www.ficm.ac.uk/sites/ficm/files/documents/2021-10/Form_for_the_Diagnosis_of_Death_using_Neurological_Criteria-long_version.pdf. Accessed 14th January 2023.

NHS Blood and Transplant. *Donation after brainstem death donor optimisation extended care bundle.* https://nhsbtdbe.blob.core.windows.net/umbraco-assets-corp/3654/dbd_care_bundle.pdf. Accessed 14th January 2023.

NHS Blood and Transplant Organ Donation and Transplantation Website. www.odt.nhs.uk. Accessed 14th January 2023.

15.12 March 2017 Acute respiratory distress syndrome

a) List three possible lung-related causes of acute respiratory distress syndrome (ARDS). (3 marks)
b) List three possible non-lung-related causes of ARDS. (3 marks)
c) List the four clinical criteria for diagnosis of ARDS. (4 marks)
d) List three clinical indices used to quantify oxygenation in ARDS and the equation used to link them. (4 marks)
e) State the appropriate tidal volume in ml/kg for ventilation of a patient with ARDS. (1 mark)
f) List three ventilatory measures that can be taken to improve oxygenation or prevent further deterioration in a patient with ARDS requiring invasive mechanical ventilation. (3 marks)
g) List two non-ventilatory measures that can be taken to improve oxygenation or prevent further deterioration in a patient with ARDS requiring invasive mechanical ventilation. (2 marks)

The Chairs' Report quoted a pass rate of 57.3% for the SAQ on this topic and said, "ARDS is a clinical condition which is seen commonly on ITU and of which candidates should have a thorough understanding. Whilst the definition was well known, the majority of candidates did not know the clinical indices used to assess oxygenation. [The sections asking about ventilatory measures that can be taken to improve oxygenation or prevent further deterioration in a patient with ARDS were] on the whole well answered but those candidates who lost marks tended to write about general ITU care rather than the specifics of care for patients with ARDS."

a) List three possible lung-related causes of acute respiratory distress syndrome (ARDS). (3 marks)

- Aspiration.
- Pneumonia or pneumonitis.
- Drowning.
- Pulmonary embolus.
- Pulmonary contusion.
- Inhalational injury.
- Reperfusion injury after cardiopulmonary bypass.

b) List three possible non-lung-related causes of ARDS. (3 marks)

- Systemic sepsis.
- Blood transfusion.
- Pancreatitis.
- Trauma.
- Burns.
- Drugs (e.g. aspirin, tricyclic antidepressants, cocaine).

c) List the four clinical criteria for diagnosis of ARDS. (4 marks)

- <u>Onset</u> within one week of known clinical insult.
- <u>Bilateral opacities</u> on CXR or CT consistent with pulmonary oedema.
- Respiratory failure <u>not fully explained by cardiac failure or fluid overload</u>. *(Need to objectively assess this with e.g. echo if there is no clear ARDS-trigger present.)*
- <u>Hypoxaemia</u>, $PaO_2/FiO_2 \leq 39.9$ kPa/300 mmHg, with PEEP 5 cmH_2O or more.

The PaO_2/FiO_2 given above is the cut-off for mild ARDS. It is easier to remember the definitions of mild, moderate and severe ARDS when using mmHg: less than 300, less than 200 and less than 100 mmHg, *instead of less than 39.9, less than 26.6 and less than 13.3 when using kPa. No doubt you will remember that 760 mmHg equates to 101 kPa, give or take a few decimal places, so you can remember the mmHg values and convert. Acute lung injury (ALI) has been redefined as mild ARDS.*

d) List three clinical indices used to quantify oxygenation in ARDS and the equation used to link them. (4 marks)

- Mean airway pressure.
- Fraction of inspired oxygen.
- Arterial partial pressure of oxygen.
- Oxygenation index = mean airway pressure × FiO_2 × $100/PaO_2$.

e) State the appropriate tidal volume in ml/kg for ventilation of a patient with ARDS. (1 mark)

- < 6 ml/kg (although 4–8 ml/kg is also quoted).

f) List three ventilatory measures that can be taken to improve oxygenation or prevent further deterioration in a patient with ARDS requiring invasive mechanical ventilation. (3 marks)

The aim of ventilation during ARDS is to maintain adequate gas exchange until cellular damage resolves without causing further lung injury due to baro-, volu-, atelec- and biotrauma. I have restricted my answers to those that reflect current evidence, excluding things such as changing ventilatory modes which is commonly done in practice but not supported by specific evidence. APRV is a favoured mode of ventilation for ARDS but lacks the necessary evidence to make it onto the list (although this is a form of "open lung" ventilation), and evidence dictates that HFOV is no longer advised in the management of ARDS. Being based on current evidence, the lists in answer to (f) and (g) are subject to change.

- Prone positioning.
- "Open lung ventilation strategy": limiting peak airway pressure < 30 cmH_2O with high PEEP ~ 15 cmH_2O OR minimising driving pressure/difference between PEEP and plateau pressures whilst achieving desired tidal volume and acceptable oxygenation.
- Recruitment manoeuvres.
- Use of NMBD to facilitate ventilation.
- Use of ventilator care bundles.
- Protocolised weaning from ventilator.

g) List two non-ventilatory measures that can be taken to improve oxygenation or prevent further deterioration in a patient with ARDS requiring invasive mechanical ventilation. (2 marks)

- Conservative fluid management.
- ECMO.
- Low-dose corticosteroid treatment.

REFERENCES

The ARDS Definition Task Force. Acute respiratory distress syndrome, the Berlin definition. *JAMA.* 2012: 307: 2526–2533.

DesPrez K et al. Oxygenation saturation index predicts clinical outcomes in ARDS. *Chest.* 2017: 152: 1151–1158.

Griffiths M et al. Guidelines on the management of acute respiratory distress syndrome. *BMJ Open Resp Res.* 2019: 6: e000420.

Liaqat A et al. Evidence-based mechanical ventilation strategies in ARDS. *J Clin Med.* 2022: 11: 319–331.

Tasaka S et al. ARDS clinical practice guideline 2021. *J Intensive Care.* 2022: 10: 32.

15.13 March 2017 Convulsive status epilepticus

The Chairs reported a pass rate of 47.1% for the SAQ on this topic. "This question was judged to be easy and is relevant to everyday practice as anaesthetists may encounter such patients in multiple areas including ITU, neurosurgery and the emergency department. Very few candidates were aware of the up-to-date definition of status epilepticus." You would have needed 14/20 to pass an "easy" SAQ. Note that new NICE guidance was issued in 2016, just before the SAQ in 2017. The topic was repeated as the focus of a question in September 2022, and so I will address it there.

15.14 September 2017 Renal replacement therapy on intensive care

This SAQ was identical to the one that appeared in September 2013. The Chairs' Report gave a pass rate of 84.9% and said, "This question had the highest pass rate in the paper. The topic is relevant to everyday practice in intensive care so it was reassuring to see that knowledge of it was generally excellent. However, a number of candidates still gave incomplete accounts of the differences between dialysis and filtration."

15.15 March 2018 Delirium

a) List four clinical features of delirium. (4 marks)
b) List two tools that may be used to diagnose delirium in the intensive care setting. (2 marks)
c) List four possible pre-existing risk factors that may predispose a patient to the development of delirium. (4 marks)
d) List two intraoperative interventions that may reduce the risk of postoperative delirium. (2 marks)
e) List three environmental issues that should be optimised to reduce the risk of development of delirium. (3 marks)
f) List four physiological or metabolic derangements that may be triggers for delirium. (4 marks)
g) Treatment of delirium focusses on management of the underlying precipitants. State when pharmacological management may be indicated. (1 mark)

When this question appeared as an SAQ, it had a pass rate of 46.5%, and the Chairs said, "This was a new and very topical ITU question. Overall the management of delirium was described well but a lot of answers lacked detail. There was poor knowledge of the definition and features of delirium. This probably reflects the fact that candidates have dealt with many patients with delirium whilst working on ITU, but have not read around the subject."

a) **List four clinical features of delirium. (4 marks)**

- Acute onset.
- Fluctuating in nature.
- Disturbance in attention.
- Disturbance in awareness/arousal/consciousness (but not severely decreased as seen in coma).
- Disturbance in cognition/disorganised thinking (e.g. memory, language, visuospatial ability, perception).
- Occurs as a direct physiological consequence of another medical condition or drug effect.

b) **List two tools that may be used to diagnose delirium in the intensive care setting. (2 marks)**

- CAM-ICU (Confusion Assessment Method for the Intensive Care Unit).
- ICDSC (Intensive Care Delirium Screening Checklist).

c) **List four possible pre-existing risk factors that may predispose a patient to the development of delirium. (4 marks)**

- Advanced age.
- Pre-existing cognitive impairment e.g. dementia.
- Pre-existing hypertension.
- Alcohol use.
- Increased ASA grade/burden of comorbidities/poorer long-term health status.
- Increased functional dependence/reduced mobility.
- Sensory impairments such as poor vision.
- Cardiac disease/cardiovascular diseases that are associated with an increased risk of stroke.
- Smoking.

d) **List two intraoperative interventions that may reduce the risk of postoperative delirium. (2 marks)**

- Use of opioid-sparing multimodal analgesia.
- Use of depth of anaesthesia monitoring to avoid excessively deep anaesthesia.

- Use of dexmedetomidine.
- Avoidance of benzodiazepines and gabapentinoids.

e) **List three environmental issues that should be optimised to reduce the risk of development of delirium. (3 marks)**

- Maintenance of orientation in time – provide access to window, clock, calendar.
- Maintenance of orientation in place – conversation to reiterate where they are, why they are there, who staff are, facilitating visits by family.
- Maintenance of mobility – ensuring mobilisation as soon as possible after illness or surgery, ensuring the correct mobility aids available, avoiding restricting patient's movement with drips, catheters, drains.
- Maintenance of sensory input by ensuring availability of patient's glasses and hearing aids.
- Maintenance of sleep by reducing noise level on ward at night, using side room, reducing unnecessary waking for medications or observations.
- Maintenance of access to hydration and nutrition – offering help with drinking and eating as necessary, providing food in a suitable consistency for the patient's needs, ensuring dentures are available, using intravenous or subcutaneous route if oral route not feasible or insufficient.

f) **List four physiological or metabolic derangements that may be triggers for delirium. (4 marks)**

- Hypoxia, hypercarbia.
- Hypotension.
- Pain.
- Infection, sepsis.
- Electrolyte imbalance.
- Hypo- or hyperglycaemia.
- Metabolic derangement due to serious illness such as acute kidney injury or acute liver failure.
- Significant inflammation/stress response to serious illness or major surgery.

g) **Treatment of delirium focusses on management of the underlying precipitants. State when pharmacological management of delirium may be indicated. (1 mark)**

Medication may be required to manage infection, cardiovascular compromise, or electrolyte imbalance, but this question has asked about treatment of the delirium itself. NICE guidance indicates that these are the indications for consideration of treatment:

- Patient's behaviour is a risk to themself or others.
- Significant patient distress.

REFERENCES

National Institute for Health and Care Excellence. *Delirium: prevention, diagnosis and management: CG103*, July 2010, last updated March 2019.

Van den Boogaard M, Slooter A. Delirium in critically ill patients: current knowledge and future perspectives. *BJA Educ.* 2019: 19: 398–404.

Zhaosheng J et al. Postoperative delirium: preoperative assessment, risk reduction and management. *BJA.* 2020: 125: 492–504.

15.16 September 2018 Ventilator-associated pneumonia

Three years after the last time, VAP was once again the focus of an SAQ with exactly the same questions asked. The pass rate was just 38.6% which left the examiners suitably "surprised," saying that the "condition is topical, important and frequently seen so candidates really should know it in more detail than was demonstrated here. Candidates lacked knowledge of definition and listed just lung protection strategies rather than protection against VAP. This question showed the closest correlation with overall performance."

15.17 September 2020 Life-threatening acute asthma

a) List five signs of life-threatening acute asthma. (5 marks)
b) List two investigation findings in life-threatening acute asthma. (2 marks)
c) Apart from oxygen, list four drugs (including their routes of administration) that may be used in the management of life-threatening acute asthma. (4 marks)
d) List three reasons for hypotension after induction of anaesthesia of a patient with life-threatening acute asthma. (3 marks)
e) List three ways in which life-threatening acute asthma may adversely affect respiratory mechanics. (3 marks)
f) List three aspects of a suitable ventilatory strategy directly after intubation of a patient with life-threatening acute asthma. (3 marks)

The CRQs are not published by the College, but much can be inferred about what the questions might have been by looking at the Chairs' Report and also by focussing on important aspects of the topic. The Chairs reported a pass rate 67.7% for the CRQ on this topic and said, "This question had a good pass rate and showed the best correlation with overall performance. In part (a) several candidates failed to read the question and gave answers such as hypoxia and low saturations when the question quite clearly asks for signs. In part (e) it appeared that many candidates did not [understand] the question. The question specifically asks for the adverse effects on respiratory mechanics. The answers given were vague such as barotrauma and pulmonary oedema. In some cases, candidates answered a completely different question explaining the physiological effects of poor gas exchange or high airway pressure."

a) List five signs of life-threatening acute asthma. (5 marks)

- Silent chest.
- Cyanosis.
- Poor respiratory effort.
- Hypotension.
- Exhaustion.
- Depressed level of consciousness.

b) List two investigation findings in life-threatening acute asthma. (2 marks)

- Peak flow < 33% predicted/best.
- PaO_2 < 8 kPa/arterial oxygen saturation < 92%.
- $PaCO_2$ in the normal range, or raised as near-fatal asthma develops.

c) Apart from oxygen, list four drugs (including their routes of administration) that may be used in the management of life-threatening acute asthma. (4 marks)

- Nebulised and intravenous salbutamol.
- Oral prednisolone or intravenous hydrocortisone or intramuscular methylprednisolone depending on ability to swallow and retain tablets.
- Nebulised ipratropium bromide.
- Intravenous magnesium sulphate.
- Nebulised or intravenous adrenaline.
- Intravenous aminophylline.

d) **List three reasons for hypotension after induction of anaesthesia of a patient with life-threatening acute asthma. (3 marks)**

- Development of tension pneumothorax due to a combination of positive pressure ventilation and gas trapping.
- Induction agents causing both direct vasodilation and negative inotropism as well as loss of the heightened sympathetic state of life-threatening acute asthma.
- Dramatic increase in intrathoracic pressure with onset of positive pressure ventilation resulting in reduction of venous return.
- Absolute hypovolaemia due to reduction in oral intake with development of severe asthma, increased evaporative respiratory losses, and the possibility of increased losses due to fever due to any associated respiratory infection.

e) **List three ways in which life-threatening acute asthma may adversely affect respiratory mechanics. (3 marks)**

- Airway narrowing due to infiltration by inflammatory cells, bronchial smooth muscle constriction, and mucus production causing an increase in resistance to expiratory gas flow.
- Rapid respiratory rate with failure to allow enough time for full exhalation especially with the increased resistance to expiratory gas flow leads to increased gas trapping with dynamic hyperinflation and therefore intrinsic PEEP.
- Increased lung volumes lead to flattening of the diaphragm and so less efficient ventilation as the intercostal (and accessory) muscles become responsible for inhalation and exhalation resulting in further failure to clear carbon dioxide and a further trigger to increase respiratory rate.

f) **List three aspects of a suitable ventilatory strategy directly after intubation of a patient with life-threatening acute asthma. (3 marks)**

- Prolonged expiratory time e.g. I:E ratio 1:4.
- Low respiratory rate, 12–14 breaths/minute.
- Minimisation of PEEP.
- Tidal volume of 6 ml/kg.
- Acceptance of low-normal oxygen saturations/PaO_2 and low-normal pH with high-normal $PaCO_2$.

REFERENCES

Demoule A et al. How to ventilate obstructive and asthmatic patients. *Intensive Care Med.* 2020: 46: 2436–2449.

National Institute for Health and Care Excellence. *Asthma, acute. Treatment summaries. British national formulary.* https://bnf.nice.org.uk/treatment-summaries/asthma-acute/. Accessed 17th January 2023.

Stanley D, Tunnicliffe W. Management of life-threatening asthma in adults. *Contin Educ Anaesth Crit Care Pain.* 2008: 8: 95–99.

15.18 March 2021 Airway pressure release ventilation

a) List the main principles of how airway pressure release ventilation (APRV) differs to conventional ventilatory modes. (2 marks)
b) List the appropriate initial settings for commencement of APRV. (4 marks)
   - P high:
   - T high:
   - P low:
   - T low:
c) Give two APRV ventilatory settings that could be changed if the patient became hypercapnic. (2 marks)
d) List four possible benefits of spontaneous ventilation in APRV. (4 marks)
e) List two possible mechanisms by which haemodynamic compromise may occur with APRV. (2 marks)
f) List two possible cardiovascular advantages associated with APRV. (2 marks)
g) List four relative contraindications to APRV. (4 marks)

The CRQ on this topic had a pass rate of 43.4%. The Chairs said that "this question was judged by the examiners to be one of the more difficult questions on the paper. The question asks about a relatively new mode of ventilation, however, given the current situation, it is a mode of ventilation that candidates would have used in their clinical practice. Candidates dropped marks throughout all the stems of this question. There was a low pass rate but the question correlated well with overall performance on the paper." CRQ papers have an even split of difficult, moderate and easy questions. APRV has actually been around since 1987 but has been used extensively during COVID. There was a comprehensive BJA Education article on the topic in January 2020 – once again, note the temporal relationship between BJA Education articles and exam questions.

a) List the main principles of how airway pressure release ventilation (APRV) differs to conventional ventilatory modes. (2 marks)

- Maintenance of prolonged periods of high airway pressure to facilitate recruitment of lung units to maximise oxygenation.
- Short periods of low pressure ("release") to facilitate carbon dioxide clearance without allowing time for decruitment, minimising lung injury associated with repetitive opening and closing of lung units.

b) List the appropriate initial settings for commencement of APRV. (4 marks)

- **P high:** patient's current plateau pressure, ideally < 30 cmH$_2$O.
- **T high:** 5 s/3–8 s.
- **P low:** 0 cmH$_2$O.
- **T low:** 0.5 s/0.3–0.8 s, ensuring that T low is short enough to terminate expiratory flow at 75% of peak expiratory flow (*T low is too long if expiratory flow continues below 75% peak expiratory flow, as it results in derecruitment and alveolar collapse*).

c) Give two APRV ventilatory settings that could be changed if the patient became hypercapnic. (2 marks)

- Decrease T high in increments of 0.2 s to a minimum of 3 s *(thus increasing the number of "releases" per minute, analogous to increasing respiratory rate in conventional ventilation modes)*.
- Increase P high *(analogous to increasing tidal volume in conventional ventilation modes)*.
- Ensuring 100% automatic tube compensation.

d) List four possible benefits of spontaneous ventilation in APRV. (4 marks)

- Reduction of respiratory muscle atrophy.
- Reduced need for sedation with consequent benefit to haemodynamic stability.
- Reduced need for neuromuscular paralysis with possible reduction in development of ICU-acquired weakness.
- Preferential opening of dependent lung units (rather than non-dependent as is seen in conventional positive pressure ventilation), thus improving ventilation-perfusion matching and reducing overdistension of non-dependent lung units.
- Promotion of venous return and consequent improvement of haemodynamic stability/reduction in need for vasopressor and inotropic support.

e) List two possible mechanisms by which haemodynamic compromise may occur with APRV. (2 marks)

- High intrathoracic pressure causing decreased right sided venous return.
- High mean airway pressure causing increased pulmonary vascular resistance.
- Reduction in right ventricular cardiac output causing reduced left sided filling and reduction in cardiac output.

f) List two possible cardiovascular advantages associated with APRV. (2 marks)

- High intrathoracic pressures resulting in reduced cardiac transmural pressure and work of systole thus maximising ejection fraction.
- Reduction in need for sedative drugs due to facilitation of spontaneous ventilation resulting in greater haemodynamic stability.
- Improvement in oxygenation may result in better myocardial oxygen delivery and therefore function and output.

g) List four relative contraindications to APRV. (4 marks)

- Significant haemodynamic instability/hypovolaemia.
- Recent pulmonary resection.
- Severe bronchospasm.
- Pulmonary hypertension with right ventricular decompensation.
- Bronchopleural fistula.
- Untreated pneumothorax.
- Restrictive lung disease.

REFERENCE

Swindin J et al. Airway pressure release ventilation. *BJA Educ.* 2020: 20: 80–88.

15.19 September 2021 Donation after neurological death

A CRQ on donation after neurological death appeared in September 2021, but this paper was withdrawn after difficulties were experienced with the online exam platform. Remember there was a question on the topic in 2016 and before that in 2008. It is an important and increasingly relevant ICU topic.

15.20 March 2022 Prone ventilation

a) State the optimum duration for a period of prone positioning in a ventilated patient with acute respiratory distress syndrome (ARDS). (1 mark)
b) Give two absolute contraindications to proning. (2 marks)
c) Give three relative contraindications to proning. (3 marks)
d) List four safety issues to be considered before proning. (4 marks)
e) Give four mechanisms by which proning improves oxygenation in a patient with ARDS. (4 marks)
f) Give three referral criteria for extracorporeal membrane oxygenation. (3 marks)
g) Apart from proning, list three ventilatory strategies for management of ARDS. (3 marks)

The Chairs reported a pass rate of 58.8% for the CRQ on this topic and said that "this is a topical question which was generally answered well. Candidates showed familiar failings, with the physiology component of the question being answered poorly. The section where candidates particularly struggled was the criteria for ECMO referral."

a) **State the optimum duration for a period of prone positioning in a ventilated patient with acute respiratory distress syndrome (ARDS). (1 mark)**

Current research has not determined the exact time for best outcomes with proning but supports a duration of 16 or more hours.

- 16 or more hours per 24-hour period.

b) **Give two absolute contraindications to proning. (2 marks)**

Veno-venous ECMO is undertaken to provide oxygenation to support lung function and is not a contraindication to prone positioning although it would be relatively unusual to perform in such circumstances. Veno-arterial ECMO is undertaken to support lung and heart function and is a contraindication to prone positioning.

- Spinal instability.
- Open chest post-cardiac surgery/trauma.
- Patient less than 24 hours post-cardiac surgery.
- Central cannulation for VA ECMO (veno-arterial extracorporeal membrane oxygenation) or BiVAD (biventricular assist device) support.

c) **Give three relative contraindications to proning. (3 marks)**

- Multiple trauma e.g. pelvic or chest fractures, pelvic fixation device.
- Severe facial fractures.
- Traumatic brain injury or raised intracranial pressure.
- Frequent seizures.
- Raised intraocular pressure.
- Tracheostomy within the preceding 24 h.
- Haemodynamic instability despite fluid and inotropic support.
- Previous poor tolerance of prone position.
- Morbid obesity.
- Pregnancy in second or third trimester.

d) List four safety issues to be considered before proning. (4 marks)

- LocSSip use.
- Adequate personnel for turning, including anaesthetist to manage airway.
- Equipment appropriate for this specific patient's reintubation if necessary.
- Preoxygenation with 100% oxygen.
- Removal of endotracheal anchor device and then securing of tube with ties.
- Chest drains to remain below the level of the patient at all times and only clamped if safe to do so.
- Availability of resuscitation drugs in case of haemodynamic instability after turning.
- Lines securely dressed and a plan for their management during turning made. Discontinuation of non-essential infusions.
- Adequate depth of sedation.
- Need for neuromuscular blockade.
- Eyes lubricated and taped.
- Nasogastric feed stopped and tube aspirated.

e) Give four mechanisms by which proning improves oxygenation in a patient with ARDS. (4 marks)

- Increase in size of functional residual capacity.
- Reduction of lung volume that is compressed by mediastinum.
- Improved V/Q matching due to more homogenous lung density and therefore homogenous ventilation in the prone position (as opposed to supine ventilation where perfusion significantly exceeds ventilation in the most dependent parts of the lungs).
- Improved homogeneity of perfusion resulting in improved perfusion of non-dependent lung units which may be the best aerated.
- Recruitment of the dorsal lung units that may have become subject to collapse.
- Attenuation of ventilator-induced lung injury, thus reducing the inflammatory response which will further contribute to lung disease and poor gas exchange.
- Improved drainage of secretions from dorsal lung areas to central airways therefore improving ventilation of diseased areas of lung.

f) Give three referral criteria for extracorporeal membrane oxygenation. (3 marks)

There are also exclusion criteria which include severe neurological injury, cardiac arrest for more than 15 minutes, refractory multiorgan failure, significant frailty, other life-limiting disease, more than seven days of mechanical ventilation, contraindication to anticoagulation, and poor recovery potential.

- Potentially reversible severe respiratory failure (e.g. PaO_2 < 10 kPa for $\geq$ 6 hours).
- Lung injury score of 3 or more (*score based on worse PaO_2/FiO_2 ratio, higher PEEP value, lower compliance, and increased numbers of lung quadrants infiltrated on chest X-ray*).
- Severe hypercapnic acidosis $\leq$ pH 7.2.
- Trial of ventilation in prone position and optimal ventilation with lung protective strategy unsuccessful in improving gas exchange.

g) Apart from proning, list three ventilatory strategies for management of ARDS. (3 marks)

- "Open lung ventilation strategy": limiting peak airway pressure < 30 cmH$_2$0 with high PEEP ~ 15 cmH$_2$O OR minimising driving pressure/difference between PEEP and plateau pressures whilst achieving desired tidal volume and acceptable oxygenation.
- Protective lung ventilation, restricting tidal volume to 6 ml/kg.
- Recruitment manoeuvres.
- Use of NMBD to facilitate ventilation.
- Use of ventilator care bundles.
- Protocolised weaning from ventilator.

REFERENCES

Bamford P et al. *Guidance for prone positioning in adult critical care.* London: Intensive Care Society, 2019. www.wyccn.org/uploads/6/5/1/9/65199375/icsficm_proning_guidance_final_2019.pdf. Accessed 18th January 2023.

Camporota L et al. Consensus on the referral and admission of patients with severe respiratory failure to the NHS ECMO service. *Lancet Respir Med.* 2021: 9: e16–e17.

Griffiths M et al. Guidelines on the management of acute respiratory distress syndrome. *BMJ Open Resp Res.* 2019: 6: e000420.

Lumb A, White A. Breathing in the prone position in health and disease. *BJA Educ.* 2021: 21: 280–283.

15.21 September 2022 Convulsive status epilepticus

a) Define convulsive status epilepticus. (1 mark)
b) List three options for immediate management of convulsive status epilepticus for a patient who does not have an individualised emergency management plan. (3 marks)
c) List three possible underlying causes of convulsive status epilepticus which will require additional pharmacological management in the acute phase. (3 marks)
d) List three drugs used as second line in the management of convulsive status epilepticus that is unresponsive to first line agents. (3 marks)
e) List two pharmacological approaches used as third line management of convulsive status epilepticus if unresponsive to second-line agents. (2 marks)
f) List three neurological complications of convulsive status epilepticus. (3 marks)
g) Give the mechanism of action of phenytoin. (1 mark)
h) List two causes of hypotension when phenytoin is administered intravenously. (2 marks)
i) List two clinical features of phenytoin toxicity. (2 marks)

The CRQ on this topic had a pass rate of 64.4%. The Chairs said, "Few candidates knew the definition of status epilepticus. In section (i) candidates failed to answer the question that was asked. The question asked for signs of toxicity yet candidates wrote about the side effects of phenytoin." Just like the close temporal relationship between new NICE guidance on epilepsy being issued in 2016 and the SAQ in 2017, this time the guidance was changed in April 2022, and the CRQ followed in September of the same year. It is really important to keep an eye out for topical national guidelines being issued in the time leading up to your exam.

a) Define convulsive status epilepticus. (1 mark)

This is the up-to-date definition as per 2022 NICE guidance.

- Seizure activity lasting more than five minutes (or recurrent seizures with failure to regain full consciousness in between, lasting more than five minutes).

b) List three options for immediate management of convulsive status epilepticus for a patient who does not have an individualised emergency management plan. (3 marks)

- Buccal midazolam.
- Rectal diazepam.
- Intravenous lorazepam if there is intravenous access and resuscitation facilities are available.

c) List three possible underlying causes of convulsive status epilepticus which will require additional pharmacological management in the acute phase. (3 marks)

- Eclampsia.
- Alcohol withdrawal.
- Hypoglycaemia or other metabolic disturbance.

d) List three drugs used as second line in the management of convulsive status epilepticus that is unresponsive to first line agents. (3 marks)

- Levetiracetam.
- Phenytoin.
- Sodium valproate.

e) List two pharmacological approaches used as third line management of convulsive status epilepticus if unresponsive to second-line agents. (2 marks)

- Phenobarbital.
- General anaesthesia.

f) List three neurological complications of convulsive status epilepticus. (3 marks)

- Cerebral hypoxia.
- Cerebral oedema.
- Cerebral haemorrhage.
- Excitotoxic CNS injury.

g) Give the mechanism of action of phenytoin. (1 mark)

- Blocks voltage gated sodium channels to reduce action potential propagation.

h) List two causes of hypotension when phenytoin is administered intravenously. (2 marks)

- Arrhythmia or bradycardia caused by phenytoin's effect on heart due to its action on voltage gated sodium channels.
- Propylene glycol solvent, which has a negatively inotropic effect and may result in bradycardia, hypotension, and asystole.

i) List two clinical features of phenytoin toxicity. (2 marks)

- Nystagmus.
- Diplopia.
- Slurred speech.
- Ataxia.
- Confusion.
- Hyperglycaemia.

REFERENCES

Carter E, Adapa R. Adult epilepsy and anaesthesia. *Contin Educ Anaesth Crit Care Pain.* 2015: 15: 111–117.

National Institute for Health and Care Excellence. *Epilepsies in children, young people and adults: NG217,* April 2022.

National Institute for Health and Care Excellence. *British national formulary.* https://bnf.nice.org.uk/drugs/phenytoin/. Accessed 16th January 2023.

Perks A et al. Anaesthesia and epilepsy. *BJA.* 2012: 108: 562–571.

15.22 February 2023 Ventilator-associated pneumonia

a) List four clinical and investigational findings that may indicate the presence of ventilator-associated pneumonia (VAP). (4 marks)
b) List four patient risk factors for development of VAP. (4 marks)
c) List two equipment-related risk factors for development of VAP. (2 marks)
d) Define the term "care bundle." (1 mark)
e) List four elements of a care bundle that may be used to minimise the risk of development of VAP. (4 marks)
f) List two other care bundles that may be used in the intensive care unit. (2 marks)
g) List three likely causative organisms for VAP in intensive care units in the UK. (3 marks)

This was the third time that ventilator-associated pneumonia formed the focus of the intensive care medicine question in the time period covered by this book. Surprisingly the pass rate was only 30.3%, the lowest of the paper, and the Chairs queried whether this "might reflect that candidates are seeing intensive care medicine as a different speciality. However, core parts of intensive care medicine are in the anaesthetic curriculum." The clinical features and risk factors for development of VAP featured in all three iterations of the question, highlighting it as key knowledge. There was an increased focus on care bundles in this year's version as well as a subsection about the microbiological causes of VAP, which are addressed here.

d) Define the term "care bundle." (1 mark)

- A group of evidence-based interventions that relate to a particular aspect of patient care. The strength of evidence supporting the individual components varies, with some elements just accepted as good practice. Implementation of all of the components together should result in better patient outcomes.

f) List two other care bundles that may be used in the intensive care unit. (2 marks)

- Central venous catheter or indwelling line care bundle.
- Sepsis care bundle.
- Tracheostomy care bundle.
- Head injury care bundle.
- Organ donor extended care bundle.

g) List three likely causative organisms for VAP in intensive care units in the UK. (3 marks)

The list of causative agents is vast and includes fungi and parasites in immunocompromised patients. Listed here are the most common ones.

- Early onset (from community): Streptococcus pneumoniae, Haemophilus influenzae, Staphylococcus aureus.
- Late onset (often multi-drug resistant): Pseudomonas aeruginosa, Methicillin-resistant Staphylococcus aureus, Enterobacteriaceae.

REFERENCES

Conway Morris A. Management of pneumonia in intensive care. *J Emerg Crit Care Med.* 2018: 2: 101.
Gunasekara P, Gratrix A. Ventilator-associated pneumonia. *BJA Educ.* 2016: 16: 198–202.
Hellyer T et al. The Intensive Care Society recommended bundle of interventions for the prevention of ventilator-associated pneumonia. *JICS.* 2016: 17: 238–243.
Kalanuria A, Zai W, Mirski M. Ventilator-associated pneumonia in the ICU. *Crit Care.* 2014: 18: 208.

16

16.1 September 2011 Amniotic fluid embolus

Amniotic fluid embolism was one of the four major causes of maternal mortality (alongside genital tract sepsis, pre-eclampsia, and eclampsia and venous thromboembolism) in the 2006–2008 report on maternal mortality from the Centre for Maternal and Child Enquiries (CMACE) and was the focus of this SAQ. The confidential enquiries into maternal deaths are now run by the collaboration MBRRACE-UK. For the sake of your obstetric practice and your exams, make sure you have looked at their website, which contains links to all their publications. The College frequently asks questions based on important recent reports and guidelines. Amniotic fluid embolism featured again in a more recent exam and so will be addressed later in this chapter.

REFERENCE

www.npeu.ox.ac.uk/mbrrace-uk.

DOI: 10.1201/9781003388494-16

16.2 March 2012 Regional anaesthesia for caesarean section

a) Give two sensory modalities that can be assessed to check the adequacy of a neuraxial block prior to caesarean section and the height of block that should be achieved for each. (4 marks)
b) State the degree of motor block that is consistent with an adequate neuraxial block for caesarean section. (I mark)
c) Give one reliable sign that indicates sympathetic block associated with neuraxial anaesthesia. (I mark)
d) State three ways in which an initially inadequate block can be improved sufficiently to allow surgery to proceed. (3 marks)
e) List five risk factors for failure of neuraxial anaesthesia for caesarean section. (5 marks)
f) Give three additional risk factors for intraoperative pain when a labour epidural has been topped up for caesarean section. (3 marks)
g) Aside from improvement of block and general anaesthesia, give three pharmacological options (with doses) appropriate for the management of pain during caesarean section under spinal anaesthesia. (3 marks)

The Chair's Report relating to this question as it first appeared as an SAQ showed a success rate of 45.7%. They said that "most candidates knew the dermatome levels and how to test the level of a block, however . . . some candidates did not read the question carefully enough or appreciated that they were required [to describe how] to improve the block itself rather than provide supplementary analgesia." I have reproduced that part of the question in part (d) of my CRQ. The long-standing lack of consensus about how the adequacy of neuraxial block should be tested prior to caesarean section is discussed in the recent OAA/AAGBI guideline referenced below.

a) Give two sensory modalities that can be assessed to check the adequacy of a neuraxial block prior to caesarean section and the height of block that should be achieved for each. (4 marks)

The guideline describes how sensory testing should be done: move from blocked to unblocked areas between midaxillary and midclavicular lines, ensuring loss of light touch (e.g. using cotton wool) up to at least T5 bilaterally. Use a second sensory modality if there is any doubt (e.g. loss of sensation to cold to a height of T4). Check the lower limit of the block, using back of leg to avoid testing near genital area.

- **Modality:** Light touch   **Height:** T5 bilaterally
- **Modality:** Cold sensation   **Height:** T4 bilaterally

b) State the degree of motor block that is consistent with an adequate neuraxial block for caesarean section. (I mark)

The guideline advises that the variability in the way anaesthetists describe their findings of a Bromage score, and the many modifications of the scale that exist, mean that a straightforward check of ensuring bilateral loss of ability to straight leg raise against gravity is "simple and reproducible."

- Inability to straight leg raise against gravity bilaterally.

c) Give one reliable sign that indicates sympathetic block associated with neuraxial anaesthesia. (1 mark)

The authors of the guideline point out that hypotension is not a reliable indicator of sympathetic block as there may be several causative mechanisms for this.

- Warm feet bilaterally.
- Dry feet bilaterally.

d) State three ways in which an initially inadequate block can be improved sufficiently to allow surgery to proceed. (3 marks)

Note that the question has not specified what sort of neuraxial anaesthesia has been used, so make sure your answer includes options for spinal and epidural.

- Positioning: flex hips to flatten lumbar lordosis, cautious head-down tilt or lateral tilt if block inadequate on one side *(remember to avoid aortocaval compression)*.
- Epidural: if using epidural or combined spinal and epidural, top up the epidural. If using spinal only, consider siting and using an epidural to raise the height of the block.
- Repeat spinal: consider reducing overall dose if some block is present. Good attention to patient positioning should help prevent high spinal.

e) List five risk factors for failure of neuraxial anaesthesia for caesarean section. (5 marks)

- Operative urgency.
- High BMI.
- Women having their first caesarean section.
- Indication for caesarean being maternal medical condition or fetal distress.
- Failure to use intrathecal opioid in spinal anaesthesia.
- Increased duration of surgery.

f) Give three additional risk factors for intraoperative pain when a labour epidural has been topped up for caesarean section. (3 marks)

- High top-up volume required.
- Adrenaline not used in top-up mixture.
- Higher numbers of clinician-administered boluses necessary in labour.
- Care by non-obstetric anaesthetist.

g) Aside from improvement of block and general anaesthesia, give three pharmacological options (with doses) appropriate for the management of pain during caesarean section under spinal anaesthesia. (3 marks)

- Nitrous oxide, although this is unlikely to help with severe pain.
- Fast-acting opioids e.g. fentanyl 25–50 mcg or alfentanil 250–500 mcg boluses.
- Ketamine 10 mg boluses.

REFERENCES

Hoyle J, Yentis, S. Assessing the height of block for caesarean section over the past three decades: trends from the literature. *Anaesthesia*. 2015: 70: 421–428.

Plaat F et al. Prevention and management of intra-operative pain during caesarean section under neuraxial anaesthesia: a technical and interpersonal approach. *Anaesthesia*. 2022: 77: 588–597.

16.3 September 2012 Intrauterine fetal death

a) Define late intrauterine fetal death (IUFD). (1 mark)
b) List five pre-existing maternal conditions or factors that are associated with an increased risk of IUFD. (5 marks)
c) List four obstetric causes of IUFD. (4 marks)
d) State four ways in which the approach to pain relief for labour with IUFD may differ compared to provision for a live birth. (4 marks)
e) Give three abnormal haematological results which may contraindicate epidural analgesia with reasons why they may be abnormal in the presence of IUFD. (6 marks)

The SAQ on this topic asked about the implications of late IUFD on overall management of the patient. The Chair's Report showed that the following should have been considered for inclusion in the answer: psychological distress, method of delivery, mandatory level 1 care (MEOWS) and possible transfer to level 2 care, exclusion of possible causes, provision of effective analgesia, and consideration of sedation. I was surprised by the inclusion of sedation in their list as this is not something that I would consider appropriate in the care of these patients, although pharmacological anxiolysis may sometimes be indicated. Delivery mode will usually be dictated by the cause for the IUFD – the majority will have a vaginal delivery, whereas IUFD caused by sepsis or abruption may necessitate caesarean delivery.

a) Define late intrauterine fetal death (IUFD). (1 mark)

- Fetal death in utero after 24 completed weeks of pregnancy.

b) List five pre-existing maternal conditions or factors that are associated with an increased risk of IUFD. (5 marks)

- Diabetes.
- Systemic lupus erythematosus.
- Advanced maternal age.
- Maternal thrombophilias.
- Rhesus D negative status.
- Obesity.
- Maternal drug use.
- Untreated maternal thyroid disease.
- Maternal infection.

c) List four obstetric causes of IUFD. (4 marks)

- Pre-eclampsia or eclampsia.
- Obstetric cholestasis.
- Uterine rupture.
- Placental abruption.
- Premature rupture of membranes.
- Cord prolapse.
- Ascending infection.

d) State four ways in which the approach to pain relief for labour with IUFD may differ compared to provision for a live birth. (4 marks)

- Maternal pain experience might be greater due to psychological distress, especially if induction and augmentation of labour is necessary – greater need for effective pain relief, an epidural may be optimal.
- Need not consider uteroplacental transfer; more effective pain-relieving opioids with lower side effects such as morphine and diamorphine may therefore be used instead of pethidine. May be given as PCA.
- Cause or consequence of IUFD may contraindicate neuraxial technique; sepsis, pre-eclampsia with deranged clotting or thrombocytopaenia, haemorrhage, or IUFD resulting in DIC.
- Remifentanil PCA relatively contraindicated according to most protocols due to lack of experience, and adverse incidents associated with use in presence of IUFD. Also, no need for a drug with rapid clearance as fetus is not living.
- Intramuscular injections contraindicated in presence of coagulopathy.

e) Give three abnormal haematological results which may contraindicate epidural analgesia with reasons why they may be abnormal in the presence of IUFD. (6 marks)

- Significantly raised white cell count; maternal sepsis as cause or effect of IUFD.
- Low platelets; may be present in severe pre-eclampsia or HELLP syndrome.
- Deranged coagulation, low fibrinogen; may accompany low platelets in the presence of DIC due to abruption, uterine rupture or occasionally because of the IUFD itself. May also occur in pre-eclampsia or HELLP syndrome. Abnormal coagulation may also be present in maternal thrombophilias.

REFERENCES

Das D, Patel N. Management of the woman with an intrauterine fetal death (IUFD). In: Fernando R, Sultan P, Phillips S (eds.), *Quick hits in obstetric anaesthesia*, 1st edition. Cham, Switzerland: Springer, 2022. Chapter 4.

Marr R, Hyams J, Bythell V. Cardiac arrest in an obstetric patient using remifentanil patient-controlled analgesia. *Anaesthesia*. 2013: 68: 283–287.

The Royal College of Obstetricians and Gynaecologists. *Late intrauterine fetal death and stillbirth: green-top guideline no. 55*, October 2010.

16.4 March 2013 Post-dural puncture headache

A woman experiences a headache 24 hours after delivery having had epidural analgesia for labour.
a) List five presenting features of a post-dural puncture headache (PDPH). (5 marks)
b) Give two risk factors for accidental dural puncture. (2 marks)
c) List five differential diagnoses of postpartum headache. (5 marks)
d) State four aspects of conservative management of PDPH. (4 marks)
e) List four risks of epidural blood patch. (4 marks)

The Chair's Report for this question in its original SAQ format stated that it was a "basic but relevant" question with a 59% success rate.

a) List five presenting features of a post-dural puncture headache (PDPH). (5 marks)

- Fronto-occipital headache developing within five days of puncture, worse on standing, improves on lying flat.
- Neck stiffness.
- Tinnitus.
- Hypacusia.
- Photophobia.
- Nausea.
- Cranial nerve palsies (blindness cranial nerve II; diplopia cranial nerves III, IV, VI; hearing loss cranial nerve VIII).
- Rarely, CSF leak from epidural puncture site.

b) Give two risk factors for accidental dural puncture. (2 marks)

- Extremes of BMI, both high and low.
- Increased depth to epidural space.
- Operator inexperience.
- Inability of patient to remain still during the procedure (e.g. due to advanced labour).

c) List five differential diagnoses of postpartum headache. (5 marks)

Infective:	Meningitis. Encephalitis. Sinusitis.
Metabolic:	Dehydration. Caffeine withdrawal.
Vascular:	Migraine. Cerebral vein thrombosis. Cerebral infarction. Subdural haematoma. Subarachnoid haemorrhage. Posterior reversible leucoencephalopathy syndrome.
Obstetric-related:	Pre-eclampsia. Lactation headache.
Neoplastic:	Primary or secondary.
Other:	Tension headache. Benign intracranial hypertension. Pneumocephalus.

d) **State four aspects of conservative management of PDPH. (4 marks)**

- Simple analgesia; paracetamol with NSAIDs if not contraindicated.
- Laxatives; straining may exacerbate CSF leak.
- Antiemetics if indicated.
- Assessment of venous thrombo-embolism risk. Encourage mobilisation, advise on use of antiembolism stockings, consider need for low molecular weight heparin *(consider implications for epidural blood patch, if required)*.
- Avoid dehydration – intravenous fluid only if unable to maintain adequate hydration orally.

e) **List four risks of epidural blood patch. (4 marks)**

- Failure: 60–70% success rate with first epidural blood patch.
- Bruising.
- Back pain and stiffness for a few days, not long term.
- Further accidental dural puncture.
- Nerve damage.
- Infection.
- Spinal canal haematoma.
- Seizure.

REFERENCES

Obstetric Anaesthetists' Association. *Treatment of obstetric post-dural puncture headache*, December 2018. www.oaa-anaes.ac.uk/assets/_managed/cms/files/Guidelines/New%20 PDPH%20Guidelines.pdf. Last accessed 28th April 2023.

Royal College of Anaesthetists and Association of Anaesthetists of Great Britain and Ireland. *Risks associated with your anaesthetic section 10: headache after a spinal or epidural injection*, 2015. www.rcoa.ac.uk/system/files/10-HeadachesSpinalEpidural2015.pdf. Accessed 4th July 2022.

Sabharwal A, Stocks G. Postpartum headache: diagnosis and management. *Contin Educ Anaesth Crit Care Pain.* 2011: 11: 181–185.

16.5 September 2013 Obesity in pregnancy

A primiparous patient with a booking BMI of 55 kg/m² presents in the high-risk obstetric anaesthetic assessment clinic at 32 weeks' gestation. She is hoping for a vaginal delivery.
a) Which specific points do you need to elicit from the history and examination? (6 marks)
b) What do you need to communicate to the patient? (7 marks)
c) Document your plan for her management on the delivery suite. (7 marks)

I have left this question here for you to see in the SAQ format as it appeared in September 2013. It was answered well with a 72.8% pass rate, according to the Chair's Report. They said that "the implications of morbid obesity on a parturient and the importance of forward planning were well appreciated by most candidates." Before the questions were presented in an SAQ format, they were a short essay style – look at this question from May 2006: "A consultant obstetrician has asked you to review a woman in her first pregnancy in the anaesthetic ante-natal assessment clinic. Her body mass index is 45 kg/m². There are no other abnormalities and at 32 weeks' gestation she is hoping for a vaginal delivery. Write a summary recording the details you would wish to cover during the appointment and your recommendations for her management when she is admitted in labour." Later in this chapter you will see a question on the same topic in CRQ format. No matter how the format of the exam changes, key topics remain important and relevant to our practice and therefore also to your revision for the Final FRCA. Below I have given answers to the SAQ question as although you won't now be asked it in SAQ style, I think the answers provide good learning about the impact of obesity in pregnancy.

a) Which specific points do you need to elicit from the history and examination? (6 marks)

Follow the alphabet to dredge the points out of your brain in a systematic manner. Remember that they have specifically asked for history and examination.

Airway:

- History of difficult airway.
- History of problems with anaesthesia in the past.
- Perform airway assessment.

Respiratory:

- History of obstructive sleep apnoea.
- History of other respiratory symptoms such as dyspnoea or asthma.
- Check oxygen saturations when supine and auscultate chest.

Cardiovascular:

- Assess exercise tolerance.
- Check for history or symptoms of ischaemic heart disease.
- Check blood pressure.
- Assess for likely ease of cannulation, consideration of need for ultrasound.

Neurological:

- Assess for likelihood of difficulty with neuraxial technique, consider ultrasound use, consider need for extra length spinal and epidural needles.

Endocrine:

- Check for history of diabetes mellitus or gestational diabetes and check medications and control.

Pharmacology:

- Document all medications.
- May be taking low molecular weight heparin, which has an impact on the timing of neuraxial techniques.

Gastrointestinal:

- History of reflux and medications to control this.

Cutaneomusculoskeletal:

- Check body mass. Consider impact on equipment need: hover mattress, bariatric bed, blood pressure cuff/need for invasive arterial monitoring, theatre table (weight limit, need for side extensions).
- Assess for ability of woman to position herself for neuraxial technique.

Obstetric:

- Check for problems with pregnancy.

b) What do you need to communicate to the patient? (7 marks)

The Obstetric Anaesthetists' Association have produced a leaflet called "Anaesthetics and pregnant women with a high BMI. What you need to know." This is another reminder to read and make use of guidelines and publications in common use.

- Reason for referral; raised BMI increases likelihood of needing caesarean or instrumental delivery and, therefore, there is an increased likelihood of an anaesthetist being involved in their care.
- Recommendation to avoid eating and to drink only clear fluids in labour in view of the increased risk of needing assistance with delivery and therefore some form of anaesthesia. This reduces the likelihood of aspiration of particulate stomach content.
- Regular antacid in labour for same reason, to reduce the risk of aspiration of highly acidic stomach content.
- Epidural and spinal may be more difficult to perform and so take longer.
- Consider early epidural, especially if labour is not progressing well; easier to perform in early rather than advanced labour and can be topped up for the purposes of caesarean or instrumental delivery, thus possibly reducing the need for general anaesthesia.
- General anaesthetic may be more difficult to perform and may have increased risks. Optimum care of mother and baby is for the mother to remain awake (with neuraxial technique if necessary) for delivery.

c) Document your plan for her management on the delivery suite. (7 marks)

My documentation would include the following points:

- BMI and body mass.
- Outcomes from clinic meeting, including any issues elicited from history and examination.
- Airway assessment, predicted difficulty with neuraxial block, and any predicted issues with cannulation.

- If the woman is currently taking low molecular weight heparin, give clear advice regarding omission of dose if any chance that she is in early labour, to consult delivery suite early for assessment and admission if indicated.
- Any specific equipment requirements.
- Instruction to alert anaesthetist on arrival in labour, junior anaesthetist to contact consultant.
- Early cannula? Depends on consultation with the woman and her individual risks.
- Early epidural? Depends on consultation with the woman.
- Instruction to restrict oral intake to clear fluids only in labour and regular antacid to be given.
- Antiembolism stockings to be worn in labour, consideration of low molecular weight heparin prophylaxis afterwards as per guidelines (ensure dose appropriate to patient weight).

REFERENCES

Centre for Maternal and Child Enquiries (CMACE). *Maternal obesity in the UK: finding from a national project.* London: CMACE, 2010.

https://www.labourpains.org/downloads/english-resources/a4-high-bmi-leaflet.pdf. Accessed 14th November 2023.

16.6 March 2014 Mitral stenosis in pregnancy

A 27-year-old woman is found to have an asymptomatic heart murmur at 13 weeks of pregnancy. A subsequent echocardiogram shows moderate mitral stenosis.
a) Give two causes of mitral stenosis. (2 marks)
b) List three normal cardiovascular changes in pregnancy (3 marks) and explain how each of these exacerbate the pathophysiology of mitral stenosis. (3 marks)
c) List two pharmacological interventions that may be required in pregnancy to manage symptomatic mitral stenosis. (2 marks)
d) Give four haemodynamic goals (4 marks) and, for each, a method by which they can be achieved (4 marks) during management of labour in a parturient with mitral stenosis.
e) State two physiological events after delivery which may predispose to development of acute pulmonary oedema. (2 marks)

The SAQ on this topic had a 65.5% pass rate. However, the Chair said, "There was a disappointing lack of knowledge of the pathology of mitral stenosis, and some candidates had no understanding at all. The physiological and clinical aspects were more soundly addressed, and the question proved a very strong discriminator between strong and weak candidates."

There is poor tolerance of an increase in circulating volume and an increase in heart rate in mitral stenosis, as this results in a shorter time period for atrial emptying with consequent atrial enlargement risking development of atrial fibrillation and pulmonary oedema.

Women with significant mitral stenosis (valve area < 1.5 cm²) should be counselled against pregnancy due to the risks to maternal health (heart failure, development of pulmonary hypertension with risk of right sided heart failure and tricuspid regurgitation, risk of thromboembolic disease secondary to the development of atrial fibrillation, and poor left atrial emptying), as well as fetal risks (premature birth, intrauterine growth retardation and fetal death). Percutaneous mitral commissurotomy may be indicated after 20 weeks' gestation in women with NYHA class III or IV and/or pulmonary artery pressure > 50 mmHg despite optimal medical therapy.

a) Give two causes of mitral stenosis. (2 marks)

- Rheumatic fever *(commonest cause worldwide but less common in developed countries)*.
- Infective endocarditis.
- Degenerative calcification.

b) List three normal cardiovascular changes in pregnancy (3 marks) and explain how each of these exacerbate the pathophysiology of mitral stenosis. (3 marks)

- 45% increase in intravascular volume: the fixed output of the left atrium is unable to cope resulting in pulmonary oedema. Increase in left atrial stretch predisposes to atrial fibrillation, which further reduces fractional left atrial emptying and increases risk of pulmonary oedema.
- 20% increase in heart rate: shorter diastole so reduced time for flow across stenosed valve, reduces left ventricular filling, reduces cardiac output (CO).
- 40% increase in CO to cope with the 40% increase in oxygen consumption caused by the fetus and raised maternal metabolism: cannot be facilitated with a significantly stenosed valve, resulting in pulmonary oedema, decreased exercise tolerance, dyspnoea, cyanosis.
- 20% reduction in systemic vascular resistance in pregnancy (alongside failure to achieve increase in CO): reduction in coronary artery perfusion, resulting in risk of ischaemia.

c) List two pharmacological interventions that may be required in pregnancy to manage symptomatic mitral stenosis. (2 marks)

- Heart rate control (both for those in sinus rhythm and those with atrial fibrillation) with β_1 blocker *(and activity limitation)*.
- Diuretics for women with congestive symptoms despite β_1 blocker.
- Anticoagulation with unfractionated or low molecular weight heparin or vitamin K antagonist, depending on the stage in pregnancy, for women at risk of or with atrial fibrillation.

d) Give four haemodynamic goals (4 marks) and, for each, a method by which they can be achieved (4 marks) during management of labour in a parturient with mitral stenosis.

- Avoidance of tachycardia: early pain management with an epidural, avoidance of drugs that stimulate tachycardia (vasopressors with β agonist effect, oxytocin boluses), prompt management of physiological tachycardia due to dehydration or blood loss.
- Maintenance of afterload: slowly incremental epidural block, α-agonist (e.g. phenylephrine) infusion to maintain afterload but avoid tachycardia.
- Avoidance of rises in pulmonary arterial pressure: assisted delivery to avoid Valsalva associated with pushing, avoidance of nitrous oxide, always ensuring adequate oxygenation, avoidance of ergometrine.
- Ensure euvolaemia: mitral stenosis is a fixed cardiac output state, so dehydration should be avoided, and any blood loss should be rapidly controlled alongside appropriate blood replacement. Ensure that positioning avoids aortocaval compression.
- Avoidance of arrhythmia: avoidance of causes of tachycardia, avoidance of acutely increasing load of left atrium (excessive fluid administration, increases in afterload), continuation of prescribed medication such as β antagonists, electrical cardioversion in event of cardiovascular instability following acute onset of atrial fibrillation.

e) State two physiological events after delivery which may predispose to development of acute pulmonary oedema. (2 marks)

- Loss of aortocaval compression.
- Autotransfusion due to contraction of uterus.

REFERENCES

Holme K, Gibbison B, Vohra H. Mitral valve and mitral valve disease. *BJA Educ.* 2017: 17: 1–9.

Regitz-Zagrosek V et al. 2018 European Society of Cardiology guidelines for the management of cardiovascular diseases in pregnancy: the task force for the management of cardiovascular diseases during pregnancy of the European Society of Cardiology (ESC). *Eur Heart J.* 2018: 39: 3165–3241.

Sayed Youssef G. Mitral stenosis in pregnant patients. *eJ Cardiol Pract.* 2018: 16: 18.

16.7 September 2014 Incidental surgery in pregnancy

a) A 28-year-old woman presents for acute appendicectomy – she is 22 weeks pregnant. Complete the following table, listing five risks to the fetus during anaesthesia for the mother (5 marks) linking them to reasons why they may occur. (5 marks)
b) List three additional pre- and intraoperative steps to maximise fetal safety if she were 27 weeks pregnant. (3 marks)
c) State two changes in maternal physiology in late pregnancy that increase the risk of maternal and therefore fetal hypoxia at induction of general anaesthesia. (2 marks)
d) Give three considerations to maximise the safety of laparoscopic surgery in a pregnant patient. (3 marks)
e) List two analgesics that are contraindicated for use when breastfeeding. (2 marks)

The Chair was concerned by the poor pass rate of 33% for the SAQ on this topic. They felt that too many candidates focussed excessively on preparing for premature delivery despite the gestational age of 22 weeks being so low as to make survival unlikely (I wonder if they repeated this question whether they would reduce the gestational age fractionally, as survival of premature babies improves as the years pass). They were also concerned that some candidates discussed the risk of teratogenesis, indicating that they do not understand the risk period for this.

Some key anaesthesia-relevant timings in obstetrics:

- *Risk of teratogenesis in first trimester (1–12/40) when main organ systems are being developed, especially 2–8/40.*
- *Consider need for antacid premedication and RSI from approximately 12/40.*
- *Risk of aortocaval compression by 18/40, may be earlier in multiple pregnancy or high BMI.*
- *Surgery and anaesthesia confer increased risk of miscarriage in second trimester (13–24/40), early labour or stillbirth after 24/40.*
- *The fetus is potentially viable from 24/40 onwards, rarely earlier.*

a) A 28-year-old woman presents for acute appendicectomy – she is 22 weeks pregnant. Complete the following table, listing five risks to the fetus during anaesthesia for the mother (5 marks), linking them to reasons why they may occur. (5 marks)

Risk to the fetus	Reasons why the risks may occur
Hypoxia with resulting fetal distress.	Failure to adequately manage maternal airway and ventilation.
Hypercarbia resulting in uterine artery constriction, fetal hypercarbia and subsequent myocardial depression.	Failure to manage maternal airway and ventilation.
Hypocarbia can cause uterine artery vasoconstriction, poor perfusion, and leftward shift of maternal oxyhaemoglobin dissociation curve.	Hyperventilation of mother causing hypocarbia.
Hypoperfusion with resulting fetal distress.	Fetoplacental unit entirely dependent on maternal perfusing pressure which may decrease due to impact of anaesthetic agents and aortocaval compression.
Possible adverse neurocognitive outcomes.	Unconfirmed/unquantified anaesthetic-induced neuronal apoptosis in developing brain.
Risk of miscarriage.	Unquantified and unlikely – more likely to relate to the disease process necessitating surgery than anaesthesia.

b) **List three additional pre- and intraoperative steps to maximise fetal safety if she were 27 weeks pregnant. (3 marks)**

- Consideration of need for fetal monitoring – liaise with obstetricians.
- Consideration of need for tocolysis – liaise with obstetricians.
- Consideration of need for steroids for fetal lung maturation – liaise with obstetricians.
- Fetus now viable so need to consider risk of premature labour; may require in utero transfer to unit with NICU if risk deemed significant – liaise with neonatologists.
- Avoid NSAIDs due to risk of premature closure of ductus arteriosus.

c) **State two changes in maternal physiology in late pregnancy that increase the risk of maternal and therefore fetal hypoxia at induction of general anaesthesia. (2 marks)**

- 20% reduction in functional residual capacity (upward pressure of gravid uterus with increased transverse diameter of the thorax).
- Increase in metabolic demand of pregnant woman (in addition to the demand of the fetoplacental unit) resulting in increased oxygen consumption.

d) **Give three considerations to maximise the safety of laparoscopic surgery in a pregnant patient. (3 marks)**

- Control of maternal end-tidal carbon dioxide.
- Use of open technique to enter abdomen.
- Low pneumoperitoneum pressure (< 12 mmHg).
- Limit Trendelenburg or reverse Trendelenburg positioning and achieve desired position slowly.
- Fetal monitoring when feasible.

e) **List two analgesics that are contraindicated for use when breastfeeding. (2 marks)**

- Codeine phosphate or tramadol *(risk of respiratory depression in the baby)*.
- Analgesic dose aspirin *(risk of Reye's syndrome in the baby)*.

REFERENCES

Delgado C et al. General anaesthesia in obstetrics. *BJA Educ.* 2020: 20: 201–207.

Haggerty E, Daly J. Anaesthesia and non-obstetric surgery in pregnancy. *BJA Educ.* 2020: 21: 42–43.

Mitchell J et al. Guideline on anaesthesia and sedation in breastfeeding women 2020. *Anaesthesia.* 2020: 75: 1482–1493.

Nejdlova M, Johnson T. Anaesthesia for non-obstetric procedures during pregnancy. *Contin Educ Anaesth Crit Care Pain.* 2012: 12: 203–206.

16.8 March 2015 Jehovah's Witness and cell salvage

You are asked to review a woman in the anaesthetic antenatal clinic. She is 30 weeks pregnant and a Jehovah's Witness. She requires an elective caesarean section at 39 weeks due to placenta praevia and a fibroid uterus.

a) State four requirements for validity of an advance decision to refuse treatment that may result in risk of death. (4 marks)

b) State four pharmacological approaches to minimising the risk or consequences of haemorrhage for this patient. (4 marks)

c) State two specific risks to be discussed with this patient before they make their advance decision. (2 marks)

d) Give five advantages of the use of intraoperative cell salvage during caesarean section. (5 marks)

e) Give five possible problems associated with the use of intraoperative cell salvage during caesarean section. (5 marks)

The Chair's Report for the SAQ on this topic showed that it had a 44.6% pass rate with 22.5% of candidates receiving a poor fail. "Candidates omitted mention of important peri-operative risks such as haemorrhage, hysterectomy and other significant morbidity and mortality. Some candidates demonstrated a worrying lack of knowledge of cell salvage and, in particular, the disadvantages of this technique." Also, note how the beginning of the question asks about management of Jehovah's Witnesses specifically but then moves on to ask about cell salvage in caesarean section more generally. Always read the question.

a) State four requirements for validity of an advance decision to refuse treatment that may result in risk of death. (4 marks)

- Patient to be over 18 years old.
- Patient to have capacity at time of writing decision.
- Patient to have lost capacity at the time of applying the advance decision.
- Written.
- Signed by patient (or on the direction of a patient unable to sign for themselves).
- Witnessed and signed by the witness.
- Specifies the treatments that the patient refuses to have.
- Acknowledges risk of death as a consequence of refusal.
- Has not been withdrawn either in writing or verbally.

b) State four pharmacological approaches to minimising the risk or consequences of haemorrhage for this patient. (4 marks)

- Preoperative optimisation of haemoglobin with iron (intravenous if necessary) and other haematinics.
- Consideration (in collaboration with haematologist) of need for erythropoietin.
- Plan for uterotonic administration following delivery – may include use of long-acting oxytocin (carbetocin) or oxytocin infusion with a step-wise plan for other uterotonics if indicated.
- Stop any drugs with an adverse effect on bleeding for an appropriate duration before surgery e.g. low molecular weight heparin, aspirin.
- Use of tranexamic acid intraoperatively to minimise blood loss.

c) State two specific risks to be discussed with this patient before they make their advance decision. (2 marks)

- Potential for haemorrhage greatly increased due to fibroids AND placenta praevia.
- Risk of death if blood not given in the event of massive haemorrhage. There are no true blood alternatives.
- Risk of major morbidity in the event of massive haemorrhage, including prolonged ICU stay, prolonged ventilation and its complications, poor wound healing, infection, hysterectomy, consequent difficulties with caring for newborn.

d) Give five advantages of the use of intraoperative cell salvage during caesarean section. (5 marks)

You need to understand the process of cell salvage in order to explain it to a patient:

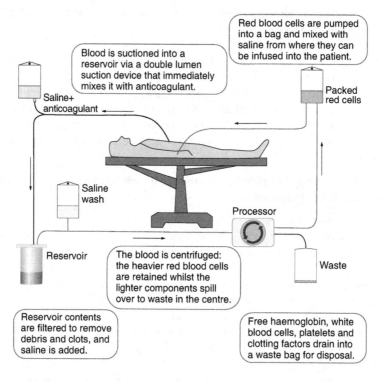

Cell salvage.

- Avoidance of risks of allogeneic transfusion; ABO incompatibility and other transfusion reactions, viral, bacterial and prion transmission, blood errors.
- Good value; consumables cost slightly more than one unit of donated blood.
- Blood reinfused at room temperature, reduces the risk of hypothermia associated with transfusion.
- Often acceptable to Jehovah's Witnesses. *(Some Witnesses would find it acceptable only when set up in continuous circulation, as in the image above, whereas others would find it acceptable even when set up to fill a bag with salvaged blood before being disconnected from the cell salvage machine and then infused.)*
- Useful in patients with atypical antibodies where crossmatch may be difficult to achieve.
- Salvaged blood has normal 2,3 DPG levels and therefore oxygen-carrying behaviour.

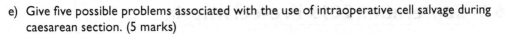

e) Give five possible problems associated with the use of intraoperative cell salvage during caesarean section. (5 marks)

- In the case of a Rhesus-positive baby with Rhesus-negative mother, there is a risk of alloimmunisation. However, this risk occurs in any delivery of positive baby to negative mother, and anti-D administration is routine in such cases.
- Leucocyte depletion filter slows infusion rate, may result in release of bradykinin causing hypotension and may become saturated requiring replacement. (*Leucocyte depletion filter use is no longer viewed as mandatory in obstetrics due to the effectiveness with which the process removes amniotic fluid from the salvaged blood. However, practice varies.*)
- Air embolism.
- High cost per use in centres where cell salvage infrequently used.
- Staff training necessary, may be difficult to maintain staff competency if infrequently used.
- Risk of bacterial contamination.
- Risk of electrolyte imbalance.
- No platelets or coagulation factors so does not eliminate need for allogeneic blood products in significant haemorrhage.
- Red cell lysis due to "skimming" (suctioning of surface of shed blood) reduces the availability of whole cells for reinfusion.
- Risk of circulatory overload.

REFERENCES

Klein A et al. Association of Anaesthetists' guidelines: cell salvage for peri-operative blood conservation 2018. *Anaesthesia.* 2018: 73: 1141–1150.

Klein A et al. Association of Anaesthetists: anaesthesia and peri-operative care for Jehovah's witnesses and patients who refuse blood. *Anaesthesia.* 2019: 74: 74–82.

Kuppurao L, Wee M. Perioperative cell salvage. *Contin Educ Anaesth Crit Care Pain.* 2010: 10: 104–108.

The Mental Capacity Act 2006. (c9): S24–S25.

National Institute for Health and Care Excellence. *Intraoperative blood cell salvage in obstetrics: IPG144,* 2005. www.jw.org.

16.9 September 2015 Pre-eclampsia

A 25-year-old woman who is 37 weeks pregnant and known to have pre-eclampsia is admitted to labour ward with a blood pressure of 160/110 mmHg on several readings.

a) State the definition of pre-eclampsia. (2 marks)
b) Give four symptoms of pre-eclampsia that women should report to a healthcare professional immediately if experienced. (4 marks)
c) Define eclampsia. (1 mark)
d) Give three risk factors for the development of pre-eclampsia. (3 marks)
e) State two drugs that may be used intravenously to control this woman's blood pressure. (2 marks)
f) State the indications for magnesium sulphate treatment in pre-eclampsia. (2 marks)
g) Give three advantages of epidural analgesia in labour for a woman with pre-eclampsia. (3 marks)
h) State two airway management issues (2 marks) and one respiratory complication (1 mark) of pre-eclampsia that may impact on the safe provision of general anaesthesia and, for each, state how the risks are mitigated.

The pass rate for the SAQ on this topic was 16.1%. The Chairs were concerned that pre-eclampsia is a common emergency condition and so candidates should know the principles of its management. They were surprised at how few candidates were able to give an acceptable definition of pre-eclampsia (note that this changed in 2019 as per NICE guidance) and how few seemed to appreciate the importance of systolic blood pressure control to prevent intracerebral haemorrhage. The abysmal pass rate made me wonder, in the previous edition of this book, whether the question would be repeated soon. The woman in this question has blood pressure at a level that qualifies as "severe" pre-eclampsia when accompanied by worsening organ dysfunction.

a) State the definition of pre-eclampsia. (2 marks)

- New onset of hypertension (two readings 4 hours apart of SBP > 140 mmHg and/or DBP> 90 mmHg) after 20 weeks of pregnancy.
- Accompanied by evidence of proteinuria or specific involvement of at least one other organ system.

b) Give four symptoms of pre-eclampsia that women should report to a healthcare professional immediately if experienced. (4 marks)

- Severe headache.
- Problems with vision, such as blurring or flashing before the eyes.
- Severe pain just below the ribs.
- Vomiting.
- Sudden swelling of the face, hands or feet.

c) Define eclampsia. (1 mark)

- Eclampsia is the occurrence of seizures on a background of pre-eclampsia (whether previously diagnosed or not).

d) Give three risk factors for the development of pre-eclampsia. (3 marks)

- Hypertensive disease in a previous pregnancy.
- Chronic kidney disease.

- Autoimmune disease.
- Type 1 or 2 diabetes mellitus.
- Chronic hypertension.
- Nulliparity.
- Age 40 years or older.
- Pregnancy interval of more than 10 years.
- BMI of 35 kg/m² or more at first antenatal assessment.
- Family history of pre-eclampsia.
- Multifetal pregnancy.

e) **State two drugs that may be used intravenously to control this woman's blood pressure. (2 marks)**

Alternatively, oral nifedipine may be used. The doses of labetalol and hydralazine quoted in different guidelines and the BNF vary, especially when it comes to increasing doses and infusion rates, but here I have given a starting point that may be considered in an emergency.

- Labetalol *(10–20 mg initially with increasing doses depending on effect).*
- Hydralazine *(5–10 mg initially with increasing doses depending on effect: fluid loading may be required due to its profound vasodilatory action).*

f) **State the indications for magnesium sulphate treatment in pre-eclampsia. (2 marks)**

Note that magnesium may also be given to women in preterm labour or having a planned preterm delivery (< 34 weeks' gestation) for fetal neuroprotection. Its use in pre-eclampsia is for its membrane stabilising effect, to reduce the risk of seizures. It has the added effect of reducing blood pressure due to its vasodilatory action but this is not an indication for its use.

- Severe pre-eclampsia for women in a critical care setting for whom delivery of the fetus is planned within 24 hours.
- For the treatment of seizures and prevention of further seizures.

g) **Give three advantages of epidural analgesia in labour for a woman with pre-eclampsia. (3 marks)**

- Vasodilation resulting in improvement in blood pressure control.
- Avoidance of opioid analgesia that might impact on alertness and thus impair ability to assess woman's condition.
- Obtundation of spikes in blood pressure associated with contraction pain.
- Ability to top-up for urgent delivery if indicated, avoiding general anaesthesia with its associated complications in pre-eclampsia.

h) **State two airway management issues (2 marks) and one respiratory complication (1 mark) of pre-eclampsia that may impact on the safe provision of general anaesthesia and, for each, state how the risks are mitigated.**

- Increased risk of difficult airway due to laryngeal oedema:
  - May require smaller tube size.
  - Use video laryngoscopy.
- Pressor response to laryngoscopy and intubation may precipitate intracranial haemorrhage:
  - Use e.g. esmolol, alfentanil or remifentanil to obtund pressor response *(paediatrician to be informed if opioid used).*
- Laryngeal oedema may worsen over duration of surgery:
  - Ensure air leak after cuff deflation before extubation.

- Pulmonary oedema resulting in hypoxia:
  - Higher airway pressures with higher PEEP than usual may be required intraoperatively.
  - Consider need for CPAP or to keep the patient intubated and ventilated postoperatively.
  - Maintain fluid restriction of 1 ml/kg/h to a limit of 80 ml/h (unless matching blood losses).

REFERENCES

American College of Obstetricians and Gynaecologists. Gestational hypertension and pre-eclampsia: ACOG practice bulletin no. 222. *Obstet Gynecol.* 2020: 135: e237–e260.

Combeer E, Sharma N. Pre-eclampsia and HELLP syndrome. In: Fernando R, Sultan P, Phillips S (eds.), *Quick hits in obstetric anaesthesia,* 1st edition. Cham, Switzerland: Springer, 2022. Chapter 39.

National Institute of Health and Care Excellence. *Preterm labour and birth: NG25,* November 2015, updated June 2022.

National Institute for Health and Care Excellence. *Hypertension in pregnancy: diagnosis and management: NG133,* June 2019, updated April 2023.

National Institute for Health and Care Excellence. *British National Formulary: labetalol hydrochloride.* https://bnf.nice.org.uk/drugs/labetalol-hydrochloride/#indications-and-dose. Accessed 6th May 2023a.

National Institute for Health and Care Excellence. *British National Formulary: hydralazine.* https://bnf.nice.org.uk/drugs/hydralazine-hydrochloride/#indications-and-dose. Accessed 6th May 2023b.

16.10 March 2016 Airway management in obstetric anaesthesia

a) Give three patient factors (3 marks) and four situational factors (4 marks) which may contribute to difficulties encountered when securing the airway under general anaesthesia in the pregnant patient.
b) List three measures that can be used to maximise oxygenation of an obstetric patient at the time of induction. (3 marks)
c) List five factors that should be considered <u>before induction</u> of an obstetric patient which would influence a decision whether to proceed with surgery, or wake the patient, in the event of a subsequent failed intubation. (5 marks)
d) Give two airway-related factors that should be considered when deciding whether to proceed with surgery or wake the patient in the event of failure to intubate an obstetric patient. (2 marks)
e) Give three recommendations of the 4th National Audit Project (Major Complications of Airway Management in the UK, NAP 4) regarding airway management in the pregnant woman. (3 marks)

When an SAQ on this topic appeared in 2016, it was five years after NAP4. NAP4 has been the basis of numerous Final FRCA questions, and its vignettes make it very readable. It is, as a report about all that can go wrong with the airway, very relevant to our practice and makes very salutary reading. In the original SAQ format all bar three of the marks could be gained by thoughtful reflection on your practice in obstetric anaesthesia and consideration of all that can go wrong. The remaining three (out of twenty) points required specific knowledge of NAP4 recommendations, reproduced here in part (e) of the reconfigured CRQ question. This exam clearly requires revision, but it also requires you to have learnt from experience and to be able to draw from that in your answers. In creating other parts to this reconfigured CRQ version, I have drawn further from NAP4 and also from the DAS/OAA obstetric airway guidelines, which are also highly relevant and worth being familiar with for the exam and for real life. The pass rate for the SAQ was 57.6% and so was higher than it had been for the mandatory obstetric question for the last several sittings. The Chairs said it was "disappointing, however, that the recommendations from NAP4 regarding the pregnant patient . . . seemed very poorly known."

a) Give three patient factors (3 marks) and four situational factors (4 marks) which may contribute to difficulties encountered when securing the airway under general anaesthesia in the pregnant patient.

Patient:

- Increased fatty tissue, breast size, tongue size associated with normal pregnancy.
- Obesity.
- Comorbidities such as asthma, PET.
- Active labour may make cooperation with assessment and pre-induction positioning difficult.
- Non-starved patient.

Situational:

- Site of obstetric theatre often isolated, away from main theatres, without the second-line airway equipment held in main theatres and rapid back-up from colleagues.
- Impact of left lateral tilt on view at laryngoscopy.
- Urgency resulting in failure to adequately assess airway, administer antacids in an appropriate time frame to take effect, position appropriately, assess for feasibility of other modes of anaesthesia.
- Intraoperative conversion of neuraxial to general anaesthesia may be challenging.

- Commonly out-of-hours, therefore often a trainee, low experience of general anaesthesia for obstetrics.
- Lack of awareness of other healthcare professionals about the potential difficulty with airway. Failure to warn, failure to assist.

b) **List three measures that can be used to maximise oxygenation of an obstetric patient at the time of induction. (3 marks)**

- Optimisation of position; head up, ramped positioning.
- Preoxygenation to F_EO_2 of 0.9 or more.
- High-flow nasal oxygen for apnoeic ventilation.
- Face mask ventilation after administration of NMBD (to a maximum peak inspiratory pressure of 20 cmH$_2$0).

c) **List five factors that should be considered <u>before induction</u> of an obstetric patient which would influence a decision whether to proceed with surgery, or wake the patient, in the event of a subsequent failed intubation. (5 marks)**

- Maternal condition; consider whether surgery is indicated for maternal health.
- Degree of fetal compromise.
- Experience of anaesthetist.
- Degree of obesity of patient.
- Degree of surgical complexity anticipated.
- Risk of aspiration (to include consideration of antacid premedication, starvation status, opioid administration, and whether previously labouring).
- Feasibility of alternative mode of anaesthesia or possibility of securing airway awake.

d) **Give two airway-related factors that should be considered when deciding whether to proceed with surgery or wake the patient in the event of failure to intubate an obstetric patient. (2 marks)**

- The rescue airway device in use.
- The degree of compromise of the maternal airway following the intubation attempts and siting of rescue device.

e) **Give three recommendations of the 4th National Audit Project (Major Complications of Airway Management in the UK, NAP 4) regarding airway management in the pregnant woman. (3 marks)**

- Difficult airway management and CICO skills must be kept up to date.
- Obstetric anaesthetists should be familiar with using second-generation SADs for airway rescue.
- Awake fibreoptic intubation should be available (skills and equipment) anywhere in the hospital.
- All recovery staff (including midwives working in recovery) should be properly trained and skills regularly updated.

REFERENCES

Cook T, Woodall N, Frerk C (eds.). *4th National Audit Project of the Royal College of Anaesthetists and the Difficult Airway Society: major complications of airway management in the United Kingdom*. London: The Royal College of Anaesthetists and Association of Anaesthetists of Great Britain and Ireland, 2011.

Mushambi M et al. Obstetric Anaesthetists' Association and Difficult Airway Society guidelines for the management of difficult and failed tracheal intubation in obstetrics. *Anaesthesia*. 2015: 70: 1286–1306.

16.11 September 2016 Regional anaesthesia for caesarean section

The SAQ on this topic focussed on assessing the adequacy of neuraxial block prior to caesarean section, actions to be taken if a spinal block proved inadequate prior to starting surgery, and steps to be taken in the event of intraoperative pain. It was therefore very similar to the question from March 2012. However it was important to read the question carefully, as is always the case in the Final FRCA, as the 2012 question asked "how might an initially inadequate block be improved sufficiently to allow surgery to proceed?" whereas the 2016 question asked you to "describe the actions you could take if your spinal block proves inadequate on testing prior to starting surgery for an elective (category 4) caesarean section." The 2016 answer would therefore include consideration of general anaesthesia, whereas the 2012 question would not. One brand-new subsection appeared in 2016, the content of which is covered below. The Chairs were "reassured" to report a 77.5% pass rate for the question.

a) Give three early symptoms (3 marks) and three signs (3 marks) of a spinal block that is ascending too high.

Symptoms:

- Difficulty breathing or taking a deep breath, difficulty speaking.
- Nausea and vomiting.
- Anxiety, feeling faint.
- Tingling and weakness of hands and arms.

Signs:

- Decreased respiratory effort, reduced saturations, weak cough.
- Cardiovascular instability: bradycardia and hypotension.
- Objective weakness of hands then arms then shoulders, high block on retesting.
- Obtundation.

16.12 March 2017 Post-dural puncture headache

The obstetric SAQ from March 2017 focussed on post-dural puncture headache, and there was considerable overlap of the subsections compared to the March 2013 version. The Chairs reported an 81.3% pass rate and said that "PDPH is a common problem in obstetric anaesthesia so it is reassuring that the question was well answered and that candidates recognised possibly serious differential diagnoses." This high pass rate may also reflect candidates looking back at the topics of previous exams and learning from them. Important clinical topics are commonly the focus of exam questions. The questions below reflect the only new subsection from the 2017 SAQ, changed somewhat into CRQ style.

a) Give three features in the history (3 marks), three features in the examination (3 marks) and two features of recent blood tests (2 marks) of this patient that would lead you to consider a serious underlying cause of the patient's headache.

History:

- Drowsiness, confusion, vomiting.
- Focal neurology.
- Seizures.
- Significant neck stiffness and photophobia *(although photophobia may also be present in PDPH).*

Examination:

- Focal neurology.
- Papilloedema.
- Hypertension.
- Hypotension and tachycardia.
- Fever.
- Reduced conscious level.
- Meningism: positive Kernig and Brudzinski's signs.
- Petechial rash.

Recent blood results:

- Features of infection: elevated CRP, raised or depressed white cell count. However, CRP and white cell count tend to be elevated after delivery anyway, so this must be viewed in the overall context.
- Features of pre-eclampsia: deranged transaminases and bilirubin, low platelets, haemolysis, elevated uric acid, proteinuria.

16.13 September 2017 Intrauterine fetal death

A woman who has had an intrauterine fetal death (IUFD) at 36 weeks' gestation in her first pregnancy is admitted to your delivery suite for induction of labour.

a) Describe the important non-clinical aspects of her management. (4 marks)

b) What are the considerations when providing pain relief for this woman? (13 marks)

c) If this patient requires a caesarean section, what are the advantages of using regional anaesthesia, other than the avoidance of the effects of general anaesthesia? (3 marks)

This is the original SAQ as it appeared in the paper, and this is the full Chairs' Report:

"Pass rate NA. This question was removed from the exam after marking but no candidates were disadvantaged by its removal. The reason for not including it in the final scores was that there was confusion amongst candidates about whether the intrauterine fetal death had occurred in the current, or a previous pregnancy. On reflection, the examiners agreed that the wording of the question did allow either interpretation. As has been outlined above, all the SAQs undergo rigorous scrutiny and are checked and rechecked for clarity and accuracy. Unfortunately, the alternative interpretation was not spotted in this case. The question will be reworded before being reused. Having said all of the above, the pass rate for this question was poor, with most marks being lost in section (b) where candidates were asked to discuss considerations for analgesia. Even those who had correctly interpreted the question tended to simply list methods of analgesia rather than outlining the advantages and disadvantages of each."

This is reassuring: whilst you MUST read the questions carefully, you do not need to waste time agonising about what they mean if it really isn't clear. If there is more than one way of interpreting the question, then there will probably be a spread of approaches amongst the candidates which will highlight to the College the lack of clarity of the question. This question is similar to that from September 2012. It would be sensible to revise all aspects of management of IUFD as it would seem likely that a question on this topic will appear again soon. Below I have changed some of the subsections from the 2017 SAQ that were not covered by the 2012 question on the same topic.

a) **Give four important non-clinical aspects of her management. (4 marks)**

- One-to-one senior midwifery care, trained in caring for women with IUFD.
- Good communication between all involved healthcare professionals to avoid possibility of lack of awareness of situation and subsequent insensitivity.
- Clear discussions with the woman regarding expectations and wishes for the delivery; pain relief, presence of friends or family, contact with the baby after birth, arrangement for mementoes to be created (photos, hair cuttings, footprints).
- Dedicated suite/room away from the noise of delivery suite, ideally with provision of non-clinical area where the woman may be with her birth partner/family/friends before delivery and may spend time with her baby, if desired, after birth. However, location for delivery is ultimately determined by maternal condition.

c) **If this patient requires a caesarean section for delivery, give three advantages of using regional anaesthesia, other than the avoidance of the effects of general anaesthesia. (3 marks)**

- Offers optimum postoperative pain relief.
- Facilitates early contact with the baby.
- Permits clearer recollection of events that may be important to the woman.
- Facilitates presence of partner at delivery.

16.14 March 2018 Pre-eclampsia

Bar a few tweaks to the layout, the SAQ in the March 2018 exam was identical to that from March 2015 (which had a really poor pass rate) apart from the fact that the patient here had a one-off blood pressure reading of 180/110 mmHg (thus severe pre-eclampsia), and there was a plan for delivery of her baby within 24 hours. Magnesium sulphate administration was therefore clearly indicated in her management. The College put some examples of CRQs on their website in the lead-up to the change of exam structure, and one of them concerned pre-eclampsia – make sure you have looked at it.

REFERENCE

Royal College of Anaesthetists Website CRQ Examples. https://rcoa.ac.uk/sites/default/files/documents/2020-02/CRQ-EXAMPLES-2018_0.pdf. Accessed 28th April 2023.

16.15 September 2018 Obesity in pregnancy

The SAQ on this topic was almost identical to that which featured in September 2013 apart from a subsection asking about the specific risks associated with a raised BMI in pregnancy. This was addressed, in a more targeted manner, in the March 2022 CRQ about obesity in pregnancy, and so you will find it later in this chapter.

16.16 March 2019 Incidental surgery in pregnancy

The SAQ on this topic was identical to that from September 2014. Despite this, the pass rate was only 32.4%. The Chairs' Report commented on how surprisingly low the pass rate was given how recently the question had been asked before. If you do no other revision for the Final FRCA, at least look at the topics that have featured before as these are the ones that are clearly considered important by the College. Again, the Chairs said that candidates focussed on conduct of anaesthesia and airway management rather than focussing on fetal safety, which was what was asked. And again, candidates discussed the risks of teratogenesis, which was not relevant to a fetus at either of the gestational ages in the question.

16.17 September 2019 Amniotic fluid embolism

Thrombosis and venous thromboembolism are the most common direct cause of maternal death (occurring within 42 days of the end of pregnancy) in the latest Mothers and Babies: Reducing Risk through Audits and Confidential Enquiries across the UK (MBRRACE-UK) report for the time period 2018–2020, published 2022.

a) State the two next most common direct causes of maternal death in the latest MBRRACE-UK report (2018–2020). (2 marks)
b) State the two leading causes of indirect maternal death in the latest MBRRACE-UK report (2018–2020). (2 marks)
c) Amniotic fluid embolism (AFE) is a direct cause of maternal mortality. Give two respiratory (2 marks), two cardiovascular (2 marks), one neurological (1 mark), one haematological (1 mark) and two obstetric (2 marks) presenting features of AFE.
d) Give three possible obstetric differential diagnoses of AFE. (3 marks)
e) Give three possible non-obstetric differential diagnoses of AFE. (3 marks)
f) State the two theories about the pathophysiology of AFE. (2 marks)

The original SAQ on this question asked about the 2018 MBRRACE Report, but I have changed it to the more recent one. National reports are often the basis of Final FRCA questions as they are clinically topical and give the examiners definitive answers. Have a look at the key messages of the report featured in this question – look at the impact of ethnicity, age, deprivation and obesity on maternal death risk and also the prevalent direct and indirect causes of death. All of this will improve your practice as well as improve your likelihood of success in the exam. There was a BJA Education article concerning amniotic fluid embolism in 2018, published 15 months before the exam. BJA Education is a great revision source and represents the College's view on topics. The pass rate for the SAQ on this topic was 51.7%.

a) State the two next most common direct causes of maternal death in the latest MBRRACE-UK report (2018–2020). (2 marks)

The overall leading cause of death was psychiatric, but MBRRACE splits this between direct psychiatric causes (suicide) and indirect (related to drugs and alcohol use). Nonetheless, death by suicide was the second leading direct cause of maternal death, sepsis third, and haemorrhage fourth.

- Suicide.
- Sepsis.

b) State the two leading causes of indirect maternal death in the latest MBRRACE-UK report (2018–2020). (2 marks)

- Cardiac disease.
- COVID-19.

c) Amniotic fluid embolism (AFE) is a direct cause of maternal mortality. Give two respiratory (2 marks), two cardiovascular (2 marks), one neurological (1 mark), one haematological (1 mark) and two obstetric (2 marks) presenting features of AFE.

I have listed the recognised presenting features of AFE but have put brackets around the ones that are less common. Maximise your chance of exam success by sticking to the more common features in your answers.

Respiratory:	Pulmonary oedema or ARDS. Cyanosis. Dyspnoea. Bronchospasm. (Cough).
Cardiovascular:	Hypotension. Cardiac arrest. (Transient hypertension). (Chest pain).
Neurological:	Seizures. Premonitory symptoms e.g. restlessness, numbness, agitation, tingling. (Headache).
Haematological:	DIC/coagulopathy.
Obstetric:	Fetal distress. Uterine atony.

d) Give three possible obstetric differential diagnoses of AFE. (3 marks)

- Eclampsia.
- Uterine rupture.
- Placental abruption.
- Acute haemorrhage.
- Peripartum cardiomyopathy.
- Uterine inversion.

e) Give three possible non-obstetric differential diagnoses of AFE. (3 marks)

- Pulmonary embolism.
- Air embolism.
- Fat embolism.
- Pulmonary oedema or heart failure.
- Tension pneumothorax.
- Myocardial infarction.
- Anaphylaxis.
- Sepsis.
- Aspiration.
- High spinal.
- Local anaesthesia toxicity.
- Transfusion reaction.
- Asthma exacerbation.
- Intracranial haemorrhage.

f) State the two theories about the pathophysiology of AFE. (2 marks)

- Mechanical theory; amniotic fluid in association with other fetal elements such as vernix and squamous cells resulting in physical obstruction of pulmonary vasculature and consequent right heart failure.
- Immune-mediated theory; immunologically active and prothrombotic contents of amniotic fluid (e.g. platelet activating factor, TNF) triggering a systemic inflammatory response.

REFERENCES

Knight M et al. (eds.). *On behalf of MBRRACE-UK: saving lives, improving mothers' care core report – lessons learned to inform maternity care from the UK and Ireland Confidential Enquires into Maternal Deaths and Morbidity 2018–2020.* Oxford: National Perinatal Epidemiology Unit, University of Oxford: 2022.

Metodiev Y et al. Amniotic fluid embolism. *BJA Educ.* 2018: 18: 234–238.

16.18 March 2020 General anaesthesia for caesarean section

The rate of accidental awareness reported during general anaesthesia (AAGA) in obstetrics was higher than in other surgical specialties in the 5th National Audit Project.

a) List four patient factors that may contribute to the increased prevalence of AAGA seen in obstetric patients. (4 marks)

b) List three situational factors which may increase the likelihood of AAGA in obstetric anaesthesia. (3 marks)

c) List four anaesthetic factors that may increase the risk of AAGA in obstetric anaesthesia. (4 marks)

d) Give two possible reasons for the association between thiopentone use in obstetric anaesthesia and the increased risk of AAGA. (2 marks)

e) Give three recommendations for obstetric anaesthesia of the 5th National Audit Project. (3 marks)

f) State four measures that can be undertaken to achieve successful intubation after a failed first attempt at intubation of the trachea of an obstetric patient. (4 marks)

The Chairs reported a 59.5% pass rate for this question, one of the lowest for the paper. They felt that it was "clear that candidates were not familiar with the 5th National Audit Project (NAP5) of the Royal College of Anaesthetists and Association of Anaesthetists. The reasons of accidental awareness under GA section [were] poorly answered. At times answers were too generalised and lacked specific detail." The rate of AAGA for caesarean section in NAP5 was reported as 1/670 which is clearly a very significant risk. It is therefore understandable that the College would want you to understand the issues that may contribute to that risk.

a) **List four patient factors that may contribute to the increased prevalence of AAGA seen in obstetric patients. (4 marks)**

- Female sex.
- Young age.
- Obesity.
- Difficult airway.
- High anxiety state of patient preceding emergency caesarean.
- Raised cardiac output of late pregnancy resulting in reduced duration of action of intravenous induction agent as well as a longer time to establish adequate partial pressure of inhalational anaesthetic agent.

b) **List three situational factors which may increase the likelihood of AAGA in obstetric anaesthesia. (3 marks)**

- Out-of-hours.
- Trainee anaesthetist as so often out-of-hours.
- Stress of emergency situation (impacting on decision-making and increasing likelihood of drug errors).
- Interval between induction and start of surgical stimulation is very brief during general anaesthesia for caesarean section (such that adequate depth of anaesthesia may not have been achieved with e.g. inhalational agent before the induction agent has started to lose effect).

c) **List four anaesthetic factors that may increase the risk of AAGA in obstetric anaesthesia. (4 marks)**

- Use of thiopentone.

- Rapid sequence induction.
- Use of neuromuscular blocking drugs.
- Omission of opioid use at induction.
- Underdosing of induction agent and/or NMBD due to failure to dose for body weight resulting in suboptimal intubating conditions, consequent difficulty, prolonged attempts, and therefore awareness.
- Intentional underdosing of inhalational agent out of concern for uterine tone.
- Unfamiliarity of using general anaesthesia for caesarean section, spinal anaesthesia being the most common mode of anaesthesia.

d) **Give two possible reasons for the association between thiopentone use in obstetric anaesthesia and the increased risk of AAGA. (2 marks)**

- Accidental unrecognised syringe swap with antibiotics.
- Unfamiliarity with thiopentone as use is declining in non-obstetric anaesthesia.
- Broad dosing range and often underdosed for patient body mass.

e) **Give three recommendations for obstetric anaesthesia of the 5th National Audit Project. (3 marks)**

- Increased risk of AAGA should be communicated to obstetric patients as part of the consent process.
- Anaesthetic technique should target adequate anaesthesia in healthy parturients by ensuring appropriate doses of induction agents, rapid attainment of adequate end-tidal inhalational agent levels after induction, use of nitrous oxide, with maintenance of uterine tone with uterotonic agents.
- Plan for management of AAGA in the event of difficult intubation, including having additional doses of hypnotic agent readily available.
- Failed neuraxial anaesthesia should be viewed as a risk factor for AAGA.
- Syringes of antibiotic at the time of induction are a risk factor for drug error and AAGA. Steps must be taken (labelling, physical separation, administration of antibiotic by non-anaesthetist, use of propofol instead of thiopentone) to minimise this risk.

f) **State four measures that can be undertaken to achieve successful intubation after a failed first attempt at intubation of the trachea of an obstetric patient. (4 marks)**

- Reduction or removal of cricoid pressure.
- External laryngeal manipulation.
- Repositioning of the head or neck.
- Use of a bougie or stylet.

REFERENCES

Chaggar R, Campbell J. The future of general anaesthesia in obstetrics. *BJA Educ.* 2017: 17: 79–83.

Mushambi M et al. Obstetric Anaesthetists' Association and Difficult Airway Society guidelines for the management of difficult and failed tracheal intubation in obstetrics. *Anaesthesia.* 2015: 70: 1286–1306.

Pandit J, Cook T (eds.). *5th National Audit Project of the Royal College of Anaesthetists and the Association of Anaesthetists of Great Britain and Ireland: accidental awareness during general anaesthesia in the United Kingdom and Ireland.* London: The Royal College of Anaesthetists and Association of Anaesthetists of Great Britain and Ireland, 2014.

16.19 September 2020 Remifentanil PCA in labour

Remifentanil patient-controlled analgesia (PCA) is a labour pain relief option for women for whom epidural analgesia is contraindicated or associated with a higher risk of complications.

a) Give three indications, apart from patient preference, where remifentanil PCA may be preferable to epidural analgesia. (4 marks)

b) Give four pharmacodynamic or pharmacokinetic properties of remifentanil that make it particularly suitable for use for analgesia in labour. (4 marks)

c) Give two other advantages of remifentanil PCA use compared to intramuscular pethidine use for labour analgesia. (2 marks)

d) Give three specific details of a typical prescription for dosing of a remifentanil PCA administration. (3 marks)

e) Apart from the availability of resuscitation equipment and routine observations, state three other measures to maximise the safety of use of remifentanil PCA. (3 marks)

f) State four actions to be taken by an anaesthetic department implementing a remifentanil PCA service for the first time. (4 marks)

This question seemed heavily based on a BJA Education article about remifentanil PCA published in November 2019, ten months before the exam. This is a reminder of how important it is to use BJA Education as a revision source. The Chairs reported a pass rate of just 29.1%, which led them to conclude that many candidates seemingly had "little knowledge or experience of PCA Remifentanil. Many did not know the dose or optimal timing, and few knew anything about the necessary protocols to ensure safe delivery of the drug in an Obstetric unit."

a) Give three indications, apart from patient preference, where remifentanil PCA may be preferable to epidural analgesia. (4 marks)

- Structural abnormality of the lumbar spine: significant scoliosis, some types of previous spinal surgery, congenital abnormality of lumbar spine.
- Acquired, congenital or pharmacological coagulation abnormalities.
- Congenital or acquired thrombocytopenia.
- Localised sepsis at the site where an epidural would be inserted.
- Local anaesthetic allergy (rare).

b) Give four pharmacodynamic or pharmacokinetic properties of remifentanil that make it particularly suitable for use for analgesia in labour. (4 marks)

- Potent mu opioid receptor agonism.
- Minimal histamine release compared to morphine resulting in reduced risk of hypotension.
- Rapid metabolism by plasma and tissue esterases in the woman and fetus so no accumulation.
- Non-saturable metabolism pathway.
- Breakdown products have negligible action.
- These last three factors result in remifentanil's short context-sensitive half-time (three minutes).

c) Give two other advantages of remifentanil PCA use compared to intramuscular pethidine use for labour analgesia. (2 marks)

- Lower subsequent requirement for epidural analgesia.

- Greater reduction in pain scores.
- Associated with a reduced rate of instrumental delivery.
- Can be used in circumstances where intramuscular injection is contraindicated e.g. significant clotting disorders.

d) **Give three specific details of a typical prescription for dosing of a remifentanil PCA administration. (3 marks)**

- 20–40 mcg bolus.
- Two-minute lockout.
- No background infusion.

e) **Apart from the availability of resuscitation equipment and routine observations, state three other measures to maximise the safety of use of remifentanil PCA. (3 marks)**

- One-to-one midwifery care in the room at all times.
- Dedicated intravenous line away from a joint to avoid drug backing up in line followed by subsequent large bolus delivery.
- Routine use of face mask or nasal oxygen.
- Instruction to ensure labouring woman is the only person to administer a dose.

f) **State four actions to be taken by an anaesthetic department implementing a remifentanil PCA service for the first time. (4 marks)**

- Establish a guideline for setting up a remifentanil PCA, monitoring of patients, equipment to be used, essential safety aspects for use, resuscitation equipment to be available etc.
- Create a patient information leaflet that explains indications, use, side effects, alternatives etc.
- Set up training for staff, including anaesthetists (setting up PCA, troubleshooting, management of complications), midwives (monitoring requirements, safety aspects of administration, need for constant one-to-one care, when to call for help), obstetricians (possible benefits of remifentanil PCA, limits of effectiveness in comparison to epidural, safety aspects), paediatricians (impact on neonates, to facilitate feedback on neonatal outcomes).
- Local patient satisfaction auditing and incident reporting.
- Input of outcomes to international registry to assist with continuous evidence sharing and quality improvement.

REFERENCES

Egan T. Remifentanil pharmacokinetics and pharmacodynamics: a preliminary appraisal. *Clin Pharmacokinet.* 1995: 29: 80–94.

Melber A. Remifentanil patient-controlled analgesia (PCA) in labour – in the eye of the storm. *Anaesthesia.* 2018: 74: 277–279.

Ronel I, Weiniger C. Non-regional analgesia for labour: remifentanil in obstetrics. *BJA Educ.* 2019: 19: 357–361.

16.20 March 2021 Adult congenital heart disease in the obstetric patient

The prevalence of adult congenital heart disease (ACHD) in the obstetric population is rising.

a) List three normal physiological changes of pregnancy that may cause decompensation in a patient with ACHD. (3 marks)

b) List two normal physiological events of labour that may cause decompensation in a patient with ACHD. (2 marks)

c) Give one normal postpartum physiological event that may cause decompensation in a patient with ACHD. (1 mark)

d) List four low-risk ACHD lesions for which delivery at a nonspecialist centre would be appropriate. (4 marks)

e) List two high-risk ACHD lesions that would necessitate delivery at a specialist cardiac centre. (2 marks)

f) List six aspects of management of labour for a patient with ACHD. (6 marks)

g) List two uterotonic drugs (with doses) which would be suitable for use in patients with ACHD. (2 marks)

The incidence of ACHD has risen in the obstetric population because of improved management of childhood lesions. Cardiac disease has remained the leading indirect cause of maternal death since 2000. It is therefore topical for the College to include a question on the impact of adult congenital heart disease on pregnancy, and an article on the subject featured in BJA Education in November 2017, just over three years before this exam. The Chairs reported a pass rate of 59.8% for the question despite it being considered "one of the harder questions in the paper" but that the "applied physiology and pharmacology components of the question saw candidates drop the most marks."

a) List three normal physiological changes of pregnancy that may cause decompensation in a patient with ACHD. (3 marks)

- Vasodilation of early pregnancy.
- Increase in total blood volume of 45% by late pregnancy.
- Increase in cardiac output of 30–50% peaking by second trimester.
- Heart rate rise of 20–25% peaking in the third trimester.
- Impaired venous return due to caval compression.

b) List two normal physiological events of labour that may cause decompensation in a patient with ACHD. (2 marks)

- Autotransfusion of blood with each uterine contraction, resulting in intermittent acute increases in preload and cardiac output.
- Rise in cardiac output in labour, increasing further during expulsive efforts.
- Valsalva manoeuvre with expulsive efforts.
- Tachycardia associated with pain of contractions.

c) Give one normal postpartum physiological event that may cause decompensation in a patient with ACHD. (1 mark)

- Autotransfusion related to uterine involution and reabsorption of oedema.
- Sudden loss of aortocaval compression resulting in acute increase in venous return.

d) List four low-risk ACHD lesions for which delivery at a nonspecialist centre would be appropriate. (4 marks)

- Mild pulmonary stenosis.
- Patent ductus arteriosus.

- Mitral valve prolapse.
- Repaired patent ductus arteriosus, atrial or ventricular septal defect.
- Anomalous pulmonary venous drainage.

e) List two high-risk ACHD lesions that would necessitate delivery at a specialist cardiac centre. (2 marks)

- Mechanical valve.
- Systemic right ventricle.
- Fontan circulation.
- Unrepaired cyanotic heart disease.
- Pulmonary hypertension.
- Left ventricular outflow tract obstruction.
- Aortopathy.

f) List six aspects of management of labour for a patient with ACHD. (6 marks)

- Consideration of induction to facilitate appropriate timing and location of delivery.
- Early venous access to allow for rapid response to blood loss.
- Consideration of continuous ECG monitoring to detect tachycardia and arrhythmias, which may cause decompensation, and ischaemia in susceptible patients.
- Consideration of need for arterial line for continuous blood pressure monitoring.
- Early epidural to reduce afterload, minimise pain-related tachycardia and increases in systemic vascular resistance, and reduce urge to push. Facilitates instrumental delivery if necessary.
- Minimisation of pushing to reduce Valsalva manoeuvre and autotransfusion – instrumental delivery with epidural may be used.
- Aim for euvolaemia – monitor and respond to fluid input and urine and blood outputs.
- Avoidance of excessive haemorrhage and ensure replacement with blood if it occurs.
- Consideration of need for antibiotics – lesion- and history-dependent.
- Avoidance of intravascular air in women with shunt. Loss of resistance to saline for epidural, meticulous care with intravenous, intra-arterial, and epidural infusion lines.

g) List two uterotonic drugs (with doses) which would be suitable for use in patients with ACHD. (2 marks)

Carbetocin 100 mcg has been found to cause identical cardiovascular changes to a bolus of oxytocin 5 IU (systemic vasodilation, tachycardia, pulmonary vasoconstriction). Ergometrine causes coronary, systemic, and pulmonary vasoconstriction. Carboprost causes systemic and pulmonary vasoconstriction.

- Vaginal, oral, sublingual or rectal misprostol 0.2–0.8 mg.
- Intravenous oxytocin 2 IU over 10 minutes (followed by an infusion if required).

REFERENCES

Bishop L et al. Adult congenital heart disease and pregnancy. *BJA Educ.* 2018: 18: 23–29.
Regitz-Zagrosek V et al. 2018 European Society of Cardiology Guidelines for the management of cardiovascular diseases in pregnancy: The Task Force for the Management of Cardiovascular Diseases during Pregnancy of the European Society of Cardiology (ESC). *Eur Heart J.* 2018; 39: 3165–3241.
Rosseland L et al. Changes in blood pressure and cardiac output during cesarean delivery: the effects of oxytocin and carbetocin compared with placebo. *Anesthesiology.* 2013: 118: 541–551.

16.21 September 2021 Pre-eclampsia

Pre-eclampsia again – unsurprising whilst it remains one of the leading causes of direct maternal death. This was the exam that was discounted due to problems with the platform used by the College for the online examination.

16.22 March 2022 Obesity in pregnancy

a) Define obesity. (1 mark)
b) Define class 3 obesity. (1 mark)
c) Give two cardiovascular complications of obesity in pregnancy. (2 marks)
d) State four neonatal complications of obesity in pregnancy. (4 marks)
e) State four peripartum complications due to obesity in pregnancy. (4 marks)
f) State four reasons why an early epidural is recommended for obese parturients. (4 marks)
g) List two infections, apart from chest and urine, that obese women are at greater risk of developing postpartum compared to non-obese women. (2 marks)
h) An obese parturient presents with a deep vein thrombosis antenatally. State how the dose of her low molecular weight heparin treatment should be calculated and the recommended duration of treatment. (2 marks)

Another question focused on the risks of obesity in pregnancy – unsurprising now that rates of obesity in the obstetric population are rising, and obesity is a common factor in deaths reported to the national enquiries, including the anaesthesia-related deaths. The referenced BJA Education article on anaesthesia for the obese parturient was published the month before this question appeared in the Final FRCA, and the majority of marks could have been gained from knowing its content. The pass rate was surprisingly low, however, at 43.6% with the Chairs commenting that "candidates demonstrated only a superficial knowledge of the obstetric complications in a patient with a high body mass index. Sections relating to neonatal and delivery complications associated with maternal obesity were particularly poorly answered."

a) Define obesity. (1 mark)

This is the World Health Organization definition.

- Excessive or abnormal fat accumulation that presents a risk to health, defined as BMI > 30 kg/m^2.

b) Define class 3 obesity. (1 mark)

- BMI > 40 kg/m^2.

c) Give two cardiovascular complications of obesity in pregnancy. (2 marks)

- Ischaemic heart disease.
- Hypertension.
- Cardiomyopathy.

d) State four neonatal complications of obesity in pregnancy. (4 marks)

- Preterm delivery.
- Small for gestational age.
- Large for gestational age.
- Macrosomia.
- Congenital abnormalities (including spina bifida, cardiac defects, cleft lip and palate).
- Stillbirth.
- Shoulder dystocia.
- Neonatal death.
- Neonatal ICU admission.

e) State four peripartum complications due to obesity in pregnancy. (4 marks)

- Thromboembolism.
- Infection and sepsis.
- Pre-eclampsia.
- Gestational diabetes.
- Anaesthetic complications.
- Dysfunctional or prolonged labour.
- Instrumental delivery.
- Failed instrumental delivery.
- Caesarean delivery.
- Postpartum haemorrhage.
- Longer hospital stay.
- Mortality.

f) State four reasons why an early epidural is recommended for obese parturients. (4 marks)

- Siting an epidural later in labour may be very challenging due to combination of high BMI and advanced labour pain resulting in inability to remain still.
- Can be topped up for instrumental or surgical delivery *(which obese parturients have a higher risk of requiring)*, thus avoiding sudden need for spinal anaesthesia, which may be challenging with added time pressure later in labour, or general anaesthesia and its attendant risks in obese parturient.
- May facilitate more effective fetal monitoring by reducing movement related to labour pain.
- Avoids need for systemic opioid analgesia with its associated risks of respiratory depression, which may be dangerous in obese parturient especially if they have a history of obstructive sleep apnoea.

g) List two infections, apart from chest and urine, that obese women are at greater risk of developing postpartum compared to non-obese women. (2 marks)

- Wound (perineum or caesarean).
- Genital tract sepsis.

h) An obese parturient presents with a deep vein thrombosis antenatally. State how the dose of her low molecular weight heparin treatment should be calculated and the recommended duration of treatment. (2 marks)

- Based on booking or early pregnancy weight.
- For the remainder of pregnancy and for at least six weeks postnatally until at least three months of treatment has been given in total.

REFERENCES

Patel S, Habib A. Anaesthesia for the parturient with obesity. *BJA Educ.* 2021: 21: 180–186.

The Royal College of Obstetricians and Gynaecologists. *Thromboembolic disease in pregnancy and the puerperium: acute management: green-top guideline no. 37b,* April 2015.

The Royal College of Obstetricians and Gynaecologists. *Care of women with obesity in pregnancy: green-top guideline no. 72,* November 2018.

16.23 September 2022 Incidental surgery in pregnancy

This is the third time incidental surgery in pregnancy featured during the time period covered by this book. However, the pass rate was 50.1%, and the Chairs said, "A theme we have seen in previous exams is that obstetrics seems to be poorly understood. The pass rate for this question was surprisingly low. This is a common clinical scenario encountered by many trainees, and a topic that they should be expected to know. Questions (c) and (d) were focused on fetal wellbeing and these sections were particularly poorly answered."

16.24 February 2023 Obstetric haemorrhage

a) List four obstetric causes of antepartum haemorrhage. (4 marks)
b) List three specific actions taken in the initial management of uterine atony after vaginal delivery. (3 marks)
c) List four drugs, with doses, that can be used in the ongoing management of uterine atony causing postpartum haemorrhage. (4 marks)
d) List five non-pharmacological approaches to management of postpartum haemorrhage due to uterine atony. (5 marks)
e) List the three most common direct causes of maternal death (occurring within 42 days of the end of pregnancy) in the latest Mothers and Babies: Reducing Risk through Audits and Confidential Enquiries across the UK (MBRRACE-UK) report for the time period 2018–2020, published 2022. (3 marks)
f) State the most common indirect cause of maternal death in the latest MBRRACE-UK report for the time period 2018–2020, published 2022. (1 mark)

Postpartum haemorrhage appeared for the first time as the main focus of a question in this year's exam, drawing on core clinical knowledge of a common obstetric complication that you should be familiar with. Indeed, the Chairs' Report stated that "most trainees will have encountered this in their day to day job" and stated a pass rate of 71.9%. The MBRRACE-UK reports are a ready source of information on which to base CRQs and have been involved in questions previously.

a) List four obstetric causes of antepartum haemorrhage. (4 marks)

- Placenta praevia.
- Placental abruption.
- Uterine rupture.
- Genital tract bleeding e.g. from the vulva, vagina or cervix.

b) List three specific actions taken in the initial management of uterine atony after vaginal delivery. (3 marks)

It is important to antenatally assess women for increased risk of uterine atony: previous postpartum haemorrhage; any cause of uterine overdistension (fetal macrosomia, multiple pregnancy, polyhydramnios); prolonged second or third stage of labour; induced, augmented or precipitous labour; abnormal placental implantation; and advanced maternal age. General anaesthesia is also associated with an increased risk of atony but is unlikely to be relevant in the case of vaginal delivery. "Active management of the third stage of labour" is the recommended approach to reducing the risk of postpartum haemorrhage due to uterine atony and involves:

- *Routine use of uterotonic on delivery of the anterior shoulder; oxytocin 10 IU intramuscularly or ergometrine 0.5 mg with oxytocin 5 IU combination (Syntometrine) intramuscularly for women at higher risk of postpartum haemorrhage (as long as there are no contraindications such as hypertensive disorders of pregnancy, essential hypertension or cardiac disease).*
- *Clamping of the cord between one and five minutes after delivery.*
- *Controlled cord traction after placental separation.*

In the past, active management involved cord clamping immediately after delivery, but this results in lower birth weight due to loss of neonatal blood volume. Current guidance is that clamping should take place between one and five minutes after delivery (unless there are indications for clamping sooner such as need for neonatal resuscitation or poor cord condition). You are likely to take other actions in the event of postpartum haemorrhage due to uterine atony, but the following actions address the atony itself.

- Fundal massage to encourage contractions.
- Catheterisation to ensure the bladder is empty.
- Oxytocin 5 IU by slow intravenous injection (even if oxytocin has previously been given).

c) **List four drugs, with doses, that can be used in the ongoing management of uterine atony causing postpartum haemorrhage. (4 marks)**

You would also use tranexamic acid, but this will not address uterine atony. Carbetocin (a long-acting oxytocic) is only licenced for use at caesarean section as prophylaxis in cases of high risk of uterine atony. I have included the mechanism of action of these drugs for completion.

Drug	Mechanism of action	Dose
Oxytocin	*Oxytocin receptor agonist.*	Repeat of 5 IU slow intravenous bolus or 40 IU infusion at a rate of 10 IU/h.
Ergometrine	*Ergot alkaloid which has multiple receptor actions including α-agonism. Contraindicated in hypertensive and cardiac disorders.*	0.5 mg intramuscular injection (or can be given slowly, after dilution, intravenously).
Carboprost	*Prostaglandin $F_{2\alpha}$ analogue. Caution with asthma.*	0.25 mg intramuscular injection repeated every 15 minutes to a maximum dose of 2 mg.
Misoprostol	*Prostaglandin E_1 analogue.*	0.8 mg sublingually, orally, vaginally or rectally.

d) **List five non-pharmacological approaches to management of postpartum haemorrhage due to uterine atony. (5 marks)**

- Bimanual uterine compression to stimulate uterine muscle contraction.
- Intrauterine balloon catheter (e.g. Bakri, Rusch, Foley) to achieve uterine tamponade.
- Haemostatic compression sutures e.g. B-Lynch.
- Ligation of blood supply to uterus (uterine or utero-ovarian arteries, or temporary cross clamp of the aorta or internal iliacs).
- Interventional radiology-guided arterial balloon occlusion or embolisation of e.g. uterine arteries, or temporary balloon occlusion of the internal iliacs (*also used prophylactically in elective cases at high risk of life-threatening postpartum haemorrhage*), or use of resuscitative endovascular balloon occlusion of the aorta (REBOA).
- Hysterectomy (*as a life-saving measure*).

e) **List the three most common direct causes of maternal death (occurring within 42 days of the end of pregnancy) in the latest Mothers and Babies: Reducing Risk through Audits and Confidential Enquiries across the UK (MBRRACE-UK) report for the time period 2018–2020, published 2022. (3 marks)**

The overall leading cause of death was psychiatric, but MBRRACE splits this between direct psychiatric causes (suicide) and indirect (related to drug and alcohol use). Nonetheless, death by suicide was the second leading direct cause of maternal death, with haemorrhage fourth.

- Thrombosis and venous thromboembolism.
- Suicide.
- Sepsis.

f) **State the most common indirect cause of maternal death in the latest MBRRACE-UK report for the time period 2018–2020, published 2022. (1 mark)**

- Cardiac disease.

REFERENCES

Drew T, Carvalho J. Major obstetric haemorrhage. *BJA Educ.* 2022: 22: 238–244.

Knight M et al. (eds.). *On behalf of MBRRACE-UK: saving lives, improving mothers' care core report – lessons learned to inform maternity care from the UK and Ireland Confidential Enquires into Maternal Deaths and Morbidity 2018–2020.* Oxford: National Perinatal Epidemiology Unit, University of Oxford, 2022.

Mavrides E, Allard S, Chandraharan E, Collins P, Green L, Hunt B, Riris S, Thomson A. On behalf of the Royal College of Obstetricians and Gynaecologists: green-top guideline no. 52: prevention and management of postpartum haemorrhage. *BJOG.* 2016: 124: 106–149.

PAEDIATRICS

17.1 September 2011 Down's syndrome

A 9-year-old child with Down's syndrome is scheduled for an adenotonsillectomy.

a) State the characteristic chromosomal abnormality that leads to Down's syndrome. (1 mark)
b) List four airway issues associated with Down's syndrome (4 marks), giving an implication for perioperative anaesthetic management for each. (4 marks)
c) List two other genetic syndromes that may predispose to a difficult airway in a child. (2 marks)
d) List two congenital cardiac conditions associated with Down's syndrome. (2 marks)
e) List three possible contributing causes for the development of pulmonary hypertension in a patient with Down's syndrome. (3 marks)
f) Give two characteristic ECG changes associated with pulmonary hypertension. (2 marks)
g) List two congenital neurological issues of relevance to anaesthesia that are associated with Down's syndrome. (2 marks)

There was no Chair's Report after the exam in September 2011. It is useful to think about the issues impacting on a patient with Down's syndrome by going through the alphabet. Aside from the problems discussed in this question, people with Down's have an increased risk of hypothyroidism, structural abnormalities of the gastrointestinal tract such as Hirschsprung's or duodenal atresia, and acute leukaemias. Their craniofacial changes impact on middle ear drainage increasing the likelihood of need for myringotomy, and impaired hearing. They are also predisposed to cataracts. These last two issues combined with the issues surrounding intellectual delay may make perioperative communication more challenging, and additionally they are at increased risk of early onset dementia.

a) State the characteristic chromosomal abnormality that leads to Down's syndrome. (1 mark)

- Trisomy 21.

b) List four airway issues associated with Down's syndrome (4 marks), giving an implication for perioperative anaesthetic management for each. (4 marks)

Depending on the age of the patient and their degree of understanding and compliance, preoperative airway assessment to assess for these issues may be challenging too. These possible airway issues, the individual patient's degree of understanding and compliance, and the tendency to increased adiposity which may make cannulation more challenging would all need to be considered when making a plan for induction.

Airway issue	Implication on perioperative anaesthetic management
Subglottic or tracheal stenosis.	• Consider need for smaller tube size (0.5–1 mm smaller than that calculated for age). • Consider risk and be alert for stridor after extubation.

(Continued)

DOI: 10.1201/9781003388494-17

(Continued)

Airway issue	Implication on perioperative anaesthetic management
Atlantoaxial instability. *(This is also very relevant to the ENT surgeons as typically the neck is extended during adenotonsillectomy).*	• Preoperative assessment for symptoms of cervical spine complications (gait abnormality, spasticity, bowel or bladder dysfunction) or head tilt or torticollis. • Maintenance of neutral cervical spine positioning for intubation – use of video laryngoscope or asleep fibreoptic intubation to help facilitate this. • Consider use of soft collar to support cervical spine positioning for prolonged procedures. • Consider preoperative assessment with flexion-extension C-spine X-rays (not accurate if < 3 years old due to lack of bone mineralisation), or MRI in symptomatic patient if extreme neck flexion required for surgery. • Postoperative clinical monitoring for signs of spinal cord compromise.
Cervical spine ankylosis (Klippel-Feil).	• Limited neck extension. Consider need for asleep videolaryngoscopy or oral fibreoptic intubation.
Craniofacial changes including macroglossia, midfacial hypoplasia, oropharyngeal hypotonia, micrognathia, small mouth, short neck, adenotonsillar hypertrophy.	• Obstructive sleep apnoea may make gas induction challenging due to loss of airway patency. • Obstructive sleep apnoea may alter drug choices e.g. avoidance of long-acting anaesthetic agents and use of multimodal analgesia with avoidance of long-acting opioids. • Severe obstructive sleep apnoea may preclude day case surgery and necessitate overnight observation with oxygen saturation monitoring.
Midfacial and mandibular hypoplasia.	• Difficult face mask ventilation may necessitate use of oropharyngeal airway.
Increased risk of GORD.	• Risk of reflux and aspiration.

c) List two other genetic syndromes that may predispose to a difficult airway in a child. (2 marks)

You only need to list the names for this question, but I have included some of the common features.

- Beckwith-Wiedemann; *macroglossia, small mid-face, OSA.*
- Pierre Robin; *micrognathia, glossoptosis, U or V shaped cleft palate. Airway management tends to become easier with age.*
- Treacher Collins; *small mid-face, high arched cleft palate, temporomandibular joint dysfunction. Airway management tends to become more difficult with age.*
- Goldenhar; *hemifacial microsomia and craniovertebral abnormalities.*
- Apert; *small mid-face, high arched palate, tracheal stenosis.*
- Mucopolysaccharidoses; *enlarged facial features, macroglossia, adenotonsillar hypertrophy.*

d) List two congenital cardiac conditions associated with Down's syndrome. (2 marks)

If a child has had corrective surgery they are at risk of conduction disturbances, and adults with Down's syndrome are predisposed to development of regurgitant valve abnormalities.

- Atrioventricular, atrial and ventricular septal defects.
- Patent ductus arteriosus.
- Tetralogy of Fallot.

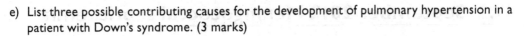

e) List three possible contributing causes for the development of pulmonary hypertension in a patient with Down's syndrome. (3 marks)

Children with Down's syndrome have reduced immunological function, an increased risk of gastro-oesophageal reflux disease, and increased tendency to hypotonia, all of which contribute to the risk of recurrent lower respiratory tract infections. The tendency to gastro-oesophageal reflux may dictate the use of rapid sequence induction and may require PPI premedication.

- Uncorrected left-to-right shunt associated with congenital cardiac defect.
- Chronic hypoxaemia due to obstructive sleep apnoea and hypoventilation due to generalised hypotonia.
- Chronic hypoxaemia due to recurrent respiratory infections.

f) Give two characteristic ECG changes associated with pulmonary hypertension. (2 marks)

- Right axis deviation.
- Right bundle branch block.
- Dominant R wave V1 (and S in V6).
- ST depression or T wave inversion in right precordial and inferior leads.
- P-pulmonale in lead II.

g) List two congenital neurological issues of relevance to anaesthesia that are associated with Down's syndrome. (2 marks)

- Epilepsy.
- Variable global developmental or intellectual delay.

REFERENCES

Allt J, Howell C. Down's syndrome. *BJA CEPD Rev.* 2003: 3: 83–86.
Raj D, Igor L. Managing the difficult airway in the syndromic child. *BJA Educ.* 2015: 15: 7–13.

17.2 September 2012 Meningococcal septicaemia

A 4-year-old child is admitted to the emergency department with suspected meningococcal septicaemia. You are asked to help resuscitate the patient prior to transfer to a tertiary centre.
a) List the clinical features of meningococcal septicaemia. (7 marks)
b) Outline the initial management of this patient. (9 marks)
c) Which investigations will guide care? (4 marks)

This is the original SAQ from September 2012. The Chair's report stated that "Although the question was answered satisfactorily, marks were lost by not calling for help and inappropriate fluid resuscitation. Many candidates failed to communicate with the tertiary centre for advice or to summon the paediatric retrieval team. This question was a very good discriminator." The pass rate was 67.6%.

Meningococcal disease may present as meningitis, septicaemia or (most commonly) as a combination of the two. NICE guidance on management of bacterial meningitis and meningococcal septicaemia was published in 2010, featured in this question in 2012, and was then updated in 2015 just in time for a slightly different version of this question to appear in the Final SAQ paper later that year. The symptoms and signs of meningococcal septicaemia, taken straight from the updated NICE guidance, are reproduced here in answer to part (a). The rest of this topic will be dealt with in the 2015 question.

a) List the clinical features of meningococcal septicaemia. (7 marks)

Nonspecific symptoms and signs:

- Fever, nausea and vomiting, lethargy, irritable/unsettled, ill-looking, anorexia, headache, muscle ache/joint pain, respiratory symptoms and difficulty breathing, chills, shivering, rapid deterioration in illness.

More specific symptoms and signs:

- Non-blanching rash, altered mental state, capillary refill time greater than two seconds, unusual skin colour, shock, hypotension, leg pain, cold hands/feet, unconsciousness, toxic/moribund state.

The guideline specifically lists the features of shock:

- Capillary refill time greater than two seconds.
- Unusual skin colour.
- Tachycardia and/or hypotension.
- Cold hands or feet.
- Toxic or moribund state.
- Altered mental state or decreased conscious level.
- Poor urine output.

REFERENCE

National Institute for Health and Care Excellence. *Meningitis (bacterial) and meningococcal septicaemia in under 16s: recognition, diagnosis and management: CG102*, June 2010, updated February 2015.

17.3 March 2013 Cerebral palsy

An 8-year-old child with severe cerebral palsy is scheduled for an elective femoral osteotomy.
a) Define cerebral palsy. (3 marks)
b) List the clinical effects of cerebral palsy on the central nervous, gastrointestinal, respiratory and musculoskeletal systems with their associated anaesthetic implications. (10 marks)
c) What are the specific issues in managing postoperative pain in this patient? (7 marks)

This is the actual SAQ from March 2015. The Chair's Report said that the pass rate was 36.4% and that the "question was poorly answered. Adult and paediatric patients with cerebral palsy presenting for surgery are not uncommon. Many examinees had little or no knowledge of the definition of cerebral palsy and could not put forward a coherent answer regarding the anaesthetic management. Awake-fibreoptic intubation was an inappropriate method of establishing the airway in this patient and the mention of sexual dysfunction was irrelevant. A snapshot from the model answer below highlights the level of knowledge that was required.

Clinical Effects: *Anaesthetic Relevance:*

Flexion deformities/spasticity   *Positioning problems; pressure sores; difficult IV access*
Scoliosis   *Restrictive respiratory pattern*
Immobility   *Unable to assess cardiopulmonary reserve*
Low muscle bulk   *Temperature control difficulties"*

Cerebral palsy was the focus of another SAQ in March 2018 and of a CRQ in September 2021, which is where you will find the answers.

17.4 September 2013 Paediatric airway

a) List five anatomical features of young children (< 3 years old) which may adversely affect upper airway management. (5 marks)
b) Give five airway problems which may occur due to these anatomical features. (5 marks)
c) Give five measures used in clinical practice to overcome these problems. (5 marks)
d) List three patient factors that increase the risk of perioperative laryngospasm in children. (3 marks)
e) List two anaesthetic factors that increase the risk of laryngospasm in paediatric patients. (2 marks)

The Chair's Report following the original SAQ acknowledged that the question was a repeat from the May 2007 paper, and stated that "each anatomical feature was linked to an airway problem and how they might be overcome in clinical practice." The pass rate was 65.4%. I have added the subsections about risk of laryngospasm.

a) List five anatomical features of young children (< 3 years old) which may adversely affect upper airway management. (5 marks)
b) Give five airway problems which may occur due to these anatomical features. (5 marks)
c) Give five measures used in clinical practice to overcome these problems. (5 marks)

I have put all of the information into one table for ease of learning. Be careful to read the question properly; it asks about airway problems that <u>affect upper airway management</u>, not a comparison of the whole respiratory system.

Anatomical feature	Problem	Overcome by
Large head with prominent occiput.	Tendency to flex neck.	Neutral position with e.g. folded towel under shoulders.
Large tongue, pliant submental tissues.	Obstruction of airway by digital pressure.	Ensure fingers applied to bony surfaces.
Absence of teeth.	Difficulty maintaining face mask ventilation.	Use of appropriately sized Guedel.
Long U-shaped epiglottis in infants, anterior funnel shaped larynx.	Difficulty with laryngoscopy, epiglottis flopping into visual field.	Straight blade may be preferred in infants, videolaryngoscopy may be required. External laryngeal pressure may be required to bring cords into view.
Narrow trachea.	Flow proportional to radius to the power of four. Small difference in radius due to trauma or oedema makes substantial difference to flow.	Careful handling of airway, select tube size carefully, minimise need for changes.
Airway functionally narrowest at level of cricoid, not vocal cords.	Cricoid is a complete ring of noncompliant cartilage so pressure of tube may cause damage.	With uncuffed tubes, a leak should be ascertained. High volume, low pressure cuffed tubes (half to one size smaller than uncuffed) are now commonly used.
Short trachea.	Risk of endobronchial intubation. Risk of accidental extubation.	Auscultate chest, vigilance. Minimisation of head movement.

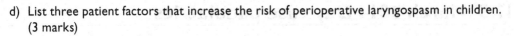

d) List three patient factors that increase the risk of perioperative laryngospasm in children. (3 marks)

- Younger age.
- Recent upper respiratory tract infection.
- Asthma.
- Structural airway abnormality.
- Gastro-oesophageal reflux disease.
- Obesity with obstructive sleep apnoea.
- Passive exposure to cigarette smoking (or active cigarette smoking).

e) List two anaesthetic factors that increase the risk of laryngospasm in paediatric patients. (2 marks)

- Inadequate depth of anaesthesia especially with acute surgical stimulation.
- Airway instrumentation.
- Inhalational anaesthetic agents especially desflurane.
- Anaesthetist with limited experience in paediatric anaesthesia.
- Intubation without use of NMBD.
- Thiopentone use.

REFERENCES

Gavel G, Walker R. Laryngospasm in anaesthesia. *Contin Educ Anaes Crit Care Pain*. 2014: 14: 47–51.
Holm-Knudsen R, Rasmussen L. Paediatric airway management: basic aspects. *Acta Anaesthesiol Scand*. 2009: 53: 1–9.

17.5 March 2014 Day case paediatrics

A 5-year-old patient presents for a myringotomy and grommet insertion as a day case. During your preoperative assessment you notice that the patient has nasal discharge.
a) Give four reasons why it would be inappropriate to cancel the operation on the basis of this information alone. (4 marks)
b) List five features in the child's history that might cause you to postpone the operation due to an increased risk of airway complications in this patient. (5 marks)
c) List four features on examination that might cause you to postpone the operation due to an increased risk of airway complications in this patient. (4 marks)
d) List four social factors that may preclude this child's treatment as a day case. (4 marks)
e) State three organisational recommendations from the Royal College of Anaesthetists regarding provision of day case surgery for children. (3 marks)

The Chair's Report of the original SAQ stated that this "question was answered poorly considering the issue is 'meat and drink' to paediatric day case practice. The majority of candidates did not mention emotional aspects, financial losses, parental work absence, school absence and inefficient use of hospital resources in the answer. The history section was poorly answered although examination features were more typically known. Surprisingly, social factors were infrequently given, although these have a major impact on suitability as a day case. Overall, there seem to be few candidates thinking about the organisational and logistical aspects of bringing a child in for day case surgery." The pass rate was 44.7%. Issues with day case paediatric surgery is a recurring topic in the Final as you will see over the course of this chapter.

a) **Give four reasons why it would be inappropriate to cancel the operation on the basis of this information alone. (4 marks)**

There is not enough information so far to determine whether the operation should be cancelled, a runny nose alone being insufficient reason. It is very common in young children and more so in children awaiting this type of surgery.

- Runny nose may be associated with the very reason the child is having surgery.
- Inefficient list usage.
- Wasted time off school for child.
- Delayed surgery resulting in ongoing hearing issues in child. May impact on education.
- Wasted parental time off work with possible financial loss.
- Loss of trust between parents, child and hospital, especially if surgery later takes place with runny nose still.

b) **List five features in the child's history that might cause you to postpone the operation due to an increased risk of airway complications in this patient. (5 marks)**

- Fever.
- Unwell in self, too unwell for school, parent states that child is unwell.
- Loss of appetite.
- Shortness of breath.
- Sore throat.
- Cough.
- Sputum production.
- Purulent nasal discharge.
- Significant cardiorespiratory comorbidities such as obstructive sleep apnoea, severe asthma, cardiac condition.

c) List four features on examination that might cause you to postpone the operation due to an increased risk of airway complications in this patient. (4 marks)

- Listless, unwell.
- Fever.
- Tachypnoea or other signs of respiratory distress.
- Purulent nasal discharge.
- Crackles on auscultation.
- Tachycardia.
- Delayed capillary refill.

d) List four social factors that may preclude this child's treatment as a day case. (4 marks)

- Poor housing conditions.
- Distance more than one hour from a hospital that could provide appropriate management of complications.
- Parents unable or unwilling to care for child postoperatively.
- No telephone.
- No access to private transport.

e) State three organisational recommendations from the Royal College of Anaesthetists regarding provision of day case surgery for children. (3 marks)

This subsection was not part of the original SAQ but is useful knowledge when discussing day case surgery in a viva scenario. The recommendations are taken from the GPAS guidelines for provision of paediatric day case anaesthesia.

- List organisation to prioritise each child according to need.
- Aim to book cases with longer recovery time earlier in the day to minimise unnecessary overnight stays.
- Minimisation of starvation time.
- Separation from adult patients by using facilities at a different time or use of a dedicated unit.
- Lower age limit for day case surgery depends on facilities, staff competencies, and medical comorbidities of the child, but significantly ex-premature babies should generally be excluded until they have reached a corrected age of 60 weeks.
- Provision of preoperative information to parents, carers, and children, including safety netting advice for postoperative complications.
- Specific guidance regarding fasting, analgesia and PONV should be discussed with parents and children.
- Clearly documented discharge criteria.

REFERENCES

Bailey C et al. Guidelines from the Association of Anaesthetists and the British Association of Day Surgery: guidelines for day-case surgery 2019. *Anaesthesia.* 2019: 74: 778–792.

Bhatia N, Barber N. Dilemmas in the preoperative assessment of children. *Contin Educ Anaesth Crit Care Pain.* 2011: 11: 214–218.

Guidelines for the Provision of Anaesthesia Services (GPAS). *Chapter 10: guidelines for the provision of paediatric anaesthesia services.* Royal College of Anaesthetists, 2023, 13–14. https://rcoa. ac.uk/sites/default/files/documents/2023-02/Chapter%2010%20Guidelines%20for%20the%20 Provision%20of%20Paediatric%20Anaesthesia%20Services%202023.pdf. Accessed 3rd February 2023.

17.6 September 2014 Atrial septal defect

A 5-year-old child presenting for day case dental surgery under general anaesthesia is found to have a heart murmur that has not been documented previously.

a) What features of the history (5 marks) and examination (5 marks) might suggest that the child has a significant congenital heart disease (CHD)?

b) If the murmur is caused by an atrial septal defect (ASD), what two ECG findings would you expect? (2 marks)

c) State two imaging modalities that may be used in the assessment of the ASD (2 marks) and what specific additional information may be obtained by these investigations? (2 marks)

d) List the current national guidelines regarding prophylaxis against infective endocarditis in children with CHD undergoing dental procedures. (4 marks)

The Chair's Report of the original SAQ, reproduced here as it appeared in the exam, said that the "question was poorly answered by many candidates who could not list the history and examination findings in such a patient. Many felt that congenital heart disease only caused left sided cardiac abnormalities and were ignorant of national guidelines on infective endocarditis prophylaxis, although the need for the latter must be encountered on a regular basis in adult subjects." The pass rate was just 39.1%.

The topic was addressed again as a CRQ in September 2020 highlighting that the College considers ASD an important specific example of congenital heart disease that may be undiagnosed at birth and therefore be first encountered in a nonspecialist centre when a child presents for incidental surgery.

17.7 March 2015 Autistic spectrum disorder

A 5-year-old boy with autistic spectrum disorder is listed for dental extractions as a day case.
a) Define autistic spectrum disorder. (1 mark).
b) List the key clinical features of autistic spectrum disorder. (5 marks)
c) List two organisational considerations when providing anaesthesia for dental extractions in children. (2 marks)
d) List four perioperative considerations when providing anaesthesia for dental extractions in children. (4 marks)
e) Describe four specific problems of providing anaesthesia for children with autistic spectrum disorder (4 marks) and outline a possible solution for each. (4 marks)

The Chair's Report of the original SAQ "anticipated that candidates would find this subject matter to be difficult and this was borne out by the pass [46.2%] and poor fail [22.1%] rates. Autistic spectrum disorder (ASD) is an important issue within paediatric anaesthetic practice, and this result suggests specific teaching on the topic needs to be undertaken in all Schools of Anaesthesia. Failure to read section [(d)] correctly led to low scores as candidates did not realise that the question referred to all children not just individuals with autistic spectrum disorder."

In the previous question, ASD meant atrial septal defect. In this question it meant autistic spectrum disorder; the question gave the name "autistic spectrum disorder" in full followed by "ASD" in brackets in the introductory statement. The College always gives the full wording of a phrase before it abbreviates it and so even in your haze of exam-induced stress you must read the questions carefully. I know one very able candidate who answered this question for a child with atrial septal defect.

a) Define autistic spectrum disorder. (1 mark)

This is in line with a recent NICE definition although I think that people on the autistic spectrum may take issue with the notion that their activities of daily living are necessarily significantly limited or impaired.

- Autistic spectrum disorder is a lifelong condition affecting brain development, present from early childhood, which significantly limits or impairs activities of daily living.

b) List the key clinical features of autistic spectrum disorder. (5 marks)

You will all have interacted with children and adults on the autistic spectrum – describe the issues of the more extreme aspects of the divergence.

- Communication problems; language delay, avoidance of conversation, failure to understand nuance, literal interpretation. Some children may be selectively mute.
- Social interaction and relationship problems; lack of eye contact, reduced use of facial expression, reduced interaction, low understanding of the usual rules of social interaction, intolerance of people entering their personal space, reduced use of gestures.
- Abstract thought difficulties; reduced ability to generalise information, reduced ability to appreciate that different people have different thoughts, knowledge, and beliefs. Reduced ability to understand metaphorical explanations.
- Adherence to routines and stereotyped behaviours; routine (and distress if routines broken), repetitive behaviours, tendency to rigid food preferences, highly specific interest for particular subjects or activities.

- Sensory issues; over and under-reactivity to some textures, noise, light.
- Association with learning difficulties in 50%.
- Associated mental health disorders; increased risk of anxiety, depression, attention deficit hyperactivity disorder.

c) **List two organisational considerations when providing anaesthesia for dental extractions in children. (2 marks)**

- Proper hospital setting required offering the same standard of care as for other cases requiring general anaesthesia.
- Availability of paediatric anaesthetic equipment.
- Staff trained in care of paediatric patients, including resuscitation.
- Facility for preoperative assessment in advance in selected cases.

d) **List four perioperative considerations when providing anaesthesia for dental extractions in children. (4 marks)**

Read the question – this is about paediatric dental surgery in general, not just for children on the autistic spectrum.

- Shared (small) airway distant to anaesthetist and anaesthetic machine.
- Blood from extractions may result in blood inhalation or laryngospasm.
- Throat pack may be used – need to have clear protocol to ensure its removal.
- Risk of dislodgement or occlusion of airway with surgery or mouth gag.
- Need for intraoperative antiemetic medication to facilitate day case – use of e.g. ondansetron as well as dexamethasone for its effects on nausea as well as effects on swelling of the operative site.
- Analgesic requirements are low, and paracetamol and NSAID preoperatively may be sufficient. Short-acting intraoperative opioid only required (longer acting opioid may contribute to postoperative nausea and vomiting and affect ability to undertake case as day case).
- Head-up positioning risks reduced cardiac output and cerebral perfusion pressure (*although often these cases are now performed on an operating table or day case trolley rather than in a dentist chair, hence putting this at the bottom of my list).*

e) **Describe four specific problems of providing anaesthesia for children with autistic spectrum disorder (4 marks) and outline a possible solution for each. (4 marks)**

Problem	Possible solution
Distress due to unfamiliar hospital setting may make it difficult to perform preoperative assessment on day of admission.	May be necessary to do this in the community, including weight measurement. Quiet, separate waiting area.
Language issues may make it difficult for the child to comprehend what is to happen.	Use of appropriate visual information, play specialist or psychologist to enhance comprehension. Information provision in advance.
Lack of familiarity with environment, out of routine, may cause distress.	Maximise the familiarity of the environment, minimise the disruption to routine by allowing e.g. own clothes, familiar objects, involvement of parent/carer, minimisation of waiting time. Give, and adhere to, a clear timetable of day.
Preoperative starvation may be poorly tolerated as it breaks routine.	First on list, clear fluids until an hour before surgery.
May dislike physical contact.	Keep to a minimum, warn first.

Problem	Possible solution
Topical local anaesthetic may not be tolerated.	Consider inhalational induction, consider staffing requirements for this.
Lack of cooperation.	Discussion regarding strategies for uncooperative child, including physical restraint, in advance. Consideration of cancelling and bringing back after premedication. Parental presence at induction.
Dysphoric response to midazolam is possible in autistic spectrum disorder.	Consider whether premedication is necessary. Consider combining midazolam with ketamine, or using oral clonidine, or intranasal dexmedetomidine.
Inability of child to communicate likes and dislikes.	Utilise parents' knowledge of child to anticipate problems; use communication passport if the child has one.

REFERENCES

Adewale L. Anaesthesia for paediatric dentistry. *Contin Educ Anaesth Crit Care Pain*. 2012: 12: 288–294.

National Institute for Health and Care Excellence. *Clinical knowledge summaries: autism in children*, Last revised August 2020.

Short J, Calder A. Anaesthesia for children with special needs, including autistic spectrum disorder. *Contin Educ Anaesth Crit Care Pain*. 2013: 13: 107–112.

17.8 September 2015 Meningococcal septicaemia

You are called to the emergency department to see a 2-year-old child who presents with a four-hour history of high temperature and drowsiness. On examination, there is prolonged capillary refill time and a non-blanching rash. A presumptive diagnosis of meningococcal septicaemia is made.

a) What are the normal weight, pulse rate, mean arterial blood pressure and capillary refill time for a child of this age? (4 marks)

b) Define appropriate resuscitation goals for this child (2 marks) and outline the management in the first 15 minutes after presentation. (7 marks)

c) After 15 minutes, the child remains shocked and is unresponsive to fluid. What is the most likely pathophysiological derangement in this child's circulation (2 marks), and what are the important further treatment options? (5 marks)

This is the second appearance of management of meningococcal septicaemia in a child in the Final exam in the time frame of this book. Again, the SAQ has been reproduced here exactly as it appeared in the exam. The Chairs' Report commented that "the pass rate for this question [56.9%] was the second highest in the paper, but the examiners still felt that it was not particularly well answered. Many candidates lost marks because they wrote similar answers for parts (b) and (c), despite the fact that in part (c), they were asked to comment on what they would do if the measures used in (b) were not successful in resuscitating the child. Incorrect dosages of drugs, particularly antibiotics, were often quoted."

Most of the subsections are repeated in the two further questions about meningococcal septicaemia that feature later in this chapter. However, I have included answers here to subsections that aren't repeated.

b) Define appropriate resuscitation goals for this child. (2 marks)

The most important aspects of initial management of a child with suspected meningococcal septicaemia and signs of shock is all about giving antibiotics early and fluid resuscitation. Targets for fluid resuscitation in a child with sepsis are addressed in the Surviving Sepsis Campaign guidelines and include the following:

- Capillary refill time less than 2 seconds.
- Normalisation of blood pressure.
- Normalisation of heart rate.
- Urine output greater than 1 ml/kg/h.
- Normal mental status or level of consciousness.
- Normalisation of lactate.

They point out that features of fluid overload in children include pulmonary oedema and new or enlarging hepatomegaly.

c) After 15 minutes, the child remains shocked and is unresponsive to fluid. What is the most likely pathophysiological derangement in this child's circulation? (2 marks)

- Septic shock: in addition to the organ dysfunction occurring as a result of the child's physiological response to infection, shock has developed due to circulatory, cellular, and metabolic dysfunction.
- Consequences include vasodilation, activation of inflammatory and coagulation cascades, capillary leak, and dysfunctional oxygen utilisation at a cellular level.

REFERENCES

Haque I, Zaritsky A. Analysis of the evidence for the lower limit of systolic and mean arterial pressure in children. *Pediat Crit Care Med.* 2007: 8: 138–144.

Luscombe M, Owens B. Weight estimation in resuscitation: is the current formula still valid? *Arch Dis Child.* 2007: 92: 412–415.

Resuscitation Council UK. *2021 resuscitation guidelines: paediatric advanced life support guidelines.* www.resus.org.uk/library/2021-resuscitation-guidelines/paediatric-advanced-life-support-guidelines#key-points. Accessed 31st March 2023.

Weiss SL et al. Surviving sepsis campaign international guidelines for the management of septic shock and sepsis-associated organ dysfunction in children. *Pediat Crit Care Med.* 2020: 21: e52–e106.

17.9 March 2016 Nonaccidental injury

You have anaesthetised a 5-year-old boy for manipulation of a forearm fracture. During the operation, you notice that he has multiple bruises on his upper arms and body that you think may indicate nonaccidental injury (NAI).

a) List six other types of physical injury that may prompt concerns of NAI in a child of this age. (6 marks)

b) Give six immediate actions that must be taken as a result of your concerns. (6 marks)

c) State five parental factors that are known to increase the risk of child abuse. (5 marks)

d) State three features of a child's past medical history that increase the risk of suffering from abuse. (3 marks)

The Chairs' Report following the original SAQ stated, "This is an important topic which is relevant to the practice of paediatric anaesthesia and forms part of mandatory training for all doctors. The question was not particularly well answered [pass rate 44.7%], with many candidates appearing not to have knowledge of the presenting signs and symptoms of child abuse. Candidates assumed that the parents were harming their child so missed important steps such as informing the senior paediatrician before contacting social services. The general lack of knowledge on this subject was reflected in the poor pass rate."

In March 2007, an intercollegiate document involving the RCoA was issued that detailed the manner in which anaesthetists may encounter child abuse and what actions should be taken in the event. Child abuse was then the focus of a question in the Final written paper in October 2008. The document was updated in July 2014, 20 months before it appeared as an SAQ in 2016. It really is important to keep an eye on the College website and be aware of topical publications and guidelines.

a) **List six other types of physical injury that may prompt concerns of NAI in a child of this age. (6 marks)**

This question is specifically about injury patterns; aspects regarding the history such as inconsistencies, multiple attendances, delayed presentation, and detached parental-child relationship on observation, even though they are all valid aspects of suspecting NAI, would not get marks.

- Unusual (strangulation bruises, ligature marks, clusters of bruises, bruises in the shape of a hand) or excessive bruising, bruises of different ages, at different stages of healing.
- Fractures of different ages.
- Cigarette burns or other thermal injury.
- Bite marks.
- Injuries in inaccessible places; neck, ear, feet, buttocks.
- Ano-genital trauma or unusual ano-genital appearance.
- Intra-abdominal, oral, or eye injuries or other trauma without adequate explanation.
- Nonfatal submersion injury without adequate explanation.

b) **Give six immediate actions that must be taken as a result of your concerns. (6 marks)**

The general principles are to act in the best interests of the child and to respect the child's right to confidentiality, if feasible.

- Check hospital notes for known safeguarding issues, details regarding other members of family.
- Inform duty/supervising anaesthetic consultant.
- Inform theatre team; surgeon, senior scrub, ODP.

- Inform child's paediatrician, on-call paediatric consultant if out of hours, or Safeguarding Team within hours.
- Ask the paediatrician to make a brief visual assessment of injuries as long as this does not excessively prolong anaesthesia.
- Full documentation of findings and actions.
- Consultant paediatrician and anaesthetist to discuss the issue with parents and child after surgery (except in unusual circumstances where this may increase risk to child).
  - If there is a fully reasonable explanation, then no further action is taken.
  - If there is continued concern, then the consultant paediatrician should refer to social care, possibly involve police if there is risk to other children at home, take full history from child and carer, consider need for forensic examination, and decide whether it is appropriate for the child to go home.

c) **State five parental factors that are known to increase the risk of child abuse. (5 marks)**

- Substance misuse.
- History of domestic abuse and/or maltreatment as a child.
- Parent within a re-ordered family.
- Single parent.
- Young parent.
- Emotional volatility, anger management problem.
- History of violent offending.
- Mental health problems which have a significant effect on parenting ability.
- Known maltreatment of animals.
- Poor education.
- Lack of parenting knowledge.
- Lack of support from family or friends.
- Poverty, financial pressures, poor housing, other causes of parental stress.

d) **State three features of a child's past medical history that increase the risk of suffering from abuse. (3 marks)**

- Chronic physical illness.
- Mental disability.
- Child from a multiple birth.
- Prematurity or low birth weight or SCBU admission.

REFERENCES

National Institute for Health and Care Excellence. *Child maltreatment: when to suspect maltreatment in under 18s: clinical guideline: CG89*, 2009.

National Institute for Health and Care Excellence. *Child maltreatment – recognition and management*, January 2019.

Royal College of Anaesthetists. *Association of Anaesthetists of Great Britain and Ireland, Association of Paediatric Anaesthetists of Great Britain and Ireland, Royal College of Paediatrics and Child Health: child protection and the anaesthetist safeguarding children in the operating theatre*, July 2014.

Royal College of Anaesthetists. *E-learning for health: safeguarding children level 3.* https://portal.e-lfh.org.uk/myElearning/Index?HierarchyId=0_25&programmeId=25. Accessed 25th April 2023.

17.10 September 2016 Down's syndrome

A 5-year-old child with Down's syndrome (trisomy 21) is scheduled for adenotonsillectomy.

a) List the cardiovascular (2 marks), airway and respiratory (5 marks) and neurological (3 marks) problems that are associated with this syndrome in children and are of relevance to the anaesthetist.

b) What are the potential problems during induction of anaesthesia and initial airway management in this patient? (6 marks)

c) What are the possible specific difficulties in the postoperative management of this child? (4 marks)

This is the original SAQ that appeared in the exam in September 2016. It was very similar to that from September 2011. The Chairs' Report commented that "Knowledge of this subject appeared to be good and the question was generally well answered [pass rate 62.1%]. However, some candidates lost marks because they did not go into enough detail regarding airway difficulties. Simply stating 'difficult airway' was not sufficient as this does not describe the specific difficulties in this case. These could be divided into those related to the presence of enlarged adenoids and tonsils and those related to a child with Down's syndrome. Candidates who scored well mentioned the possibility of airway obstruction after induction of anaesthesia, the need for airway adjuncts, possible subglottic stenosis and/or atlanto-axial instability, amongst other things."

17.11 March 2017 Anaesthesia in the ex-preterm baby

A 12-week-old male baby presents for a unilateral inguinal hernia repair. He was born at 30 weeks' gestation.

a) At what gestational age at birth would a baby be classified as preterm? (1 mark)
b) At what birth weight (kg) would a baby be classified as having low birth weight? (1 mark)
c) List five airway and respiratory concerns when anaesthetising an ex-preterm baby. (5 marks)
d) List five other complications of prematurity which may need to be considered when planning anaesthesia for this baby. (5 marks)
e) List two pharmacokinetic differences that may be observed in a preterm baby. (2 marks)
f) Give two advantages and two disadvantages of general anaesthesia for inguinal hernia repair for this baby. (4 marks)
g) Give two alternatives to general anaesthesia as the sole anaesthetic approach for inguinal hernia repair in this baby. (2 marks)

The Chairs' Report following the original SAQ stated that "knowledge of the anaesthetic issues surrounding prematurity and the very young is important. . . . Candidates who scored poorly tended to give generic answers about physiological problems in any paediatric patient rather than specific perioperative problems for this particular ex-premature neonate."

The pass rate for this question was 28.0%, and it has not been re-examined since. I would recommend reading the recent BJA article, referenced below, which provides a good summary of the pertinent issues.

a) At what gestational age at birth would a baby be classified as preterm? (1 mark)

The WHO defines babies born before 28 weeks as "extremely preterm" and babies born before 32 weeks as "very preterm."

- Preterm < 37 weeks gestational age.

b) At what birth weight (kg) would a baby be classified as having low birth weight? (1 mark)

Again, WHO classification states that babies weighing less than 1 kg at birth have an "extremely low birth weight" and babies under 1.5 kg have a "very low birth weight."

- Low birth weight < 2.5 kg.

c) List five specific airway and respiratory concerns when anaesthetising an ex-preterm baby. (5 marks)

Apart from the fact that he was very preterm, you have no other information about the baby's condition or when he left the neonatal intensive care unit. He was born at a stage when organogenesis was ongoing and is therefore at risk of immature physiology. Keep your answers specific to those of a preterm baby. You would not get marks for generic issues affecting all babies. The issues below contribute to the risk of central, obstructive and mixed apnoeas, which is when breathing ceases for 20 seconds or more with associated bradycardia. The risk of apnoeas continues until 60 weeks corrected age and would necessitate postoperative monitoring, including oxygen saturations, impedance pneumography and heart rate. Factors associated with anaesthesia and surgery, including hypoxia, hypoglycaemia, hypo- or hyperthermia, anaemia, sedative drugs, the stress response to surgery, and pain, all increase the risk of apnoeas.

- Complications of previous prolonged intubation, such as laryngo- and tracheomalacia, or subglottic stenosis, increase the risk of difficult intubation or need for smaller tube diameter.

- Increased upper airway soft tissue compliance and poor muscle coordination increase the risk of airway obstruction on induction of anaesthesia. Contributes to obstructive apnoeas.
- Disrupted vasculogenesis causes abnormal distribution of pulmonary capillaries and thickened pulmonary arterioles which results in reduced lung compliance, atelectasis, and V/Q mismatching.
- Reduced type I muscle fibres in the intercostal muscles and diaphragm, low glycogen stores, and inefficient chest wall mechanics (horizontally aligned ribs; compliant chest wall, which reduces the efficiency of inhalation; and low elastic recoil, which limits the efficiency of exhalation) resulting in risk of respiratory fatigue.
- Low lung elasticity leads to collapse of small airways and gas trapping even with normal breathing, with closing capacity encroaching on FRC.
- Immature control of ventilation with attenuated chemoreceptor and central responses, and a biphasic response to hypoxia with initial hyperventilation followed by hypoventilation and apnoea. Causes central apnoeas.
- Long-term ventilation with barotrauma, volutrauma, and excessive fraction of inspired oxygen on a background of immature lung development contribute to the development of bronchopulmonary dysplasia, a situation of poor lung compliance and hyper-reactivity with increased risk of perioperative bronchospasm. *(Risks reduced by antenatal steroids, surfactant, lung protective ventilation, and lower inspired oxygen concentrations.)*

d) List five other complications of prematurity which may need to be considered when planning anaesthesia for this baby. (5 marks)

I have grouped these by body system to aid recall and learning, but each bullet point should achieve a mark.

Cardiovascular:

- Increased risk of all congenital cardiac defects and delayed closure of ductus arteriosus (hypoxia and acidosis may prompt reopening of the ductus arteriosus).
- Difficulty cannulating due to multiple previous cannulations.
- High ratio of fibrous to contractile tissue resulting in noncompliant ventricles and fixed stroke volume. Cardiac output can be raised with increased heart rate only (this is seen in term neonates but is exaggerated with prematurity).

Neurological:

- Premature babies at significant risk of intraventricular haemorrhage due to structural immaturity and inadequate autoregulation with consequences such as cerebral palsy or hydrocephalus.

Endocrine:

- Reduced glycogen stores in conjunction with preoperative starvation may result in hypoglycaemia. Excessive starvation must be avoided, and consideration given to glucose supplementation.
- Hyperglycaemia may result from defective glucose regulation, including impaired insulin secretion, exacerbated by stress response to surgery, pain and mechanical ventilation.

Gastrointestinal:

- Reflux is common due to underdevelopment of the gastro-oesophageal sphincter, reduced oesophageal motility and delayed gastric emptying, thus increasing the risk of aspiration and apnoeas.

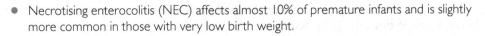

- Necrotising enterocolitis (NEC) affects almost 10% of premature infants and is slightly more common in those with very low birth weight.

Haematological:

- Risk of anaemia related to lower baseline haemoglobin and previous frequent blood sampling.
- Coagulopathy may occur due to deficiency of clotting factor production and low platelet count.

Renal:

- Immature nephron function with risk of abnormal electrolyte, acid and water handling.

Metabolic:

- All babies have high risk of hypothermia, but an ex-preterm baby is at even greater risk due to paucity of subcutaneous fat, immature thermogenesis due to reduced brown fat and increased surface-area-to-volume ratio.

e) List two pharmacokinetic differences that may be observed in a preterm baby. (2 marks)

- Absorption of oral drugs may be reduced due to reflux.
- Distribution:
  - Relative increase in total body water will increase volume of distribution of water-soluble drugs.
  - Reduced plasma protein binding increases the availability of free drug, potentially leading to toxicity or excessive effect.
- Metabolism may be slower due to immature liver enzyme systems.
- Excretion may be slower due to immaturity of kidneys.

f) Give two advantages and two disadvantages of general anaesthesia for inguinal hernia repair for this baby. (4 marks)

Advantages:

- Optimum operating conditions with still baby.
- Use of sedatives to improve operating conditions when using regional anaesthesia may increase the risk of postoperative apnoeas in an ex-preterm baby.
- Avoids failed regional technique with need for on-table conversion to general anaesthesia.

Disadvantages:

- Possible difficult airway management due to anatomy and previous intubations.
- Risk of desaturation at induction, with consequent risks of hypoxaemia.
- Risk of apnoeas increased following general anaesthesia.
- General anaesthesia does not have the inherent postoperative analgesic effects of a regional technique, therefore increasing the need for opioid analgesia, which may contribute to the risk of apnoeas.
- Positive pressure ventilation may contribute to right-to-left shunt or further barotrauma in already damaged lungs.
- Possible increased risk of neurotoxicity in ex-preterm babies (although problems unlikely after a single, brief anaesthetic if baby otherwise well).

g) Give two alternatives to general anaesthesia as the sole anaesthetic approach for inguinal hernia repair in this baby. (2 marks)

- Spinal anaesthesia.
- Caudal anaesthesia.
- Epidural anaesthesia with plain local anaesthetic infusion to avoid opioids.
- General anaesthesia with neuraxial technique to avoid postoperative opioid need.
- General anaesthesia with regional technique such as ilioinguinal or TAP block to minimise the need for postoperative opioids.

REFERENCES

Jones L et al. Regional (spinal, epidural, caudal) versus general anaesthesia in preterm infants undergoing inguinal herniorrhaphy in early infancy. *Cochrane Database Syst Rev.* 2015: 6: Article No. CD003669.

Macrae J, Ng E, Whyte H. Anaesthesia for premature infants. *BJA Educ.* 2021: 21: 355–363.

Peiris K, Fell D. The prematurely born infant and anaesthesia. *Contin Educ Anaesth Crit Care Pain.* 2009: 9: 73–77.

17.12 September 2017 Day case paediatrics

A 5-year-old boy presents for a myringotomy and grommet insertion as a day case. During your preoperative assessment, you notice that he has nasal discharge.

a) List the features in the history (5 marks) and examination (6 marks) that would potentially cause an increased risk of airway complications.

b) Why would it be inappropriate to cancel the operation? (6 marks)

c) What social factors would prevent this child being treated as a day case? (3 marks)

The Chairs' Report following the original SAQ, reproduced here exactly as it was in the exam, acknowledged that "this question had been used before and was thought to be moderately difficult. It had the highest correlation with overall performance. Candidates generally did better on this occasion than when it was last used, so it seems that knowledge of this important and frequently seen scenario has improved." The pass rate was 74%.

This SAQ was almost identical to the question from March 2014. Basing revision on past questions makes sense because it means that you will revise topics that the College considers important. The paediatric anaesthesia curriculum is not vast; it is inevitable that there will be themes that repeat.

17.13 March 2018 Cerebral palsy

An 8-year-old child is scheduled for an elective right femoral osteotomy due to impending dislocation of the hip. She has severe cerebral palsy.

a) What is cerebral palsy? (3 marks)
b) List the typical clinical features of severe cerebral palsy, with their associated anaesthetic implications. Do this for the central nervous system (3 marks), respiratory system (2 marks), musculoskeletal system (3 marks) and gastrointestinal system. (2 marks)
c) What are the expected problems in providing adequate postoperative analgesia in this patient? (2 marks)
d) Outline a management plan to optimise analgesia in this patient. (5 marks)

This SAQ from March 2018, reproduced exactly as it appeared in the exam paper, covered mostly the same content as that from March 2013. The Chairs' Report said that "the pass rate is encouraging with candidates demonstrating knowledge of the difficulties of dealing with such patients." The topic was then the focus of a CRQ in September 2021, where you will find the answers.

17.14 September 2018 Meningococcal septicaemia

You are called to the emergency department to see a 2-year-old child who presents with a 4-hour history of high temperature and drowsiness. On examination there is prolonged capillary refill time and a non-blanching rash. A presumptive diagnosis of meningococcal septicaemia is made.

a) What are the normal weight and capillary refill time for a child of this age? (2 marks). Describe how you would perform an assessment of capillary refill time. (2 marks)

b) List appropriate resuscitation goals for this child (2 marks) and outline the management in the first 15 minutes after presentation. (7 marks)

c) After 15 minutes, the child remains shocked and is unresponsive to fluid. What are the most likely pathophysiological derangements in this child's circulation? (2 marks)

d) What are the important further treatment options? (5 marks)

Another SAQ, reproduced as it appeared in the exam, on meningococcal septicaemia. It was almost identical to that from 2015, but this time it also asked for a description of how to assess capillary refill time. Pressure is exerted with finger or thumb on the child's sternum for five seconds to cause blanching and the time taken for colour to return to normal after pressure is released is noted. Peripheral perfusion can be gauged by similarly testing the child's fingertip. The Chairs' Report said, "This was well answered [pass rate was 64.2%] with candidates exhibiting good knowledge. The examiners were aware that management of this condition can vary and took this into account in the marking." It is reassuring to read that they do this.

17.15 March 2019 Strabismus surgery

You are asked to assess a 15 kg 4-year-old child who is scheduled for a strabismus (squint) correction as a day case procedure.

a) List the anaesthetic considerations of this case with regards to the age of the patient. (4 marks)

b) List the anaesthetic considerations of this case with regards to day case surgery. (3 marks)

c) Give four specific anaesthetic considerations for strabismus surgery. (4 marks)

d) During the operation, the patient suddenly develops a profound bradycardia. Give two steps in your immediate management of this situation. (2 marks)

e) Give four elements of your strategy to reduce the risk of postoperative nausea and vomiting. (4 marks)

f) Give three elements of your postoperative analgesic plan. (3 marks)

The Chairs' Report following the original SAQ stated that "knowledge of day case surgery in the paediatric population is an important topic. So it was disappointing that this question was answered so poorly [pass rate 51.6%] . . . very few candidates could give suitable options for analgesia, failing to mention local anaesthetic techniques."

a) **List the anaesthetic considerations of this case with regards to the age of the patient. (4 marks)**

- Must ensure availability of correct paediatric equipment, drug doses, staff training, recovery, and resuscitation facilities.
- Play therapist, parent, techniques for maximising cooperation at induction.
- Preoperative assessment often takes place on the day of surgery for paediatric patients – thorough assessment still necessary especially as squint is associated with some congenital disorders, some of which may impact on airway management.
- Consideration of need for premedication; anxiolysis in selected cases, topical local anaesthetic for cannulation.
- This child is small for age, which may be indicative of comorbidity, associated syndrome, or even neglect.

b) **List the anaesthetic considerations of this case with regards to day case surgery. (3 marks)**

- Adequate management of pain and postoperative nausea and vomiting to allow return to normal function and diet before discharge.
- Use of short-acting agents where choices exist.
- Absence of major comorbidities that would contraindicate day case surgery.
- Assurance of adequate social factors for day case; access to phone and private transport, within one hour of a hospital with capabilities of managing complications, parents able and willing to care for child postoperatively, adequate housing conditions.
- Surgery itself should have low risk of serious complications, minimal expected blood loss and be associated with postoperative pain that can be managed at home.

c) **Give four specific anaesthetic considerations for strabismus surgery. (4 marks)**

Some congenital syndromes associated with squint in children include trisomy 21, Pierre Robin sequence, Marfan syndrome, craniofacial syndromes and mucopolysaccharidoses.

- Oculocardiac reflex is a significant risk with strabismus surgery. Consideration of pre-treatment with atropine or glycopyrrolate, or having the drugs ready in case of bradycardia.

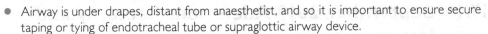

- Airway is under drapes, distant from anaesthetist, and so it is important to ensure secure taping or tying of endotracheal tube or supraglottic airway device.
- Still, soft eyes with neutral gaze required for surgery and so anaesthesia should be sufficiently deep and gas exchange adequately controlled.
- Postoperative nausea and vomiting is a common issue in eye surgery and especially strabismus surgery. Adequate control necessary to avoid vomiting and retching after wake up.
- Potentially difficult airway if coexisting congenital syndrome.

d) During the operation, the patient suddenly develops a profound bradycardia. Give two steps in your immediate management of this situation. (2 marks)

Only two points are available here (both in my CRQ and the original SAQ), and so my steps are aimed at interrupting the oculocardiac reflex. However, in a viva situation, make sure you mention the general points of being a safe anaesthetist, including an A to E assessment. Hypoxia also presents with bradycardia in children and so, in reality, checking for this would be undertaken simultaneously.

- Ask surgeon to stop surgical stimulus (pressure on globe, traction on extraocular muscles).
- Intravenous atropine 20 mcg/kg or glycopyrrolate 10 mcg/kg if it doesn't resolve.
- (Ensure full oxygenation, no break in circuit, airway patency, 100% oxygen.)

e) Give four elements of your strategy to reduce the risk of postoperative nausea and vomiting. (4 marks)

- Consider TIVA technique for maintenance.
- Minimisation of preoperative fasting time, ensuring clear fluids are given until one hour preoperatively.
- Multimodal analgesia to minimise long-acting opioid use.
- Intravenous fluid bolus for maintenance of hydration if preoperative intake inadequate.
- Multimodal antiemetic use, including ondansetron and dexamethasone intraoperatively and rescue options for postoperatively.
- Avoidance of nitrous oxide.

f) Give three elements of your postoperative analgesic plan. (3 marks)

- Multimodal analgesia including paracetamol and NSAID (unless contraindicated) given as premedication and continued postoperatively.
- Topical local anaesthetic drops by surgeon e.g. tetracaine.
- Sub-Tenon's block by surgeon.
- A dose of long-acting opioid i.e. morphine intraoperatively.

REFERENCE

Lewis H, James I. Update on anaesthesia for paediatric ophthalmic surgery. *BJA Educ.* 2021: 21: 32–38.

17.16 September 2019 Adenotonsillectomy and laryngospasm

A 4-year-old child presents for elective day case adenotonsillectomy.
a) Give two indications for adenotonsillectomy in children. (2 marks)
b) Give three approaches to managing anxiety in a child preoperatively. (3 marks)
c) Give two medical, two surgical and two social factors that determine suitability for day case surgery in paediatrics. (6 marks)
d) Give four elements of your analgesic strategy for this case. (4 marks)
e) The child develops airway obstruction after tracheal extubation at the end of the case. You suspect laryngospasm. Give four sequential steps you would take after calling for help and alerting the theatre team. (4 marks)
f) State the dose of suxamethonium that may be given intramuscularly (including into the tongue) in the event of laryngospasm occurring in the absence of intravenous access. (1 mark)

The Chairs' Report of the original CRQ stated that this is an "important topic and was well answered [with a pass rate of 92.3%]. The pass rate was the highest on the paper. It is reassuring that candidates have sound knowledge of the management of laryngospasm."

a) Give two indications for adenotonsillectomy in children. (2 marks)

- Frequent tonsillitis or severe (requiring hospitalisation) recurrent tonsillitis.
- Obstructive sleep apnoea or sleep disordered breathing due to enlarged tonsils.
- Peritonsillar abscess (quinsy).
- Chronic tonsillitis.
- Guttate psoriasis exacerbated by recurrent tonsillitis.
- Concern regarding histology of tonsil.

b) Give three approaches to managing anxiety in a child preoperatively. (3 marks)

- Giving age-appropriate information.
- Pharmacological anxiolysis e.g. oral midazolam or ketamine, or intranasal dexmedetomidine.
- Psychological input prior to admission in severe cases.
- Involvement of play therapist or distraction techniques.
- Active involvement of parents or carers.
- Engagement with anaesthetic technique e.g. handling the mask, "blowing up the balloon."
- Optimisation of environment e.g. minimisation of staff numbers in room, minimisation of noise levels.

c) Give two medical, two surgical and two social factors that determine suitability for day case surgery in paediatrics. (6 marks)

The need for overnight admission of children with OSA presenting for adenotonsillectomy is assessed on a case-by-case basis, with high apnoea-hypopnoea index score on sleep study, severe airway obstruction, witnessed desaturations, cyanosis, floppy episodes, or apnoeas all increasing the likelihood of need for admission. Presence of a congenital syndrome would also reduce the threshold for considering overnight stay.

- Medical: more than 60 weeks corrected age, absence of significant chronic comorbidities (e.g. chronic lung disease, congenital heart disease, other congenital syndromes) that increase perioperative risk or necessitate more prolonged monitoring (e.g. severe or poorly controlled OSA).
- Surgical: minimal risk of serious complications, low risk of significant blood loss, postoperative pain should be manageable at home with oral medications, the procedure must be one that does not prohibit return to normal oral intake beyond a few hours.
- Social: parents willing and able to care for child postoperatively, access to a telephone, living within an hour of a hospital with the capabilities of managing complications, access to private transport, adequate housing conditions.

d) **Give four elements of your analgesic strategy for this case. (4 marks)**

- Paracetamol and ibuprofen (if NSAIDs not contraindicated) commenced preoperatively and continued postoperatively.
- Dexamethasone (also useful in the prevention of postoperative nausea and vomiting) as a single intraoperative dose.
- Consideration of intraoperative ketamine, dexmedetomidine or preoperative gabapentinoid in patients with contraindications to simple analgesics.
- Short-acting intraoperative opioids e.g. fentanyl only, to minimise postoperative respiratory depression, complications in patients with OSA, postoperative nausea and vomiting and postoperative opioids as rescue only.
- Acupuncture.
- Honey may offer a small improvement in postoperative pain.

e) **The child develops airway obstruction after tracheal extubation at the end of the case. You suspect laryngospasm. Give four sequential steps you would take after calling for help and alerting the theatre team. (4 marks)**

This is an anaesthetic emergency and is included in the Association of Anaesthetists' Quick Reference Handbook.

- Direct visualisation and suction to remove contaminants e.g. blood that may be stimulating the airway.
- Give CPAP with 100% oxygen and face mask by circle system or T-piece depending on the patient's weight.
- Deepen anaesthesia if volatile agent still on or give propofol intravenously.
- Give NMBD intravenously.

f) **State the dose of suxamethonium that may be given intramuscularly (including into the tongue) in the event of laryngospasm occurring in the absence of intravenous access. (1 mark)**

- 4 mg/kg.

REFERENCES

Aldamluji N et al. PROSPECT guideline for tonsillectomy: systematic review and procedure-specific postoperative pain management recommendations. *Anaesthesia*. 2021: 76: 947–961.

Association of Anaesthetists. *Quick reference handbook: 3.6 laryngospasm and stridor*, 2018. https://anaesthetists.org/Portals/0/PDFs/QRH/QRH_3-6_Laryngospasm_and_stridor_v1.pdf?ver=2018-07-25-112714-407. Accessed 2nd April 2023.

Bailey C et al. Guidelines from the Association of Anaesthetists and the British Association of Day Surgery: guidelines for day-case surgery 2019. *Anaesthesia*. 2019: 74: 778–792.

Heikal S, Stuart G. Anxiolytic premedication for children. *BJA Educ*. 2020: 20: 220–225.

National Health Service. *Clinical pathways: tonsillitis and tonsillectomy*. https://clinical-pathways.org.uk/clinical-pathways/tonsillitis-and-tonsillectomy. Accessed 2nd April 2023.

Zalan J, Vaccani J, Murto K. Paediatric adenotonsillectomy: part 2: considerations for anaesthesia. *BJA Educ*. 2020: 20: 193–200.

17.17 March 2020 Anterior mediastinal mass

An 8-year-old child with an anterior mediastinal mass presents for diagnostic lymph node biopsy under general anaesthesia.

a) List three contents of the anterior mediastinum. (3 marks)
b) List five symptoms and signs relating to the mediastinal mass that are suggestive of significant perioperative risk. (5 marks)
c) List three findings on imaging that are predictive of significant perioperative risk in this child. (3 marks)
d) List three possible causes of anterior mediastinal mass in children. (3 marks)
e) Give two possible approaches to reducing the size of this child's mass to improve the safety of anaesthesia. (2 marks)
f) After induction of anaesthesia and despite maintaining spontaneous ventilation, the patient shows signs of respiratory compromise. After calling for help and commencing 100% oxygen, list two options to try to improve respiratory function. (2 marks)
g) Give two options if cardiovascular compromise has occurred after induction of anaesthesia. (2 marks)

The original CRQ was withdrawn from the exam and no further comment given. However, this remains an important topic and the principles of anaesthesia for a child with a mediastinal mass can also be applied to adult practice. Mediastinal masses can cause tracheal and superior vena caval compression and may even obstruct cardiac output. Patients may therefore complain of dynamic obstructive symptoms and may have a position in which they are least symptomatic. Maintenance of spontaneous ventilation during anaesthesia preserves the transmural pressure gradient that is maintaining airway patency, and so rendering the patient apnoeic may result in complete loss of airway with inability to pass an endotracheal tube through the compressed part of the airway.

Mediastinal anatomy is a common viva question. It is the area bounded by the two pleural sacs.

- *Superior mediastinum: from thoracic inlet to the top of the pericardium at T4, contains major thoracic blood vessels, oesophagus, trachea.*
- *Posterior mediastinum: between the posterior pericardium and vertebrae, contains oesophagus, thoracic duct, descending aorta, azygous vein, vagus nerve, lymph nodes.*
- *Middle mediastinum: between the anterior and posterior mediastinum – contains the heart, origins of the major vessels, phrenic nerves.*
- *Anterior mediastinum: small space between the anterior aspect of the pericardium and the underside of the sternum.*

a) List three contents of the anterior mediastinum. (3 marks)

- Connective tissue.
- Thymus (or remnants of thymus).
- Lymph nodes.

b) List five symptoms and signs relating to the mediastinal mass that are suggestive of significant perioperative risk. (5 marks)

The child may have other symptoms relating to the underlying cause of the anterior mediastinal mass such as night sweats and generalised lymphadenopathy.

- Orthopnoea.
- Cough when supine.

- Stridor.
- Wheeze.
- Syncopal symptoms.
- Upper body oedema.

c) List three findings on imaging that are predictive of significant perioperative risk in this child. (3 marks)

- Reduction (< 70%) in tracheal cross-sectional area.
- Carinal or bronchial compression.
- Great vessel compression.
- Pericardial effusion.

d) List three possible causes of anterior mediastinal mass in children. (3 marks)

- Lymphoma, both Hodgkin's and non-Hodgkin's.
- Acute lymphoblastic leukaemia.
- Vascular malformations.
- Non-haematological malignancies, including germ cell tumours.

e) Give two possible approaches to reducing the size of this child's mass to improve the safety of anaesthesia. (2 marks)

- Preoperative chest radiotherapy.
- Steroid treatment.

f) After induction of anaesthesia and despite maintaining spontaneous ventilation, the patient shows signs of respiratory compromise. After calling for help and commencing 100% oxygen, list two options to try to improve respiratory function. (2 marks)

In some cases, anaesthesia for lymph node biopsy can be avoided if imaging has returned sufficiently detailed information to start a treatment plan, or if the child is able to tolerate a biopsy under local or regional anaesthesia. In very severe cases, cardiopulmonary bypass may be necessary if the risks of anaesthesia are deemed too high.

- CPAP.
- Repositioning of patient to position that they were most comfortable in preoperatively.
- Positive pressure ventilation with PEEP.
- One-lung ventilation.
- Rigid bronchoscopy.

g) Give two options if cardiovascular compromise has occurred after induction of anaesthesia. (2 marks)

- Ensure adequate intravenous filling with fluid bolus.
- Reduce anaesthetic depth.
- Reposition patient.
- Sternotomy and elevation of mass.

REFERENCES

Ellis H, Feldman S. *Anatomy for anaesthetists*, 7th edition. Blackwell Science, 1997.
Mcleod M, Dobbie M. Anterior mediastinal masses in children. *BJA Educ.* 2019: 19: 21–26.

17.18 September 2020 Atrial septal defect

A 4-year-old child presents for dental extraction under general anaesthesia. A heart murmur is heard on auscultation.

a) List five features in the patient history that might suggest significant congenital heart disease (CHD). (5 marks)
b) List five findings on examination of the child that might suggest significant congenital heart disease. (5 marks)
c) Give two ECG findings that may be expected in a child with an atrial septal defect (ASD). (2 marks)
d) State two further investigations that would be useful in a child with suspected ASD and what information each would give about the defect. (4 marks)
e) Describe the current guidelines regarding prophylactic antibiotics against endocarditis in patients with congenital heart disease undergoing dental extraction. (3 marks)
f) Give one possible long-term consequence of an unrepaired atrial septal defect. (1 mark)

The Chairs' Report of the original CRQ stated that this is "an important topic, as children with congenital heart disease are susceptible to the same ailments as healthy children, and so can present to their local hospital for emergency and elective surgery. There was a lot of repetition of answers in sections (a) and (b). Section (a) asked for features in the history whereas section (b) asked for features of the examination. Though the words history and examination were in bold, several candidates wrote about clinical signs in the history section." The pass rate was 51.3%. The low pass rate is disappointing, particularly given that the knowledge tested is exactly the same as that for the SAQ in September 2014.

a) **List five features in the patient history that might suggest significant congenital heart disease (CHD). (5 marks)**

- Failure to thrive, falling centiles, small for age.
- Difficulty feeding as a neonate.
- Recurrent chest infections.
- Cough.
- Poor exercise tolerance.
- Squatting.
- Parental report of cyanosis, "funny turns."
- Syndrome known to be associated with congenital cardiac disease e.g. Down's syndrome, VATER, Turner's.
- Family history of congenital cardiac disease.

b) **List five findings on examination of the child that might suggest significant congenital heart disease. (5 marks)**

- Irregular pulse.
- Features of the murmur; harsh, variable sound intensity, presence of precordial thrill, diastolic, pansystolic ("innocent murmurs" will be early systolic murmur or continuous venous hum although these features do not rule out a pathological cause).
- Cyanosis.
- Signs of respiratory distress due to heart failure; tachypnoea, accessory muscle use, crackles on auscultation.
- Other features of heart failure; cool peripheries, sweating, tachycardia, hepatomegaly.
- Features suggestive of a syndrome associated with congenital cardiac defects.

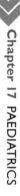
c) Give two ECG findings that may be expected in a child with an atrial septal defect (ASD). (2 marks)

You either know it or you don't, but it is only 2 marks.

- Prolonged PR interval.
- Right bundle branch block.
- Left axis deviation if primum defect, right axis deviation if secundum defect.

d) State two further investigations that would be useful in a child with suspected ASD and what information each would give about the defect. (4 marks)

- Echocardiogram (transthoracic or transoesophageal):
  — To determine whether secundum or primum defect and for assessment of involvement of tricuspid and mitral valves, and shunt between ventricles.
  — Assess the direction of the shunt.
  — Assess for the presence of pulmonary hypertension.
- Cardiac MRI:
  — 3D structure of heart lesion, valvular involvement, shunt volume.
- Cardiac CT:
  — 3D structure of heart lesion, chamber size.
- Chest X-ray:
  — Assess for presence of pulmonary oedema.

e) Describe the current guidelines regarding prophylactic antibiotics against endocarditis in patients with congenital heart disease undergoing dental extraction. (3 marks)

This question featured in the 2014 SAQ, and I don't know if it made a reappearance in 2020. NICE guidance from 2008 (updated in 2016) advised not to give antibiotic prophylaxis to patients at risk of endocarditis due to perception of lack of benefit in the face of risks of anaphylaxis and antibiotic resistance. However, over subsequent years there has been a move towards giving prophylaxis in selected circumstances (see ESC guidelines referenced below) for dental procedures involving manipulation of the gingival or periapical aspects of the teeth or where there will be perforation of the oral mucosa. Antibiotic prophylaxis is not required for any other procedure, although the usual prophylactic antibiotics should be given for perioperative cover for surgery where antibiotics are indicated for any patient. Maintenance of good oral and skin hygiene, avoidance of tattoos and piercings, prompt disinfection of wounds, prompt bacterial infection treatment, avoidance, where possible, of central venous access using peripheral access in preference, and care to manage all lines appropriately are included in the guidance.

- Antibiotic prophylaxis should be considered for those at highest risk of infective endocarditis; prosthetic heart valves or valve repair with prosthetic material, previous infective endocarditis, cyanotic CHD, repaired CHD using prosthetic material for six months after surgery or lifelong if shunt or valvular regurgitation persists.
- Given 30–60 minutes prior to treatment.
- Amoxicillin or ampicillin, with use of clindamycin for penicillin-allergic patients.

f) Give one possible long-term consequence of an unrepaired atrial septal defect. (1 mark)

- Supraventricular tachycardias.
- Heart failure.
- Frequent chest infections.
- Pulmonary hypertension, right heart failure.
- Paradoxical embolism.

REFERENCES

Baumgartner H et al. 2020 ESC guidelines for the management of adult congenital heart disease: the task force for the management of adult congenital heart disease of the European Society of Cardiology (ESC): endorsed by: Association for European Paediatric and Congenital Cardiology (AEPC), International Society for Adult Congenital Heart Disease (ISACHD). *Eur Heart J*. 2021: 42: 563–645.

Habib G et al. 2015 ESC guidelines for the management of infective endocarditis: the task force for the management of infective endocarditis of the European Society of Cardiology (ESC): endorsed by: European Association for Cardio-Thoracic Surgery (EACTS), the European Association of Nuclear Medicine (EANM). *Eur Heart J*. 2015: 36: 3075–3128.

National Institute for Health and Care Excellence. *Prophylaxis against infective endocarditis: antimicrobial prophylaxis against infective endocarditis in adults and children undergoing interventional procedures: clinical guideline: CG64*, March 2008, updated July 2016.

17.19 March 2021 Adenotonsillectomy and post-tonsillectomy bleeding

A 6-year-old child presents for elective adenotonsillectomy following recurrent tonsillitis.

a) Give two advantages and two disadvantages of a supraglottic airway device, in comparison to an endotracheal tube, when managing the airway for elective tonsillectomy. (4 marks)

b) The patient suffers a post-tonsillectomy bleed on the ward. Describe four signs or symptoms of blood loss. (4 marks)

c) Give the blood volume (in litres) of this child and the equations used to determine this. (3 marks)

d) List three specific concerns when assessing this child. (3 marks)

e) Describe two actions you would take on the ward. (2 marks)

f) The patient returns to theatre for ongoing bleeding. What position would you choose for airway management and why? (2 marks)

g) List two additional precautions you would take at induction of general anaesthesia. (2 marks)

The Chairs' Report following the original CRQ commented that this is "an area of the syllabus that candidates would be expected to know. The question was deemed by the examiners to be one of the easier questions on the paper and this was reflected in the highest pass rate for this paper," 89.5%. An SAQ that covered the same key issues, primary bleeding after tonsillectomy (bleeding that happens within 24 hours of the original surgery), featured in the Final written paper in March 2010. Secondary bleeding occurs up to 28 days after surgery and may be associated with infection.

a) **Give two advantages and two disadvantages of a supraglottic airway device, in comparison to an endotracheal tube, when managing the airway for elective tonsillectomy. (4 marks)**

Advantages:

- Straightforward to site.
- Good protection of airway from blood.
- Smooth emergence.
- Paralysis not required.
- Airway protection until awake.
- Avoids trauma of laryngoscopy and intubation.

Disadvantages:

- Surgical access may be more limited.
- Less secure than endotracheal intubation – may become dislodged by the Boyle Davis gag.

b) **The patient suffers a post-tonsillectomy bleed on the ward. Describe four signs or symptoms of blood loss. (4 marks)**

- Tachycardia.
- Tachypnoea.
- Prolonged capillary refill.
- Reduced urine output.
- Cool peripheries.
- Mottled skin.

- Altered mentation – initially anxious, latterly reduced consciousness.
- Hypotension – late sign.
- Evidence of blood loss as emesis of swallowed blood or bleeding from mouth.

c) Give the blood volume (in litres) of this child and the equations used to determine this. (3 marks)

In a 6-year-old child the expected blood volume would be 70 ml/kg. Infants have a blood volume of 80 ml/kg, and preterm infants 90 ml/kg.

- 1.4 litres.
- Estimated weight = (Age in years + 4) × 2 = 20 kg.
- Blood volume = 70 ml/kg = 70 × 20 ml.

d) List three specific concerns when assessing this child. (3 marks)

- Ongoing blood loss causing hypovolaemia or shock.
- Swallowed blood causing a full stomach.
- Aspirated blood into pulmonary tree.
- Possibility of difficult airway due to ongoing bleeding, oedema from previous intubation.
- Potential need for urgent surgery, with concomitant parental and child anxiety.

e) Describe two actions you would take on the ward. (2 marks)

Two actions, when there are so many you would undertake. I haven't stuck to the usual ABC approach as I have tried to put them in order of specificity to the situation. Usually bleeding is venous, and therefore resuscitation is the primary aim before definitive surgical intervention.

- Arrange for urgent contact with ENT, theatres, and senior anaesthetist.
- Ensure intravenous or intraosseous access and commence intravenous resuscitation if compromised.
- Send blood for point-of-care haemoglobin as well as laboratory full blood count, coagulation and cross match.
- Ensure child is positioned to allow blood to drain from mouth.
- Apply oxygen if the child is shocked.

f) The patient returns to theatre for ongoing bleeding. What position would you choose for airway management and why? (2 marks)

- Sitting or ramped positioning to facilitate patient comfort during preoxygenation as blood will continue to be swallowed rather than pooling in the oropharynx.
- Supine with head-down tilt to minimise risk of aspiration of blood into pulmonary tree, but this will result in pooling of blood in oropharynx during preoxygenation and may not be tolerated by patient.
- Head-down lateral decubitus positioning allows drainage of blood during preoxygenation or during gas induction, but anatomy will be unfamiliar for intubation and may make a difficult intubation even more challenging.

g) List two additional precautions you would take at induction of general anaesthesia. (2 marks)

- Two functioning suction devices available as any component of suction equipment may become blocked with clots at critical moment.

- Variety of endotracheal tubes, same size and smaller size compared to that used for the original surgery, due to likelihood of oedema and risk of tube becoming blocked by blood.
- Second-line airway equipment availability, including video laryngoscope.
- Consideration of use of high-flow nasal oxygen to prolong time to hypoxia at induction.
- Ensure surgical team is prepared and scrubbed ready for operation.
- Patient may become hypotensive on induction due to concomitant shock – ensure blood available, prepare vasopressors.

REFERENCES

Lee A, Hache M. Pediatric anaesthesia management for post-tonsillectomy bleed: current status and future directions. *Int J Gen Med.* 2022: 15: 63–69.

Ravi R, Howell T. Anaesthesia for paediatric ear, nose and throat surgery. *Contin Educ Anaes Crit Care Pain.* 2007: 7: 33–37.

17.20 September 2021 Cerebral palsy

A 6-year-old who has cerebral palsy presents for bilateral femoral osteotomy.
a) Define cerebral palsy. (1 mark)
b) List the most common types of cerebral palsy. (3 marks)
c) Give two respiratory effects and two central nervous system effects of cerebral palsy, giving an anaesthetic implication for each. (4 marks)
d) State three difficulties that may be encountered during endotracheal intubation for a child with cerebral palsy. (3 marks)
e) List three classes of medication that the patient may already be taking. (3 marks)
f) List three other pharmacological considerations when anaesthetising a patient for cerebral palsy. (3 marks)
g) Describe how you would manage postoperative pain in this patient. (3 marks)

The third appearance of cerebral palsy as the focus of a paediatric exam question, the first time as a CRQ, and generally the same sorts of issues were addressed but sometimes in a slightly different way. This was the exam paper that was voided due to problems with the online platform.

a) Define cerebral palsy. (1 mark)

A group of permanent, activity-limiting movement and posture disorders caused by acquired pathology to the developing brain during the antenatal, intrapartum, postnatal, or early infancy stages.

Antenatal (70–80%):

- *Maternal antenatal infections (TORCH: toxoplasma, other, rubella, cytomegalovirus, herpes simplex).*
- *Teratogen exposure.*
- *Premature birth.*
- *Low socioeconomic status resulting in a range of environmental risk factors.*
- *Multiple gestation.*
- *Genetic and metabolic disorders.*

Perinatal (10%):

- *Non-vertex presentation.*
- *Placental abruption.*
- *Ruptured uterus.*
- *Prolonged or obstructed labour.*
- *Post-maturity.*

Postnatal (10%):

- *Sepsis or meningitis.*
- *Head injury.*
- *Intraventricular haemorrhage.*
- *Hyperbilirubinaemia.*
- *Respiratory distress.*

b) **List the most common types of cerebral palsy. (3 marks)**

All of these can be hemiplegic, diplegic, or quadriplegic.

- Spastic.
- Dyskinetic.
- Ataxic.

c) **Give two respiratory effects and two central nervous system effects of cerebral palsy, giving an anaesthetic implication for each. (4 marks)**

This question is only asking about the impact of cerebral palsy on the respiratory and central nervous systems, but the effects on other systems were questioned in the previous SAQs on cerebral palsy, and so I have included its impact on a range of other body systems in this table. The severity of presentation of cerebral palsy is very variable, and so the issues listed below represent the more severe end of the spectrum.

	Clinical effects	Anaesthetic implications
Respiratory:	History of premature birth, previous ventilation, recurrent pneumonia, and gastro-oesophageal reflux predispose to chronic lung disease.	Assess for acute infection. Consider need for respiratory assessment, physiotherapy. May still require long-term oxygen therapy or CPAP.
	Weak cough, respiratory muscle hypotonia, reduced immunity due to malnutrition.	Increased propensity to lung infection – check for acute infection preoperatively.
	Long term truncal spasticity results in scoliosis.	Restrictive defect, pulmonary hypertension, cor pulmonale, respiratory and cardiac failure.
Central nervous system:	Epilepsy.	Ensure medication is not missed when nil by mouth. Ensure drug levels are checked if there is a recent change in seizure frequency. Consider the impact of enzyme inducers and inhibitors.
	Cognition or communication problems.	May increase child's anxiety. Involve carers, play specialist. Consider individual need for sedative/anxiolytic premedication but caution is required if the child has respiratory compromise.
Airway:	*Hypersalivation.*	*May make face mask ventilation and visualisation on laryngoscopy challenging. Consider antisialagogue.*
	Poor dentition.	*May complicate airway management. Loose or decayed teeth should be managed in advance.*
	Risk of temporomandibular joint dislocation if affected by muscle spasticity.	*Possibility of difficult intubation – difficult airway equipment, asleep fibreoptic or video laryngoscopy may be indicated.*

	Clinical effects	Anaesthetic implications
Cardiovascular:	Pulmonary hypertension or right heart failure may exist in patients with chronic lung disease.	Preoperative echo and cardiology review in patients with severe lung disease. Blood loss may be tolerated poorly. Intraoperative management to include lowest possible airway pressures, optimisation of gas exchange, maintenance of intravascular volume and of vascular tone.
Gastrointestinal:	Swallowing difficulties, oesophageal dysmotility, abnormal lower oesophageal sphincter tone.	Increased risk of reflux, consider need for rapid sequence induction.
	Swallowing difficulty	Poor nutrition, low weight, need to calculate drug doses based on weight not age. Consider the possibility of anaemia, dehydration or electrolyte disturbance and treat preoperatively (may have PEG). Difficulty with oral medications.
	Chronic constipation.	Avoid exacerbation with excessive opioid administration.
Cutaneomusculoskeletal:	Spasticity causes fixed flexion deformities, joint dislocations.	Cannulation, monitoring and positioning problems. Risk of spasticity and dystonia postoperatively, may cause pain and surgical complications.
	Thin skin, little subcutaneous fat, atrophic musculature (large surface-area-to-weight ratio).	Prone to pressure sores, poor heat conservation, poor wound healing. Need for careful padding and active warming at all times.
	Immobility.	Cannot assess cardiopulmonary reserve.
	Non-weight-bearing long bones become osteopenic, especially in association with low vitamin D levels and anticonvulsant medication.	Bone fragility, risk of fracture.
Urological:	Neuropathic bladder, communication difficulties, and immobility contribute to incontinence.	Long term catheterisation, risk of urinary tract infection. Latex catheters are avoided to stop repeated latex exposure triggering allergy.

d) **State three difficulties that may be encountered during endotracheal intubation for a child with cerebral palsy. (3 marks)**

- Difficulty with positioning due to kyphoscoliosis and contractures.
- Difficulty with preoxygenation due to patient compliance.
- Poor dentition due to chronic reflux and difficulties with complying with dental hygiene (mouth opening limited by spasticity, poor compliance due to learning difficulties) may increase risk of dental damage.
- Excessive oral secretions may impair view of direct or indirect laryngoscopy.
- Spasticity of muscles around the temporomandibular joint may lead to reduced mouth opening.
- Risk of reflux and aspiration.
- Desaturation during intubation attempts due to chronic lung disease.

e) **List three classes of medication that the patient may already be taking. (3 marks)**

To think about what drugs the patient may be on, I have first thought about how their condition affects them long term.

Pathology	Medication classes
Chronic pain.	Analgesics including simple analgesics (paracetamol), gabapentinoids.
Spasticity.	Benzodiazepines or antispasmodic medications (baclofen).
Oral secretions.	Antimuscarinics (hyoscine patch).
Gastro-oesophageal reflux disease.	Proton pump inhibitors.
Seizures.	Anticonvulsants.
Mental health changes.	Antidepressants.

f) **List three other pharmacological considerations when anaesthetising a patient for cerebral palsy. (3 marks)**

Although not strictly a pharmacological consideration, some patients with spasticity may have an intrathecal drug delivery device fitted (for continuous administration of analgesia and/or antispasmodic). These have their own specific perioperative considerations.

- Pharmacokinetics:
  - Absorption; GORD may reduce absorption of orally or enterally administered medications – may have implications for postoperative analgesia.
  - Distribution; may have low body weight due to difficulties with oral intake – malnourishment results in a proportional increase in total body water and a reduction in body fat, causing an increase in volume of distribution of hydrophilic drugs such as NMBDs and a reduction in volume of distribution of lipophilic drugs such as propofol.
  - Metabolism; anticonvulsants generally induce cytochrome P450 enzymes (except valproate) and so may increase the rate of metabolism of perioperative drugs.
  - Excretion; renal excretion of drugs may be impaired by chronic kidney disease related to neurogenic bladder dysfunction.
- Pharmacodynamics:
  - Upregulation of acetylcholine receptors means non-depolarising NMBDs are less potent and have shorter duration of action; caution with use of suxamethonium.
  - Obstructive sleep apnoea; use of long-acting opioids and anaesthetic agents should be avoided where possible.
  - Proconvulsant drugs e.g. alfentanil, pethidine, should be avoided or used with caution if the child has epilepsy.

g) **Describe how you would manage postoperative pain in this patient. (3 marks)**

A subsection on postoperative analgesia or the issues associated with managing it has been included in all three questions on management of a child with cerebral palsy.

- Neuraxial technique including the possibility of epidural infusion with local anaesthesia only (or with clonidine to reduce spasm) to avoid the respiratory depressant and constipating effects of opioids. May need escalated level of postoperative care to facilitate epidural use.
- Multimodal analgesia to include regular paracetamol and NSAIDs if not contraindicated in a formulation that can be taken orally, if feasible, by the child or via PEG if applicable.
- Continue antispasmodic medications and avoid triggers of spasms e.g. cold, pain, anxiety.

- Involvement of parents or caregivers in pain assessment, if there are communication difficulties, and use presence of familiar adults to improve pain experience.
- Consideration of continuous opioid infusion if neuraxial technique not possible as child may not have the physical or intellectual capability to use a PCA – would need escalated level of care to manage this safely.

REFERENCES

Hayakawa H, Pincott E, Ali U. Anaesthesia and cerebral palsy. *BJA Educ.* 2022: 22: 26–32.

Parry Prosser D, Sharma N. Cerebral palsy and anaesthesia. *Contin Educ Anaesth Crit Care Pain.* 2010: 10: 72–76.

17.21 March 2022 Meningococcal septicaemia

You are called to the emergency department to review a 2-year-old baby who is unwell with suspected meningococcal septicaemia.

a) State the normal weight, heart rate, mean arterial pressure and capillary refill time in a child of this age. (4 marks)

b) The mean arterial pressure is 50 mmHg. State how you would restore the circulation. (3 marks)

c) Name the antibiotic and its dose (per kilogram body weight) that should be given immediately. (1 mark)

d) List four indications for intubation, apart from those relating to airway or respiratory concerns. (4 marks)

e) State three abnormalities that you might see on the patient's blood tests. (3 marks)

f) The child continues to be hypotensive despite resuscitation with intravenous fluids. State a further five steps in your ongoing management. (5 marks)

The Chairs' Report stated that the pass rate for the original CRQ on this topic was the highest in the paper, 82.8%, and commented that "some candidates dropped marks in section (b) by not answering what was asked. The question asked for steps to restore the circulation, but some candidates offered temporising measures to elevate the blood pressure. The last section asked for 5 further steps in the management of septic shock and some candidates lost marks by repeating answers from previous sections."

This is the fourth time meningococcal sepsis has appeared in the Final exam in the time frame of this book. Several of the subsections of the question have been asked before – subsection (a) in the September 2015 paper (they kept the child the same age just for added convenience) and subsections (c), (e), and (f) are reworded from the September 2012 question.

a) State the normal weight, heart rate, mean arterial pressure and capillary refill time in a child of this age. (4 marks)

It is difficult to give a definitive answer for part (a) as there is such a variety of ranges and calculations in use. I would hope that the College would recognise a range of values. Also, average _mean_ *arterial blood pressure is rarely quoted for children in the literature.*

Weight	12 kg.	2 × (age in years + 4) according to the Resuscitation Council UK and tradition. A newer calculation is (3 × age in years) + 7.
Pulse rate	95–140 bpm.	
Mean arterial blood pressure	58 mmHg.	(1.5 × age in years) + 55 gives the 50th centile. *However, according to Resuscitation Council UK, MAP 50th centile is 70 mmHg for a 1-year-old and 75 mmHg for a 5-year-old, the 5th centiles being 55 mmHg and 50 mmHg respectively. Tables give different ranges for boys and girls, and it also varies according to a child's height.*
Capillary refill time	Less than two seconds.	

b) The mean arterial pressure is 50 mmHg. State how you would restore the circulation. (3 marks)

I don't really like the wording of this question. Antibiotics will stop the fluid leak, ultimately, and restore the circulation, but antibiotics are asked about in the next subsection. Inotropic support will restore circulation by enhancing pump function and by treating vasoplegia. However, I _think_ *they are just* *wanting to know how you'd restore circulatory <u>volume</u>. The most recent Surviving Sepsis Campaign guidelines for children has moved away from recommending using blood for fluid resuscitation of children in septic shock – they suggest against using blood if the haemoglobin is > 70 g/dl in a haemodynamically stable child, and feel unable to make a recommendation of transfusion threshold for children who are unstable with septic shock. NICE guidance talked about use of 0.9% saline and then 4.5% human albumin solution, but the Surviving Sepsis Campaign guidelines advise the use of a balanced crystalloid and could not see convincing evidence of any advantage of albumin use.*

- Give an intravenous or intraosseous bolus of balanced crystalloid 10 ml/kg.
- Repeat up to 60 ml/kg titrating against markers of restoration of circulating volume such as:
  — Capillary refill time less than two seconds.
  — Normalisation of blood pressure.
  — Normalisation of heart rate < 140 bpm.
  — Urine output greater than 1 ml/kg/h.
  — Normal mental status or level of consciousness.
  — Normalisation of lactate.
- Assess repeatedly for markers of fluid overload as an indication of when to stop further fluid boluses: new or worsening hepatomegaly, signs of pulmonary oedema.

c) Name the antibiotic and its dose (per kilogram body weight) that should be given immediately. (1 mark)

This should cover Haemophilus influenzae and Streptococcus pneumoniae. Different antibiotics are advised in babies under three months.

- Ceftriaxone 80–100 mg/kg to a maximum of 4 g.

d) List four indications for intubation, apart from those relating to airway or respiratory concerns. (4 marks)

The answer to this is stated in the NICE guidance referenced, but being logical should allow you get four marks in this question without knowing the exact criteria.

- Circulatory:
  — Ongoing shock despite 40+ ml/kg fluid resuscitation.
  — Post-cardiorespiratory arrest.
- Neurological:
  — Reduction in, or fluctuations of, GCS.
  — Need to control intractable seizures.
  — Evidence of raised intracranial pressure.
  — To facilitate safe transfer for neuroimaging or to tertiary centre.

e) State three abnormalities that you might see on the patient's blood tests. (3 marks)

Straight out of NICE guidance, a list of metabolic disturbances that secondary care should "anticipate, monitor and correct." Additionally, there is raised white cell count and raised CRP which will be corrected by the treatment of the underlying condition.

- Hypoglycaemia.
- Acidosis.
- Hypokalaemia.
- Hypocalcaemia.
- Hypomagnesaemia.
- Anaemia.
- Coagulopathy.

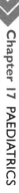

f) The child continues to be hypotensive despite resuscitation with intravenous fluids. State a further five steps in your ongoing management. (5 marks)

This is taken from both NICE and the Surviving Sepsis Campaign. NICE also recommends checking for errors such as extravasation of drug or wrong dilution if catecholamine infusions do not have the desired effect.

- Adrenaline or noradrenaline infusion (via a peripheral cannula if central access not available).
- Vasopressin infusion if high-dose catecholamine infusion required.
- Consideration of intravenous hydrocortisone.
- Correction of acidosis.
- Correction of hypocalcaemia.
- Advice from paediatric intensivist or retrieval service.

REFERENCES

National Institute for Health and Care Excellence. *Meningitis (bacterial) and meningococcal septicaemia in under 16s: recognition, diagnosis and management: CG102*, June 2010, updated February 2015.

National Institute for Health and Care Excellence. *British National Formulary for Children.* https://bnfc.nice.org.uk/drugs/ceftriaxone/#indications-and-dose. Accessed 28th April 2023.

Weiss SL et al. Surviving sepsis campaign international guidelines for the management of septic shock and sepsis-associated organ dysfunction in children. *Pediat Crit Care Med.* 2020: 21: e52–e106.

17.22 September 2022 Inhaled foreign body

You are asked to pre-assess a 10-month-old baby who has presented with a suspected inhaled foreign body.

a) Give five signs and symptoms that may indicate that this child needs immediate surgical management. (5 marks)
b) What is the most important thing to maintain during induction and why? (2 marks)
c) How can oxygenation be maintained during the procedure? (3 marks)
d) Describe an analgesic strategy for rigid bronchoscopy. (2 marks)
e) List four specific complications that may occur during the provision of anaesthesia for inhaled foreign body removal. (4 marks)
f) What drug at what dosage would you use to reduce the risk of post-extubation airway swelling? (2 marks)
g) You are called to recovery because the patient has developed stridor. State a pharmacological therapy, with dose, that may be useful in reducing airway oedema. (2 marks)

The Chairs' Report of the original CRQ stated that "knowledge of this subject appeared to be good and the question was generally well answered [with a pass rate of 60.1%]. However, some candidates lost marks because they didn't know the specific complications when anaesthetising this type of case."

a) **Give five signs and symptoms that may indicate that this child needs immediate surgical management. (5 marks)**

Coughing and choking at the time of the inhalation of the foreign body are common, but often the child then settles. The following symptoms and signs would raise the concern that urgent surgical intervention is required. A history of inhalation of dangerous objects such as button battery or multiple magnets would also warrant urgent surgical management.

- Change in voice, hoarse voice.
- Difficulty swallowing, drooling.
- Stridor.
- Respiratory distress, tripod posturing.
- Low oxygen saturations, cyanosis.
- Obtundation.

b) **What is the most important thing to maintain during induction and why? (2 marks)**

- Spontaneous respiration; maintenance of respiratory mechanics and muscle tone, avoiding positive pressure ventilation, which risks the foreign body moving further down the airway and becoming more difficult to retrieve or causing complete obstruction.

c) **How can oxygenation be maintained during the procedure? (3 marks)**

If the foreign body is proximal, the case should be quick and the patient can remain spontaneously ventilating. However, if the obstruction is in the smaller airways, the procedure can be very prolonged and muscle relaxation and positive pressure ventilation may be required.

- Attachment of breathing circuit to the 22 mm side port of ventilating bronchoscope for spontaneous ventilation or IPPV.
- High-flow nasal oxygenation for intermittent oxygenation if procedure is brief and a short period of apnoea when the rigid bronchoscope is in place can be tolerated.

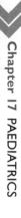

- Face mask oxygenation followed by brief intubation with rigid bronchoscope for retrieval of straightforward obstruction followed by reoxygenation by face mask.
- Attachment of oxygen tubing to side port of surgical laryngoscope for more proximal foreign bodies.

d) Describe an analgesic strategy for rigid bronchoscopy. (2 marks)

Managing analgesia and sedation is a fine balance in this type of case. Too little risks complications associated with surgical stimulation and light plane of anaesthesia. Too much risks apnoea and requirement of IPPV to maintain oxygenation.

- Topicalisation of airway under direct vision with lidocaine up to 4 mg/kg via a mucosal atomisation device once patient is sufficiently deeply anaesthetised to tolerate laryngoscopy.
- Paracetamol and ibuprofen (after checking for contraindications).
- Short-acting opioids (e.g. fentanyl boluses 0.5 mcg/kg) intraoperatively titrated to effect, taking care to avoid apnoea.

e) List four specific complications that may occur during the provision of anaesthesia for inhaled foreign body removal. (4 marks)

- Complete airway obstruction due to dislodgement of foreign body.
- Anaesthetic:
  - Hypoxaemia and hypercapnia.
  - Laryngospasm, bronchospasm.
  - Regurgitation and aspiration.
  - Loss of airway.
- Surgical:
  - Dental, lip, or tongue damage by rigid bronchoscope.
  - Trauma to airways by bronchoscope, including haemorrhage, bronchial or tracheal perforation, pneumothorax, or pneumomediastinum.

f) What drug at what dosage would you use to reduce the risk of post-extubation airway swelling? (2 marks)

The dose range quoted exceeds BNF advice but is common in the literature regarding the specific issue of post-extubation stridor risk reduction.

- Intravenous dexamethasone.
- 0.25–0.5 mg/kg.

g) You are called to recovery because the patient has developed stridor. State a pharmacological therapy, with dose, that may be useful in reducing airway oedema. (2 marks)

Nebulised budesonide is also used in the management of croup and so would be an option here if dexamethasone had not already been given intraoperatively.

- Nebulised adrenaline (0.5 mg/kg of 1:1000 solution, to a maximum of 5 mg).

REFERENCES

Bould, M. Essential notes: the anaesthetic management of an inhaled foreign body in a child. *BJA Educ.* 2019: 19: 66–67.

Iyer N et al. A network meta-analysis of dexamethasone for preventing postextubation upper airway obstruction in children. *Annals ATS.* 2023: 20: 118–130.

Kendigelan P. The anaesthetic consideration of tracheobronchial foreign body aspiration in children. *J Thorac Dis.* 2016: 3803–3807.

Sutherland J, Bowen L. Ingestion of foreign bodies and caustic substances in children. *BJA Educ.* 2023: 23: 2–7.

17.23 February 2023 Pyloric stenosis

A 4-week-old term baby presents for surgery for pyloric stenosis.
a) Give three differential diagnoses for regurgitation and vomiting in this baby. (3 marks)
b) List three mechanisms of potassium loss in pyloric stenosis. (3 marks)
c) State the initial approach to fluid resuscitation in a shocked baby with pyloric stenosis. (1 mark)
d) List three factors to consider regarding ongoing fluid requirements in a patient with pyloric stenosis, following acute resuscitation. (3 marks)
e) Why does metabolic alkalosis need to be corrected prior to surgery? (1 mark)
f) How may the risk of aspiration be reduced before induction of anaesthesia? (1 mark)
g) List two possible techniques using local anaesthesia that may be used as part of the anaesthetic and analgesic approach for pyloromyotomy. (2 marks)
h) List three postoperative complications following general anaesthesia that neonates are at increased susceptibility to (3 marks), stating for each the physiological or anatomical underlying reason. (3 marks)

The Chairs' Report stated that the question was "well answered" with a pass rate of 70.8%. However, "many candidates did not know why preoperative alkalosis needs to be corrected prior to surgery." Although it hasn't previously featured as a question in the Final FRCA written paper over the time period of this book, the pathophysiology of pyloric stenosis in causing a hypochloraemic hypokalaemic metabolic alkalosis is a common question to encounter during the viva.

a) **Give three differential diagnoses for regurgitation and vomiting in this baby. (3 marks)**

- Medical causes:
  — Gastro-oesophageal reflux.
  — Milk intolerance.
  — Gastroenteritis.
  — Sepsis of any cause.
  — Congenital metabolic disease.
- Surgical causes:
  — Raised intracranial pressure.
  — Duodenal or oesophageal atresia.
  — Bowel obstruction due to malrotation, obstructed hernia, intussusception, Hirschsprung's disease, volvulus.

b) **List three mechanisms of potassium loss in pyloric stenosis. (3 marks)**

- Gastrointestinal loss; vomiting leads to loss of water, hydrochloric acid, and sodium and potassium ions resulting in a hypokalaemic, hypochloraemic metabolic alkalosis.
- Intracellular movement; buffering of intravascular alkalosis by movement of hydrogen ions out of the cells in exchange for potassium ions into the cells.
- Renal loss; hypovolaemia triggers aldosterone release, which retains sodium in exchange for urinary potassium loss in an attempt to restore blood volume. *Initially bicarbonate is excreted in the urine in exchange for hydrogen ions in an attempt to restore acid-base status but worsening of hypovolaemia causes excretion of hydrogen in exchange for sodium retention in an attempt to boost intravascular volume, resulting in a paradoxically acid urine, and worsening of systemic alkalosis.*

c) **State the initial approach to fluid resuscitation in a shocked baby with pyloric stenosis. (1 mark)**

- 20 ml/kg bolus isotonic crystalloid (0.9% saline or Hartmann's solution) and reassess volume status clinically.

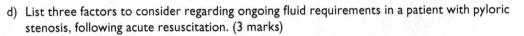

d) List three factors to consider regarding ongoing fluid requirements in a patient with pyloric stenosis, following acute resuscitation. (3 marks)

- Maintenance fluids corrected for body mass.
- Compensation for ongoing losses.
- Electrolyte needs, especially potassium, based on ongoing reassessment of blood tests.
- Need for glucose substrate whilst not being fed.
- Clinical response in terms of signs of dehydration or fluid overload.

e) Why does metabolic alkalosis need to be corrected prior to surgery? (1 mark)

Alkalosis leads to reduced hydrogen ion concentration in the CSF therefore reducing respiratory drive, increasing the likelihood of apnoeas to which babies of this age are already susceptible especially in conjunction with anaesthetic agents and opioids.

- Reduced respiratory drive or apnoea.

f) How may the risk of aspiration be reduced before induction of anaesthesia? (1 mark)

- Nasogastric tube insertion and "four quadrant" aspiration prior to induction (*aspiration of the tube with the baby in supine, left lateral, prone and then right lateral positions*).
- Point-of-care gastric antrum ultrasound may be used to assess for the presence of gastric contents.

g) List two possible techniques using local anaesthesia that may be used as part of the anaesthetic and analgesic approach for pyloromyotomy. (2 marks)

Surgery may be undertaken laparoscopically or as an open technique, usually with a curved circum-umbilical incision. Paracetamol is the mainstay of postoperative analgesia, and there are good reasons to avoid opioids in patients of this age.

- Local anaesthesia infiltration by the surgeon.
- Transversus abdominis plane blocks.
- Rectus sheath blocks.

h) List three postoperative complications following general anaesthesia that neonates are at increased susceptibility to (3 marks), stating for each the physiological or anatomical underlying reason. (3 marks)

- Perioperative adverse airway events such as laryngospasm; airway is narrower so small reductions in diameter due to e.g. post-extubation oedema or airway secretions can lead to significant reduction in air flow.
- Apnoeas; incompletely developed chemoreceptor and central respiratory responses to hypoxia and hypercapnia.
- Hypothermia; thin skin, high surface-area-to-volume ratio, immature thermogenesis.
- Hypoglycaemia; limited glycogen stores so reduced capacity to cope with periods of starvation.

REFERENCES

Craig R, Deeley A. Anaesthesia for pyloromyotomy. *BJA Educ.* 2018: 18: 173–177.
Macrae J, Ng E, Whyte H. Anaesthesia for premature infants. *BJA Educ.* 2021: 21: 355–363.

PAIN MEDICINE

18.1 September 2011 Back pain

A 68-year-old woman attends the Pain Management Clinic with a two-year history of pain in her back and legs.

a) List nine factors in the presentation of back pain that would alert you to the need for further investigation or referral. (9 marks)
b) List four conservative options for the management of low back pain. (4 marks)
c) Give three pharmacological options for the management of low back pain. (3 marks)
d) Radiofrequency denervation may be considered if conservative and pharmacological options have not been effective. State two further prerequisites for this treatment. (2 marks)
e) State the indication for considering caudal epidural for low back pain management. (1 mark)
f) State a surgical option that may be considered when radiological findings are consistent with sciatic symptoms and nonsurgical management has failed to improve the patient's function or pain. (1 mark)

Back pain is a common reason for attendance at pain clinics and you should have a clear idea of what the underlying causes are, how to distinguish them, and how they can be managed. There are three main causes of back pain:

Musculoskeletal: 95% (sacroiliac joint, facet joint, discogenic pain, ligamental injury, myofascial pain).

Features: dull, mechanical ache, lumbosacral and buttocks. Referred pain to legs is common but not below knee. Those aged 20–55 years most affected.

Nerve root (radicular) pain: 4% (due to disc herniation, spinal stenosis, and epidural adhesions).

Features: well localised, sharp electric shock pain, typically radiating below the knee. Exacerbated by coughing, straining, sneezing. Straight leg raise or femoral stretch test will reveal nerve root irritation. Neurological examination may show sensory, motor, and reflex abnormalities.

Serious spinal pathology: 1% (due to trauma, malignancy, inflammatory conditions, infection).

a) **List nine factors in the presentation of back pain that would alert you to the need for further investigation or referral. (9 marks)**

This is asking you for the factors that might indicate to you that the patient has serious spinal pathology, the "red flags." If you can remember the possible causes of serious spinal pathology, then you will be able to list the symptoms and signs that would raise your suspicions. This list is taken from NICE guidance and indicates the red flags for cauda equina, spinal fracture, cancer, and infective causes.

- Severe progressive bilateral neurological deficit of the legs.
- Urinary retention or incontinence.
- Faecal incontinence.

DOI: 10.1201/9781003388494-18

- Perianal or perineal loss of sensation OR laxity of anal sphincter.
- Sudden onset severe central spinal pain relieved by lying down.
- History of major trauma or lesser trauma in people with osteoporosis or corticosteroid use.
- Structural deformity of the spine.
- Spinal tenderness.
- Age over 50 years.
- Gradual onset of symptoms.
- Severe unremitting pain that persists on lying.
- No improvement after six weeks of conservative management.
- Unexplained weight loss.
- Fever.
- Tuberculosis.
- Recent urinary tract infection.
- Diabetes.
- History of intravenous drug use.
- HIV infection, immunosuppressant use, other reason for immunocompromise.

b) **List four conservative options for the management of low back pain. (4 marks)**

- Self-management; reassurance, information, advice to continue usual activities, and exercise.
- Exercise, including group NHS classes.
- Manual therapy as part of an overall management package.
- Psychological therapy; cognitive behavioural therapy to be used within a pain management programme.
- Pain management programme (PMP); all interventions combined into one package of care; education, exercise, relaxation techniques, goal setting, pacing, psychological therapy.

c) **Give three pharmacological options for the management of low back pain. (3 marks)**

- Paracetamol, but not to be used alone.
- NSAIDs – assess risks and benefits, consider need for gastric protection, lowest dose for shortest duration possible.
- Short course of weak opioid (codeine, dihydrocodeine, tramadol) for acute management if NSAIDs not tolerated, contraindicated, or ineffective.

d) **Radiofrequency denervation may be considered if conservative and pharmacological options have not been effective. State two further prerequisites for this treatment. (2 marks)**

- Main source of pain confirmed to be coming from structures supplied by the medial branch nerve/after positive response to diagnostic medial branch block.
- Moderate to severe levels of localised back pain.

e) **State the indication for considering caudal epidural for low back pain management. (1 mark)**

- If the pain is accompanied by severe pain in the sciatic nerve territory.

f) State a surgical option that may be considered when radiological findings are consistent with sciatic symptoms and nonsurgical management has failed to improve the patient's function or pain. (1 mark)

- Spinal decompression.

REFERENCES

Jackson M, Simpson K. Chronic back pain. *Contin Educ Anaesth Crit Care Pain*. 2006: 6: 152–155.

National Institute for Health and Care Excellence. *Neuropathic pain in adults: pharmacological management in non-specialist settings: CG173*, November 2013, updated February 2017.

National Institute for Health and Care Excellence. *Low back pain and sciatica in over 16s: assessment and management: NG59*, November 2016.

National Institute for Health and Care Excellence. *Clinical knowledge summaries: back pain – low (without radiculopathy)*, February 2022.

18.2 March 2013 Coeliac plexus block

a) Give the names of the three nerves that contribute to the coeliac plexus. (3 marks)
b) Give four anatomical relations of the coeliac plexus. (4 marks)
c) Give three indications for coeliac plexus block. (3 marks)
d) Give two anatomical approaches used for coeliac plexus block. (2 marks)
e) State eight specific complications associated with coeliac plexus block. (8 marks)

When this question appeared as an SAQ in 2013, it had a 36.4% pass rate. The Chair's Report revealed that questioning on the anatomy of the coeliac plexus was poorly answered, one candidate wrote about the cervical plexus (always read the questions carefully), and that generic answers to complications of coeliac plexus block (local anaesthesia toxicity, pain, infection, bleeding) would not be accepted.

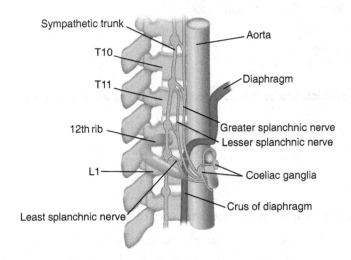

Coeliac plexus anatomy.

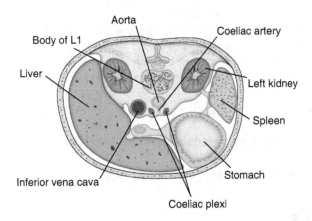

Cross-section of the coeliac plexi.

a) Give the names of the three nerves that contribute to the coeliac plexus. (3 marks)

- Greater splanchnic *(T5–10)*.
- Lesser splanchnic *(T10–11)*.
- Least splanchnic *(T11–12)*.

b) Give four anatomical relations of the coeliac plexus. (4 marks)

- Retroperitoneal.
- Anterolateral to the body of LI bilaterally.
- Anterior to the aorta and crura of diaphragm.
- Either side of the origin of the coeliac artery.
- Medial to the inferior vena cava.
- Posterior to the stomach and pancreas.

c) Give three indications for coeliac plexus block. (3 marks)

The coeliac plexus supplies the liver, gall bladder, spleen, stomach, pancreas, kidneys, adrenals, small intestine, and large intestine proximal to splenic flexure. Any cause of intractable pain involving these organs can be managed with coeliac plexus block.

- Pancreatic cancer pain.
- Stomach cancer pain.
- Chronic pancreatitis pain.

d) Give two anatomical approaches used for coeliac plexus block. (2 marks)

- Posterior approach.
- Anterior (retro- or transcrural).
- Transaortic.
- Transdiscal.
- Paramedian.

e) State eight specific complications associated with coeliac plexus block. (8 marks)

- Retroperitoneal bleeding due to injury of the aorta or inferior vena cava by the needle.
- Intravascular injection into great vessels (should be prevented by checking the needle position with radio-opaque dye).
- Paraplegia secondary to phenol injection into arterial supply of spinal cord.
- Direct spinal cord or nerve root damage.
- Retrocrural spread of phenol, causing spinal nerve root damage.
- Intrathecal or epidural injection.
- Visceral puncture, damage, abscess or cyst formation (stomach or kidney).
- Injection into psoas muscle with risk of cyst or abscess formation.
- Pneumothorax.
- Chylothorax.
- Thrombosis.
- Sexual dysfunction (phenol spread along sympathetic chain).
- Leg warmth.
- Hypotension (dilatation of upper abdominal vessels).

REFERENCES

Menon R, Swanepoel A. Sympathetic blocks. *Contin Educ Anaesth Crit Care Pain*. 2010: 10: 88–92.
Scott-Warren J, Bhaskar A. Cancer pain management: part II: interventional techniques. *Contin Educ Anaesth Crit Care Pain*. 2015: 15: 68–72.

18.3 September 2013 Continuous epidural analgesia

a) State five complications that should be rapidly recognisable by healthcare professionals caring for patients having continuous epidural analgesia (CEA). (5 marks)
b) Give four organisational factors that are necessary to ensure safe management of CEA in the ward setting. (4 marks)
c) State two aspects of equipment monitoring that must be undertaken regularly throughout the duration of CEA. (2 marks)
d) State four aspects of patient monitoring that must be undertaken regularly throughout the duration of CEA. (4 marks)
e) State three safety features of the pump used for CEA. (3 marks)
f) State two safety features of the epidural infusion system used for CEA. (2 marks)

The Chair's Report for this question when it appeared as an SAQ stated that it was based on "Best Practice in the Management of Epidural Analgesia in the Hospital Setting," published by the Faculty of Pain Medicine of the Royal College of Anaesthetists three years before the exam question, and so knowledge of this guidance would have made answering very straightforward. However, I think that any anaesthetist who regularly cares for patients with epidurals should be able to answer this question well and this was reflected by a good pass rate of 70.4%. The guideline has since been updated in 2020.

a) **State five complications that should be rapidly recognisable by healthcare professionals caring for patients having continuous epidural analgesia (CEA). (5 marks)**

- Hypotension.
- Spinal canal space-occupying lesions (epidural haematoma or abscess), which may present with lower limb neurology.
- Total spinal.
- Post-dural puncture headache.
- Local anaesthetic toxicity.
- Nerve damage.

b) **Give four organisational factors that are necessary to ensure safe management of CEA in the ward setting. (4 marks)**

- Adequate staff training; anaesthetists, specialist pain nurses, and ward nursing staff.
- Inpatient pain service led by consultant or SAS anaesthetist.
- Protocols for all aspects of CEA management including identification and management of complications.
- Twenty-four-hour anaesthetic service to manage problems out of hours.
- Handover of ongoing CEAs for at least daily review.
- Resuscitation equipment, Intralipid, and naloxone should be readily available.

c) **State two aspects of equipment monitoring that must be undertaken regularly throughout the duration of CEA. (2 marks)**

- Venous cannula patency.
- Pump infusion rate, name, and concentration of drugs used.

d) State four aspects of patient monitoring that must be undertaken regularly throughout the duration of CEA. (4 marks)

- Heart rate.
- Blood pressure.
- Respiratory rate.
- Sedation score.
- Temperature.
- Pain score at rest and on movement.
- Motor and sensory block.
- National Early Warning Score 2 (NEWS2)/paediatric alternative.
- Epidural insertion site checking for inflammation and leakage.

e) State three safety features of the pump used for CEA. (3 marks)

- Configured for epidural analgesia only, in millilitres.
- Pre-set limits for maximum infusion rate and bolus size.
- Lock-out time if used for PCEA.
- Alarms (air, end of infusion, high pressure).
- Locked box (but able to see fluid without unlocking).
- Lock/code required for programming/bolus administration.
- Documented maintenance programme.

f) State two safety features of the epidural infusion system used for CEA. (2 marks)

- Closed, no injection ports.
- Antibacterial filter.
- Yellow stripe to infusion system.
- NRFit connections.

REFERENCE

Faculty of Pain Medicine of the Royal College of Anaesthetists et al. *Best practice in the management of epidural analgesia in the hospital setting.* London: The Royal College of Anaesthetists, 2020.

18.4 March 2014 Back pain

A 68-year-old patient attends the Pain Management Clinic with a history of intractable low back pain.

a) What symptoms and signs would alert you to the need for urgent investigation and referral? (10 marks)

b) List recommended treatment options that may be considered (with examples) if a magnetic resonance imaging (MRI) scan has excluded significant pathology. (10 marks)

This SAQ appeared in March 2014 and was virtually identical to the one from September 2011. I have left it here for you in its old SAQ format along with this extract from the Chair's Report, which gives insight to the aspects of answering that would have scored marks: "68.9% pass rate. Generally well answered. Most candidates understood the importance of 'red flags' in this clinical scenario. Some candidates ignored the result of the MRI scan and gave treatment options which referred to abnormal imaging (e.g. surgical approaches) and consequently detracted from their score. Reference to psychological and alternate/complementary therapies contributed to a high scoring answer."

18.5 September 2014 Rib fractures

You are called to the emergency department to assess a 63-year-old man with known chronic respiratory disease. He has sustained unilateral fractures to his 9th, 10th, and 11th ribs but has no other injuries. Regular administration of paracetamol and codeine phosphate have not provided adequate pain relief.

a) Give four respiratory problems which could result from inadequate pain relief in this patient. (4 marks)
b) State two ways in which the effectiveness of his pain relief can be assessed. (2 marks)
c) List four factors, relating to the patient or their rib fracture injuries at the point of presentation, that are predictive of an increased risk of mortality. (4 marks)
d) State two other pharmacological approaches to management of this patient's pain. (2 marks)
e) List four regional analgesia options which may be considered for management of rib fracture pain and, for each, comment on what anatomical locations of the fractures would indicate use of that technique. (4 marks)
f) Give three indications for consideration of surgical fixation of fractured ribs. (3 marks)
g) State which ribs are most likely to be fractured as a consequence of trauma. (1 mark)

The Chair's Report for the SAQ on this topic stated that it had been thought to be too easy when discussed at the Standards Setting Day. They were therefore surprised when the pass rate was only 43.7%. They commented that "many candidates were unable to suggest how the effectiveness of analgesic interventions could be assessed, and few offered regional techniques in their answer. It was surprising that a number suggested codeine/paracetamol compounds in their answer despite the question indicating that these agents had been unhelpful. This emphasises the need to read the question thoroughly." However, I know if I had been answering this question as an SAQ, I would have felt that it was important to state that codeine and paracetamol should be given regularly as it did not say so in the original question (I have changed it so that it now does in its CRQ form). Many hospitals will have a guideline for the management of rib fractures, reiterating just how much of the revision for this exam can be done just by maximising your clinical learning opportunities.

a) **Give four respiratory problems which could result from inadequate pain relief in this patient. (4 marks)**

- Inadequate ventilation due to pain, reduced PaO_2, increased $PaCO_2$ OR respiratory failure.
- Basal atelectasis.
- V/Q mismatch.
- Failure of secretion clearance.
- Pneumonia.

b) **State two ways in which the effectiveness of his pain relief can be assessed. (2 marks)**

- Pain scores, either VAS (visual analogue scores) or matching face to pain.
- Assessment of pain at rest, on movement, when deep breathing, when coughing, on incentive spirometry, and ability to comply with respiratory physiotherapy.
- Frequency of use of breakthrough pain medication.

c) List four factors, relating to the patient or their rib fracture injuries at the point of presentation, that are predictive of an increased risk of mortality. (4 marks)

There are likely to be other factors that are associated with an increased risk of mortality, but these ones have been proven and incorporated into a risk-prediction tool.

- Increasing patient age.
- Increasing numbers of rib fractures (*each actual fracture being counted rather than the number of individual ribs that have fractures*).
- Pre-existing chronic lung condition.
- Use of anticoagulants before the injury.
- Lower oxygen saturations.

d) State two other pharmacological approaches to management of this patient's pain. (2 marks)

There are some small-scale studies that have assessed the use of lidocaine patches and have shown some improvements in pain scores or opioid usage, but their use has not been adopted in the guidelines featured in the BJA Education articles referenced. There is also the option to try ketamine or gabapentinoids for their opioid-sparing effect, but if a patient is not controlled on the simple multimodal approaches detailed in this answer, then they need a regional analgesic technique.

- Consider NSAIDs; must actively seek contraindications, limit duration, and consider gastrointestinal protection.
- Add oral morphine sulphate immediate release solution (or oxycodone immediate release if reduced renal function) as required to the regular codeine, and then change to modified release oral morphine once total daily opioid dose required is known.
- Opioid PCA (morphine, fentanyl or oxycodone). However, if the patient already has compromised respiratory function, beware of causing further deterioration.

e) List four regional analgesia options which may be considered for management of rib fracture pain and, for each, comment on what anatomical locations of the fractures would indicate use of that technique. (4 marks)

- Thoracic epidural for bilateral fractures (*offers excellent analgesia for both unilateral and bilateral fractures but might be limited by hypotensive effect and can usually only be managed in specific wards*).
- Erector spinae catheter for posterior fractures.
- Serratus anterior plane catheter for anterior or lateral fractures.
- Thoracic paravertebral catheter for unilateral fractures, or can be performed bilaterally.

f) Give three indications for consideration of surgical fixation of fractured ribs. (3 marks)

- Flail chest or other severe chest wall deformity.
- Failure to wean from artificial ventilation due to rib fractures.
- Problems with pain management in non-intubated patients despite appropriate analgesic and regional technique use.
- Patients undergoing thoracotomy for associated thoracic injury.
- Problematic rib fracture non-union.
- Scoring predictive of respiratory compromise or increased mortality.

Chapter 18 PAIN MEDICINE

457

g) State which ribs are most likely to be fractured as a consequence of trauma. (1 mark)

Ribs 1–3 are relatively protected by the clavicle and shoulder girdle, and ribs 11 and 12 are "floating" and so are more mobile and less likely to be fractured.

- Ribs 4–10 are most likely to be fractured.

REFERENCES

Battle C et al. Predicting outcomes after blunt chest wall trauma: development and external validation of a new prognostic model. *Crit Care.* 2014: 18: R98.

May L, Hillermann C, Patil S. Rib fracture management. *BJA Educ.* 2016: 16: 26–32.

Williams A, Bighma C, Marchbank A. Anaesthetic and surgical management of rib fractures. *BJA Educ.* 2020: 20: 332–340.

18.6 March 2015 Post-amputation pain syndrome

You are called to see a 25-year-old man who suffered a traumatic below knee amputation 24 hours ago. He is using a morphine patient-controlled analgesia (PCA) and was comfortable until two hours ago, when he started to experience severe pain.

a) Give four reasons why his pain control may be inadequate. (4 marks)
b) List four measures that could be considered to re-establish pain control. (4 marks)
c) List three features of the patient's pain that would suggest that he has post-amputation pain syndrome. (3 marks)
d) List three first-line oral pharmacological options available for long term management of post-amputation pain syndrome. (3 marks)
e) List two non-orally administered pharmacological options available for long-term management of post-amputation pain syndrome in the event of failure of effect or lack of patient tolerance of first line agents. (2 marks)
f) Give four risk factors for the development of post-amputation pain syndrome. (4 marks)

The Chair's Report for the SAQ on this subject revealed that this was a very discriminatory question with a 53.6% pass rate and 10% of candidates receiving a poor fail: "weak candidates simply wrote 'neuropathic pain' as the answer and did not describe what they meant by the term." Post-amputation pain syndrome occurs because of nerve damage, resulting in changes to the nervous system at multiple locations, causing dysfunctional transmission of sensory information and abnormal pain perception.

Peripheral nerves:

- *Upregulation of sodium and calcium channels – spontaneous firing of damaged nerves peripherally or in dorsal root ganglion (DRG).*
- *Neuroma development in damaged nerves that are sensitive to chemical or mechanical stimuli.*
- *Neural injury due to amputation causes release of pro-inflammatory mediators that lower the activation thresholds of nociceptors.*

Spinal cord:

- *Aβ fibres from Rexed's laminae III and IV sprout into Rexed's laminae I and II due to the absence of input from C fibres from amputated limb – therefore, touch and pressure may be interpreted as pain (allodynia). NMDA receptors are thought to have a critical role in this phenotypic change.*
- *Sympathetic nerves sprout into the dorsal root ganglion, again stimulating pain pathways.*

Somatosensory cortex:

- *Errors in cortical remapping of the homunculus – over-amplification of pain experience, touch being interpreted as pain, pain being felt when other structures touched. Increased activity in a number of brain centres involved in the emotional and autonomic response to pain.*

a) Give four reasons why his pain control may be inadequate. (4 marks)

Imagine yourself being called to the ward to see this patient – what would your thought processes be? It has not stated where the pain is, so consider other causes.

- Failure of morphine delivery; check syringe full, pump working well, patient using pump well, cannula patent.

- Nociceptive pain problem; e.g. development of infection, wound dehiscence, haematoma formation in stump.
- Neuropathic pain problem; development of phantom limb pain due to nerve damage resulting in changes to the nervous system at multiple locations, causing dysfunctional transmission of sensory information and abnormal pain perception.
- Other pain source; major trauma victim – check for coexisting injuries.
- Loss of effect from any regional or neuraxial blocks used at time of management of his traumatic limb amputation.

b) **List four measures that could be considered to re-establish pain control. (4 marks)**

- Intravenous morphine titrated to effect (with oxygen saturations, respiratory rate, heart rate, and blood pressure monitoring) and consideration of increasing PCA bolus dose and hourly limit if considered safe to do so (may need HDU admission).
- Multimodal approach; check that the patient is receiving regular paracetamol and NSAIDs if appropriate.
- Initiate antineuropathic agent if indicated.
- Ketamine infusion.
- Sciatic nerve block or catheter *(as this is a below knee amputation. Femoral and sciatic nerve blocks or catheters should be considered for above knee amputation).*
- Epidural analgesia.

c) **List three features of the patient's pain that would suggest that he has post-amputation pain syndrome. (3 marks)**

- Nature of pain: shooting, burning, cramping, aching.
- Location of pain: distal to stump, associated with the missing leg.
- Degree of pain: apparent disproportion between pain experienced and stimulus applied.

d) **List three first-line oral pharmacological options available for long-term management of post-amputation pain syndrome. (3 marks)**

As per NICE CG173 and IASP NeuPSIG 2015 guidelines:

- Amitriptyline (TCA).
- Duloxetine or venlafaxine (SNRIs).
- Gabapentin OR gabapentin enacarbil/gabapentin extended release.
- Pregabalin.

e) **List two non-orally administered pharmacological options available for long-term management of post-amputation pain syndrome in the event of failure of effect or lack of patient tolerance of first line agents. (2 marks)**

As per NICE CG173 and IASP NeuPSIG 2015 guidelines:

- Capsaicin 8% patches.
- Lidocaine 5% patches.
- Botulinum toxin A.

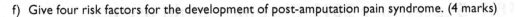

f) Give four risk factors for the development of post-amputation pain syndrome. (4 marks)

- Severe preoperative pain.
- Bilateral amputation.
- Severe nociceptive stump pain.
- Repeated limb surgeries.
- Increasing age.

REFERENCES

Finnerup N et al. Pharmacotherapy for neuropathic pain in adults: a systematic review, meta-analysis and updated NeuPSIG recommendations. *Lancet Neurol*. 2015: 14: 162–173.

Fitzmaurice B, Rayen A. Treatments for neuropathic pain: up-to-date evidence and recommendations. *BJA Educ*. 2018: 18: 277–283.

National Institute for Health and Care Excellence. *Neuropathic pain in adults: pharmacological management in non-specialist settings: CG173*, November 2013, updated September 2020. www.nice.org.uk/guidance/cg173/ifp/chapter/About-this-information. Last accessed 29th September 2022.

Neil M. Pain after amputation. *BJA Educ*. 2016: 16: 107–112.

18.7 September 2015 Chronic opioid use and surgical pain, spinal cord stimulators, and intrathecal drug delivery systems

a) List four opioid-sparing techniques that can be considered as part of the postoperative pain management plan for a patient taking regular opioids for non-malignant pain. (4 marks)

b) List three clinical features of opioid withdrawal. (3 marks)

c) List three clinical features of opioid overdose. (3 marks)

d) State the equianalgesic doses of oral tramadol, codeine, and oxycodone compared to 10 mg oral morphine. (3 marks)

e) List four perioperative implications of an existing spinal cord stimulator (SCS). (4 marks)

f) List three perioperative considerations for a patient who has an intrathecal drug delivery (ITDD) system. (3 marks)

The Chairs reported a 25% pass rate for the SAQ on this topic and said that it was considered a difficult question (which would therefore have meant that only 10–11 marks out of 20 would have been required to pass). The first part of the SAQ asked, for 8 marks, how you would manage the perioperative opioid requirements of a patient who is having elective surgery and who takes regular opioids for non-malignant pain. This clearly requires a much more freehand answer than is feasible in a CRQ, but I have reproduced an answer here as I think it contains useful knowledge about perioperative opioid management for such a patient. Interestingly, the Chairs said that "very few candidates gave any information about management of transdermal pain patches in the perioperative period. There are differing opinions as to whether patches should be continued, particularly in the case of buprenorphine, but candidates were able to gain marks for either opinion provided they showed that they were aware of the potential problems of altered absorption and partial antagonism." It is good to know the College will give marks for either stance where both are recognised approaches.

Perioperative ≐ preoperative + intraoperative + immediately postoperative.

Preoperative:

- *Involve chronic pain team for complex patients. Ensure the preoperative pain is as optimised as possible (consider use of non-opioids as a method of reducing opioid requirement).*

- *Establish the reason for the patient's opioid analgesia use. This may have implications for the perioperative period e.g. positioning limitations, may be the reason for the surgery.*

- *Establish drug, dose, duration of use, route of administration.*

- *Formulate plan for postoperative pain relief depending on the nature of surgery e.g. degree of pain likely to be involved, whether patient will be able to take medications via oral route, make calculations of opioid equivalence if patient's condition will dictate conversion to intravenous analgesia postoperatively. Need to ensure usual 24-hour dose PLUS extra to manage the pain from surgery.*

- *Normal doses of oral slow release and immediate release opioids to be taken on day of surgery.*

Intraoperative:

- *The decision as to whether to continue opioid patches depends on the nature of surgery. For example, it may be appropriate to continue patch with non-opioid analgesics and immediate-release oral morphine for breakthrough if day case surgery with low predicted*

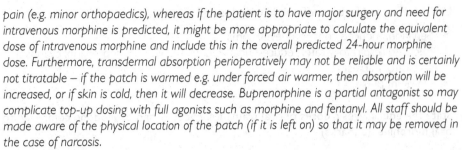

pain (e.g. minor orthopaedics), whereas if the patient is to have major surgery and need for intravenous morphine is predicted, it might be more appropriate to calculate the equivalent dose of intravenous morphine and include this in the overall predicted 24-hour morphine dose. Furthermore, transdermal absorption perioperatively may not be reliable and is certainly not titratable – if the patch is warmed e.g. under forced air warmer, then absorption will be increased, or if skin is cold, then it will decrease. Buprenorphine is a partial antagonist so may complicate top-up dosing with full agonists such as morphine and fentanyl. All staff should be made aware of the physical location of the patch (if it is left on) so that it may be removed in the case of narcosis.

- Awareness that larger doses of morphine intraoperatively will be required to achieve the same effect compared with opioid-naïve patients.
- Use of other analgesics such as paracetamol, NSAIDs (unless contraindicated), ketamine, neuraxial, and regional techniques to reduce overall opioid requirement.

Postoperative:

- Regular input from inpatient acute pain team.
- Higher bolus doses of morphine in PCA will need to be kept under review regularly as equivalence calculations are approximate; the patient is therefore at risk of both unrelieved pain and narcosis.
- Use pain scores to assess for unrelieved pain – aim to facilitate deep breathing, movement, physiotherapy.
- Be aware of signs of withdrawal or overdose.
- In view of the risks of either overdosing or withdrawal, it may be appropriate to manage the patient in a higher dependency setting than would normally be dictated by the nature of surgery, or extended recovery may be required.
- If intravenous morphine is used, convert back to oral dosing as soon as is feasible (consider any change in renal function postoperatively and its impact on opioid clearance).
- Make plan for de-escalation of opioids postoperatively and include this in discharge paperwork.

a) List four opioid-sparing techniques that can be considered as part of the postoperative pain management plan for a patient taking regular opioids for non-malignant pain. (4 marks)

- Regular paracetamol and NSAIDs (unless contraindicated).
- Regional analgesia – block or ongoing catheter technique.
- Neuraxial analgesia – spinal, spinal catheter, or epidural.
- Ketamine infusion.
- Gabapentinoids.
- Lidocaine infusion.
- Magnesium infusion.

b) List three clinical features of opioid withdrawal. (3 marks)

- Adrenergic hyperactivity (tachycardia, palpitations, sweating, hypertension, hyperthermia, piloerection, sweating).
- Generalised malaise, flu-like symptoms, myalgia.
- Abdominal cramps, diarrhoea, nausea, and vomiting.
- Lacrimation and rhinorrhoea.
- Yawning.

c) List three clinical features of opioid overdose. (3 marks)

- Sedation, reduced conscious level, coma.
- Reduced respiratory rate, reduced tidal volume, respiratory depression, cyanosis, respiratory arrest.
- Pin-point pupils.

d) State the equianalgesic doses of oral tramadol, codeine, and oxycodone compared to 10 mg oral morphine. (3 marks)

There is a useful guideline by the Faculty of Pain Medicine that details the conversion ratios for oral and transdermal opioids. Their conversion ratios are based on BNF data, but some of the other College publications give slightly different values.

Opioid	Equivalent dose to 10 mg oral morphine
Tramadol	100 mg
Codeine	100 mg
Oxycodone	6.6 mg

e) List four perioperative implications of an existing spinal cord stimulator (SCS). (4 marks)

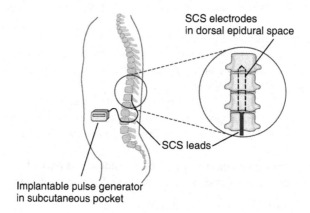

Spinal cord stimulator.

Spinal cord stimulators are used for neuropathic pain, CRPS, and ischaemic pain due to angina or peripheral vascular disease. They achieve their effect through gate control theory and modulation of release of other neurotransmitters. Leads are surgically placed in the dorsal epidural space (usually requires laminotomy) or percutaneously via a Tuohy needle. The leads are commonly placed at T8 or T9 level. The pulse generator can be left external to the body initially to check efficacy and then placed in a subcutaneous pocket (e.g. upper back, abdomen, gluteal) and the leads tunnelled to it subcutaneously.

- Seek advice from team that manages the patient's SCS.
- SCS turned off during surgery to avoid accidental reprogramming or activation by electromagnetic interference.
- Care with positioning. Device may have pressure area implications. Avoid excessive flexion, extension or rotational movements of the spine which increases risk of lead migration, especially in the early weeks after insertion.

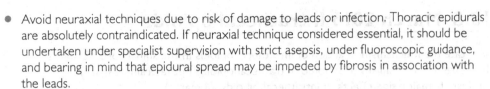

- Avoid neuraxial techniques due to risk of damage to leads or infection. Thoracic epidurals are absolutely contraindicated. If neuraxial technique considered essential, it should be undertaken under specialist supervision with strict asepsis, under fluoroscopic guidance, and bearing in mind that epidural spread may be impeded by fibrosis in association with the leads.
- Bipolar diathermy should be used wherever possible. If unipolar absolutely necessary, position the return plate to avoid electrical passage through the SCS.

f) List three perioperative considerations for a patient who has an intrathecal drug delivery (ITDD) system. (3 marks)

ITDD systems deliver drugs into the CSF and thus directly to the dorsal horn, meaning much smaller doses are required; opioids, local anaesthetic, clonidine or ziconotide for refractory pain, or baclofen for spasticity. The pump may be external or fully implanted with reservoir filling performed percutaneously. It may have a fixed rate or be programmable (beware – some will have their delivery rates affected by MRI). It may be sited anywhere from thoracic level to the second sacral segment. Risks: dural granuloma formation, leg oedema, infection, CSF leak, drug errors, complications and issues associated with the pump or catheter itself, human factor errors relating to lack of familiarity with ITDD systems.

- Should only be accessed/used/filled by clinicians experienced in their use.
- Significant risk of infection so spinal anaesthesia only if benefits considered to outweigh risks – consider location of ITDD system as this must be avoided. Intrathecal bolus may be given via the device if it is at a suitable level. However, the system will be primed with the usual drug it delivers, so beware delivering a large bolus along with the intended bolus.
- Meticulous aseptic technique when utilising the ITDD system to avoid risk of infection.
- Epidural catheter insertion is feasible above or below the ITDD system site but only if benefits considered by experts to outweigh risks.
- Opioid dosing as for opioid-naïve patient (unless patient also takes oral opioids).
- No diathermy within 30 cm of pump or catheter.

REFERENCES

British Pain Society. *Intrathecal drug delivery for the management of pain and spasticity in adults: recommendations for best clinical practice.* British Pain Society, 2015.

Bull C, Baranidharan G. Spinal cord stimulation and implications for anaesthesia. *BJA Educ.* 2020: 20: 182–183.

Faculty of Pain Medicine, Royal College of Anaesthetists. *Surgery and opioids: best practice guidelines,* 2021. https://fpm.ac.uk/sites/fpm/files/documents/2021-03/surgery-and-opioids-2021_4.pdf. Accessed 27th February 2023.

Lynch L. Intrathecal drug delivery systems. *Contin Educ Anaesth Crit Care Pain.* 2014: 14: 27–31.

National Institute for Health and Care Excellence. *Spinal cord stimulation for chronic pain of neuropathic or ischaemic origin: TA159,* October 2008.

Simpson G, Jackson M. Perioperative management of opioid-tolerant patients. *BJA Educ.* 2017: 17: 124–128.

18.8 March 2016 Intrathecal opioids

a) State the mechanism of action of intrathecal opioids in the spinal cord. (2 marks)
b) State the mechanism of action of intrathecal opioids in the brain. (1 mark)
c) List six major side effects of intrathecal opioids. (6 marks)
d) List five factors that may increase the risk of postoperative respiratory depression following administration of intrathecal opioids. (5 marks)
e) List four regional anaesthesia techniques that may be used to support the postoperative pain management of a patient undergoing an elective laparotomy for resection of colonic tumour. (4 marks)
f) List two intravenous options that may be used to further reduce opioid requirements, apart from paracetamol and NSAIDs. (2 marks)

The SAQ on this topic had just a 31.7% pass rate. The Chairs reported, "It was anticipated that candidates would find this question difficult and this proved to be the case. Intrathecal opioids are used widely in anaesthetic practice, but candidates' knowledge of their use was poor. Advanced sciences are part of the intermediate curriculum, so knowledge of applied pharmacology is expected. Some candidates failed to read . . . the question and gave the side effects of intravenous opioids or intrathecal local anaesthetic in their answer." Once again, this question reiterated the importance of using College publications in your revision – I have reproduced the subsections (c) and (d) almost exactly as they appeared in the original SAQ format, and their answers were given in list form in a CEACCP article, "Intrathecal opioids in the management of acute postoperative pain," referenced below.

a) State the mechanism of action of intrathecal opioids in the spinal cord. (2 marks)

- Opioid receptors are located in Rexed's laminae I and II, presynaptically on C and Aδ fibres. Stimulation causes inactivation of voltage sensitive calcium channels (KOP) or potassium channel opening (DOP and MOP), resulting in hyperpolarisation of the cell membrane and so reduced release of excitatory neurotransmitters glutamate and substance P.
- To a lesser extent, opioid receptors are located postsynaptically where their activation causes potassium channel opening and indirect activation of descending inhibitory pathways from brainstem.

b) State the mechanism of action of intrathecal opioids in the brain. (1 mark)

- Intrathecal opioids spread in a cephalad direction (pumped upwards by effect of respiration and pulsation of brain with heartbeat) to cause central effects: stimulation of receptors in nucleus raphe magnus and periaqueductal grey results in reduced GABAergic tone on the descending inhibitory pathways, thus allowing them to exert an antinociceptive effect at spinal level.

c) List six major side effects of intrathecal opioids. (6 marks)

- Nausea and vomiting.
- Respiratory depression.
- Pruritus.
- Sedation.
- Delayed gastric emptying.
- Urinary retention.
- Sweating.

d) List five factors that may increase the risk of postoperative respiratory depression following administration of intrathecal opioids. (5 marks)

- Hydrophilic opioid use. *(Lipophilic opioids rapidly partition to receptor and non-receptor sites, i.e. epidural fat, myelin, white matter. CSF concentration reduces rapidly and so the peak in plasma concentration occurs rapidly. Therefore, centrally mediated respiratory depression and that mediated by decreased sensitivity of peripheral chemoreceptors happens early. Hydrophilic opioids, e.g. morphine, maintain a high CSF concentration for longer, allowing more drug to spread in a cephalad direction with time and for the peak plasma concentration, and thus respiratory depression, to occur much later.)*
- Increasing age.
- Concomitant use of long-acting sedatives.
- Coexisting respiratory disease.
- Positive pressure ventilation.
- Obstructive sleep apnoea.
- Obesity.

e) List four regional anaesthesia techniques that may be used to support the postoperative pain management of a patient undergoing an elective laparotomy for resection of colonic tumour. (4 marks)

- Single shot spinal or spinal catheter.
- Rectus sheath blocks or catheters.
- Transversus abdominis plane blocks.
- Thoracic epidural.
- Quadratus lumborum blocks.
- Transversalis fascia plane blocks.

f) List two intravenous options that may be used to further reduce opioid requirements, apart from paracetamol and NSAIDs. (2 marks)

- Intravenous lidocaine.
- Intravenous magnesium.
- Intravenous ketamine.

REFERENCES

Hindle A. Intrathecal opioids in the management of acute postoperative pain. *Contin Educ Anaesth Crit Care Pain.* 2008: 8: 81–85.

lilyas C, Jones J, Forley S. Management of the patient presenting for emergency laparotomy. *BJA Educ.* 2019: 19: 113–118.

McDonald J, Lambert G. Opioid receptors. *Contin Educ Anaesth Crit Care Pain.* 2005: 5: 22–25.

Onwochei D, Borglum J, Pawa A. Abdominal wall blocks for intra-abdominal surgery. *BJA Educ.* 2018: 18: 317–322.

Rucklidge M, Beattie E. Rectus sheath catheters for patients undergoing laparotomy. *BJA Educ.* 2018: 18: 166–172.

18.9 September 2016 Complex regional pain syndrome

a) Complete the following table listing the four main categories of symptoms and signs used to establish a diagnosis of complex regional pain syndrome (CRPS) and give an example of each. (4 marks)
b) List two other criteria, apart from symptoms and signs, that are required for the diagnosis of CRPS. (2 marks)
c) List two possible preventative measures that may protect against the development of CRPS. (2 marks)
d) List four conservative treatment options that may be important in the holistic management of a patient with CRPS. (4 marks)
e) List five pharmacological options for the management of symptoms of CRPS. (5 marks)
f) List three interventional techniques that may be considered in the management of CRPS. (3 marks)

When an SAQ on this topic appeared in 2016, the Chairs' Report stated a pass rate of 75.2% saying, "This question had the greatest predictive value of the 12, which means that candidates who scored highly in this question tended to do well overall. Most marks were gained in [the part] which dealt with treatment options for complex regional pain syndrome. The signs and symptoms of the syndrome are based on the Budapest criteria and knowledge of these appeared to be patchy." There was a very similar question in 2008 asking about the symptoms and signs of CRPS, how many of each are required to make a diagnosis (according to the Budapest Criteria of the IASP, the answer is at least one symptom in three or more of the four categories and at least one sign in two or more of the categories, although it is now appreciated that a person who has symptoms and signs that don't quite reach the threshold for diagnosis should still be considered for treatment for CRPS) and what the other prerequisites are for diagnosis. Note that the College added some CRQs to their website as examples of the new exam format in the lead-up to the change; one of them is on the topic of CRPS.

a) Complete the following table listing the four main categories of symptoms and signs used to establish a diagnosis of complex regional pain syndrome (CRPS) and give an example of each. (4 marks)

Category	Symptoms	Signs
Sensory	Hyperaesthesia. Allodynia.	Hyperalgesia to pinprick testing. Allodynia.
Vasomotor	Temperature asymmetry. Skin colour changes. Skin colour asymmetry.	Temperature asymmetry. Skin colour changes. Skin colour asymmetry.
Sudomotor/oedema	Oedema. Sweating changes. Sweating asymmetry.	Oedema. Sweating changes. Sweating asymmetry.
Motor/trophic	Decreased range of motion. Motor dysfunction (weakness, tremor, dystonia). Trophic changes (hair, nail, skin).	Decreased range of motion. Motor dysfunction (weakness, tremor, dystonia). Trophic changes (hair, nail, skin).

b) List two other criteria, apart from symptoms and signs, that are required for the diagnosis of CRPS. (2 marks)

- Continuing pain disproportionate to inciting event.
- No other diagnosis that can better explain the symptoms and signs.

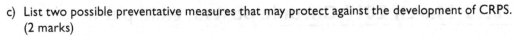

c) List two possible preventative measures that may protect against the development of CRPS. (2 marks)

- Vitamin C 500 mg once a day for 50 days after wrist fracture has been shown to reduce development of CRPS.
- Early rehabilitation after trauma with vigilance for development of abnormal pain responses.

d) List four conservative treatment options that may be important in the holistic management of a patient with CRPS. (4 marks)

- Patient education.
- Physical therapies including desensitisation, gradual weight bearing, fine motor exercises, aerobic conditioning, TENS, hydrotherapy, mirror visual feedback.
- Oedema control strategies.
- Occupational therapy; pacing, prioritising, planning, vocational support, relaxation techniques.
- Psychological interventions; psychologist input as part of multidisciplinary pain management programme, cognitive behavioural therapy.

e) List five pharmacological options for the management of symptoms of CRPS. (5 marks)

- Tricyclic antidepressant e.g. amitriptyline.
- Gabapentinoids e.g. gabapentin or pregabalin.
- Selective serotonin and noradrenaline reuptake inhibitors e.g. duloxetine.
- TRPV1 receptor agonist i.e. capsaicin cream.
- Opioids e.g. tramadol for rescue therapy only.
- Vasodilator e.g. calcium channel antagonist or alpha-1 adrenoceptor antagonists for symptoms of redness and heat of the affected part.
- NMDA receptor antagonism e.g. ketamine intravenous infusion – weak evidence.
- Oral baclofen for dystonia.

f) List three interventional techniques that may be considered in the management of CRPS. (3 marks)

- Spinal cord stimulation.
- Dorsal ganglion stimulation.
- Intrathecal baclofen administration for dystonia.
- Sympathetic nerve blocks *(weak evidence)*.
- Targeted botulinum toxin injection for dystonia *(weak evidence)*.

REFERENCES

Bharwani K et al. Complex regional pain syndrome: diagnosis and treatment. *BJA Educ.* 2017: 17: 262–268.

Ganty P, Chawla R. Complex regional pain syndrome: recent updates. *Contin Educ Anaesth Crit Care Pain.* 2014: 14: 79–84.

Goebel A et al. *Complex regional pain syndrome in adults: UK guidelines for diagnosis, referral and management in primary and secondary care.* London: Royal College of Physicians, 2018.

National Institute for Health and Care Excellence. *Neuropathic pain – drug treatment,* August 2022. https://cks.nice.org.uk/topics/neuropathic-pain-drug-treatment/management/neuropathic-pain-drug-treatment/. Last accessed 29th September 2022.

18.10 March 2017 Chronic postsurgical pain

a) List the diagnostic features of chronic postsurgical pain. (3 marks)
b) List five surgical procedures commonly associated with chronic postsurgical pain. (5 marks)
c) List four patient-related risk factors for the development of chronic postsurgical pain. (4 marks)
d) Apart from the risk attributed to specific procedures, list four risk factors for the development of chronic postsurgical pain related to the surgery itself or associated perioperative treatment. (4 marks)
e) List two possible anaesthetic interventions that may be employed to minimise the risk of chronic postsurgical pain. (2 marks)
f) State the peripheral and central nervous system changes that occur in the development of chronic postsurgical pain. (2 marks)

The Chairs' Report for the SAQ on this topic said that it had been judged to be a "hard" question (thus requiring 10–11/20 to pass). They said that "global knowledge of this syndrome was poor," and the section on pathophysiology was "particularly badly answered" resulting in a pass rate of just 37.4%.

a) List the diagnostic features of chronic postsurgical pain. (3 marks)

- Pain developing or increasing after surgical procedure.
- Pain persisting beyond healing process (> 3 months).
- Pain localised to surgical area or area (dermatome or Head's zone) with related innervation.
- Other causes excluded.
- May be neuropathic in nature.

b) List five surgical procedures commonly associated with chronic postsurgical pain. (5 marks)

It is difficult to give a definitive list as different studies have assessed different operations, based on differing definitions. There is also likely to be a reporting bias for operations performed at high volume and therefore more readily studied. These procedures seem to feature most commonly.

- Amputation.
- Thoracotomy.
- Craniotomy.
- Inguinal hernia repair.
- Mastectomy.
- Cholecystectomy.
- Caesarean section.
- Sternotomy.
- Knee arthroplasty.
- Vasectomy.

c) List four patient-related risk factors for the development of chronic postsurgical pain. (4 marks)

- Younger age.
- Lower educational level.
- Psychological factors: anxiety, fear of surgery, depression.
- Genetic susceptibility.
- Higher BMI.

- Female sex.
- Poor social support, unemployment.
- Preoperative pain either at the surgical site or other chronic pain conditions such as fibromyalgia or preoperative opioid use.

d) **Apart from the risk attributed to specific procedures, list four risk factors for the development of chronic postsurgical pain related to the surgery itself or associated perioperative treatment. (4 marks)**

- Procedures that involve significant nerve and tissue damage.
- Longer duration of surgery.
- Surgical complications.
- Repeated surgery.
- Poor pain control postoperatively, days of poor control being worse than a single episode of severe pain.
- Adjuvant radiotherapy.
- Adjuvant neurotoxic chemotherapy.

e) **List two anaesthetic interventions that may be employed to minimise the risk of chronic postsurgical pain. (2 marks)**

The two interventions listed in the answer are the only ones for which there is reasonable evidence. A number of agents have been investigated for their possible effect on reduction of development of chronic postsurgical pain, but conclusive data is lacking. Such agents include ketamine, magnesium, clonidine, dexmedetomidine, gabapentinoids, and intravenous lidocaine. NSAIDs and COX-2 inhibitors reduce inflammation and so would remove some of the trigger to the peripheral changes in the nervous system that occur with transition to chronic pain. Some of these agents may, of course, be a useful aspect of effective multimodal analgesia.

- Use of regional anaesthesia.
- Reduction of opioid dose through use of multimodal analgesia.

f) **State the peripheral and central nervous system changes that occur in the development of chronic postsurgical pain. (2 marks)**

This is clearly a very simplified answer. I include this question here more for education than because I think the College could ask it in this style. A subsection of the original SAQ asked about changes at spinal cord level for 4 marks.

- Peripheral: repeated peripheral nerve stimulation or nerve damage causes inflammation with activation of lymphocytes and release of inflammatory mediators. Leads to increased sodium and calcium channel expression resulting in reduced threshold for, or spontaneous, firing of peripheral nerves. Abnormal neuronal sprouting at the neurone terminals results in enlargement of the receptive field.
- Central: increased glutamate release from first-order neurones at the dorsal horn increases glutamate (NMDA) receptor density at postsynaptic membranes on second-order neurones, increasing transmission. Transmission occurs in previously inactive second-order neurones, neurones that do not normally transmit pain information, and may persist beyond duration of initial input. There may be loss of inhibitory neurones and reduction in descending inhibitory pathway activity. Microglia, activated by nerve damage, release substances that further sensitise and excite neurones. Increased activity in a number of brain centres associated with the perception and emotional and autonomic responses to pain e.g. thalamus, periaqueductal grey.

REFERENCES

Feizerfan A, Sheh G. Transition from acute to chronic pain. *Contin Educ Anaesth Crit Care Pain*. 2015: 15: 98–102.

International Classification of Diseases 11th Revision. *World Health Organisation*, Version February 2022. https://icd.who.int/browse11/l-m/en#/http://id.who.int/icd/entity/302680255. Accessed 16th September 2022.

Niraj G, Rowbotham D. Persistent postoperative pain: where are we now? *BJA*. 2011: 107: 25–29.

Rosenberger D, Pogatzki-Zahn E. Chronic post-surgical pain – update on incidence, risk factors and preventive treatment options. *BJA Educ*. 2022: 22: 190–196.

Werner M, Kongsgaard U. Defining persistent post-surgical pain: is an update required? *BJA*. 2014: 113: 1–4.

18.11 September 2017 Rib fractures

You are called to the emergency department to assess a 63-year-old man with known chronic obstructive pulmonary disease (COPD). He has sustained fractures to his 9th, 10th, and 11th ribs but has no other injuries. Paracetamol and codeine phosphate have not provided adequate pain relief.

a) What are the possible effects on the respiratory system of inadequate pain relief in this patient? (6 marks)

b) How can the effectiveness of his pain relief be monitored? (5 marks)

c) What methods, other than the drugs that have already been given, are available to improve management of this patient's pain? (9 marks)

This question, left here unchanged from its original SAQ format, was virtually identical to that from September 2014. The Chairs reported a 74.8% pass rate and were reassured "to see such widespread appreciation of how to monitor and manage a common but potentially serious condition." I wonder if the good success rate relates partly to the repetition of questions based on important and commonly encountered topics.

18.12 March 2018 Cancer pain

a) List six possible causes of pain in a patient with advanced cancer. (6 marks)
b) List three approaches to minimise side effects from opioid medications in patients with advanced cancer. (3 marks)
c) State the method by which the dose of a modified-release morphine preparation can be established in a patient who has been receiving immediate-release morphine for cancer pain. (2 marks)
d) List five pharmacological approaches to managing advanced cancer pain apart from the use of opioid medications. (5 marks)
e) List four non-pharmacological approaches to managing advanced cancer pain. (4 marks)

When an SAQ on this topic appeared in 2018, the Chairs' Report reflected that this question was new and that the pass mark was high at 85.5%. It was almost as if the questions related directly to the content of two articles on cancer pain management from CEACCP articles in 2014 and 2015. CEACCP and BJA Education articles really are a great source of Final FRCA revision.

a) List six possible causes of pain in a patient with advanced cancer. (6 marks)

- Local mass effect causing inflammation, compression, oedema, ischaemia, visceral stretch, bowel-obstruction, necrosis – affects neural and non-neural tissue.
- Pain-inducing chemical release by tumour including prostaglandins, interleukins, leukotrienes that sensitise nerve endings to painful stimuli.
- Treatment-associated causes including acute or chronic postsurgical pain, radiation-induced neuritis or plexopathy, chemotherapy-induced neuropathy.
- Chronic pain development consequent to any of the primary causes of pain.
- Paraneoplastic phenomena; anti-Hu and Yo neuronal antibodies causing peripheral neuropathy, or mono- or polyneuropathy.
- Associated conditions; infection, immunosuppression-induced herpetic reactivation, hypercalcaemia, osteoporosis, pathological fracture, immobility.
- Exacerbation of pre-existing conditions.
- Psychological state of patient exacerbating experience of all of the above.

b) List three approaches to minimise side effects from opioid medications in patients with advanced cancer. (3 marks)

- Minimise overall opioid dose by using the WHO analgesia ladder and adjuvant therapies (pharmacological, interventional, psychological, complementary).
- Targeted management of specific side effects (laxatives for constipation, antiemetics for nausea and vomiting).
- Co-administration with a specific antagonist such as naloxone.
- Rotation of opioid type to minimise side effect profile for individual patient.
- Experienced clinician managing prescription to maintain lowest possible dosage and convert to use of long-acting preparation to reduce risk of addiction.

c) State the method by which the dose of a modified-release morphine preparation can be established in a patient who has been receiving immediate-release morphine for cancer pain. (2 marks)

- Ensure control is adequate and daily usage is stable, total the doses of immediate-release preparation excluding the doses used for pain control due to specific triggers such as movement ("incident pain").
- Give this dose as a single dose if a 24 hour preparation is selected or divide into two for a 12-hour preparation. *Continue to offer immediate-release morphine for breakthrough and incident pain.*

d) List five pharmacological approaches to managing advanced cancer pain apart from the use of opioid medications. (5 marks)

- WHO analgesic ladder; regular paracetamol, NSAIDs if not contraindicated.
- Neuropathic pain medications; gabapentinoids, tricyclics, lidocaine.
- Other adjuvant pain-relieving treatments; ketamine, cannabinoids.
- Treatment of underlying cause; antispasmodics for colic pain, bisphosphonates for bone pain, steroids for spinal cord compression, pain of raised intracranial pressure, or for acute shrinkage of susceptible tumours.
- Nerve blocks; somatic or visceral, using local anaesthetic with or without steroid.
- Oncological treatments; chemotherapy may achieve rapid reduction in tumour size and therefore reduction in mass-effect-induced pain; hormone therapy for susceptible tumours, immunotherapy.
- Management of associated depression or anxiety with e.g. SSRI.

e) List four non-pharmacological approaches to managing advanced cancer pain. (4 marks)

- Surgery; management of pathological fractures, bowel surgery alleviating obstruction.
- Radiotherapy.
- Physical therapies; graded exercise, physiotherapy.
- Psychological therapies; CBT, counselling.
- Complementary therapies; acupuncture, aromatherapy, reflexology.
- Interventional treatments; neurolytic nerve blocks (somatic, visceral, or intrathecal).

REFERENCES

National Institute for Health and Care Excellence. *Palliative cancer care – pain*, March 2021. https://cks.nice.org.uk/topics/palliative-cancer-care-pain/management/.

Scott-Warren J, Bhaskar A. Cancer pain management: part I: general principles. *Contin Educ Anaesth Crit Care Pain.* 2014: 14: 278–284.

Scott-Warren J, Bhaskar A. Cancer pain management: part II: interventional techniques. *Contin Educ Anaesth Crit Care Pain.* 2015: 15: 68–72.

18.13 September 2018 Chronic opioid use and surgical pain, spinal cord stimulators

The SAQ on this topic was very similar in content to that from September 2015 except it did not ask about intrathecal drug delivery devices and asked very specifically about how buprenorphine should be managed in the perioperative period. The pass rate of the question was 73.9%, the highest of the paper, but the Chairs stated that "there was a lack of knowledge [of] problems with buprenorphine treatment." The subsections of the SAQ about buprenorphine are the only part of the question that I address here as all other sections have been covered previously.

a) **What possible pain control issues might chronic buprenorphine use cause perioperatively? (2 marks)**

   - Buprenorphine is a partial agonist at MOP but is an antagonist at KOP and DOP and has high affinity for receptors resulting in prolonged duration of action. Continued buprenorphine may reduce the maximal effect of other opioids administered perioperatively causing analgesic failure.

b) **What are the options for managing the chronic use of sublingual buprenorphine perioperatively? (2 marks)**

   - Rotate to full agonist well in advance of surgery.
   - Continue sublingual buprenorphine and give full analgesic doses of other opioid perioperatively OR supplemental buprenorphine.
   - Ensure maximal opioid-sparing analgesia given.

REFERENCE

Simpson G, Jackson M. Perioperative management of opioid-tolerant patients. *BJA Educ.* 2017: 17: 124–128.

18.14 March 2019 Post-amputation pain syndrome

This SAQ was identical to that from March 2015 except that it used the term post-amputation pain syndrome rather than phantom limb pain. The pass rate was only 52.7%. The Chairs' Report stated that "examiners were surprised at the lack of knowledge on this topic particularly as this question had been used recently. The condition is important and frequently seen, so candidates should know it in more detail than was demonstrated here. Poorer candidates were unable to describe the features or management of phantom limb pain." This really highlights the importance of looking at past papers and addressing topics that the College, very fairly, believe to be important due to the frequency with which they are encountered in the clinical setting.

18.15 September 2019 Intrathecal opioids

The September 2019 exam was a hybrid of six SAQs and six CRQs, and this question was one of the SAQs. Its content overlapped almost entirely with that from March 2016. The pass rate was 57.3% with the Chairs commenting that "this question had been used previously and this was reflected by an improvement in the pass rate. Candidates scored well in sections (a) and (c) but the mechanism of action of intrathecal opioids was answered poorly. Pain management requires a knowledge of advanced pharmacology and this is an area of the curriculum that is consistently neglected by candidates." This should further reinforce to you how important it is to revise topics that have featured previously and topics that reflect common clinical practice.

18.16 March 2020 Chronic opioid use and surgical pain

This was the first paper made up entirely of CRQs. The focus of the CRQ on this topic was on the acute pain management of a patient taking long-term opioids, the perioperative issues of opioid patches, and the specific issues with buprenorphine use. It would therefore all be familiar content to anyone who had had a look at past papers as it was covered by the pain module questions from September 2018 and September 2015. The Chairs commented that the pass rate was 70.7% but that "it was the feeling of the examiners that candidates lacked knowledge in the management and implications of analgesic patches. . . Candidates focused on comparing a buprenorphine patch and fentanyl patch rather than mentioning the peri-operative implications."

18.17 September 2020 Chronic postsurgical pain

There is a variety of terminology used to describe this syndrome, and the Chairs' Report for this paper calls it persistent postoperative pain. However, I'm sticking to chronic postsurgical pain as this is how it is described in the ICD-11. As in the question on this topic in March 2017, the focus was on the types of surgery that are associated with a higher risk of chronic postsurgical pain, the factors that seem to predispose to it, methods that may be employed to reduce its incidence, and the changes in the nervous system that occur with its development. It is important, for this exam and the viva, that you have a brief but comprehensible explanation ready of the normal pathways involved in pain sensation and how these change in the development of chronic pain. The Chairs reported a pass rate of 61.4% and said, "The management of patients with persistent post-operative pain is becoming a common clinical problem and this was reflected in a good pass rate for this question."

18.18 March 2021 Trigeminal neuralgia

a) List six clinical features of trigeminal neuralgia. (6 marks)
b) List five differential diagnoses of trigeminal neuralgia. (5 marks)
c) What is the cause of classical trigeminal neuralgia, and how is it diagnosed? (2 marks)
d) List four red flags that might indicate a serious underlying cause of trigeminal neuralgia. (4 marks)
e) State the first- and second-line drug treatment options for trigeminal neuralgia. (2 marks)
f) Give one non-pharmacological treatment option for classical trigeminal neuralgia. (1 mark)

The Chairs' Report said that the success rate of the CRQ on this topic was 67.5%. They reiterated the fact that you will only achieve one mark per line so not to waste time trying to cram more in: "Some candidates disadvantaged themselves and wrote as much as they could in the space provided. As per the candidate instructions, only the first distinct answer per line is marked." If there are more points that you want to write than lines available, aim to give as diverse a range of points as possible.

a) List six clinical features of trigeminal neuralgia. (6 marks)

- Unilateral facial pain affecting one or more divisions of the trigeminal nerve.
- Recurrent paroxysms of pain.
- Pain lasting from a fraction of a second to two minutes each time.
- Severe intensity.
- Electric shock-like, shooting, stabbing nature of pain.
- Precipitated by innocuous stimulation within the affected trigeminal distribution.

b) List five differential diagnoses of trigeminal neuralgia. (5 marks)

- Headache disorders such as cluster headache.
- Dental pain due to cracked tooth or abscess.
- Temporomandibular joint disorders.
- Sinusitis.
- Other neuralgias such a post-herpetic neuralgia, glossopharyngeal neuralgia.
- Tolosa-Hunt syndrome.
- Salivary gland disorders.

c) What is the cause of classical trigeminal neuralgia, and how is it diagnosed? (2 marks)

- Cause; compression of the nerve root by a nearby vascular structure resulting in morphological change to the nerve such as atrophy, displacement, distortion, or localised demyelination.
- Diagnosis; as per the clinical characteristics listed above in conjunction with MRI demonstrating compression of the nerve with morphological changes, not just contact with a vascular structure (or as seen during surgery).

d) List four red flags that might indicate a serious underlying cause of trigeminal neuralgia. (4 marks)

- Sensory changes.
- Deafness.
- History of skin or oral lesions that may spread perineurally.
- Pain only present in the ophthalmic division or bilateral pain.

- Optic neuritis.
- Family history of multiple sclerosis.
- Age of onset less than 40 years.

e) **State the first- and second-line drug treatment options for trigeminal neuralgia. (2 marks)**

- First-line; carbamazepine.
- Second-line; one of gabapentinoids, amitriptyline, phenytoin, topiramate, lamotrigine, baclofen. Oxcarbazepine if carbamazepine not used as first-line. *None of the second-line drugs are licenced for this use.*

f) **Give one non-pharmacological interventional treatment option for classical trigeminal neuralgia. (1 mark)**

- Microvascular decompression of the trigeminal nerve root in the posterior fossa.
- Stereotactic radiosurgery delivering focused radiation to the nerve root at the point of proven compression.
- Thermal, chemical, or mechanical ablation of the Gasserian ganglion.

REFERENCES

Headache Classification Committee of the International Headache Society. The International Classification of Headache Disorders. 3rd edition. 2018. https://ichd-3.org/13-painful-cranial-neuropathies-and-other-facial-pains/13–1-trigeminal-neuralgia/13–1–1-classical-trigeminal-neuralgia/13-1-1-1-classical-trigeminal-neuralgia-purely-paroxysmal/. Last accessed 26th September 2022.

National Institute for Health and Care Excellence. Clinical Knowledge Summaries: Trigeminal neuralgia. January 2022. https://cks.nice.org.uk/topics/trigeminal-neuralgia/ Last accessed 26th September 2022.

Vasappa C, Kapur S, Krovvidi H. Trigeminal neuralgia. *BJA Educ.* 2016: 16: 353–356.

Yao A, Barad M. Diagnosis and management of chronic facial pain. *BJA Educ.* 2020: 20(4): 120–125.

18.19 September 2021 Neuropathic pain and diabetic neuropathy

A 64-year-old man with a 20-year history of type 2 diabetes presents with pain and paraesthesia affecting his feet.

a) Define neuropathic pain. (1 mark)
b) List four characteristic features of neuropathic pain. (4 marks)
c) Apart from his diabetes, list five possible causes for neuropathic pain in the distribution described that should be considered. (5 marks)
d) List five risk factors for development of peripheral neuropathy in patients affected by diabetes. (5 marks)
e) List the two main mechanisms that result in peripheral nerve damage in diabetes. (2 marks)
f) What is the first line treatment of this patient's painful diabetic peripheral neuropathic pain? (1 mark)
g) In what circumstances would capsaicin be indicated in the management of this patient's neuropathic pain? (1 mark)
h) What is the mechanism of action of capsaicin in the management of neuropathic pain? (1 mark)

There was no Chairs' Report for the September 2021 sitting of the CRQ paper. However, the focus of this question reiterates the importance of a thorough understanding of the diagnosis and management of neuropathic pain.

a) Define neuropathic pain. (1 mark)

- Pain that arises as a direct consequence of a lesion or diseases affecting the somatosensory system.

b) List four characteristic features of neuropathic pain. (4 marks)

- Paraesthesia – prickling, tingling, pins-and-needles sensations in the absence of stimulation.
- Spontaneous episodes of pain.
- Allodynia – painful sensation in response to usually innocuous stimulation.
- Pain is shooting, electric shock, burning in nature.
- Hyper- or hypoalgesia (exaggerated or lack of response to a mildly painful stimulus e.g. pinprick).

c) Apart from his diabetes, list five possible causes for neuropathic pain in the distribution described that should be considered. (5 marks)

- Hypothyroidism.
- Vitamin B12 deficiency.
- Alcohol excess.
- HIV infection.
- Syphilis infection.
- Spinal stenosis.
- Cancer e.g. oat cell carcinoma of the lung, lymphoma.
- Autoimmune conditions such as SLE, rheumatoid arthritis.
- Benign monoclonal gammopathy.

d) List five risk factors for development of peripheral neuropathy in patients affected by diabetes. (5 marks)

- Longer duration of diabetes.
- Poor glycaemic control.
- Hypertension.
- Smoking.
- Hyperlipidaemia.
- High BMI.

e) List the two main mechanisms that result in peripheral nerve damage in diabetes. (2 marks)

- Hyperglycaemia resulting in damage to and impairment of repair of microvascular supply to nervous tissue causing nerve tissue damage.
- Hyperglycaemia causing direct damage and damage via the generation of inflammatory mediators to nervous tissue.

f) What is the first line treatment of this patient's painful diabetic peripheral neuropathic pain? (1 mark)

- Amitriptyline, duloxetine, gabapentin or pregabalin.

g) In what circumstances would capsaicin be indicated in the management of this patient's neuropathic pain? (1 mark)

- If oral medications were not tolerated or if the patient did not want to take oral medications and pain is localised.

h) What is the mechanism of action of capsaicin in the management of neuropathic pain? (1 mark)

- Stimulation of TRPVI receptors (a type of calcium ion channel) in C-fibres causing initial release and subsequent depletion and reduction in release of substance P, thus reducing pain sensation transmission.

REFERENCES

Bennett M. The LANSS pain scale: the Leeds assessment of neuropathic symptoms and signs. *Pain.* 2001: 92: 147–157.

Fitzmaurice B, Rayen A. Treatments for neuropathic pain: up-to-date evidence and recommendations. *BJA Educ.* 2018: 18: 277–283.

International Association for the Study of Pain. www.iasp-pain.org/advocacy/global-year/neuropathic-pain/. Last accessed 29th September 2022.

National Institute for Health and Care Excellence. *Neuropathic pain – drug treatment*, August 2022. https://cks.nice.org.uk/topics/neuropathic-pain-drug-treatment/management/neuropathic-pain-drug-treatment/. Last accessed 29th September 2022.

Rajan R, de Gray L, George E. Painful diabetic neuropathy. *BJA Educ.* 2014: 14: 230–235.

18.20 March 2022 Post-amputation pain syndrome

This was the third appearance of this topic over the time frame covered by this book. The Chairs' Report stated a pass rate of just 46.9% with which they were rightly disappointed given the frequency of the topic's appearance in the exam. "No sections were answered particularly well, however, question performance correlated well with overall performance. Candidates struggled with the practical aspects of pain management . . . weaker candidates were unable to describe the features of phantom limb pain. A number of candidates listed the names of drugs as opposed to classes of drugs in section (d)." The wording of section (d) was new, as previous SAQs asked for "pharmacological options," which I would have answered with the usual options detailed in NICE guidance for management of neuropathic pain. However, if considering classes, I would have listed tricyclic antidepressants (i.e. amitriptyline), gabapentinoids (i.e. gabapentin, pregabalin), selective serotonin and noradrenaline reuptake inhibitors (SNRIs, i.e. duloxetine), TRPVI receptor agonist (i.e. capsaicin cream or patch), and opioids (tramadol is indicated for acute control whilst awaiting specialist input). However, the BJA Education article from 2016 that focuses on this topic also mentions NMDA antagonists.

REFERENCES

National Institute for Health and Care Excellence. *Neuropathic pain in adults: pharmacological management in non-specialist settings: CG173*, November 2013, updated September 2020. www.nice.org.uk/guidance/cg173/ifp/chapter/About-this-information. Last accessed 29th September 2022.

Neil M. Pain after amputation. *BJA Educ*. 2016: 16: 107–112.

18.21 September 2022 Rib fractures

This is the third appearance of this topic over the time frame of this book; it is a common clinical condition. The focus was on the respiratory complications of rib fractures, which ribs are most likely to be fractured and why, and the regional techniques that may be employed in the management of the associated pain. The Chairs reported a pass rate of 57.1% for the CRQ and said that the "analgesic components of this question were answered well. Candidates tended to drop marks on the stems relating to anatomy."

18.22 February 2023 Chronic postsurgical pain

This is the third time that chronic postsurgical pain has been the subject of the pain medicine question over the time frame of this book. The same knowledge was required to pass this question as those from 2017 and 2020, and the Chairs reported a pass rate of 65.5% saying that it "was a well answered question. As well as the definition, most candidates had a good idea about the risk factors and treatments."

19 OPHTHALMIC

19.1 September 2013 Regional anaesthesia for eye surgery

A 76-year-old man is scheduled for elective cataract surgery under local anaesthesia.
a) List three goals of local anaesthesia (LA) for this procedure. (3 marks)
b) State four LA techniques that may be used for cataract surgery. (4 marks)
c) List five contraindications to the use of LA as the sole technique for the procedure. (5 marks)
d) State four details specific to an LA block that should be documented in the anaesthetic record. (4 marks)
e) State four specific complications of performing a sub-Tenon's block. (4 marks)

The Chair's Report of the original SAQ found it to be "answered well and a good discriminator. The question was based on the document entitled 'Local Anaesthesia for Ophthalmic Surgery: joint guidelines from the Royal College of Anaesthetists and the Royal College of Ophthalmologists' (February 2012)." The pass rate was 81.5%.

I wouldn't have liked to find a question on ophthalmology in my Final. However, keeping an eye on the RCoA website in the months leading up to the exam should have alerted candidates to the publication of this guideline (a time lag like this is typical). Also, once the panic subsides, it's clear that even if the guideline hasn't been read, the points for parts (a) and (c) are readily achievable through application of common sense. For part (d), writing down the list of points you would record for any block would gain most of the points available – there is very little that is ophthalmic-specific in the answer I have given that comes directly from the guideline. After that, all you have to do is remember the names of some blocks that are specifically used in ophthalmic surgery.

a) List three goals of local anaesthesia (LA) for this procedure. (3 marks)

- To provide pain-free surgery.
- To facilitate the surgical procedure.
- To minimise the risk of systemic and local complications.
- To reduce the risk of surgical complications.

b) State four LA techniques that may be used for cataract surgery. (4 marks)

- Topical (with or without intracameral local anaesthesia).
- Subconjunctival.
- Sub-Tenon's.
- Peribulbar (extraconal).
- Retrobulbar (intraconal).

DOI: 10.1201/9781003388494-19

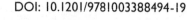

c) **List five contraindications to the use of LA as the sole technique for the procedure. (5 marks)**

- Patient refusal.
- Allergy to LA.
- Localised sepsis.
- Inability to cooperate due to anxiety, confusion, learning difficulties.
- Inability to lie flat and still due to musculoskeletal, respiratory or cardiac conditions, or significant cough.
- Inability to tolerate ocular manipulation without blepharospasm.
- Grossly abnormal coagulation.

d) **State four details specific to an LA block that should be documented in the anaesthetic record. (4 marks)**

More generically, you would need to include the name, job role, and GMC number of the person performing the block and the use of monitoring techniques, frequency, and recordings. Although not mentioned in the 2012 document, the use of "Prep, Stop, Block; Stop Before You Block" should be part of your answer if asked again.

The exact technique employed, including the following:

- Prep, Stop, Block; Stop Before You Block.
- Asepsis.
- Entry site/s.
- Length and type of needle/cannula.
- Volume and concentration of LA agent and adjuvant.
- Requirement for supplemental LA.
- Use of oculo-compression.
- Use of systemic analgesia or sedation.
- Quality of block.
- Complications.

e) **State four specific complications of performing a sub-Tenon's block. (4 marks)**

- Chemosis (conjunctival swelling).
- Subconjunctival haemorrhage.
- Orbital haemorrhage with risk of optic nerve and central retinal artery compression with risk of blindness.
- Retrobulbar haematoma.
- Globe perforation – risk is increased if length of eye is > 26 mm.
- Neuraxial LA spread/total spinal.
- Corneal abrasion.
- Prolonged muscular palsy causing diplopia.
- Allergy to hyaluronidase.

REFERENCES

Anker R, Kaur N. Regional anaesthesia for ophthalmic surgery. *BJA Educ.* 2017: 17: 221–227.

Royal College of Anaesthetists and the Royal College of Ophthalmologists. *Local anaesthesia for ophthalmic surgery: joint guidelines from the Royal College of Anaesthetists and the Royal College of Ophthalmologists*, 2012.

19.2 September 2018 Penetrating eye injury

An otherwise healthy, ASA 1, 32-year-old man who was involved in a road traffic accident has suffered a penetrating eye injury.

a) What factors determine the intraocular pressure in a healthy eye? (3 marks)

b) What key points would you need to know when assessing this patient preoperatively? (5 marks)

c) The patient requires urgent surgery. Discuss your specific intraoperative management. (4 marks)

d) What contraindications are there to performing a regional block in elective ophthalmic surgery? (5 marks)

e) What different types of regional block are suitable for ophthalmic surgery? (3 marks)

This SAQ was repeated almost identically as a CRQ in 2021, right down to the patient details! Even though you may have little experience of managing penetrating eye injuries, application of physiology and having some knowledge about regional ophthalmic blocks would get you most of the marks here. However, the pass rate was 41.9%, and the Chairs' Report said the "question was not well answered and possibly demonstrated a lack of experience in traumatic eye injuries. The examiners felt that the candidates failed to appreciate that this was an isolated injury in an otherwise fit patient. Some candidates also failed to appreciate the degree of neuromuscular block required." I am not clear that the question assures you that "this was an isolated injury," and I would definitely want to know about the possibility of associated injuries given there has been sufficient impact to have caused a penetrating eye injury.

19.3 March 2021 Penetrating eye injury

An ASA 1, 32-year-old man was involved in a road traffic accident and has suffered a penetrating eye injury.

a) Name the structure that separates the anterior and posterior chambers of the eye. (1 mark)
b) Name the transparent covering of the anterior aspect of the globe. (1 mark)
c) List three factors that determine the intraocular pressure in a healthy eye. (3 marks)
d) What key points would you need to know when assessing this patient preoperatively? (4 marks)
e) The patient requires urgent surgery. List five specific aspects of your intraoperative management. (5 marks)
f) List four contraindications to performing a regional block in elective ophthalmic surgery. (4 marks)
g) List two regional block techniques suitable for ophthalmic surgery. (2 marks)

The Chairs' Report on the original CRQ on this topic acknowledged that it "had previously been used in the SAQs and has been adapted for the CRQ format. The pass rate for this question was poor [33.2%] with many candidates not displaying much knowledge about the clinical aspects of anaesthetising a patient for an emergency eye operation. Additionally, candidates failed to answer the question asked, for example, [when] asked about factors controlling intraocular pressure … a number of candidates discussed factors controlling blood flow to the eye."

a) Name the structure that separates the anterior and posterior chambers of the eye. (1 mark)

- Iris.

b) Name the transparent covering of the anterior aspect of the globe. (1 mark)

- Cornea.

c) List three factors that determine the intraocular pressure in a healthy eye. (3 marks)

- Active secretion of aqueous humour by ciliary bodies.
- Passive secretion by ultrafiltration of aqueous humour, influenced by blood pressure, plasma oncotic pressure and intraocular pressure.
- Drainage via the trabecular network and canal of Schlemm dependent on balance between intraocular pressure and episcleral venous pressure.
- Reverse ultrafiltration into interstitium of sclera, dependent on pressure difference between it and the anterior chamber of the eye.

d) What key points would you need to know when assessing this patient preoperatively? (4 marks)

Tricky. It is hard to give a definitive list here, especially if the College are taking the view, as in the 2018 question, that this is an isolated injury in an otherwise well patient.

- Any associated injuries, especially brain and cervical spine, that would impact on prioritisation of issues or on conduct of anaesthesia.
- Fasting status in relation to timing of incident.
- Airway assessment.
- History of complications with anaesthesia, including tendency to postoperative nausea and vomiting.

- Size of perforation, with a larger hole leading to greater risk of extrusion of globe contents.
- Whether surgery is intended to be sight-saving, therefore impacting on the degree of urgency.

e) **The patient requires urgent surgery. List five specific aspects of your intraoperative management. (5 marks)**

- Rapid sequence induction for securing of the airway if the patient is not starved.
- Minimisation of rises in intraocular pressure: minimise sympathetic stimulation due to inadequate pain relief, ensure normalisation of PaO_2 and $PaCO_2$.
- Full muscle relaxation with monitoring of train-of-four to ensure full relaxation of extraocular muscles and also to facilitate optimum ventilation. Nerve stimulator can also be used to assure adequate relaxation before intubation attempts if rapid sequence induction is performed with rocuronium.
- Consideration of deep extubation or extubation facilitated by remifentanil if starvation status allows, to minimise coughing and straining at extubation which will cause spikes in intraocular pressure.
- Adequate antiemesis to minimise the rise in intraocular pressure caused by vomiting.
- Consideration of impact of drug choices on intraocular pressure (e.g. transient rise due to suxamethonium and ketamine, reduction with use of inhalational and most other intravenous agents) but ensuring that safely securing the airway takes priority.
- Avoidance of positional or mechanical causes of raised intraocular pressure; avoid tight tube ties, ensure head is in neutral position, make slight head-up tilt to operating table.

f) **List four contraindications to performing a regional block in elective ophthalmic surgery. (4 marks)**

This is a similar question to that asked in 2013 and 2018. Clearly, it's a list worth knowing.

- Patient refusal.
- Allergy to LA.
- Localised sepsis.
- Inability to cooperate due to anxiety, confusion, learning difficulties.
- Inability to lie flat and still due to musculoskeletal, respiratory or cardiac conditions, or significant cough.
- Inability to tolerate ocular manipulation without blepharospasm.
- Grossly abnormal coagulation.

g) **List two regional block techniques suitable for ophthalmic surgery. (2 marks)**

This is a slightly different question compared to that asked in 2013, specifying "regional block," rather than local anaesthetic techniques.

- Sub-Tenon's.
- Peribulbar (extraconal).
- Retrobulbar (intraconal).

REFERENCES

Anker R, Kaur N. Regional anaesthesia for ophthalmic surgery. *BJA Educ.* 2017: 17: 221–227.
Murgatroyd H, Bembridge J. Intraocular pressure. *Contin Educ Anaes Crit Care Pain.* 2008: 8: 100–103.

19.4 February 2023 Ophthalmic surgery

a) Describe the sensory innervation of the eye. (2 marks)
b) State normal intra-ocular pressure (mmHg) in an adult. (1 mark)
c) State the afferent and efferent pathways that mediate the oculo-cardiac reflex. (2 marks)
d) What part of the cardiac conduction pathway does the oculo-cardiac reflex affect? (1 mark)
e) List two possible perioperative triggers of the oculo-cardiac reflex. (2 marks)
f) State the anterior and posterior attachments of the Tenon's fascia. (2 marks)
g) List three benefits of sub-Tenon's block for ophthalmic surgery. (3 marks)
h) List two anaesthetic drugs that can cause a rise in intraocular pressure. (2 marks)
i) List five specific intraoperative aims when providing general anaesthesia for isolated penetrating eye injury. (5 marks)

The Chairs said that "despite being thought to be a difficult question this had the highest pass rate [of the paper]. The only poorly answered [subsections] were about the anatomy of Tenon's fascia – a small proportion of the overall marks for the question." The pass rate was 77.3%. The clinical principles of anaesthesia for penetrating eye injury, as addressed in subsections (h) and (i), have been previously assessed in questions on the same topic in March 2021 and September 2013. The remainder of the question involves a reasonably thorough knowledge of anatomy and physiology which reiterates the importance of basic sciences in the Final.

a) **Describe the sensory innervation of the eye. (2 marks)**

- Optic nerve for light perception *(leaves the globe posteriomedially, passes though orbit, and exits via optic foramen)*.
- Branches of the ophthalmic branch of the trigeminal nerve (V_1) for sensation *(lacrimal, frontal, and nasociliary branches, pass through superior orbital fissure)*.

b) **State normal intra-ocular pressure (mmHg) in an adult. (1 mark)**

- 10–21 mmHg.

c) **State the afferent and efferent pathways that mediate the oculo-cardiac reflex. (2 marks)**

The reflex occurs via synapses in the ciliary ganglion.

- Afferent: ophthalmic branch of the trigeminal nerve (V_1).
- Efferent: vagus nerve.

d) **What part of the cardiac conduction pathway does the oculo-cardiac reflex affect? (1 mark)**

- Sinoatrial node.

e) **List two possible perioperative triggers of the oculo-cardiac reflex. (2 marks)**

- Pressure in globe e.g. hydrostatic pressure of injectate of regional anaesthetic technique, pressure applied to encourage local anaesthesia spread (manually or with use of Honan balloon), pressure applied by surgeon during surgery.
- Traction on extra-ocular muscles e.g. in the performance of squint surgery.

f) **State the anterior and posterior attachments of the Tenon's fascia. (2 marks)**

- Anterior: the limbus, which is the corneoscleral junction.
- Posterior: dural sheath around optic nerve.

g) List three benefits of sub-Tenon's block for ophthalmic surgery. (3 marks)

- Provides an akinetic globe for surgery.
- It is considered to be the least painful of the regional anaesthetic techniques for eye surgery.
- Provides good analgesia.
- Good sensory block reduces the risk of oculo-cardiac reflex by blocking the afferent limb of the pathway.
- Uses a blunt cannula and so reduces the risk of harm associated with techniques involving sharp needles.
- If used in place of general anaesthesia, avoids related complications including those of airway management.

REFERENCE

Anker R, Kaur N. Regional anaesthesia for ophthalmic surgery. *BJA Educ.* 2017: 17: 221–227.

PLASTICS AND BURNS

20.1 March 2013 Burns and smoke inhalation injury

You are asked to assess a 24-year-old male who has been admitted to the emergency department with 30% burns from a house fire.

a) State four aspects of the history that would lead you to suspect significant inhalational injury. (4 marks)
b) List four examination findings that would lead you to suspect significant inhalational injury. (4 marks)
c) List three investigations that may be useful in the assessment of inhalational injury and the findings for each that might indicate severity. (6 marks)
d) List four indications for early tracheal intubation to secure the airway. (4 marks)
e) Explain how burns injuries influence the safety of use of suxamethonium and give the time period of this effect. (2 marks)

In the original SAQ, subsection (a) asked, for 8 marks, "What would lead you to suspect significant inhalational injury?" The Chair said, "Section (a) required details of the history (burn received in enclosed space/delayed escape), general observations, features of upper and lower airway injury and harm from noxious gases." The pass rate was 64.2%.

a) **State four aspects of the history that would lead you to suspect significant inhalational injury. (4 marks)**

- Fire in enclosed space.
- Flames/fumes/smoke/steam/superheated gases and liquids.
- Delayed escape.
- Loss of consciousness at scene due to drugs/alcohol/head injury/hypoxia/carbon monoxide poisoning/cyanide poisoning.
- Fatalities in the same incident.

b) **List four examination findings that would lead you to suspect significant inhalational injury. (4 marks)**

The problems with inhalational injury stem from the effects of heat, inhalation of particulate matter and respiratory irritants, and inhalation of chemicals that cause cytotoxic hypoxia.

- Voice change, stridor, hoarseness.
- Cough.
- Burns to face, lips, tongue, pharynx, nasal mucosa.
- Soot in sputum, nose, mouth.
- Crackles on chest auscultation consistent with pulmonary oedema.
- Respiratory distress, increased respiratory rate, cyanosis, reduced oxygen saturations.
- Reduced level of consciousness, agitation.

DOI: 10.1201/9781003388494-20 495

c) List three investigations that may be useful in the assessment of inhalational injury and the findings for each that might indicate severity. (6 marks)

The question didn't specify whether this is to assess the awake or anaesthetised patient, so I have included both to be on the safe side.

- Arterial blood gas analysis; hypoxaemia, raised carboxyhaemoglobin level, lactic acidosis.
- Poor PaO_2:FiO_2 in ventilated patient.
- Venous blood gas; decreased arteriovenous oxygen difference (*due to inability to utilise oxygen following carbon monoxide and cyanide poisoning*).
- Chest X-ray; may be normal, may show atelectasis, pulmonary oedema, ARDS.
- Fibreoptic laryngoscopy (awake patient); laryngeal oedema, mucosal pallor or erythema and ulceration.
- Bronchoscopy (anaesthetised patient); carbonaceous deposits, mucosal pallor or erythema and ulceration.

d) List four indications for early tracheal intubation to secure the airway. (4 marks)

Facial swelling and oedema are likely to be significant following severe inhalational injury. Use uncut tube to accommodate this swelling and ensure tube fixation is monitored to ensure that the swelling does not cause the tube to migrate up and out of the airway. A large diameter tube is also useful to facilitate bronchoscopy.

- Stridor (indicating impending airway obstruction) or actual airway obstruction.
- Respiratory distress causing inadequate gas exchange.
- Hypoxaemia or hypercapnia.
- Full-thickness neck burns.
- Oropharyngeal oedema.
- Low GCS.
- Cardiac arrest.
- Imminent transfer required and risk of deterioration en route.

e) Explain how burns injuries influence the safety of use of suxamethonium and give the time period of this effect. (2 marks)

Some sources say that it is safe to use suxamethonium up to 48 hours or even longer after burns but my answer is erring on the side of caution.

- Upregulation of nicotinic receptors causes risk of hyperkalaemia.
- Suxamethonium can be used within the first 24 hours following a significant burn (*unless the patient is already hyperkalaemic from rhabdomyolysis due to associated muscle damage and compartment syndrome*) and then not for a year.

REFERENCES

Gill P, Martin R. Smoke inhalation injury. *Contin Educ Anaesth Crit Care Pain.* 2015: 15: 143–148.
McCann C, Watson A, Barnes D. Major burns: part 1: epidemiology, pathophysiology and initial management. *BJA Educ.* 2022: 22: 94–103.
McGovern C, Puxty K, Paton L. Major burns: part 2: anaesthesia, intensive care and pain management. *BJA Educ.* 2022: 22: 138–145.

20.2 March 2017 Burns and smoke inhalation injury

You are asked to assess a 24-year-old male who has been admitted to the emergency department with 30% burns from a house fire.

a) What clinical features would lead you to suspect significant inhalational injury? (10 marks)

b) List the indications for early tracheal intubation to secure the airway. (4 marks)

c) Which investigations would you use to assess the severity of the inhalational injury (3 marks) and what are the likely findings? (3 marks)

The SAQ, reproduced here as it appeared in the exam, was almost identical to that from March 2013. The pass rate this time was 57.9%.

20.3 March 2018 Free flap surgery

A 55-year-old woman is listed for a mastectomy and free-flap breast reconstruction for breast cancer.

a) Give an example of a pedicled flap donor site and a free flap donor site used in reconstructive breast surgery. (2 marks)

b) Give four factors that influence perfusion in a free flap (4 marks), giving an example of how anaesthetic technique can be used to manipulate each. (4 marks)

c) List three surgical causes of flap failure. (3 marks)

d) List three preoperative patient factors that may increase the risk of flap failure. (3 marks)

e) List four specific elements of postoperative free flap monitoring. (4 marks)

The Chairs' Report of the original SAQ stated that this was a "well answered question [pass rate 64.3%] and candidates gave very comprehensive answers, giving almost too much information in some cases by including very general considerations, rather than simply those specific to free flap surgery. However, the poorer candidates struggled to score marks and this may reflect lack of clinical exposure to such cases."

Sometimes reconstructive surgery is deferred until a later date, and at other times it is performed at the same time as the cancer surgery itself. Either way, the dissection of the flap and its anastomosis to recipient site is a prolonged process sometimes involving a change in the patient's position. Think of the list of issues that need to be addressed for any prolonged surgery. It may be a shared case involving breast and plastic surgeons – all relevant personnel should be involved in the team brief.

a) **Give an example of a pedicled flap donor site and a free flap donor site used in reconstructive breast surgery. (2 marks)**

Breast reconstruction may be implant based or performed with the use of a flap of the patient's own tissue. A free flap is when that tissue is removed entirely from the body and anastomosed elsewhere, whereas a pedicled flap involves retaining the primary vascular and neurological supply for the tissue but moving it on a pedicle to cover another area of the body. Free flaps consisting of just skin and fat are less at risk of ischaemia than those that contain muscle, as muscle is more metabolically active. Flap reconstruction is also performed after major head and neck surgery – see the question from September 2014 in that chapter.

- Pedicled flap:
  - Latissimus dorsi flap.

- Free flap:
  - Transverse rectus abdominis myocutaneous (TRAM) free flap *(skin, fat, and muscle – risk of decrease in abdominal wall strength; can also be used as a pedicled flap).*
  - Deep inferior epigastric perforator (DIEP) free flap *(skin and fat).*
  - Superior (SGAP) or inferior (IGAP) gluteal flaps *(skin and fat).*
  - Transverse myocutaneous gracilis (TMG) flap *(skin, fat, and muscle).*

b) Give four factors that influence perfusion in a free flap (4 marks), giving an example of how anaesthetic technique can be used to manipulate each. (4 marks)

Blood flow in a free flap is denervated and therefore is largely influenced by the perfusion pressure and humoral factors that can regulate the tone of the feeding artery and draining vein. Think of Hagen-Poiseuille's law any time you think about flow. Poor oxygen delivery to a flap (due to heart or lung disease) can also increase the risk of flap failure, but this question asks specifically about determinants of flow, rather than oxygen delivery.

- Maintenance of arterial pressure:
  - Cardiac output directed fluid therapy to ensure appropriate filling.
  - Monitoring of anaesthesia depth to avoid excessive depth, which has a detrimental effect on blood pressure.
  - Consideration of withholding of on-the-day antihypertensive drugs such as ACE inhibitors and angiotensin-2 receptor blockers.
  - Use of vasopressors guided by cardiac output monitoring.

- Minimisation of venous pressure:
  - Ensuring adequately deep anaesthesia with no straining or lack of coordination with ventilator by using remifentanil infusion or muscle relaxant, and monitoring depth of anaesthesia and/or train-of-four.
  - Use of cardiac output monitoring to avoid excessive fluid therapy, which will risk flap oedema and extramural pressure, which may impede venous outflow.

- Ensuring adequate blood vessel radius:
  - Using temperature monitoring to ensure that the surface to core body temperature difference (skin surface and core e.g. bladder, oesophageal) does not exceed 1.5°C to minimise risk of vasoconstriction, and use of forced air warmers, fluid warmers, and resistive heating mat.
  - Ensuring that pain is adequately controlled to minimise risk of sympathetically mediated vasoconstriction.
  - Use of cardiac output monitoring to avoid inappropriate vasopressor use.
  - Monitoring of and responding to arterial blood gas to avoid alkalosis.

- Optimisation of blood viscosity:
  - Aim for haematocrit of 0.3–0.35 as this offers optimum balance between oxygen delivery and blood flow, using arterial blood gas monitoring and cardiac output monitoring to guide fluid management and blood transfusion as required.
  - Maintenance of normothermia.

c) List three surgical causes of flap failure. (3 marks)

Free flap failure is most often due to surgical complications, despite the focus in the RCoA syllabus on physiological goals of anaesthesia for free flap surgery.

- Insufficient arterial supply:
  - Kinking at anastomosis site, anastomotic failure.
  - Thrombosis.
  - Vasospasm.

- Insufficient venous drainage:
  - Anastomotic kinking.
  - Compression due to haematoma.
  - Thrombosis.
  - Excessive flap handling causing oedema and impaired venous outflow.

- Reperfusion injury to flap tissue:
  - Excessive warm ischaemic time of flap tissue resulting in release of inflammatory mediators causing microvascular failure.

- Infection.

d) List three preoperative patient factors that may increase the risk of flap failure. (3 marks)

This is a list of issues that predispose to the possible reasons for surgical flap failure, or problems that will result in impaired oxygen delivery despite adequate perfusion. I have put more than one issue per bullet point in order to group them – you would be able to separate these points out in the exam. Some flaps are performed at the same time as the surgery to treat cancer and at other times it is delayed. Consideration should be given to deferring reconstructive surgery for a patient who is significantly affected by cancer or the effects of its treatment.

- Poorly controlled diabetes, chemotherapy (or other pharmacologically) induced immunosuppression increase the risk of infection.
- Haematological problems such as polycythaemia or a prothrombotic state associated with cancer or cancer treatment will increase risk of poor blood flow or thrombosis. Anaemia will result in impaired oxygen-carrying capacity.
- Cigarette smoking causes vasoconstriction, tissue hypoxia due to the toxins in inhaled tobacco smoke, and lung or heart disease causing impaired oxygenation and possible atherosclerosis, which could impair the anastomosis.
- Microvascular damage following radiotherapy may impair blood flow at the anastomosis site.
- Poor nutrition following cancer symptoms and treatment may result in poor wound healing.

e) List four specific elements of postoperative free flap monitoring. (4 marks)

Failed flaps normally need urgent (< 6 h) reoperation to identify and manage the reason for failure. A flap that has poor arterial supply will be pale, cool, have delayed capillary refill, will lack normal tissue turgor, and have a lack of bleeding on pinprick. A flap that has impaired venous drainage will be warm, purple-blue colour, swollen, with venous bleeding on pinprick. Some flaps will have a Doppler probe implanted during surgery, or the site for external Doppler monitoring will be marked by the surgeon at the end of surgery. Normal arterial flow is identified by a triphasic Doppler sound.

- Flap colour.
- Capillary refill.
- Oedema/turgor.
- Temperature.
- Doppler.
- Bleeding on pinprick (usually assessed by surgeons if concerns about other aspects of monitoring).

REFERENCE

Nimalan N, Branford O, Stocks G. Anaesthesia for free flap breast reconstruction. *BJA Educ.* 2016: 16: 162–166.

20.4 March 2020 Burns

You are called to the emergency department to assess a woman who has suffered major burns affecting the front of her torso and the whole of her left arm. She weighs approximately 60 kg.
a) List three functions of the skin. (3 marks)
b) Estimate the percentage body surface area of burns of this patient. (1 mark)
c) State the Parkland formula for estimating fluid requirements of this patient and the timing over which it is given. (2 marks)
d) Give three reasons why additional fluids in excess of the volume predicted may be required. (3 marks)
e) Give three approaches to monitoring the effectiveness of fluid rehydration of this patient. (3 marks)
f) List four indications for transfer to a major burns centre. (4 marks)
g) Describe one indication for escharotomy prior to transfer. (1 mark)
h) List two approaches to reducing heat loss in theatre during debridement procedures. (2 marks)
i) Give an approach to reducing blood loss during debridement surgery. (1 mark)

The Chairs said the pass rate for the CRQ on this topic was 61.1% and that the "question was answered well. It was reassuring that candidates were able to assess the airway in a patient with burns and were aware of the concerns of anaesthetising such patients. Candidates knew the Parkland formula, but it was disappointing that many candidates could not apply their knowledge and calculate the correct fluid requirements." There are two really useful articles (referenced below) that featured as a pair in BJA Education concerning initial and later management of burns and one focussing on inhalational injury that would give you the syllabus knowledge required for the Final FRCA. Make sure you read them.

a) List three functions of the skin. (3 marks)

Think of the complications of burns management, many of which relate to loss of skin function. Full thickness burns destroy down to the dermis, causing destruction of nerve endings (therefore making them less painful), and making them non-blanching (due to destruction of the dermal vascular plexus). The epidermis cannot regenerate if the dermis is badly damaged, meaning these burns are more severe in terms of complications, and management will involve skin grafting.

I have related the functions to the layers of the skin below:

- Epidermis (outer five layers of skin):
  - Innate immunity, barrier function.
  - Prevention of fluid loss.
  - Melanocytes in basal layer account for skin pigmentation.
  - Sensory function including light touch and pain.
- Dermis (inner two layers):
  - Thermoregulation (dermal vascular plexus, piloerection, sweat glands).
  - Flexibility.

b) Estimate the percentage body surface area of burns of this patient. (1 mark)

Using the Lund-Browder chart ("rule of nines") for adults, her anterior torso is 18%, and the anterior and posterior aspects of her arm are 4.5% each. The Mersey Burns App will help calculate the percentage of body surface area burned and also calculate fluid requirements. Areas that are just erythematous should be excluded from calculation.

- 27%.

c) **State the Parkland formula for estimating fluid requirements of this patient and the timing over which it is given. (2 marks)**

This formula applies to adults with over 15% body surface area burns – below this, the fluid shifts are less, and oral rehydration should be adequate (unless there are associated injuries that dictate otherwise). Traditionally, Ringer's lactate was the fluid of choice, but Hartmann's is commonly used, and some sources describe the use of colloids or albumin. There is a recent movement for more conservative fluid resuscitation in burns, using a modified Parkland formula of 2–4 ml/kg x percentage of total body surface area burned, because of evidence of fluid overload when using the traditional Parkland formula. However, there is no consensus at the time of writing so if asked to calculate the initial fluid requirements of a burns patient, stick to 4 ml/kg.

- Fluid requirement = 4 ml × weight (kg) × percentage of total body surface area burned.
- Half of the total requirement calculated by the above formula is given in the first 8 hours from the time of the burn, the remaining half in the subsequent 16 hours.

d) **Give three reasons why additional fluids in excess of the volume predicted may be required. (3 marks)**

Debridement of deep partial and full thickness burns should take place early, ideally within 48 hours, to reduce the necrotic load that drives the inflammatory response, to remove a site for infection development, and to decrease overall blood loss.

- Blood loss due to associated injuries.
- Blood loss due to debridement of burned areas (up to 3–4% blood volume loss per % BSA excised).
- Evaporative losses from debrided areas.
- Inhalational injury.
- Electrical burns.
- Maintenance requirements in a patient not having oral intake.
- Significant fluid shifts due to SIRS response.

e) **Give three approaches to monitoring the effectiveness of fluid rehydration of this patient. (3 marks)**

- Ensuring urine output > 0.5–1 ml/kg/h.
- Monitoring serum lactate as this reflects tissue perfusion.
- Minimising core-peripheral temperature difference.
- Serial haematocrit assessment.
- Cardiac output monitoring or stroke volume variation monitoring.

f) **List four indications for referral for consideration of transfer to a specialised burn care service. (4 marks)**

The National Network for Burn Care (NNBC) has published national guidance regarding the referral criteria, but there may be regional differences depending on your local burns service. There are a variety of care providers with a range of specialism from plastics facility to burns unit to burns centre, but it is important to have an idea of the severity of burn that should make you consider discussing the case with experts.

- All burns ≥ 2% TBSA in children or ≥ 3% in adults.
- All full thickness burns.
- All circumferential burns.
- Any burn not healed in two weeks, or concerns regarding healing such as infection.

- Suspicion of burns due to nonaccidental injury.
- Burns to hands, feet, face, perineum, or genitalia.
- Chemical, electrical, or cold injury burns.
- Smoke inhalational injury.
- Febrile or unwell child with burns.
- Medical comorbidities that may impede burns wound healing.
- Suspicion of toxic shock syndrome.

g) Describe one indication for escharotomy prior to transfer. (1 mark)

An escharotomy is a surgical incision through noncompliant, full thickness burn tissue. Patients with significant burns may also require fasciotomies as part of their management if they have significant muscle injury and raised compartment pressures.

- Chest or abdominal burns that restrict ventilation.
- Circumferential burns on limbs which restrict perfusion distally.

h) List two approaches to reducing heat loss in theatre during debridement procedures. (2 marks)

- Minimising patient exposure.
- Maintaining theatre temperature at 28–33°C.
- Forced air warmers.
- Intravenous fluid warmers.
- Use of heat lamps.
- Under body resistive heating mat use.
- Use of heat and moisture exchange filter or other method to humidify anaesthetic gases.

i) Give an approach to reducing blood loss during debridement surgery. (1 mark)

- Use of limb tourniquets.
- Use of topical adrenaline.
- Near patient coagulation testing to address coagulation deficiencies rapidly.

REFERENCES

Barnes J et al. The Mersey burns app: evolving a model of validation. *Emerg Med J.* 2015: 32: 637–641.

British Burn Association. *National burn care referral guidance*, 2012. www.britishburnassociation. org/wp-content/uploads/2018/02/National-Burn-Care-Referral-Guidance-2012.pdf. Accessed 27th January 2022.

Gill P, Martin R. Smoke inhalation injury. *Contin Educ Anaesth Crit Care Pain.* 2015: 15: 143–148.

McCann C, Watson A, Barnes D. Major burns: part 1: epidemiology, pathophysiology and initial management. *BJA Educ.* 2022: 22: 94–103.

McGovern C, Puxty K, Paton L. Major burns: part 2: anaesthesia, intensive care and pain management. *BJA Educ.* 2022: 22: 138–145.

VASCULAR SURGERY

21.1 March 2012 Ruptured abdominal aortic aneurysm

A 79-year-old patient presents with a leaking abdominal aortic aneurysm (AAA). The vascular surgery and radiology teams decide to undertake an endovascular aneurysm repair (EVAR) procedure.

a) List four risk factors which predispose to the development of AAA. (4 marks)
b) List three clinical features or investigations that may be used to help assess the degree of blood loss. (3 marks)
c) List two elements of your approach to intravascular resuscitation prior to surgery. (2 marks)
d) List three reasons why a local anaesthetic approach may not be feasible for this patient. (3 marks)
e) Give three reasons for the risk of cardiovascular instability at the point of induction of general anaesthesia. (3 marks)
f) List three reasons for ongoing bleeding intraoperatively. (3 marks)
g) Give two postoperative complications for which vigilance should be maintained following EVAR. (2 marks)

The Chair's Report for the original SAQ said that there was a 54.1% pass rate and that "many candidates missed the point of the question and launched into the detailed anaesthetic management, not mentioning many of the organisational issues. It appeared from the answers that many candidates had not seen elective or emergency EVAR." The subsection of question that this comment relates to asked, for 11 marks, "What are the main preoperative anaesthetic considerations for this procedure?" The answer should therefore have included details of a focussed preassessment specifically looking for the likely comorbidities and medications of a patient presenting for ruptured AAA and issues concerning poor cardiorespiratory reserve or frailty; initial resuscitation; liaising with the vascular, radiology, and theatre teams to plan transfer; ensuring communication with your ODP to plan anaesthesia and monitoring; initiating the major haemorrhage protocol and communicating with blood bank; principles of preoperative resuscitation; planning for postoperative care; and discussion with patient (if feasible) and family and allowing the family brief contact before proceeding urgently to surgery. This is the sort of conversation you may now have in a viva, but a CRQ will target its questions more specifically.

It really is easier to describe something that you have seen rather than just read about. Look at the exam syllabus and try to address your blind spots by arranging to go to some specific lists either in your own hospital or elsewhere within your school of anaesthesia. Issues surrounding the endovascular nature of this surgery include the increased need for careful communication due to the involvement of both the vascular surgical and radiological teams, the remote site of the interventional radiology suite with its attendant risks of suboptimal equipment and support, the non-tipping radiology table for induction of

DOI: 10.1201/9781003388494-21

anaesthesia (if GA is used then preparations must be such that surgery can proceed immediately after induction to facilitate rupture control, in the same manner as category 1 caesarean section), low light levels, restricted access to the patient due to the presence of the C arm, and minimal ability to warm the patient as warming mattresses may obscure the radiological view and a forced air warmer may be used on only the very uppermost part of the patient therefore with limited effect.

a) List four risk factors which predispose to the development of AAA. (4 marks)

These associated comorbidities should be actively sought in your focussed preoperative assessment as they are very significant in terms of physiological ability to tolerate major surgery and haemorrhage. Some of these diseases increase the likelihood of the patient taking long term anticoagulants or antiplatelets which may impact on control of bleeding. An assessment of frailty, exercise tolerance, and symptoms of significant cardiac or respiratory disease should be included in the overall assessment of whether to proceed with surgery.

- Age > 65 years.
- Male sex.
- Cigarette smoking.
- Chronic obstructive pulmonary disease.
- Coronary, cerebrovascular, or peripheral vascular disease.
- Family history of AAA.
- Hyperlipidaemia.
- Hypertension.

b) List three clinical features or simple investigations that may be used to help assess the degree of blood loss. (3 marks)

Blood loss is concealed, and the volume of loss is difficult to quantify radiologically. These surrogates are used to help assess the degree of patient compromise.

- Cardiovascular instability i.e. hypotension and tachycardia.
- Reduced peripheral perfusion, capillary refill time, mottled skin.
- Decrease in GCS.
- Acid-base status with development of lactic acidosis.
- Haematology with reduction of haemoglobin.
- Blood clotting studies with development of coagulopathy.
- Blood biochemistry studies or oligoanuria may indicate development of AKI.
- ECG may indicate ischaemia due to poor perfusion.

c) List two elements of your approach to intravascular resuscitation prior to surgery. (2 marks)

In the past, permissive hypotension to as low as 70 mmHg systolic was advised to minimise the risk of disruption of any protective clot that had developed. However, very low systolic blood pressure preoperatively is associated with a greater risk of poor outcome; it is not known whether low blood pressure is just a marker of significant bleeding and whether the risk can be modified by increasing the preoperative blood pressure with resuscitation.

- Toleration of below normal blood pressure, guided by GCS/avoidance of excessive fluid administration to minimise risk of clot disruption.
- Use of red cells, fresh frozen plasma and platelets in a 1:1:1 ratio.
- Minimisation of use of non-blood fluids as they are not helpful for oxygen carriage or coagulation.
- Establish large bore intravenous access for intraoperative use.

d) List three reasons why a local anaesthetic approach may not be feasible for this patient. (3 marks)

Local anaesthesia offers the benefit of avoiding a general anaesthetic in an already cardiovascularly compromised patient. Light sedative or analgesic infusions such as propofol or remifentanil TCI may be required to make the procedure tolerable for the patient and reduce the risk of stent malposition due to patient agitation and movement. Commonly, the initial phase of achieving rupture control may be undertaken under local anaesthesia and then surgery continued under general anaesthesia once better cardiovascular stability has been achieved. A bifurcated graft may be sited percutaneously with local anaesthesia alone. An aorto-uni-iliac is, as the name suggests, one sided only and will therefore occlude all supply to the contralateral leg. A femoro-femoral crossover operation will therefore be necessary, and this usually requires general anaesthesia. Its advantage is that it is quicker to achieve control of the rupture with an aorto-uni-iliac stent.

- Back and abdominal pain associated with leaking aneurysm may be severe and therefore not tolerated by the patient, resulting in movement.
- Patient agitation due to cerebral hypoperfusion may result in a moving and uncooperative patient.
- Use of resuscitative endovascular balloon occlusion of the aorta (REBOA) may cause acute lower body ischemia with intolerable pain.
- Ischaemic buttock pain due to internal iliac occlusion may be intolerable and result in movement.
- Use of aorto-uni-iliac graft necessitating femoro-femoral crossover afterwards for which general anaesthesia is likely to be needed.
- Respiratory insufficiency due to expanding retroperitoneal haematoma.
- Associated chronic conditions such as COPD with long-term cough may make lying still for prolonged periods unfeasible.

e) Give three reasons for the risk of cardiovascular instability at the point of induction of general anaesthesia. (3 marks)

These reasons are why induction of anaesthesia takes place on the radiology table with the surgical and radiological teams scrubbed and patient prepped.

- Loss of the profound sympathetic tone associated with the pain of aneurysmal leak.
- Relaxation of abdominal muscles due to loss of consciousness and use of NMBD resulting in reduction of tamponade of the retroperitoneal clot.
- Initiation of intermittent positive pressure ventilation in an under-resuscitated patient causing reduction in venous return.
- Cardio-depressant effects of intravenous and inhalational anaesthetic agents.

f) List three reasons for ongoing bleeding intraoperatively. (3 marks)

- Type I endoleak (failure to adequately create a seal of either the proximal or distal ends of the stent with the vessel wall resulting in ongoing bleeding into the rupture).
- Insidious bleeding from the groin entry sites during a prolonged procedure.
- Endovascular arterial injury during guidewire or stent manipulations.
- Failure to control coagulopathy due to inability to adequately warm the patient or address coagulopathy.

g) Give two postoperative complications for which vigilance should be maintained following EVAR. (2 marks)

- Abdominal compartment syndrome.
- Ischaemic colitis.

- Acute kidney injury.
- Cholesterol embolisation syndrome.
- Lower limb ischaemia due to distal dislodgement of thrombus.

REFERENCES

Berry K, Gudgeon J, Taylor J. Anaesthesia for endovascular repair of ruptured abdominal aortic aneurysms. *BJA Educ*. 2022: 22: 208–215.

Leonard A, Thompson J. Anaesthesia for ruptured abdominal aortic aneurysm. *BJA Educ*. 2008: 8: 11–15.

National Institute for Health and Care Excellence. *Abdominal aortic aneurysm: diagnosis and management: NG156*, March 2020.

21.2 March 2016 Carotid endarterectomy

A 56-year-old man is listed for carotid endarterectomy ten days after suffering an acute, non-disabling stroke.

a) Give three local or regional anaesthesia techniques for carotid endarterectomy. (3 marks)
b) List four potential advantages to regional anaesthesia for carotid endarterectomy. (4 marks)
c) List four specific problems associated with regional anaesthesia for carotid endarterectomy. (4 marks)
d) List three possible reasons for haemodynamic instability during carotid endarterectomy. (3 marks)
e) List three aspects of minimisation of the patient's perioperative stroke risk. (3 marks)
f) The patient has straightforward surgery but becomes confused and agitated in the Post-Anaesthetic Care Unit four hours postoperatively. List three specific differential diagnoses. (3 marks)

The Chair's Report of the original SAQ said that "this question had one of the highest correlations with overall performance; i.e. candidates who did well in this question performed well in the SAQ overall. As mentioned above, some candidates did not read the question properly but fortunately did not lose too many marks as a result."

Carotid endarterectomy improves outcomes (reduces risk of fatal or disabling stroke) of symptomatic patients with 50%–99% carotid stenosis (according to North American Symptomatic Carotid Endarterectomy Trial, NASCET, criteria) compared with the best medical management (control of hypertension, antiplatelet drugs, statins or diet to reduce serum cholesterol, stopping smoking, controlling diabetes, and reducing alcohol intake). Neurologically stable patients who have had a transient ischaemic attack or stroke should ideally have carotid endarterectomy within two weeks if stenosis is 50%–99%.

A very brief description of the surgical approach to carotid endarterectomy:

- *Exposure of carotid.*
- *Cross-clamping above and below the area of stenosis (heparin given just prior to this).*
- *Vertical (sometimes transverse – "eversion") incision.*
- *Cerebral blood flow reduced whilst cross-clamp on, dependent on the collateral flow via Circle of Willis. Ipsilateral blood flow can be improved with a shunt from below to above cross-clamp. Some surgeons use shunts routinely, some only in patients under general anaesthesia (as neurological status cannot be monitored), some only if perfusion appears inadequate.*
- *Atheroma removed, defect closed by primary closure or using a patch (synthetic or autologous vein graft). Using a patch reduces the risk of re-stenosis.*

a) **Give three local or regional anaesthesia techniques for carotid endarterectomy. (3 marks)**

- Local anaesthetic infiltration.
- Superficial cervical plexus block.
- Deep cervical plexus block.
- Combined superficial and deep cervical plexus blocks.
- Intermediate cervical plexus block.

b) List four potential advantages to regional anaesthesia for carotid endarterectomy. (4 marks)

c) List four specific problems associated with regional anaesthesia for carotid endarterectomy. (4 marks)

For the sake of learning, I have grouped these into a table.

Advantages	Specific problems
Responsive patient can be monitored continuously for any change in neurological functioning intraoperatively.	Risks associated with blocks: intravascular/epidural/subarachnoid injection, local anaesthetic toxicity, phrenic nerve damage etc.
Monitoring in the early postoperative period improved as not recovering from general anaesthetic.	Risk of need to convert to GA with restricted airway access intraoperatively.
Lower need for shunt with its attendant risks: particulate or bubble embolisation, arterial wall dissection, kinking, thrombosis.	Needs cooperative patient: surgery may be prolonged, claustrophobia from drapes, overheating, full bladder.
Artery is closed at normal patient blood pressure: may reduce postoperative haematoma. Possibly more stable blood pressure throughout.	Potential for patient movement causing surgical difficulty.
Avoids airway instrumentation (with associated risk of spike in blood pressure), general anaesthetic, and their associated risks (everything from sore throat to failed intubation).	Potential for patient stress/pain causing myocardial ischaemia.

d) **List three possible reasons for haemodynamic instability during carotid endarterectomy. (3 marks)**

- Surgical manipulation of the vagus nerve resulting in profound bradycardia and hypotension.
- Impaired carotid baroreceptor reflex due to damage to the receptor fibres due to surgical incision or due to the removal of plaque resulting in periods of hypertension (*carotid sinus baroreceptors are located in the carotid sinus, at the bifurcation of the common carotid artery*).
- Carotid cross-clamping results in cerebral hypoperfusion and a reflex, sympathetically mediated, compensatory increase in arterial blood pressure. There is the reverse effect on removal of cross-clamp.
- Impaired carotid baroreceptor reflex due to carotid plaque disease (worse if bilateral), recent stroke (blood pressure more labile for two weeks), hypertension, and diabetes, in association with use of inhalational and intravenous anaesthetic medications which further impair baroreceptor response, may result in variable blood pressure.
- Patients with significant carotid artery disease are at increased risk of major adverse cardiovascular events perioperatively which may result in haemodynamic instability.
- Intraoperative agitation caused by overly distended bladder resulting in hypertension.

e) **List three aspects of minimisation of the patient's perioperative stroke risk. (3 marks)**

This question, which was included in the original SAQ, did not specify which type of stroke. I have subdivided my answer to help organise my thoughts, but this would not be necessary in the exam.

Embolic (biggest risk):

- Avoid shunt use where possible, or meticulous surgical technique to avoid thromboembolism or air embolism when using a shunt.
- Meticulous surgical technique to avoid dislodgement of atheroma.
- Perioperative administration of antiplatelets, usually dual antiplatelet therapy (DAPT).
- Heparin before cross-clamping.

Ischaemic:

- Use of a shunt during cross-clamp if collateral circulation is inadequate.
- Pharmacological management of perioperative hypotension.

Haemorrhagic:

- Pharmacological management of perioperative hypertension.

f) **The patient has straightforward surgery but becomes confused and agitated in the Post-Anaesthetic Care Unit 4 hours postoperatively. List three specific differential diagnoses. (3 marks)**

Three marks, three complications. You wouldn't need all the detail given on cerebral hyperperfusion syndrome. I have just included it here as an explanation. The list of differential diagnoses for a confused patient in PACU would also include urinary retention, delirium due to alveolar hypoventilation, hypotension, the effects of sedative, long-acting opioid or centrally acting anticholinergic drugs, or withdrawal from alcohol. However, these are much lower down the exam answer list as they are less specific to a patient who has had a carotid endarterectomy.

- Stroke.
- Cerebral hyperperfusion syndrome, occurs from immediately postoperatively until a month later. Chronic hypoperfusion results in areas of impaired autoregulation. Increased microvascular permeability occurs on reperfusion of previously underperfused areas of brain, increasing vulnerability to oedema. This is ischaemia-reperfusion injury. Extreme hypertension resulting from impaired carotid baroreceptor function postoperatively, in combination with the previous changes, may result in oedema and haemorrhage. This results in hypertensive encephalopathy, severe headache, variable neurological deficits, seizures, cerebral oedema, cerebral haemorrhage.
- Carotid artery dissection or restenosis.
- Myocardial infarction or failure.
- Hypoxia due to postoperative haematoma compromising the airway.

REFERENCES

Ladak N, Thompson J. General or local anaesthesia for carotid endarterectomy? *Contin Educ Anaesth Crit Care Pain.* 2012: 12: 92–96.

National Institute for Health and Care Excellence. *Stroke and transient ischaemic attack in over 16s: diagnosis and initial management: NG128,* Published May 2019, updated April 2022.

Stoneham M, Thompson J. Arterial pressure management and carotid enterectomy. *BJA.* 2009: 102: 442–452.

Stoneham M et al. Regional anaesthesia for carotid endarterectomy. *BJA.* 2015: 114: 372–383.

21.3 September 2016 Endovascular aneurysm repair

A 79-year-old man with a 6 cm infra-renal abdominal aortic aneurysm is to undergo an endovascular aneurysm repair (EVAR). He is known to have chronic obstructive pulmonary disease.
a) List eight advantages of an EVAR compared to an open repair of the aneurysm for this patient. (8 marks)
b) List five preoperative patient risk factors for acute kidney injury (AKI) associated with any EVAR procedure. (5 marks)
c) List three surgical risk factors for AKI associated with any EVAR procedure. (3 marks)
d) List four perioperative measures to minimise the risk of AKI following EVAR. (4 marks)

The Chairs said that the pass rate for the original SAQ was 57.2% and that "there were no major themes that emerged in the answers to this question. It was presumably easier to answer for those who had had the chance to see the procedure during their training."

a) List eight advantages of an EVAR compared to an open repair of the aneurysm for this patient. (8 marks)

They are specifically asking about <u>this patient.</u> The issues to focus on are that the patient is elderly, that he has chronic obstructive pulmonary disease, and that the aneurysm is infra-renal.

- Open repair may be optimal in younger patients with few comorbidities as although the intraoperative risks are higher, there are fewer long-term problems with the graft e.g. endoleak. This gentleman is elderly and has comorbidities that mean that the risk of long-term problems is less of an issue when compared to the intraoperative risks to him of an open repair.
- In view of the patient's age, he is likely to have other comorbidities, including cardiovascular and renal disease, increasing the need for a minimally invasive technique with fewer perioperative complications and less metabolic and haemodynamic stress.
- EVAR can be performed with a neuraxial technique or just local anaesthesia to the groins, thus offering potential for avoidance of intubation, effects of positive pressure ventilation on diseased lungs, risk of pneumonia.
- Avoids presence of large abdominal wound, the pain of which can cause difficulty achieving deep breathing and adequate cough postoperatively, thus increasing the risk of respiratory complications.
- Reduces the possible need for opioid analgesia postoperatively with its respiratory depressant effect.
- Infra-renal aneurysms tend to be technically the most straightforward AAA to be done by EVAR and so operating time for an awake technique should be tolerable.
- Early ambulation (next day) facilitated, helping to maintain muscle strength and reducing risks of deep vein thrombosis, deconditioning, and pneumonia in vulnerable individual.
- Reduced risk of large blood loss and coagulopathy, important in a patient with limited reserve to tolerate it.

b) List five preoperative patient risk factors for acute kidney injury (AKI) associated with any EVAR procedure. (5 marks)

We've moved on from the specific patient to more general issues. This often happens in Final questions and is a source of error when candidates fail to notice the shift in focus.

- Advanced age.
- Pre-existing renal impairment, or history of AKI.

- Diabetes mellitus.
- Cardiac failure.
- Liver disease.
- Preoperative dehydration.
- Hypertension.
- High body mass index.
- Peripheral arterial disease.
- Immunocompromise.

c) **List three surgical risk factors for AKI associated with any EVAR procedure. (3 marks)**

Previously, I would have included complex and prolonged surgery hence high contrast load near the top of my list. However, the risks associated with contrast are more in doubt now, so it has moved further down:

- Embolisation of atheromatous plaque into renal arteries.
- Obstruction of, or damage to, renal arteries by stent maldeployment, especially associated with fenestrated and branched EVARs.
- Surgical complications resulting in bleeding and hypotension.
- Ischaemia and then reperfusion of lower limbs resulting in inflammatory response – exacerbated by prolonged ischaemia time due to complex or complications of surgery.
- Complex and prolonged surgery necessitating high contrast load.

d) **List four perioperative measures to minimise the risk of AKI following EVAR. (4 marks)**

- Avoid perioperative dehydration; minimise preoperative starvation time, cardiac output monitoring to guide fluid replacement intraoperatively (and possibly postoperatively), start fluids pre-procedure, ensure full circulation, monitor urine output, monitor blood loss and replace as indicated by near patient testing.
- Avoid perioperative hypotension; management of fluid status as above, with use of vasopressor if indicated by cardiac output monitoring.
- Avoid nephrotoxic drugs perioperatively; omission of ACE inhibitors and angiotensin-2 receptor blockers on day of surgery, care with repeat doses of aminoglycosides and ensure patient is fluid replete when administered, NSAIDs not a suitable choice for pain control.
- Glucose control; maintain normal range in diabetic patients, consider use of variable rate insulin infusion in type I diabetes.
- Minimise surgical complications with meticulous technique.
- Limitation of contrast load, especially in patients with pre-existing chronic kidney disease or risk of acute kidney injury. Scheduling of surgery so that kidneys have a week to recover from any preoperative contrast. Intravascular fluid expansion at time of contrast use, using low or iso-osmolar formulations and non-iodinated media are all thought to reduce risk. *Some centres use sodium bicarbonate or N-acetylcysteine, although evidence for this is absent. Recent evidence has questioned the association between contrast and AKI.*

REFERENCES

Ehmann M. Renal outcomes following intravenous contrast administration in patients with acute kidney injury: a multi-site retrospective propensity-adjusted analysis. *Intensive Care Med.* 2023: 49: 205–215.

Everson M et al. Contrast-associated acute kidney injury. *BJA Educ.* 2020: 20: 417–423.

National Institute for Health and Care Excellence. *Abdominal aortic aneurysm: diagnosis and management: NG156*, March 2020.

National Institute for Health and Care Excellence. *Clinical knowledge summaries: acute kidney injury*, Last revised August 2021.

Webb S, Allen S. Perioperative renal protection. *Contin Educ Anaesth Crit Care Pain.* 2008: 8: 176–180.

21.4 September 2019 Carotid endarterectomy

The CRQ on carotid endarterectomy in this hybrid paper addressed the same sorts of themes as the SAQ from 2016. The pass rate was a fantastic 87.7%. A reminder to keep your answers specific at all times, the Chairs said, "In this question, weak candidates performed poorly in part (c) by answering in general terms and failing to give specific reasons why there may be cardiovascular instability during this operation."

21.5 September 2021 Open aortic aneurysm repair

A 75-year-old gentleman presents for open repair of a 6 cm abdominal aortic aneurysm.
a) List three possible immediate effects of aortic cross-clamping. (3 marks)
b) Give three approaches to mitigating these effects of aortic cross-clamping. (3 marks)
c) Give three causes of hypotension upon removal of the aortic cross-clamp. (3 marks)
d) Give three approaches to mitigation of hypotension upon removal of the aortic cross-clamp. (3 marks)
e) Give two approaches for maintaining distal perfusion during cross-clamp for thoracic descending aortic aneurysm repair. (2 marks)
f) Describe the blood supply to the lumbosacral segments of the spinal cord. (3 marks)
g) How can spinal cord ischaemia be minimised in patients undergoing thoracic aortic surgery? (3 marks)

Cross-clamp physiology is a common viva question and allows examiners to question cardiovascular physiology and anatomy in parallel. There was no Chairs' Report for this sitting of the exam.

a) List three possible immediate effects of aortic cross-clamping. (3 marks)

The majority of the physiological changes can be described in terms of the cardiovascular system or changes in regional blood flow.

- Acute increase in afterload, increases myocardial wall tension and oxygen requirement and may precipitate myocardial ischaemia, failure, or even cardiac arrest.
- Loss of venous capacitance of distal part of body with increase in central circulating volume with risk of pulmonary oedema and raised intracranial blood flow.
- Impaired blood flow distal to the cross-clamp risking mesenteric, hepatic, renal, lower limb, and spinal cord ischaemia.
- Development of thrombosis at site of vascular damage due to cross-clamp with risk of subsequent embolisation.
- Cross-clamp application over an area of atheromatous plaque can lead to embolic phenomena.

b) Give three approaches to mitigating these effects of aortic cross-clamping. (3 marks)

- Deepening of anaesthesia to vasodilate arterial tree proximal to clamp.
- Use of vasodilatory infusions e.g. GTN, remifentanil.
- Anticoagulation with heparin prior to cross-clamp application.
- Maintenance of adequate gas exchange to ensure sufficient oxygen delivery to myocardium and avoid cardio-depressant effect of hypercapnia.
- Avoidance of siting clamp at heavily atheromatous parts of the aorta.

c) Give three causes of hypotension upon removal of the aortic cross-clamp. (3 marks)

- Sudden and profound decrease in afterload directly causes hypotension.
- Reduction in perfusion pressure at aortic root due to drop in afterload will reduce coronary perfusion pressure and may precipitate myocardial ischaemia, failure, or cardiac arrest.
- Reperfusion of lower body causes recirculation of ischaemic metabolites and inflammatory mediators of ischaemia-reperfusion injury, which have a cardio-depressant effect.

- Sequestration of circulating volume in capacitance vessels causes relative hypovolaemia reducing venous return.
- Failure to adequately address fluid losses during cross-clamp time will exacerbate all of these issues.

d) **Give three approaches to mitigation of hypotension upon removal of the aortic cross-clamp. (3 marks)**

- Gradual release of cross-clamp with brief re-application if necessary.
- Adequate intravascular filling prior to cross-clamp removal.
- Use of vasoconstrictors and inotropes.
- Cessation of vasodilatory infusions, ensuring depth of anaesthesia is not excessive.
- Increase minute ventilation aiming for normocapnia to minimise any vasodilatory effect of respiratory acidosis compounding the inevitable metabolic acidosis.
- Treatment of any electrolyte imbalance to minimise risk of arrhythmia and to maintain cardiac contractility.

e) **Give two approaches for maintaining distal perfusion during cross-clamp for thoracic descending aortic aneurysm repair. (2 marks)**

- Partial left heart bypass – proximal cannulation of left atrium or pulmonary vein, via bypass machine (no oxygenator required, just pump), return cannulation in aorta distal to clamp or common femoral artery.
- Gott shunt – cannula connecting proximal aorta and distal aorta.
- Partial femoro-femoral bypass – proximal cannulation of femoral vein, via bypass machine (with or without oxygenator), return cannulation to femoral artery

f) **Describe the blood supply to the lumbosacral segments of the spinal cord. (3 marks)**

The following is the same answer to the question given in the March 2021 question in neuroanaesthesia. It is a common topic in the Final – do not neglect it! The artery of Adamkiewicz has an origin that is variable between individuals. If an individual has an unusually low origin, then there can be unexpected effect on their spinal cord of an aortic cross-clamp at a level not usually associated with poor spinal cord perfusion.

- Anterior spinal artery; formed by the union of branches from the two vertebral arteries at the foramen magnum and supply the anterior 2/3 of the cord (*spinothalamic and corticospinal tracts*).
- Two posterior spinal arteries; formed from each of the vertebral arteries or the posterior inferior cerebellar arteries and supply the posterior 1/3 of the cord (*dorsal columns*).
- Segmental arterial supply; numerous paired branches perfuse the spinal cord along its length, arising from vertebral, deep cervical, intercostal, aortic, and pelvic vessels. Arteria radicularis magna/artery of Adamkiewicz is the biggest segmental artery and forms a major supply to the lumbosacral spinal cord, arising at a variable vertebral level between T8–L4, but typically at T12–L1. It usually originates from an intercostal or, less commonly, a lumbar artery.

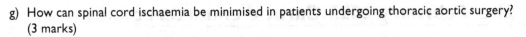

g) **How can spinal cord ischaemia be minimised in patients undergoing thoracic aortic surgery? (3 marks)**

The usual approaches to minimising the risk of secondary neurological damage are important perioperatively, but the question asks specifically how the risk of ischaemia, the primary insult, can be minimised.

Spinal cord perfusion pressure (SCPP) = mean arterial pressure (MAP) – CSF pressure.

SCPP should be at least 70 mmHg.

- Spinal drain to minimise CSF pressure (< 15 mmHg).
- Maintenance of MAP with use of adequate volume replenishment and vasoconstrictor or vasopressor as required.
- Lowest possible site for aortic clamping that can facilitate the intended surgery *(to minimise clamping above significant segmental arteries)*.
- Sequential clamping of aorta with neurophysiological monitoring to detect which of the segmental arteries are important for cord perfusion, thus identifying those that must be reimplanted into the graft.
- Minimisation of clamp time.

REFERENCES

Agarwal S, Kendall J, Quarterman C. Perioperative management of thoracic and thoracoabdominal aneurysms. *BJA Educ.* 2019: 19: 119–125.

Hashimi M, Thompson J. Anaesthesia for elective open abdominal aortic aneurysm repair. *Contin Educ Anaesth Crit Care Pain.* 2013: 13: 208–212.

21.6 February 2023 Carotid endarterectomy

This is the third time that carotid endarterectomy has been the focus of a question in the time frame of this book. Again, the lines of questioning were on advantages and disadvantages of regional versus general anaesthesia, the options for local or regional anaesthesia and specific complications, consequences of haemodynamic instability, and specific causes of agitation and confusion in PACU. The Chairs reported that the question was "well answered" with a pass rate of 69.7%.

ANATOMY

22.1 March 2014 Vagus nerve

a) State two nuclei of the vagus nerve. (2 marks)
b) Describe how the right vagus nerve reaches the thoracic inlet. (3 marks)
c) List two posterior relations of the right vagus nerve in the neck at C6. (2 marks)
d) State two posterior relations of the right vagus nerve in the thorax at T4. (2 marks)
e) List four branches of the vagus nerve in the head and neck. (4 marks)
f) List three branches of the vagus nerve in the thorax and/or abdomen. (3 marks)
g) List four clinical situations that may produce vagal reflex bradycardia. (4 marks)

The Chair's Report following the original SAQ highlighted a pass rate of 44.4% and commented on generally poor anatomical knowledge, with better performance in the latter parts of the question which were more clinically orientated. Although anatomy is uncommon as the sole focus of a SAQ or CRQ historically, the CRQ format of the exam makes it easier to ask anatomy-based questions for all clinical topics, especially regional anaesthesia. This Chair's Report stated, "Candidates must understand that relevant anatomy will be tested throughout all parts of the Final FRCA examination and should not write the subject off."

a) **List two nuclei of the vagus nerve. (2 marks)**

- Dorsal (vagal) nucleus *(parasympathetic innervation for thoracic and abdominal viscera)*.
- Nucleus ambiguus *(motor to muscles of the larynx and oropharynx and parasympathetic innervation for the heart)*.
- Solitary nucleus/nucleus of the tractus solitarius *(viscerosensory fibres from pharynx, larynx, oesophagus, thoracic and abdominal viscera, and chemosensory fibres from epiglottis)*.
- Spinal trigeminal nucleus *(somatosensory fibres from outer ear canal, pinna, dura)*.

b) **Describe how the right vagus nerve reaches the thoracic inlet. (3 marks)**

- The vagus nerve leaves the skull via the jugular foramen *(along with the glossopharyngeal and accessory nerves and internal jugular vein)*.
- Travels in the carotid sheath, running between sternocleidomastoid anterolaterally and anterior scalene posteriorly.
- Within the carotid sheath, it is posterolateral to the carotid artery and posteromedial to the internal jugular vein.
- It enters the thorax anterior to the right subclavian artery and posterior to the superior vena cava.

DOI: 10.1201/9781003388494-22

c) List two posterior relations of the right vagus nerve in the neck at C6. (2 marks)

Cross-sectional anatomy at T4 and C6 are important areas of anatomy to revise for every stage of the exam.

- Anterior scalene.
- Phrenic nerve.
- Longus coli.

Other relations of the vagus nerve at C6 include the following:

- *Anteriorly: omohyoid and thyroid gland.*
- *Medially: sympathetic trunk.*
- *Laterally: sternocleidomastoid.*

d) State two posterior relations of the right vagus nerve in the thorax at T4. (2 marks)

- Oesophagus.
- Right lung.

Other relations of the <u>right</u> vagus nerve at T4 include the following:

- *Anteriorly: phrenic nerve, superior vena cava.*
- *Medially: trachea.*
- *Laterally: azygos vein and right lung.*

Conversely the <u>left</u> vagus nerve descends anterior to the aortic arch.

e) List four branches of the vagus nerve in the head and neck. (4 marks)

Jugular fossa:

- Meningeal branch.
- Auricular nerve.

Neck:

- Pharyngeal nerve.
- Superior laryngeal nerve.
- Right recurrent laryngeal nerve.
- Cardiac branches.

f) List three branches of the vagus nerve in the thorax and/or abdomen. (3 marks)

Thorax:

- Oesophageal branches.
- Pericardial branches.
- Left recurrent laryngeal nerve.
- Branches to cardiac plexus.
- Branches to pulmonary plexus.

Abdomen:

- Gastric branches.
- Hepatic branch.
- Coeliac branches.

g) **List four clinical situations that may produce vagal reflex bradycardia. (4 marks)**

- Central afferent pathway triggered by stress or pain.
- Oculocardiac reflex caused by traction on extra-ocular muscles during surgery.
- Trigeminocardiac reflex during maxillofacial surgery.
- Stimulation of larynx during intubation, laryngoscopy, or with suctioning.
- Peritoneal stretch during laparoscopic surgery.
- Manipulation of abdominal and pelvic organs.
- Cervical or anal dilatation during surgery or examination.
- As part of the baroreceptor reflex to systemic hypertension.

REFERENCE

Ellis H, Feldman S, Lawson S. *Anatomy for anaesthetists*, 7th edition. Oxford: Blackwell Science, 1997.

APPLIED CLINICAL PHARMACOLOGY

23.1 March 2013 Antiplatelet drugs

a) Name four indications for antiplatelet drugs in clinical practice. (4 marks)
b) List five antiplatelet agents in clinical use and their underlying mechanisms of action. (10 marks)
c) List three possible causes of thrombocytosis. (3 marks)
d) List three possible causes of thrombocytopenia. (3 marks)

The Chair's Report for the original SAQ showed a 66.1% pass rate for a "straightforward question that is very topical." The original SAQ asked how active bleeding may be managed following administration of an antiplatelet agent. This is the same as bleeding under any other circumstances except that the antiplatelet should be stopped if the balance of risks makes it safer to do so, the effects of some are much longer lasting than others, ticagrelor has a specific antagonist, and large quantities of platelet transfusions may be required due to their rapid inactivation by any remaining antiplatelet in circulation. Discussion with a haematologist would be important.

a) Name four indications for antiplatelet drugs in clinical practice. (4 marks)

- Cardiovascular disease:
  - Primary prevention in at risk patients.
  - Secondary prevention in patients who have had myocardial infarction, any percutaneous coronary intervention including coronary stent, or bypass surgery.

- Cerebrovascular disease:
  - Primary prevention in patients at risk of thrombotic cerebrovascular events.
  - Secondary prevention of thrombotic events in patients who have had transient ischaemic attacks or thrombotic stroke.

- Peripheral vascular disease.

- Obstetric disease:
  - Prevention of pre-eclampsia and eclampsia.
  - Reduction of risk of stillbirth, fetal growth restriction, preterm birth, and early pregnancy loss.

- Haematological conditions:
  - Essential thrombocythaemia.

- In place of an anticoagulant where anticoagulant is contraindicated e.g. in haemofiltration circuits when heparin cannot be used.

- Side effect of a drug's intended use e.g. antipyretics, analgesics.

DOI: 10.1201/9781003388494-23

b) **List five antiplatelet agents in clinical use and their underlying mechanisms of action. (10 marks)**

What follows is an incredibly simplified version of platelet activation. I have focused on the aspects of the pathway that antiplatelet medications act upon to achieve their effect:

- *Platelets stay inactive by release of chemicals such as prostacyclin and nitric oxide from intact endothelium.*
- *Inactive platelets maintain calcium efflux out of the platelet and into tubular system via a cAMP-driven pump.*
- *Platelets are activated by exposed collagen or von Willebrand's factor (due to damage to the endothelium) or thrombin in the blood (due to activation of the coagulation pathways).*
- *The activated platelets release ADP from platelet dense granules and make thromboxane A_2 via the COX-1 pathway.*
- *ADP reduces cAMP thus inactivating the outward pump of calcium and allowing release of calcium from the tubular system, causing a conformational change in the platelet, resulting in degranulation and release of further proaggregatory mediators. It activates the platelet's GPIIb/IIIa receptors and also activates other platelets via $P2Y_{12}$ ADP receptors.*
- *Thromboxane A_2 also causes release of calcium from the tubular system resulting in a conformational change of the platelet causing degranulation and release of further proaggregatory mediators. It also activates the platelet's GPIIb/IIIa receptors.*
- *Fibrinogen will crosslink platelets by binding with activated GPIIb/IIIa receptors at each end, or bind to von Willebrand's factor exposed in the damaged endothelium, thus anchoring the platelet plug in place.*
- *This process takes place alongside the clotting cascade, which results in creation of further thrombin for further platelet activation. The result is a thrombus of activated crosslinked platelets and fibrin.*

The question asks for a list of five drugs and their mechanisms of action. I have put them into a table for the purposes of including some other detail that may be useful for the exam, but you should give the information the question asks for.

Aspirin			Irreversible cyclo-oxygenase inhibitor, which at low doses is more active on the COX-1 pathway, stopping thromboxane A_2 production.
$P2Y_{12}$ ADP receptor antagonists	Thienopyridines	Clopidogrel	Irreversible inhibition of $P2Y_{12}$ ADP receptor to prevent platelet aggregation. Is a prodrug, metabolised to active form by (mainly) CYP2C19 of the CYP450 enzyme group. This results in a time lag in efficacy, causes inter-individual variation in efficacy due to genetic variation, and formation of active drug inhibited by drugs that inhibit CYP2C19 e.g. omeprazole and esomeprazole.
		Prasugrel	Irreversible inhibition of $P2Y_{12}$ ADP receptor to prevent platelet aggregation. Prodrug (no reported genetic variation in efficacy).
	Cyclopentyl-triazolopyrimidine	Ticagrelor	Reversible $P2Y_{12}$ ADP receptor antagonist – causes conformational change in the receptor inhibiting its ADP signalling. Can be reversed with bentracimab.
	ATP analogue	Cangrelor	Intravenous short-acting $P2Y_{12}$ ADP receptor antagonist. Metabolism through dephosphorylation, not dependent on liver or kidneys. Platelet function returns to normal in 60 min.

(Continued)

(Continued)

Glycoprotein IIb/IIIa receptor inhibitors	Abciximab (a monoclonal antibody), eptifibatide, tirofiban	Intravenously administered, binds to the GPIIb/IIIa receptors preventing platelet crosslinking via fibrinogen, or anchoring of platelet to endothelial wall via von Willebrand's factor.
Dipyridamole, cilostazol		Phosphodiesterase inhibition reducing breakdown of cAMP therefore helping maintain platelets in their inactive state. (Both also cause vasodilation.)
Prostacyclin		Binds to platelet G-protein coupled receptor, increasing cAMP production by adenylate cyclase, helping maintain platelets in their inactive state.

c) List three possible causes of thrombocytosis. (3 marks)

Primary thrombocytosis:

- Essential thrombocythaemia.
- Polycythaemia vera.
- Myelofibrosis.
- Leukaemia.

Reactive thrombobocytosis:

- Disseminated malignancy.
- Inflammation.
- Surgery.
- Iron deficiency.
- Blood loss or haemolysis.

d) List three possible causes of thrombocytopenia. (3 marks)

Decreased platelet production:

- B12 or folic acid deficiency.
- Bone marrow failure.
- Leukaemia.
- Radiation.
- Aplastic anaemia.
- Myeloma.
- HIV.

Increased platelet destruction:

- Immune-mediated:
  - Idiopathic thrombocytopenic purpura.
  - Autoimmune conditions.
  - HIV, Dengue.
  - Heparin.
  - Post-transfusion purpura.

- Non-immune-mediated:

  - Disseminated intravascular coagulation.
  - Thrombotic thrombocytopenic purpura.
  - Splenic sequestration.
  - HELLP.

REFERENCES

Ramalingam G, Jones N, Besser M. Platelets for anaesthetists: part 1: physiology and pathology. *BJA Educ*. 2016a: 16: 134–139.

Ramalingam G, Jones N, Besser M. Platelets for anaesthetists: part 2: pharmacology. *BJA Educ*. 2016b: 16: 140–145.

Smart S, Aragola S, Hutton P. Antiplatelet agents and anaesthesia. *Contin Educ Anaesth Crit Care Pain*. 2007: 7: 157–161.

23.2 March 2014 Total intravenous anaesthesia

An adult patient is to receive a target-controlled infusion (TCI) of propofol.

a) What is the volume of distribution (l/kg), pKa, and clearance (ml/kg/min) of propofol? (3 marks)

b) With reference to the three-compartment model, what is represented by V_1? (1 mark)

c) Describe how TCI devices ensure a steady-state blood concentration. (4 marks)

d) Give two pharmacological properties of a drug that will affect equilibration with the effect site. (2 marks)

e) Describe the pharmacokinetic principles that allow effect-site targeting when using TCI propofol. (3 marks)

f) Define context sensitive half time. (1 mark)

g) Give two pharmacokinetic properties of propofol that account for its fast offset time when given by infusion. (2 marks)

h) List four advantages of using a TCI device for infusion of propofol compared to a manual propofol infusion regimen. (4 marks)

The Chair's Report after the original SAQ in 2014 commented on "widely distributed ignorance of the subject matter within the cohort" and a "'black-box' mentality from the majority of candidates with little real understanding of how infusion devices work or the underlying pharmacokinetics." The pass mark was just 17.5%. TIVA has been the focus of some questions in the physics and clinical measurement chapter, propofol features in a question regarding its complications in the intensive care medicine chapter, and TIVA was the focus of another applied clinical pharmacology question in a CRQ in 2022. There is an even greater focus now on TIVA since the 2021 RCoA curriculum, and so if you were thinking you could leave pharmacology behind now that you have done your Primary, think again! Remember the three-compartment model?

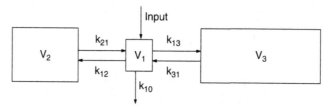

Three-compartment model.

a) Give the volume of distribution of a bolus dose (l/kg), pKa, and clearance (ml/kg/min) of propofol. (3 marks)

The pharmacokinetic properties of commonly used induction agents, neuromuscular blocking drugs, and opioids are frequently encountered topics in the Final – don't neglect them!

- Volume of distribution of a bolus dose: 4 l/kg.
- pKa: 11.
- Clearance: 25–60 ml/kg/min.

b) With reference to the three-compartment model, what is represented by V_1? (1 mark)

- V_1 is the central compartment into which the drug is injected and cleared. It represents plasma and any tissues that behave like plasma in respect to that particular drug.

c) Describe how TCI devices ensure a steady-state blood concentration. (4 marks)

Bolus, elimination, transfer (BET).

- TCI devices and programmes rely on the concept of a three-compartmental model of the way in which a specific drug behaves within the body. The sizes of the different compartments and the rate constants between them depend upon the model and drug being used. They also depend on certain patient characteristics such as height, weight, and age, which will require inputting into the administration device being used.
- To achieve a desired drug concentration rapidly, a bolus is given that is equal to the desired concentration multiplied by the volume of V_1 ($Cp \times V_1$).
- Drug leaves this central compartment down its concentration gradient initially to vessel-rich tissues (V_2) and then to tissues with poorer blood supplies (V_3). There are therefore two superimposed reducing infusion rates that allow for this loss from the central compartment. These superimposed rates stop once full distribution is assumed to have occurred.
- Elimination of the drug occurs from the central compartment and a constant infusion rate is required to account for this – this will be the steady-state infusion rate once equilibrium is reached.

d) Give two pharmacological properties of a drug that will affect equilibration with the effect site. (2 marks)

- Degree of drug ionisation at physiological pH, or pKa.
- Lipid solubility.
- Plasma protein binding.

e) Describe the pharmacokinetic principles that allow effect-site targeting when using TCI propofol. (3 marks)

Targeting the effect-site concentration aims to eliminate the hysteresis observed between plasma concentration and actual drug effect that takes place in the brain. The effect-site compartment volume is negligibly small, and so the rate constant determining movement of drug to effect site (K_{eo}) is one way only, from plasma to effect site, unlike the rate constants determining movement between other compartments. K_{eo} is not known and must be determined through experiment. Different, hypothetical, K_{eo} values are used to plot effect-site concentration curves, and the one that results in a concentration matching plasma concentration at peak observed drug effect is then determined as the actual K_{eo}. Peak drug effect will occur when the curve of the declining plasma concentration of the drug after bolus injection crosses the peak of the curve of the rising effect-site concentration.

- Assumption that effect site volume is negligible.
- Assumption that there is a rate constant (K_{eo}) that determines movement of drug to the effect site but not a reciprocal one, as the effect site size is negligible.
- Assumption that the rate constant can be determined by modelling different K_{eo} values and their effect-site concentration (Ce) curves and picking the one where peak Ce matches the declining plasma concentration after a bolus at the same point in time as the peak effect of the anaesthetic agent occurring clinically.

f) Define context sensitive half time. (1 mark)

- The time taken for a concentration of drug to reduce by half once an infusion at steady state is stopped.

g) Give two pharmacokinetic properties of propofol that account for its fast offset time when given by infusion. (2 marks)

- Rapid metabolism in the liver at a rate that exceeds redistribution back from V_2 and V_3.
- Propofol has no active metabolites.

h) List four advantages of using a TCI device for infusion of propofol compared to a manual propofol infusion regimen. (4 marks)

- The bolus dose and infusion rate are determined by computer models based on patient and drug characteristics, not guess-work.
- Theoretically, correct dosing therefore reduces risk of awareness on the one hand, and excessive cardiovascular and respiratory effects on the other.
- Theoretically, TCI can achieve steady state more rapidly. If a propofol infusion is initiated at a fixed rate, it takes five half-lives to reach steady state.
- Changing infusion rate with TCI results in pause or bolus as well, to achieve desired effect more rapidly – not so with manual.
- Using TCI is less labour-intensive than repeatedly checking and changing the rate manually.
- More rapid wake-up at end of surgery by avoiding excessive dosing during the preceding infusion.

REFERENCES

Absalom A, Mani V, De Smet T, Struys M. Pharmacokinetic models for propofol – defining and illuminating the devil in the detail. *BJA*. 2009: 10: 26–37.

Al-Rifai Z, Mulvey D. Principles of total intravenous anaesthesia: practical aspects of using total intravenous anaesthesia. *BJA Educ*. 2016: 16: 276–280.

Hill S. Pharmacokinetics of drug infusions. *Contin Educ Anaesth Crit Care Pain*. 2004: 4: 76–80.

23.3 March 2015 Reversal of neuromuscular blockade

a) Outline two mechanisms of spontaneous recovery from neuromuscular blockade following the administration of rocuronium. (2 marks)
b) Which class of drug does neostigmine belong to? (1 mark)
c) Describe the mechanism of action of neostigmine in reversing neuromuscular blockade. (2 marks)
d) Give two advantages and three disadvantages of using neostigmine for reversal of neuromuscular blockade. (5 marks)
e) Which class of drug does sugammadex belong to? (1 mark)
f) Describe the mechanism of action of sugammadex in reversing neuromuscular blockade. (2 marks)
g) Give three advantages and two disadvantages of using sugammadex for reversal of neuromuscular blockade. (5 marks)
h) List two postoperative pulmonary complications associated with inadequate reversal of neuromuscular blockade. (2 marks)

The Chair's Report following the original SAQ said that the 52.7% pass rate was "disappointing," pointing out that "these agents are 'meat and drink' to the profession." With increasing focus on safe intraoperative monitoring of neuromuscular blockade, risks of awareness, and increasing availability of quantitative train of four monitoring, they remain a key part of anaesthetic practice.

a) Outline two mechanisms of spontaneous recovery from neuromuscular blockade following the administration of rocuronium. (2 marks)

After the administration of rocuronium, there is a dynamic association and dissociation of the rocuronium with the nicotinic receptors. Concentration gradients will therefore determine where the drug goes.

- Redistribution of the drug occurs down its concentration gradient into the plasma, once plasma levels start to decrease.
- The reduction in plasma concentration is driven by biliary and renal excretion as well as by a small proportion of liver metabolism.

b) Which class of drug does neostigmine belong to? (1 mark)

- Reversible acetylcholinesterase inhibitor.

c) Describe the mechanism of action of neostigmine in reversing neuromuscular blockade. (2 marks)

- Neostigmine binds to the esteratic site of acetylcholinesterase to form a carbamylated complex. As such it is a non-competitive antagonist of the enzyme.
- This increases the amount of acetylcholine at the neuromuscular junction, competing with residual rocuronium for postsynaptic acetylcholine receptors.

Other drugs that share this mechanism are the following:

- *Edrophonium – short-acting, competitive antagonist of acetylcholinesterase (binds to anionic site).*
- *Organophosphate compounds – irreversibly phosphorylates the esteratic site – can lead to a cholinergic syndrome due to excess acetylcholine.*

d) **Give two advantages and three disadvantages of using neostigmine for reversal of neuromuscular blockade. (5 marks)**

Advantages:

- Cheap.
- Familiar.
- Anaphylaxis is rare.

Disadvantages:

- Unwanted muscarinic receptor action causing bradycardia, gut stimulation (possibly with implications on anastomotic integrity), secretions, bronchospasm, urinary retention.
- Co-administration of glycopyrrolate to mitigate muscarinic effects results in dry mouth, tachycardia.
- No use in "can't intubate, can't oxygenate" situations when neuromuscular blocking drug has just been given.
- Not appropriate for use in deep neuromuscular blockade; observer error in train-of-four monitoring may lead to overestimation of level of reversibility, resulting in ineffective administration or premature administration with the possibility of recurarisation.
- Ceiling of effect – increasing its dose does not necessarily increase its efficacy.
- May cause depolarising block if given in excessive quantities.
- Slow onset of action with peak effect reached after eight minutes, which may not be reached prior to patient waking if given at the end of the case.
- Renally excreted and therefore may have prolonged effects in renal failure.

e) **Which class of drug does sugammadex belong to? (1 mark)**

- (Gamma) cyclodextrins.

f) **Describe the mechanism of action of sugammadex in reversing neuromuscular blockade. (2 marks)**

- Ring-like structure with a negatively charged hydrophilic outer surface that attracts the positively charged aminosteroid and draws it in to the lipophilic inner surface, thus encapsulating it.
- The rocuronium-sugammadex complex is renally cleared at a rate similar to glomerular filtration rate.

g) **Give three advantages and two disadvantages of using sugammadex for reversal of neuromuscular blockade. (5 marks)**

Advantages:

- With appropriate dosing, reverses from full paralysis with rocuronium, useful in "can't intubate, can't oxygenate" (CICO) situations.
- In typical circumstances, no risk of recurarisation due to irreversible encapsulation of neuromuscular blocking drug.
- No significant cardiovascular effects.
- May be used to temporarily reverse neuromuscular block intraoperatively (e.g. to facilitate peripheral nerve monitoring or neurophysiological testing).

Disadvantages:

- Flucloxacillin and fusidic acid may displace neuromuscular blocking drug from sugammadex, potentiating block.

- Sugammadex will encapsulate progesterone, reducing the efficacy of hormonal contraceptives – women of childbearing age should be given "missed pill" advice.
- High cost in some countries.
- Potential for allergic reactions greater than neostigmine.
- Not effective against benzylisoquinoliniums.
- Not approved for use in patients with renal failure due to inability to excrete the complex.
- Vagal side effect with risk of profound bradycardia or cardiac arrest – rare.

h) **List two postoperative pulmonary complications associated with inadequate reversal of neuromuscular blockade. (2 marks)**

- Impaired respiratory effort leading to alveolar hypoventilation causing hypoxia and hypercapnia.
- Desaturation and respiratory failure.
- Airway obstruction.
- Pulmonary aspiration.
- Need for reintubation (+/– unexpected admission to intensive care).

REFERENCES

Hunter J. Reversal of neuromuscular block. *BJA Educ.* 2020: 20: 259–265.

Khirwadkar R, Hunter J. Neuromuscular physiology and pharmacology: an update. *Contin Ed Anaesth Crit Care Pain.* 2012: 12: 237–244.

23.4 September 2016 Diabetes management

a) In a patient with diabetes mellitus, what clinical features may indicate autonomic involvement? (4 marks)
b) What are the other microvascular (3 marks) and macrovascular (3 marks) complications of diabetes mellitus?
c) List the classes of oral hypoglycaemic agents that are available (5 marks). Describe their mechanisms of action. (5 marks)

Above is the SAQ as it appeared in the exam. The Chairs' Report following the SAQ commented that "very few candidates knew about any oral hypoglycaemic drugs other than sulphonylureas and biguanides. The other classes of drugs are now quite frequently used and should therefore be known about." The pass rate was only 38.4%. The SAQ was repeated in an almost identical manner in September 2019, and I will answer the question there.

23.5 March 2017 Postoperative nausea and vomiting

a) List the patient-related (7 marks) and anaesthetic-related (3 marks) risk factors for postoperative nausea and vomiting (PONV) in adult patients.

b) What are the unwanted effects of PONV in adults? (6 marks)

c) Which non-pharmacological interventions have been shown to be effective in reducing PONV in adults? (2 marks)

d) Briefly explain the proposed mechanisms of action of $5HT_3$ antagonists such as ondansetron when used as anti-emetics. (2 marks)

The Chairs' Report following this original SAQ said that the pass rate was 68.3%. "This was one of the two easy questions and the pass rate was the second highest overall [for the paper], as might be expected given the frequency with which PONV occurs. Despite this, many candidates had insufficient knowledge of risk factors for PONV and of the non-pharmacological methods that may be used to reduce it. Candidates who scored well had a sensible structured approach to this common problem." A score of 14/20 was required to pass an easy question. The topic was repeated as the focus of a CRQ in September 2020 with very similar themes questioned, so I have answered it there.

23.6 September 2019 Diabetes management

a) List four clinical features that may indicate autonomic involvement in a patient with diabetes mellitus. (4 marks)
b) List three other microvascular complications of diabetes mellitus. (3 marks)
c) List three macrovascular complications of diabetes mellitus. (3 marks)
d) What is the recommended upper limit of HbA1c for elective surgery? (1 mark)
e) State the Association of Anaesthetists of Great Britain & Ireland (AABGI) guidance for perioperative blood glucose monitoring in diabetic patients. (3 marks)
f) List three classes of oral hypoglycaemic agents that are available (3 marks) and describe the mechanism of action of each. (3 marks)

This exam paper was hybrid; six CRQs and six SAQs. This topic was questioned as an SAQ, and I have changed it minimally to make it into more of a CRQ style. The Chairs said that the pass rate for the SAQ was 71.5% and that "This question had been used previously and this was reflected in the improved pass rate. Knowledge of the complications of diabetes and the features of autonomic involvement was well answered and probably reflects that we see many diabetic patients in our clinical practice. Marks were lost in [section (e)] as very few candidates were aware of the AAGBI guidelines on blood glucose monitoring. The last part of the question was poorly answered. Candidates did not read the question, listing drugs as opposed to giving the classes of oral hypoglycaemic drugs." In fact, when they last used a version of this question in September 2016, they attributed 5 marks to the question about classes of oral hypoglycaemics and 5 marks to the mechanisms of actions rather than the 3 marks each in this paper. However, better to learn all of them and not get caught out, either in the exam or in real life.

a) **List four clinical features that may indicate autonomic involvement in a patient with diabetes mellitus. (4 marks)**

It has asked for four clinical features so I have put down too much here, but that is for the sake of you learning a more complete list. The nerve damage in diabetes is thought to relate to the direct damage caused by diabetes to the nerve tissue but also indirect damage due to blood supply being reduced due to microvascular damage.

- Cardiovascular; resting tachycardia, arrhythmias, orthostatic hypotension.
- Gastrointestinal; bloating after meals, constipation, and diarrhoea.
- Genitourinary; impotence, loss of bladder control.
- Sweating; gustatory sweating or reduced ability to sweat.

b) **List three other microvascular complications of diabetes mellitus. (3 marks)**

- Retinopathy.
- Nephropathy.
- Neuropathy (*usually mixed sensory and motor polyneuropathy, glove-and-stocking distribution, but also mononeuritis multiplex as well as the autonomic involvement already described*).
- Microvascular cardiac disease.

c) **List three macrovascular complications of diabetes mellitus. (3 marks)**

- Coronary artery disease.
- Cerebrovascular disease.
- Hypertension.
- Peripheral vascular disease.

d) What is the recommended upper limit of HbA1c for elective surgery? (1 mark)

- < 69 mmol/mol.

e) State the Association of Anaesthetists of Great Britain & Ireland (AABGI) guidance for perioperative blood glucose monitoring in diabetic patients. (3 marks)

- Target CBG 6–10 mmol/l (increase upper limit to 12 in poorly controlled diabetics or those being managed by modification of usual treatment rather than VRIII).
- Check pre-induction and at least hourly thereafter.
- Reduce time interval between checks if results are outside of acceptable range.

f) List three classes of oral hypoglycaemic agents that are available (3 marks) and describe the mechanism of action of each. (3 marks)

GLP1 analogues were for subcutaneous administration only until relatively recently when an oral formulation was made. There is a reasonable amount of interest in it as an approach for assisting with weight loss in non-diabetics. I have included a name from each class in the hope of assisting with learning, but the question does not ask for this, as the Chairs' Report pointed out.

Class	Mechanism of action
Biguanides (e.g. metformin).	Decreases hepatic gluconeogenesis, improves peripheral insulin sensitivity.
Sulphonylureas (e.g. gliclazide).	Stimulates pancreatic insulin secretion.
Thiazolidinediones (e.g. pioglitazone).	Improves peripheral insulin sensitivity.
Alpha-glucosidase inhibitors (e.g. acarbose).	Inhibits enzymatic breakdown of disaccharides to monosaccharides in the gut therefore inhibiting carbohydrate absorption.
Meglitinides (e.g. repaglinide).	Stimulates pancreatic insulin excretion.
SGLT-2 (sodium-glucose linked-transporter) inhibitors (e.g. canagliflozin).	Inhibits reuptake of glucose from the kidney thus increasing its excretion.
DPP4 inhibitors (gliptins) (e.g. sitagliptin).	Inhibits DPP4 from breaking down endogenous GLP1, which is a peptide released by the gut after meals to enhance insulin secretion and reduce glucagon release.
GLP1 analogues (Glucagon-like peptide analogues/incretin mimetics/incretins) (e.g. semaglutide).	Mimics the action of endogenous GLP1 to enhance insulin secretion and reduce glucagon release in a glucose-dependent manner.

REFERENCES

Association of Anaesthetists of Great Britain and Ireland. Peri-operative management of the surgical patient with diabetes. *Anaesth.* 2015: 70: 1427–1440.

Nicholson G, Hall G. Diabetes and adult surgical inpatients. *Contin Educ Anaesth Crit Care Pain.* 2011: 11: 234–238.

23.7 September 2020 Postoperative nausea and vomiting

a) List four patient-related risk factors for postoperative nausea and vomiting (PONV) in adults. (4 marks)
b) Give two complications of PONV in adults. (2 marks)
c) State the location of the vomiting centre. (1 mark)
d) List three inputs to the vomiting centre. (3 marks)
e) For the following four drugs, state the receptor that they target and the locations of action of each in the control of nausea and vomiting: cyclizine, hyoscine, ondansetron, and prochlorperazine. (8 marks)
f) Give two non-pharmacological interventions that have been shown to be effective in reducing PONV in adults. (2 marks)

Despite being very similar to the 2017 SAQ, the CRQ in 2020 only had a pass rate of 36.2% with the Chairs' Report commenting on poor CRQ technique: "Some candidates continued to write as much as they could and adopted a scattergun approach to their answers. As per candidate instructions, only the first distinct answer per line was marked. Part (a) asked for patient-related risk factors, but many answers were not specific and included anaesthetic factors such as drugs and bag mask ventilation. The pharmacology of anti-emetics was surprisingly poorly answered."

a) List four patient-related risk factors for postoperative nausea and vomiting (PONV) in adults. (4 marks)

- Female gender.
- History of PONV.
- History of motion sickness.
- Non-smoker.
- Younger age.

Other risk factors can be classified into anaesthetic or surgical risk factors:

Anaesthetic factors: volatile use, nitrous oxide use, postoperative opioid use, increased duration of anaesthesia, neostigmine use, stomach distension due to bag-valve-mask ventilation.

Surgical factors: middle ear surgery, strabismus surgery, laparoscopic surgery, neurosurgery.

The APFEL score is a risk stratification tool that identifies four major risk factors for PONV (female gender, non-smoker, history of PONV, and postoperative opioid use) and attributes a risk of PONV of 20% for each factor present.

b) Give two complications of PONV in adults. (2 marks)

- Reduced patient satisfaction.
- Delayed discharge from PACU.
- Delayed discharge from hospital/unexpected hospital stay in day case patients (with the implications of cost, inconvenience, poor bed usage).
- Delayed return to oral intake (especially important in diabetic patients).
- Suture/wound dehiscence.
- Aspiration of gastric contents.
- Dehydration.
- Electrolyte imbalance.

- Metabolic alkalosis.
- Oesophageal rupture.
- Raised intracranial and intraocular pressure.

c) **State the location of the vomiting centre. (1 mark)**

- Medulla (brainstem).

d) **List three inputs to the vomiting centre. (3 marks)**

- Cerebral cortex (emotions, fear).
- Other sensory inputs (pain, smell, sight).
- Vestibular centre.
- Chemoreceptive trigger zone.
- Gastrointestinal; chemoreceptors, mechanoreceptors, vagal afferents.
- Baroreceptors.

e) **For the following four drugs, state the receptor that they target and the locations of action of each in the control of nausea and vomiting: cyclizine, hyoscine, ondansetron, and prochlorperazine. (8 marks)**

I have included drugs from the other classes of antiemetics in the table below for completeness.

Drug	Receptor antagonism	Location
Cyclizine	Histamine H_1 (also with antimuscarinic effect).	Vestibular centre. Vomiting centre.
Hyoscine	Muscarinic acetylcholine.	Vestibular centre. Vomiting centre. Chemoreceptive trigger zone.
Ondansetron	$5HT_3$.	GI tract; impacting motility, secretion. Chemoreceptive trigger zone. Vomiting centre.
Prochlorperazine	Dopamine D_2.	Chemoreceptive trigger zone. Vomiting centre. GI tract; impacting secretion, motility, mucosal blood flow. *(Domperidone is a D2 receptor antagonist that does not cross the blood-brain-barrier and so is safer for use in Parkinson's.)*
Dexamethasone	*Intracellular corticosteroid.*	*Mechanism of action unclear, may involve reduction in inflammatory response to surgery, including reduction in serotonin release in gut, altered substance P production and reduced pain response.*
Aprepitant	*Neurokinin-1 receptor.*	*Chemoreceptor trigger zone. GI tract; impacts motility and inflammation.*
Nabilone, a cannabinoid	*CB1 receptors.*	*Chemoreceptor trigger zone: presynaptic stimulation of CB1 receptors reduces release of $5HT_3$ (reducing input to the vomiting centre). GI tract; reduces motility.*

f) **Give two non-pharmacological interventions that have been shown to be effective in reducing PONV in adults. (2 marks)**

- Acupressure, acupuncture.
- Aromatherapy.
- Avoidance of dehydration (avoid excessive starvation period).
- Gum chewing.

Understanding of the mechanisms involved in stimulating emesis are complex and incompletely understood, but the vomiting pathway is a common viva topic and being able to draw a diagram to illustrate it should help in remembering the mechanism of action of the commonly used antiemetics.

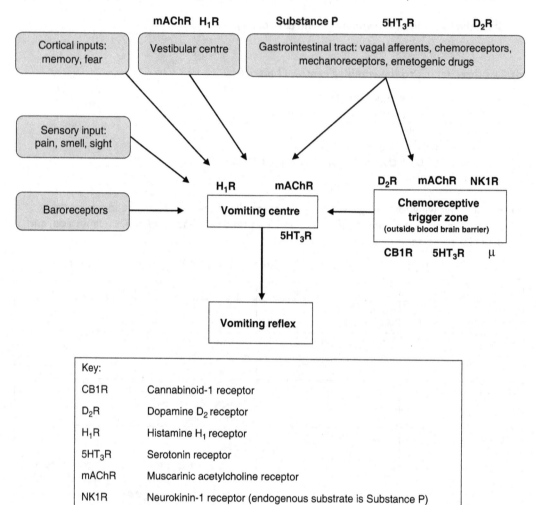

Vomiting pathway.

REFERENCES

Pierre S, Whelan R. Nausea and vomiting after surgery. *Contin Educ Anaesth Crit Care Pain*. 2013: 13: 28–32.

Tong G et al. Fourth consensus guidelines for the management of postoperative nausea and vomiting. *Anesth Analg*. 2020: 131: 411–448.

23.8 September 2021 Diabetes management

a) List four classes of oral hypoglycaemic medication (4 marks), giving a side effect other than hypoglycaemia for each. (4 marks)
b) Give the target intraoperative blood glucose range (mmol/l) in a diabetic patient undergoing surgery. (1 mark)
c) Give the three diagnostic criteria for diabetic ketoacidosis (DKA). (3 marks)
d) State the treatment of hypoglycaemia in a diabetic patient under general anaesthesia. (2 marks)
e) Give two indications for the perioperative use of a variable rate intravenous insulin infusion (VRIII) for patients with type 2 diabetes. (2 marks)
f) List four perioperative complications associated with poor long-term diabetes control. (4 marks)

The original CRQ contained a large amount of material from the 2015 Association of Anaesthetists' guideline on perioperative management of patients with diabetes, and I have also added content from the more recent Centre for Perioperative Care diabetes management guideline. This highlights again the importance of reading clinical guidelines as part of your revision for the Final.

a) **List four classes of oral hypoglycaemic medication (4 marks), giving a side effect other than hypoglycaemia for each. (4 marks)**

If you can't remember the mechanisms of action of these drugs, flick back to the September 2019 question to remind yourself. Sulphonylureas and meglitinides should not be taken when starving due to risk of hypoglycaemia, SGLT-2 inhibitors should not be taken when starving because of the risk of DKA or euglycaemic ketoacidosis, and metformin should not be taken for 48 hours from the day of any procedure involving use of contrast media if eGFR < 60 ml/min for fear of increasing the risk of lactic acidosis in the presence of impaired kidney function.

Class	Side effect
Biguanides (e.g. *metformin*).	Lactic acidosis, GI side effects.
Sulphonylureas (e.g. *gliclazide*).	Weight gain, increased risk of cardiovascular harm if used long term.
Thiazolidinediones (e.g. *pioglitazone*).	Increased risk of cardiovascular death, macular oedema, and bladder cancer.
Alpha-glucosidase inhibitors (e.g. *acarbose*).	Fermentation of carbohydrate by gut flora causing bloating, diarrhoea, abdominal pain, nausea. Contraindicated in inflammatory bowel disease.
Meglitinides (e.g. *repaglinide*).	Weight gain, GI upset.
SGLT-2 (sodium-glucose linked-transporter) inhibitors (e.g. *canagliflozin*).	Polyuria, dehydration, polydipsia, increased risk of genital candidiasis and urinary tract infection. Rarely, Fournier's gangrene. Risk of DKA or euglycaemic ketoacidosis if taken when starving.
DPP4 inhibitors *(gliptins)* (e.g. *sitagliptin*).	Pancreatitis, pancreatic cancer.
GLP1 analogues (*Glucagon-like peptide analogues/incretin mimetics/ incretins*) (e.g. *semaglutide*).	Reduced gastric emptying, weight loss.

b) Give the target intraoperative blood glucose range (mmol/l) in a diabetic patient undergoing surgery. (1 mark)

- 6–10 mmol/l.

c) Give the three diagnostic criteria for diabetic ketoacidosis (DKA). (3 marks)

- Blood glucose concentration >11 mmol/l OR known to be diabetic.
- Blood or capillary ketone concentration > 3 mmol/l OR ketonuria 2+ on urine dip.
- Bicarbonate concentration of < 15 mmol/l AND/OR pH <7.3.

d) State the treatment of hypoglycaemia in a diabetic patient under general anaesthesia. (2 marks)

- Blood glucose 4–6 mmol/l: give 10 g glucose, equivalent to an intravenous bolus of 50 ml 20% glucose.
- Blood glucose < 4 mmol/l: give 20 g glucose, equivalent to an intravenous bolus of 100 ml 20% glucose.

e) Give two indications for the perioperative use of a variable rate intravenous insulin infusion (VRIII) for patients with type 2 diabetes. (2 marks)

- Patients who are taking insulin and will miss more than one meal.
- Poorly controlled diabetes with HbA1c > 69 mmol/mol.
- Patients with recurrent hyperglycaemias.
- Patients requiring emergency surgery who have a blood glucose > 10 mmol/l.

f) List four perioperative complications associated with poor long-term diabetes control. (4 marks)

Studies have shown variable outcomes, but these are the risks listed in the Association of Anaesthetists' guideline of 2015.

- 50% increase in mortality.
- More than doubling of risk of postoperative respiratory infections.
- Doubling of risk of surgical site infections.
- Threefold risk of urinary tract infections.
- Doubling of risk of perioperative myocardial infarction.
- Almost twofold increase in risk of perioperative acute kidney injury.
- Perioperative hypoglycaemia.
- Perioperative hyperglycaemia or ketoacidosis.

REFERENCES

Association of Anaesthetists of Great Britain and Ireland. Peri-operative management of the surgical patient with diabetes. *Anaesth.* 2015: 70: 1427–1440.

Centre for Perioperative Care. *Guideline for perioperative care for people with diabetes mellitus undergoing elective and emergency surgery.* London, 2021, updated December 2022.

National Confidential Enquiry into Patient Outcome and Death. *Highs and lows.* London: National Confidential Enquiry into Patient Outcome and Death, 2018.

Stubbs D, Levy N, Dhatariya K. Diabetes medication pharmacology. *BJA Educ.* 2017: 17: 198–207.

23.9 September 2022 Total intravenous anaesthesia

a) State three components of a total intravenous anaesthesia (TIVA) giving set that facilitate safe drug delivery. (3 marks)
b) List four factors that may influence the choice of target concentration value when using target-controlled infusion (TCI) of propofol. (4 marks)
c) List three methods of monitoring depth of anaesthesia when using TIVA. (3 marks)
d) Two hours after the start of uneventful surgery with TIVA anaesthesia, the patient moves during a point of high surgical stimulation. Describe four aspects of immediate management. (4 marks)
e) List three causes of accidental awareness under anaesthesia specifically when using TIVA. (3 marks)
f) List three differences between the Marsh and Schnider models for TCI propofol. (3 marks)

The Chairs' Report following the original CRQ commented that "This was the worst performing question on the paper. The question referenced the Joint Guidelines from the Association of Anaesthetists and the Society for Intravenous Anaesthesia, as well as the 5th National Audit Project. Candidates tended to answer in general terms as opposed to referencing these documents in their answers. The last question was poorly answered as candidates showed a lack of understanding of the Marsh and Schnider models." The pass rate was just 22.2%. The question contained elements of pharmacology and physics, as well as a strong focus on critical incident triggers. This once again reiterates the need to read key guidelines issued by our main educational bodies.

a) **State three components of a total intravenous anaesthesia (TIVA) giving set that facilitate safe drug delivery. (3 marks)**

This question specifically asks about the giving set but don't forget that ensuring TIVA safety starts with the operator and continues with safe drug preparation and labelling, presence of functioning infusion pumps with alarms, and ends with a visible cannula.

- Luer-lock connections at each end to reduce the risk of accidental disconnection.
- Anti-siphon valve at drug syringe connector points – reduces risk of uncontrolled drug infusion.
- Anti-reflux valve at fluid line connector point to reduce the risk of backward flow of drug up infusion tubing resulting in failure to deliver the drug or delivery of a bolus of the drug subsequently.
- Drug and fluid lines should join together as close as possible to the patient to minimise dead space in which a drug may accumulate.
- Extra connections or three-way taps should not be added to the drug delivery lines.

b) **List four factors that may influence the choice of target plasma concentration value when using target-controlled infusion (TCI) of propofol. (4 marks)**

Patient factors:

- Cardiovascularly compromised patients (due to e.g. sepsis, haemorrhage, cardiovascular pathology) will require lower concentration.
- Age; elderly patients will require lower concentrations.
- Preoperative patient anxiety may make required concentration higher.

Anaesthetic factors:

- More rapid speed of induction will require higher initial target concentration.
- Co-administration of CNS depressants (e.g. opioids and benzodiazepines) will allow reduction in the target concentration required to produce anaesthesia, due to additive or synergistic drug effects.
- Regional anaesthesia will reduce the strength of surgical stimulus and thus reduce required target concentration.
- Processed EEG or other depth of anaesthesia monitoring outputs may result in change of target.

Surgical factors:

- Intense surgical stimulation is likely to require higher target concentration (e.g. Mayfield pin insertion during neurosurgery), whereas minimal stimulation (e.g. endoscopy) is likely to require lower target concentrations akin to sedation.

c) **List three methods of monitoring depth of anaesthesia when using TIVA. (3 marks)**

- Clinical signs; sweating, lacrimation, facial grimacing, movement (especially to command) in an unparalysed patient.
- Association of Anaesthetists' standards of monitoring of anaesthetised patients; heart rate, blood pressure, respiratory rate and volume if spontaneously ventilating. Nonspecific and can be altered by the pharmacodynamic side effects of drugs used in TIVA.
- Processed EEG most commonly used and, as per the Association of Anaesthetists' guidelines 2021, should be monitored before administration of neuromuscular blocking drug, and continue until reversal is confirmed by peripheral nerve stimulation.
- Raw EEG is sometimes used in clinical practice. Raw analysis of EEG waveforms is used to determine wakefulness.
- Auditory evoked and somatosensory evoked potentials.
- Isolated forearm technique, mostly a research-based technique where a neuromuscular blocking drug is administered after the application of an inflated tourniquet to one arm (so it does not circulate to muscles distal to tourniquet). Movement of the arm either intentionally, in response to command, or unintentionally may indicate lighter planes of anaesthesia.

d) **Two hours after the start of uneventful surgery with TIVA anaesthesia, the patient moves during a point of high surgical stimulation. Describe four aspects of immediate management. (4 marks)**

The Association of Anaesthetists produced a NAP5 Handbook which included a guide as to what to do if awareness is suspected. Verbal reassurance is a key part of their recommendations at every stage.

- Pause surgery.
- Verbal reassurance to the patient.
- Ensure analgesia, checking for patency of TIVA lines, cannula, and pump function etc.
- Deepen anaesthesia, checking for patency of TIVA lines, cannula, and pump function etc., adding volatile agent if indicated.
- Document events on anaesthetic chart.

e) **List three causes of accidental awareness under anaesthesia specifically when using TIVA. (3 marks)**

Read the question – this is not looking for patient or surgical factors, but rather factors specific to TIVA. In NAP5, the two commonest causes of accidental awareness during TIVA were failure to deliver the *intended dose of drug and poor understanding of the underlying pharmacological principles, and so I have grouped my answers here according to these two headings although each one is a separate point. Bear in mind that TIVA is different to TCI, the former being any anaesthetic achieved by intravenous agents alone and the latter including the use of a programmed pump to target a specific plasma or effect-site concentration.*

- Failure to give intended dose of drug:
  - Equipment failure including pump failure, failure to connect to mains and battery exhausted, accidental disconnection, fault in giving set, tissued or disconnected cannula.
  - Human error resulting in incorrect concentration of drug selected, wrong drug in wrong preprogrammed pump, wrong patient demographics inputted.

- Poor understanding of underlying pharmacology:
  - Failure to give an initial bolus dose *(although a TCI pump will do this for you)*.
  - Change from volatile to TIVA e.g. for transfer to ICU and failure to establish adequate concentrations of intravenous agent before stopping inhalational.
  - Administration of excessively low fixed infusion rate instead of TCI.
  - Generalised lack of education or training in TIVA.

g) List three differences between the Marsh and Schnider models for TCI propofol. (3 marks)

Marsh	Schnider
Requires patient body mass to be inputted.	Requires patient sex, mass and height (to calculate lean body mass), and age to be inputted.
Compartment sizes are proportional to body mass.	V1 and V3 are of fixed size, V2 influenced by age (smaller if older).
Rate constants for slow and fast redistribution are fixed.	Rate constants for fast redistribution are influenced by age, and rate constants for slow redistribution are fixed.
Larger V1, 0.028 l/kg so 16 l for a 70 kg patient, so larger initial bolus dose to achieve desired concentration resulting in risk of cardiovascular instability (especially in older patient who will be delivered the same bolus dose as a 20-year-old of the same body mass).	Smaller V1, fixed at 4.27 l, so fixed bolus dose for given desired concentration so risk of underdosing of younger and obese patients.
Elimination rate constant fixed.	Elimination rate constant adjusted by lean body mass, mass, height.
Initially designed as a plasma-site targeted programme although effect-site targeting now feasible.	Initially designed as an effect-site targeted programme although plasma-site targeting now feasible.

REFERENCES

Absalom A, Mani V, De Smet T, Struys M. Pharmacokinetic models for propofol – defining and illuminating the devil in the detail. *BJA*. 2009: 10: 26–37.

Association of Anaesthetists, London, UK. *The 'NAP5 handbook': concise practice guidance on the prevention and management of accidental awareness during general anaesthesia*, 2019. https://anaesthetists.org/Home/Resources-publications/Guidelines/The-NAP5-Handbook. Accessed 27th March 2023.

Klein AA et al. Recommendations for standards of monitoring during anaesthesia and recovery 2021. *Anaesthesia*. 2021: 76: 1212–1223.

Nimmo AF et al. Joint guidelines from the Association of Anaesthetists and the Society for Intravenous Anaesthesia: guidelines for the safe practice of total intravenous anaesthesia (TIVA). *Anaesthesia*. 2018: 74: 211–224.

Pandit J, Cook T (eds.). *5th National Audit Project of the Royal College of Anaesthetists and the Association of Anaesthetists of Great Britain and Ireland: accidental awareness during general anaesthesia in the United Kingdom and Ireland*. London: The Royal College of Anaesthetists and Association of Anaesthetists of Great Britain and Ireland, 2014.

APPLIED PHYSIOLOGY AND BIOCHEMISTRY

24.1 March 2012 Preoxygenation

a) Define functional residual capacity (FRC). (2 marks)
b) List four factors that reduce FRC. (4 marks)
c) Apart from FRC, give three factors that determine how long oxygen saturation can be maintained in an apnoeic patient. (3 marks)
d) State five practical aspects of performing successful preoxygenation. (5 marks)
e) How can the adequacy of preoxygenation be assessed? (1 mark)
f) Give two clinical advantages of preoxygenating a fit adult prior to anaesthesia. (2 marks)
g) Give three clinical disadvantages of preoxygenating a fit adult prior to anaesthesia. (3 marks)

The Chair's Report following the original SAQ said that it was "poorly answered," and this was reflected by the 50.5% pass rate. They noted that "words such as FRC, oxygen consumption, carbon dioxide production, alveolar ventilation, alveolar gas equation and wash-in" are key in describing preoxygenation physiology and were missing from many answers. This question is almost identical to one that featured in 2008, four years previously. It's fair game, as it's pretty central to our practice!

a) Define functional residual capacity (FRC). (2 marks)

The FRC is largely composed of nitrogen under normal conditions, and so preoxygenation increases the oxygen content of the FRC by washing out nitrogen, otherwise called denitrogenation.

- The <u>volume</u> of gas/air present in the lungs at the end of <u>normal/tidal</u> expiration.

b) List four factors that reduce FRC. (4 marks)

- Supine posture *(improved by ramping)*.
- Anaesthesia.
- Encroachment on FRC by obesity, pregnancy, ascites, bowel obstruction, kyphoscoliosis.
- Young age; children have lower FRC per unit body mass.

c) Apart from FRC, give three factors that determine how long oxygen saturation can be maintained in an apnoeic patient. (3 marks)

This depends upon the balance between how quickly the oxygen is being used, how much of a reservoir there is to use, and whether there is a way to keep topping up that reservoir. The reservoir is the product of the functional residual capacity and its oxygen content.

Remember the alveolar gas equation?

$PAO_2 = PiO_2 - PaCO_2/RQ$

It demonstrates that increasing PiO_2 increases PAO_2 and how a raised $PaCO_2$ has a negative impact on PAO_2.

DOI: 10.1201/9781003388494-24   545

- Oxygen reservoir available: this is the product of the FRC and its oxygen content. The determinants of FRC are listed above, whereas oxygen content can be determined by the following:
  - Fraction of inspired oxygen preceding apnoea *(the alveolar gas equation determines that breathing 100% oxygen increases the available reservoir by a factor of nearly 5, compared to room air)*.
  - Respiratory or cardiac disease causing shunt, reducing the effectiveness of preoxygenation.
  - $PaCO_2$ (according to the alveolar gas equation, an elevated $PaCO_2$ results in a reduced PAO_2).

- Rate of oxygen consumption – increased by the following:
  - Sepsis.
  - Thyrotoxicosis.
  - Pregnancy.
  - Critical illness.
  - Fasciculations secondary to suxamethonium.
  - Childhood – greater oxygen consumption per unit weight.

- Patency of airway:
  - *At normal steady state, oxygen is removed from the lungs at the rate of its consumption (approximately 250 ml/min in a textbook adult). Carbon dioxide delivery to the lungs is 80% of this, as determined by a respiratory quotient of 0.8. After apnoea, oxygen removal from the lungs persists at the same rate. However, as the partial pressure of carbon dioxide in the alveoli starts to rise, the concentration gradient between blood and alveoli reduces, negatively impacting on further movement of carbon dioxide into the lungs. Lung volume consequently falls. If the airway is patent, this results in apnoeic mass movement of gas (oxygen, if the anaesthetic mask is still firmly held in place) into the lungs, significantly extending the time to desaturation (although the negative consequences of acidosis and hypercapnia will not be addressed by this).*

d) **State five practical aspects of performing successful preoxygenation. (5 marks)**

- Explanation to, and consent from patient to improve compliance.
- Ramped positioning to increase the size of FRC.
- Consider other measures to improve FRC in specific circumstances such as nasogastric drainage of stomach contents in patients with bowel obstruction or ascitic drainage in patients with significant ascites or preoperative management of pleural effusion.
- Tight-fitting mask (anaesthetic machine circuit) avoids entrainment of room air.
- High-flow nasal oxygen can be used as an alternative to face mask.
- Use of FiO_2 1.0.
- Gas flow to exceed patient's minute ventilation to ensure gas in circuit remains as close as possible to 100% oxygen while patient is still breathing.
- Continue high-flow oxygen after patient has stopped breathing to facilitate apnoeic mass movement of oxygen.
- Three to five minutes duration.
- Tidal breathing.

e) How can the adequacy of preoxygenation be assessed? (1 mark)

- Monitor fraction of expired oxygen (F_EO_2), to target greater than 0.9.

f) Give two clinical advantages of preoxygenating a fit adult prior to anaesthesia. (2 marks)

g) Give three clinical disadvantages of preoxygenating a fit adult prior to anaesthesia. (3 marks)

Advantages	Disadvantages
Difficult to predict difficult intubation, therefore provides a margin of safety in unpredicted difficulties.	Risk of respiratory incident during induction in fit patients is low, so may be unnecessary.
Cannot predict severe laryngospasm.	Prolongs induction by five minutes.
	Intolerance of tight-fitting mask, sense of claustrophobia.
	Increases alveolar collapse at induction resulting in risk of atelectasis and postoperative hypoxia.
	Adverse consequences of hyperoxia in certain patients e.g. after myocardial infarction or stroke.

REFERENCES

Ashrad-Kashani N, Kumar R. High-flow nasal oxygen therapy. *BJA Educ.* 2017: 17: 63–67.

Patel A, Nouraei S. Transnasal humidified rapid-insufflation ventilatory exchange (THRIVE): a physiological method of increasing apnoea time in patients with difficult airways. *Anaesthesia.* 2015: 70: 323–329.

Sirian R, Wills J. Physiology of apnoea and the benefits of preoxygenation. *Contin Educ Anaesth Crit Care Pain.* 2009: 9: 105–108.

24.2 September 2012 Elderly physiology

a) Outline the major changes in the cardiovascular system of elderly patients. (7 marks)
b) What are the perioperative implications of each change? (13 marks)

I have reproduced, above, the SAQ exactly how it appeared in the exam. In 2012 the SAQs had fewer subdivisions than they did latterly, just before the change to the very targeted CRQ format. Even then, however, the College demonstrated they were happy to have quite brief answers as reflected in the Chair's Report: "This question was set to explore the knowledge of both the physiological and pathological changes that occur as a result of ageing. Many of the answers were insufficiently detailed and not systematic. It is acceptable to structure your answers in tabulated form if the sections of a question are linked. In this case, the answers to (a) and (b) were associated.

For example:

(a) Cardiovascular change	(b) Anaesthetic implication
Increased systemic vascular resistance Hypertension Left ventricular hypertrophy	Cardiovascular instability May need to obtund pressor responses Antihypertensive medication
Beta receptor down-regulation	Reduced responsiveness to catecholamines and sympathomimetic agents
Etc.	

Other cardiovascular changes include reduced autonomic responsiveness, reduced cardiac output secondary to reduced stroke volume, degeneration of SA and AV nodes and conducting system, increased incidence of valvular heart disease and ischaemic heart disease. Similar questions in the future might feature changes in the respiratory or central nervous systems of the elderly." However, the pass mark was only 46.9%. Physiology of the elderly reappeared as a topic in March 2020, and so there is a CRQ-style question later in this chapter.

24.3 September 2012 Hyperparathyroidism

a) List two causes of primary hyperparathyroidism. (2 marks)
b) State three biochemical abnormalities seen in primary hyperparathyroidism. (3 marks)
c) List five systemic effects of hyperparathyroidism, other than biochemical abnormalities. (5 marks)
d) State two specific preoperative concerns when providing anaesthesia for parathyroidectomy. (2 marks)
e) List five specific intraoperative anaesthetic considerations when providing anaesthesia for parathyroidectomy. (5 marks)
f) List three specific postoperative complications following parathyroidectomy. (3 marks)

The Chair's Report of the original SAQ stated a 46.1% pass rate, commenting that "candidates appeared to have little idea of the anaesthetic issues and often wrote generic answers with little or no focus on the specifics of parathyroid surgery. It was a common misconception that parathyroid adenomas are large and will obstruct the airway. Hardly any candidates mentioned gland localisation techniques (methylene blue), and a significant number did not include hypocalcaemia as an important postoperative problem. Many failed to mention optimal patient positioning and the fact that the surgeon may wish to use a peripheral nerve stimulator."

There are four parathyroid glands, located at the poles of the thyroid gland. However, there is great variation in their location. They are small, 3 × 6 × 2 mm. Blood supply is from the inferior thyroid artery. Their secretion is inhibited by high parathyroid hormone and calcium levels and stimulated by high phosphate levels.

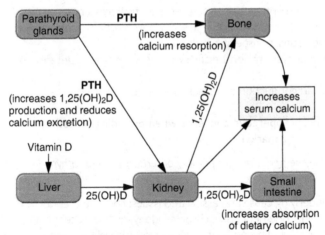

Calcium regulation.

a) List two causes of primary hyperparathyroidism. (2 marks)

Secondary hyperparathyroidism occurs in chronic kidney disease; the failing kidney does not excrete phosphate efficiently and does not hydroxylate vitamin D, reducing calcium absorption from the gastrointestinal tract. After a prolonged period of secondary hyperparathyroidism, tertiary hyperparathyroidism may develop. Here, even once calcium and phosphate levels return to normal (e.g. after a renal transplant), the parathyroid glands continue to oversecrete.

- Parathyroid adenoma.
- Gland hyperplasia.
- Parathyroid cancer.

b) State three biochemical abnormalities seen in primary hyperparathyroidism. (3 marks)

- Elevated parathyroid hormone.
- Elevated calcium.
- Reduced phosphate.
- Elevated alkaline phosphatase.

c) Name five systemic effects of hyperparathyroidism (other than electrolyte abnormalities). (5 marks)

"Stones, bones, abdominal groans, psychic moans." Take your pick from any of the systemic effects grouped below.

- Renal: stones, impaired concentrating ability, polyuria, renal failure.
- Skeletal: bone resorption, pain, fractures, osteitis fibrosis cystica.
- Gastrointestinal: calcium-induced gastric hypersecretion, peptic ulceration, acute and chronic pancreatitis, nonspecific abdominal pain.
- Central nervous system: nonspecific symptoms, weakness, deterioration in memory and cerebration.
- Cardiovascular: conduction defects, hypertension.

d) State two specific preoperative concerns when providing anaesthesia for parathyroidectomy. (2 marks)

Parathyroidectomy may be performed for primary or tertiary hyperparathyroidism for example in patients with end-stage renal failure.

- Consider underlying cause and associated issues; coexistent endocrine disease (e.g. as part of multiple endocrine neoplasia), chronic kidney disease, recent transplant.
- Consider the impact of hyperparathyroidism; calcium level (may need correction preoperatively, bisphosphonate treatment, and fluids), renal function, cardiac rhythm (check ECG).

e) List five specific intraoperative anaesthetic considerations when providing anaesthesia for parathyroidectomy. (5 marks)

- Surgical field is near airway. Reinforced tube or LMA may be used.
- Positioning is supine, head up to optimise surgical field, sandbag under shoulders to improve access; care is needed as patient may have osteoporosis and is therefore at risk of pathological fracture.
- Potentially prolonged surgery especially if checking with frozen sections for completeness of adenoma resection or on-table parathyroid hormone assays; need for warming, pressure area care, and mechanical thromboprophylaxis.

- Methylene blue used to identify glands causes risk of anaphylaxis and interference with oxygen saturations monitoring.
- Recurrent laryngeal nerve monitoring may be required by surgeon. Short-acting NMBD may be used for intubation, or longer acting agent with immediate reversal after securing airway. Remifentanil infusion may be considered to obtund the cough reflex and reduce the need for ongoing NMBD use.
- Can feasibly be performed with regional anaesthetic technique using bilateral superficial cervical plexus blocks with supplementation (although this is rare).
- A smooth emergence profile with minimal coughing is required to ensure haemostasis. Use of remifentanil infusion and adequate antiemesis can help with this.

f) **List three specific postoperative complications following parathyroidectomy. (3 marks)**

- Hypocalcaemia; check at 6 hours and 24 hours. May need oral or intravenous supplementation.
- Recurrent laryngeal nerve palsy; voice change, difficulty breathing, airway obstruction.
- Haematoma causing airway obstruction (rare in comparison to post-thyroidectomy).
- Incomplete resection (resulting in failure to resolve the abnormal biochemistry associated with hyperparathyroidism).

REFERENCE

Malhotra S, Sodhi V. Anaesthesia for thyroid and parathyroid surgery. *Contin Educ Anaesth Crit Care Pain.* 2007: 7: 55–58.

24.4 March 2013 Physiology after heart transplant

A 56-year-old man is listed for elective surgery. He received an orthotopic heart transplant 12 years before.

a) What key alterations in cardiac physiology and function must be considered when planning general anaesthesia? (10 marks)

b) What are the implications of the patient's immunosuppressant therapy for perioperative care? (6 marks)

c) What long-term health issues may occur in this type of patient? (4 marks)

The SAQ, reproduced here in its original form, had a 27% pass rate with the Chair reporting that it was "the most difficult question on the paper." They said that "A majority of the candidates demonstrated poor understanding of the physiology of a transplanted heart and the side effects of immunosuppressive therapy of relevance to the anaesthetist:

- *Increased infection risk – may need antibiotic prophylaxis/strict asepsis.*
- *Common agents cause a degree of chronic kidney disease.*
- *Avoid NSAIDs – enhanced side effects.*
- *Important to maintain stable plasma levels – ensure drugs taken/given.*
- *IV steroid cover may be required.*
- *Cyclosporin enhances and azathioprine reduces aminosteroid NMBD action."*

Physiology of the transplanted heart was the focus of a CRQ in September 2021, and I have addressed the topic there.

24.5 September 2015 Cerebrospinal fluid

a) Outline the production and circulation of cerebrospinal fluid (CSF). (3 marks)
b) How does intracranial pressure affect production and absorption of CSF? (2 marks)
c) List four differences between the biochemistry of CSF and plasma. (4 marks)
d) State three diagnostic indications for lumbar puncture. (3 marks)
e) State three therapeutic indications for lumbar puncture. (3 marks)
f) List two procedural factors that predispose to the development of a post-dural puncture headache after lumbar puncture. (2 marks)
g) List three patient factors that predispose to the development of a post-dural puncture headache after lumbar puncture. (3 marks)

The Chairs' Report following the original SAQ commented that they would have expected the pass rate (50.9%) to have been a little higher as this was one of the easy questions in the paper. Specifically, regarding the part asking about the risk factors that predispose to post-dural puncture headache after lumbar puncture, they commented that "many candidates talked about the factors that increase the risk of accidental dural puncture and, whilst the information they gave on that topic was correct, it was not what was asked for so they could not be given any marks." Read the questions carefully!

a) Outline the production and circulation of cerebrospinal fluid (CSF). (3 marks)

- Choroid plexuses (tufts of capillaries) secrete sodium into the lateral and fourth ventricles, creating osmotic pressure that draws water with it, thus creating CSF.
- Production rate of 500 ml/day, but constant reabsorption means volume present is only approximately 150 ml.
- Lateral ventricles drain into third ventricle via foramen of Monro. Third ventricle drains into fourth ventricle via aqueduct of Sylvius, from which it can circulate to the spinal canal.
- It enters the subarachnoid space from the fourth ventricle via the foramina of Luschka (lateral) and Magendie (medial).
- Absorption is via arachnoid granulations, outpouchings of the arachnoid through the dura that exist in close proximity to venous sinuses.

b) How does intracranial pressure affect production and absorption of CSF? (2 marks)

- Production is opposed if intracranial pressure rises, as CSF hydrostatic pressure opposes the osmotic pressure generated by sodium secretion.
- Absorption via arachnoid granulations is dependent on CSF pressure being higher than venous pressure – higher CSF pressure will increase absorption rate.
- Small increases in ICP can be "buffered" by movement of CSF out of the ventricles and down to the spinal cord – this initially helps to keep brain volume constant as per the Monro-Kellie doctrine.

c) List four differences between the biochemistry of CSF and plasma. (4 marks)

I would hope that a description of the differences would suffice here, rather than actual values. I don't think I would be prepared to give brain space to memorising the actual values.

- CSF sodium levels are higher than plasma due to active secretion.
- CSF chloride is also higher as it accompanies sodium to maintain electrical neutrality.
- CSF pH is lower (more acidic) than plasma, owing in part to higher pCO_2 (which ultimately sensitises central chemoreceptors).
- All other ions found in plasma are also found in the CSF but at a lower level.

- CSF glucose is approximately two-thirds of the level of plasma or more.
- CSF protein content is very low in disease-free state.
- Osmolarity of CSF and serum is equal.

d) State three diagnostic indications for lumbar puncture. (3 marks)

It's easy to just list our specialty's encounters with lumbar puncture, but just as with indications for arterial cannulation, try to think of other specialties' indications.

- Central nervous system (CNS) infections such as meningitis or encephalitis due to viral, bacterial, fungal, or mycobacterial causes.
- Subarachnoid haemorrhage (detection of xanthochromia).
- CNS diseases such as Guillain-Barré, multiple sclerosis.
- Carcinomatous meningitis.
- Intrathecal administration of contrast media for myelography or cisternography.

e) State three therapeutic indications for lumbar puncture. (3 marks)

- Intrathecal administration of chemotherapy or antibiotics.
- Therapeutic relief of idiopathic intracranial hypertension.
- Spinal drain insertion to mitigate against perioperative spinal cord ischaemia.
- Neuraxial anaesthesia.
- As part of siting an intrathecal drug delivery device (for management of chronic pain or spasticity).

f) List two procedural factors that predispose to the development of a post-dural puncture headache after lumbar puncture. (2 marks)

- Multiple punctures.
- Larger-gauge needle.
- Use of traumatic, cutting needle rather than pencil-point.

g) List three patient factors that predispose to the development of a post-dural puncture headache after lumbar puncture. (3 marks)

- Increased incidence in young adults, lower incidence in older adults, lower perceived rate in children but probably due to failure to report.
- Female sex.
- Pregnancy.
- Lower body mass index.

REFERENCES

Aitkenhead A, Moppet I, Thompson J. *Smith and Aitkenhead's textbook of anaesthesia*, 6th edition. Churchill Livingstone, 2013.

Turnbull D, Shepherd D. Post-dural puncture headache: pathogenesis, prevention and treatment. *BJA*. 2003: 91: 718–729.

Wrobel M, Volk T. Post-dural puncture headache. *Anesth Pain*. 2012: 1: 273–274.

24.6 September 2015 Smoking

a) List four effects of cigarette smoking on the cardiovascular system, and give the underlying mechanism of each. (4 marks)
b) Describe three pathophysiological mechanisms by which cigarette smoking can impair systemic oxygen delivery. (3 marks)
c) List five effects of cigarette smoking on the respiratory system that are relevant to the conduct of general anaesthesia. (5 marks)
d) List three other perioperative complications that cigarette smokers are at increased risk of. (3 marks)
e) List three physiological benefits of smoking cessation 24 hours prior to surgery. (3 marks)
f) Give two drug classes that may be used to aid smoking cessation. (2 marks)

The Chairs' Report of the original SAQ reflected a good pass rate of 55.5% but commented that "candidates who lost marks generally did so because they did not know the pathophysiological mechanisms involved in the difficulties caused by smoking. Remember that applied physiology is also part of the syllabus."

a) List four effects of cigarette smoking on the cardiovascular system, and give the underlying mechanism of each. (4 marks)

- Hypertension; raised circulating catecholamine levels and accelerated atherosclerosis formation increase left ventricular afterload, resulting in left ventricular hypertrophy, diastolic dysfunction and, ultimately, heart failure.
- Tachycardia; raised circulating catecholamine levels due to stimulation of nicotinic receptors.
- Peripheral vascular disease; accelerated atherosclerosis formation.
- Ischaemic heart disease; due to combination of accelerated atherosclerosis formation and prothrombotic state (due to carbon monoxide, nicotine, and other chemicals in cigarette smoke causing polycythaemia, enhanced platelet action, increased fibrinogen levels).
- Heart failure; subsequent to infarction, ischaemia, and cardiac muscle damage, as well as due to pathophysiological response to chronically elevated afterload.
- Pulmonary embolism.

b) Describe three pathophysiological mechanisms by which cigarette smoking can impair systemic oxygen delivery. (3 marks)

The combined effect is reduced oxygen delivery to the myocardium during a time of increased need, resulting in increased risk of ischaemia, which further promotes carboxyhaemoglobin formation, further reducing myocardial oxygen delivery, increasing the risk of perioperative ischaemia and infarction.

- Hypoxic hypoxia; airway and respiratory conditions related to smoking that result in reduced oxygen availability within the alveolus and reduced effective gas exchange.
- Anaemic hypoxia; haemoglobin has a 250-fold increased affinity for carbon monoxide compared to oxygen, thus creating carboxyhaemoglobin and reducing availability for oxygen carriage.
- Anaemic hypoxia; shift of oxygen dissociation curve to left due to presence of carbon monoxide, reducing the ability of haemoglobin to release oxygen.
- Histotoxic hypoxia; inhibition of cytochrome oxidase by carbon monoxide, reducing oxygen-dependent synthesis of ATP in mitochondria.

c) **List five effects of cigarette smoking on the respiratory system that are relevant to the conduct of general anaesthesia. (5 marks)**

- Pre-existing airways disease as a result of smoking such as cancer and chronic obstructive pulmonary disease with risk of consequent infection and vulnerability to the effects of positive pressure ventilation.
- Increased upper airway irritability; breath-holding, laryngospasm at induction and instrumentation.
- Increased lower airway reactivity, bronchospasm, mucus secretion.
- Impaired mucociliary transport and secretion clearance; risk of atelectasis, lobar collapse, postoperative pneumonia, shunt.
- Accelerated rate of FEV_1 reduction with age; significantly reduced level is predictive of postoperative respiratory complications.
- Increased closing capacity.
- Increased risk of pulmonary embolism due to hypercoagulability.

d) **List three other perioperative complications that cigarette smokers are at increased risk of. (3 marks)**

- Surgical site and organ space infections, sepsis and septic shock.
- Anastomotic breakdown.
- Increased risk of ICU admission.
- Longer postoperative stay.
- Increased risk of death.

e) **List three physiological benefits of smoking cessation 24 hours prior to surgery. (3 marks)**

The longer the time period of smoking cessation, the better, but even 24 hours can make a difference.

- Reduced circulating nicotine level (half-life in air of 30 minutes) and thus circulating catecholamine levels return to normal within one hour, reducing myocardial oxygen demand.
- Reduced circulating carbon monoxide (half-life in air of four hours) leads to carboxyhaemoglobin clearance within 24 hours, improving oxygen delivery to all tissues including the myocardium, reducing the risk of perioperative ischaemic event.
- Blood hypercoagulability will start to improve as carbon monoxide levels fall, reducing the risk of perioperative thrombotic events.
- As oxygen carriage improves, physiological reserve to cope with perioperative periods of inadvertent hypoxia improves.
- Postoperatively, ongoing smoking is known to be associated with poor tissue healing including wounds, anastomoses, flaps.

f) **Give two drug classes that may be used to aid smoking cessation. (2 marks)**

- Nicotine receptor agonist (*e.g. lozenges, patches, nasal spray, or gum*).
- Nicotinic receptor antagonist (*e.g. bupropion*).
- Nicotinic receptor partial agonist (*e.g. varenicline*).

Use of electronic cigarettes, or vaping, is a commonly used approach to smoking cessation but also is being used more commonly by people who have never smoked.

- *These contain nicotine and therefore confer a degree of cardiovascular risk but have negligible carbon monoxide production.*

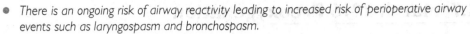

- There is an ongoing risk of airway reactivity leading to increased risk of perioperative airway events such as laryngospasm and bronchospasm.
- There are concerns about additive substances, especially in flavoured vapes, for which there is little long-term risk data.
- There is little evidence currently regarding the overall safety profile and risk reduction (if any) of postoperative complications in comparison to cigarette smoking.

REFERENCES

Carrick M, Robson J, Thomas C. Smoking and anaesthesia. *BJA Educ.* 2019: 19: 1–6.

Cutts T, O'Donnell A. The implications of vaping for the anaesthetist. *BJA Educ.* 2021: 21: 243–249.

Moppett I, Curran J. Smoking and the surgical patient. *CEPD Rev.* 2001: 1: 122–124.

24.7 March 2016 Preoxygenation

a) What physiological factors determine the rate of fall in arterial oxygen saturation in an apnoeic patient (3 marks) and which patient groups are most likely to show a rapid fall? (4 marks)

b) How may oxygenation, prior to intubation, be optimised during a rapid sequence induction (8 marks) and how can its progress be measured? (1 mark)

c) What are the possible respiratory complications of prolonged delivery of 100% oxygen? (4 marks)

This SAQ, reproduced here as it appeared in the exam, was very similar in content to that from March 2012. However, the pass rate was only 44.4% with the Chairs commenting that the "physiology surrounding oxygenation and the practice of preoxygenation should be well understood by candidates as this subject is very relevant to every day clinical practice ... applied physiology is part of the syllabus, yet many candidates had no knowledge of the physiology in part (a)."

There is a slight change of wording to part (b), compared to the 2012 question. Now it wants to know how oxygenation can be improved up until the point of intubation, not just during preoxygenation. Factors to include would therefore be the use of standard nasal cannulae with low-flow nasal oxygen fixed in place before preoxygenation (as long as mask seal is not affected), use of high-flow nasal oxygen, the maintenance of face mask positioning and seal until the moment of intubation, and ensuring that the airway is supported to maintain its patency in conjunction with any of these techniques. As for the consequences of prolonged administration of 100% oxygen – there is an entire question on hyperoxia coming up!

24.8 September 2017 Pulmonary hypertension

a) Define pulmonary hypertension. (2 marks)
b) List the five categories of pulmonary hypertension. (5 marks)
c) Give three cardiovascular consequences of chronic pulmonary hypertension. (3 marks)
d) Give four specific goals of anaesthesia management for a patient with pulmonary hypertension. (4 marks)
e) List four classes of medication that may be used in the management of chronic pulmonary hypertension. (4 marks)
f) List two pharmacological agents which may be used in the management of acute pulmonary hypertension. (2 marks)

The Chairs took the view that the original SAQ had a "respectable pass rate" (53.7%), but that "some candidates displayed a poor understanding of cardiac physiology in answering this, seemingly confusing the right and left sides of the heart . . . some gave very generic answers related to cardiac disease in general, rather than outlining specific goals for this condition." The examiners thought this was a difficult question and so only 10–11/20 would have been required to pass.

a) Define pulmonary hypertension. (2 marks)

- <u>Mean</u> pulmonary artery pressure of 25 mmHg or greater at rest or 30 mmHg on exercising (measured by right heart catheterisation).

b) List the five categories of pulmonary hypertension. (5 marks)

The WHO classification identifies five groups of pulmonary hypertension with common pathophysiological features:

- Group 1 pulmonary arterial hypertension:
  - Idiopathic (may be familial, abnormal genes have been identified).
  - Associated with systemic disease such as connective tissue diseases, HIV, chronic haemolytic anaemia.
  - Drug and toxin associated.
  - Persistent pulmonary hypertension of the newborn.
- Group 2 left heart disease (due to consequences of raised left atrial pressure).
- Group 3 chronic lung disease (e.g. COPD, interstitial lung disease, OSA).
- Group 4 chronic thromboembolic disease.
- Group 5 other multisystemic disorders or multiple or unknown mechanisms (e.g. sarcoidosis or myeloproliferative disease).

c) Give three cardiovascular consequences of chronic pulmonary hypertension. (3 marks)

- Chronic pulmonary hypertension results in hypertrophy of the right ventricle.
- Increased oxygen demand of the right ventricle can lead to ischaemia, fibrosis, and diastolic dysfunction. Untreated this will progress to systolic dysfunction.
- Increased pressure within and remodelling of the right ventricle can lead to tricuspid regurgitation.
- Under normal circumstances, coronary blood flow to the right ventricle occurs throughout the cardiac cycle. However, as it hypertrophies, right ventricular intramural pressure rises, and thus coronary perfusion mimics that of the left ventricle, occurring predominantly in diastole. As such, coronary perfusion of the right ventricle reduces as it hypertrophies (when its need is increased).

- Reduced right ventricular output and deviation of the interventricular septum to the left can lead to left ventricular failure.

Acute pulmonary hypertension (which may be seen in massive pulmonary embolus, venous air embolus or bone cement implantation syndrome) causes a sudden rise in right ventricular afterload and bowing of the septum to the left, with the risk of causing acute heart failure and cardiac arrest.

d) Give four specific goals of anaesthesia management for a patient with pulmonary hypertension. (4 marks)

The principles of management are to minimise right ventricular afterload, and maintain right ventricular preload, coronary perfusion pressure and contractility. A patient with significantly raised pulmonary artery pressure is at high risk for anaesthesia.

- Minimise increase in pulmonary vascular resistance (and thus right ventricular afterload) by avoiding the following:
  - Hypoxaemia.
  - Hypercarbia.
  - Hypothermia.
  - Pain/sympathetic stimulation.
  - Acidaemia.
  - High airway pressures and PEEP.
  - Use of nitrous oxide.

- Avoid falls in systemic vascular resistance to maintain coronary perfusion pressure:
  - Invasive blood pressure monitoring starting prior to induction to facilitate rapid response to a decrease in blood pressure; aim to maintain BP at preoperative values.
  - Cardiostable induction using increased opioid dose, reduced induction agent dose.
  - Use of vasoconstrictor to mitigate vasodilatory effects of commonly used anaesthetic agents or neuraxial anaesthesia.

- Maintenance of optimum right ventricular preload:
  - Treat blood loss rapidly.
  - Appropriate fluid loading in response to vasodilatory effects of general or neuraxial anaesthetic techniques.
  - Avoidance of excessive fluid loading.
  - Consideration of cardiac output monitoring to guide fluid administration.

- Maintenance of sinus rhythm, normal rate:
  - Avoidance of causes of tachycardia (which impairs diastolic filling time); pain, light anaesthesia, drugs.
  - Avoidance of bradycardia (which impairs forward flow); prompt management of reflex bradycardia due to vagal stimulation, beware of effect of loss of thoracic sympathetic stimulation associated with high spinal blockade.
  - Maintain contractility, specifically of the right ventricle (this may include use of inotropes or inodilators).

e) List four classes of medication that may be used in the management of chronic pulmonary hypertension. (4 marks)

I have not laid out my answers here as would be appropriate in the exam but in a way that I hope helps understanding and learning.

- Treatment of the underlying condition:
  - Long-term anticoagulation with warfarin to reduce thromboembolic risk.
  - Inhaled beta-2 agonists and steroid treatment as part of the management of chronic lung disease.

— Diuretics and ACE inhibitor or angiotensin-2 receptor blocker as part of the management of left heart disease.

- General treatment for patients with pulmonary hypertension:
  — Warfarin or direct oral anticoagulants (*abnormal vasculature may predispose to clots in the pulmonary vessels causing further deterioration*).
  — Diuretics to reduce fluid retention associated with right heart failure.
  — Oxygen to raise oxygen saturations and cause pulmonary vasodilation.

- Targeted treatment to cause pulmonary vasodilation in pulmonary arterial hypertension (i.e. the first of the WHO categories) and those with pulmonary hypertension related to chronic thromboembolic disease (*although treatment of choice for these patients is pulmonary endarterectomy*):
  — Calcium channel blockers (*e.g. amlodipine, nifedipine*).
  — Endothelin receptor antagonists (*e.g. bosentan, ambrisentan*).
  — Phosphodiesterase-5 inhibitors (*e.g. sildenafil, tadalafil*).
  — Prostaglandins (*e.g. inhaled iloprost, long-term infusion epoprostenol*).
  — Soluble guanylate cyclase stimulators (*e.g. riociguat*).

f) List two pharmacological agents which may be used in the management of acute pulmonary hypertension. (2 marks)

Again, I have not answered as would be required in the exam, but hopefully the list below is a clearer way for you to understand the approach to management of acute pulmonary hypertension. The approaches below are in addition to establishing and managing the precipitating event that has caused the acute deterioration.

- Reduction of right ventricular afterload:
  — Nebulised prostacyclin.
  — Intravenous sildenafil.
  — Inhaled nitric oxide.

- Improvement of right ventricular contractility:
  — Inodilators (milrinone, enoximenone, levosimendan) (*may cause hypotension*).
  — Inotropes (dobutamine, dopamine, noradrenaline).

- Maintenance of systemic vascular resistance:
  — Vasoconstrictors (noradrenaline, vasopressin, metaraminol, phenylephrine).

- Optimisation of right ventricular preload:
  — Diuretics.
  — Fluids.

REFERENCES

Condliffe R. Critical care management of pulmonary hypertension. *BJA Educ.* 2017: 17: 228–234.
Elliot C, Kiely D. Pulmonary hypertension. *Contin Educ Anaesth Crit Care Pain.* 2006: 6: 17–22.
Pilkington S, Taboada D, Martinez G. Pulmonary hypertension and its management in patients undergoing non-cardiac surgery. *Anaesthesia.* 2015: 70: 56–70.
Price L et al. Perioperative management of patients with pulmonary hypertension undergoing non-cardiothoracic, non-obstetric surgery: a systematic review and expert consensus statement. *BJA.* 2021: 126: 774–790.

24.9 March 2018 Preoxygenation

a) What are three physiological factors that determine the rate of fall in arterial oxygen saturation in an apnoeic patient? (3 marks)

b) Which patient groups are most likely to desaturate rapidly? (4 marks)

c) How may oxygenation, prior to intubation, be optimised during a rapid sequence induction? (8 marks)

d) How can the progress of preoxygenation be measured? (1 mark)

e) What are four possible respiratory complications of prolonged delivery of 100% oxygen? (4 marks)

The Chairs' Report stated that this SAQ, an exact repeat from March 2016, was generally well answered, and "it was good to see that basic physiological knowledge is maintained." The pass rate was 67.5%.

24.10 March 2019 Smoking

a) List the effects of cigarette smoking on the cardiovascular system and on oxygen delivery (6 marks), outlining the pathophysiological mechanisms for each. (6 marks)
b) Give the respiratory system effects of cigarette smoking, other than those you have outlined above, that are relevant to general anaesthesia. (5 marks)
c) What advice would you give a smoker the day before a scheduled procedure under general anaesthesia (1 mark) and why? (2 marks)

The Chairs' Report of this unchanged SAQ stated that "candidates showed a good understanding of the effects of smoking, its pathophysiology and anaesthetic implications. This question had been used previously so it was satisfying to see that candidates had learned more about the topic in the interim." The pass rate was 69.6%. As acknowledged by the Chairs, this question is exactly the same as, was used in September 2015 and if your revision had included past papers, you would have been well placed to get maximum marks in this year's edition.

24.11 March 2020 Elderly physiology

a) Define the term frailty. (1 mark)
b) List four cardiovascular changes that occur in elderly patients and an anaesthetic implication of each. (8 marks)
c) State three reasons why the elderly may be more susceptible to hypotension associated with neuraxial anaesthesia. (3 marks)
d) Give three pharmacokinetic changes in the elderly that may impact on response to or handling of intravenous anaesthetic agents. (3 marks)
e) Define the term postoperative cognitive dysfunction (POCD). (1 mark)
f) List four risk factors for the development of POCD. (4 marks)

The Chairs' Report following the original CRQ commented that "candidates continue to underestimate the importance of basic sciences and how they underpin anaesthesia." I have added content regarding postoperative cognitive dysfunction in creating this CRQ, as it is an increasingly discussed topic given the ageing population. You should be able to rattle through a systems-based approach to the physiological and anatomical differences between paediatric and adult patients. Similarly, you should be able to list the major systems-based changes that occur with ageing. The pass rate for the question was 61.5%.

a) Define the term frailty. (1 mark)

This would be a good opening viva question, and there are several different definitions which reflect the decreased physiological reserve that occurs with age. You wouldn't have to give one of these precise definitions, but you would need to make it clear that you understand the concept.

- Loss of resilience that means people don't bounce back quickly after a physical or mental illness, an accident, or other stressful event *(NICE)*.
- A state of increased vulnerability to poor resolution of homoeostasis after a stressor event *(British Geriatric Society)*.

b) List four cardiovascular changes that occur in elderly patients and an anaesthetic implication of each. (8 marks)

Cardiovascular change	Anaesthetic implication
Reduced arterial elasticity and arteriosclerosis causing raised systemic vascular resistance, long-standing hypertension, and consequent left ventricular hypertrophy.	Cardiovascular instability. Liable to excessive pressor responses which may need obtunding. Need to maintain blood pressure at usual levels to ensure cerebral perfusion. Antihypertensive medication may result in electrolyte imbalance or perioperative hypotension. Diastolic dysfunction, reduced ability to cope with fluid load.
Loss of atrial pacemaker cells.	Lower intrinsic heart rate. In conjunction with reduced ability to increase stroke volume, there is less ability to respond to reduced blood pressure caused by vasodilation caused by anaesthetic agents.
Loss of cells of atrioventricular node and conduction pathways.	Susceptible to arrhythmias.

Cardiovascular change	Anaesthetic implication
Increased risk of valvular disease.	Depends on valve and problem with valve. Issues include reduced ability to cope with fluid loads or losses and fixed cardiac output state which may contraindicate neuraxial techniques.
Decreased beta receptor function and numbers.	Impaired response to catecholamines and sympathomimetics, hypotension more difficult to treat.
Reduced carotid baroreceptor response to hypotension.	Impaired response to hypotension.
Increased risk of ischaemic heart disease.	Increased risk of perioperative acute coronary syndrome.

c) **State three reasons why the elderly may be more susceptible to hypotension associated with neuraxial anaesthesia. (3 marks)**

- Reduced carotid baroreceptor response to decrease in blood pressure.
- Reduced beta receptor function and number limits the cardiac response to decrease in blood pressure (as well as increased probability of taking regular beta-blocker).
- Ventricular wall thickening due to hypertrophy and diastolic dysfunction will lead to reduced ability to increase stroke volume in response to hypotension.
- Aortic sclerosis or stenosis will limit ability to increase cardiac output and may lead to myocardial ischaemia as a consequence of significant drop in systemic vascular resistance, exacerbating hypotension.
- Common pre-existing arrhythmias such as atrial fibrillation will reduce the ability to increase stroke volume in the presence of reduced blood pressure.
- Impaired response to approaches to limit hypotension; fluid boluses may be poorly tolerated in diastolic dysfunction, exogenous beta agonism has limited effect (although response to alpha agonism is preserved).

d) **Give three pharmacokinetic changes in the elderly that may impact on response to or handling of intravenous anaesthetic agents. (3 marks)**

If you didn't know the answers, think through the four elements of pharmacokinetics – absorption (not relevant to the question), distribution, metabolism, excretion – and extrapolate from the physiological changes that you are aware of in the elderly.

- Overall reduced protein production may lead to reduced binding, causing a higher active drug concentration.
- Contracted blood volume may lead to increased drug concentration after bolus administration.
- Reduced cardiac output and so prolonged arm-brain circulation time may lead to an excessive bolus dose being administered with consequent negative cardiovascular response if clinical effect is used as a guide to determine dose required.
- Reduced total body water leads to increased concentration of water-soluble drugs.
- Increased proportional body fat content leads to increased volume of distribution of lipid-soluble drugs with consequent prolonged effect (e.g. propofol).
- Decreased hepatic mass, blood flow, and enzymatic action results in reduced hepatic clearance, prolonging drug effect.
- Decreased glomerular filtration rate and renal blood flow results in slower excretion, prolonging drug (and metabolite) effects.

e) Define the term postoperative cognitive dysfunction (POCD). (1 mark)

POCD is distinct from delirium, and may be seen as a decline in function from an already depressed baseline in patients with dementia.

- Decline in cognition compared to baseline following surgery.

f) List four risk factors for the development of POCD. (4 marks)

The evidence for risks for POCD remains incomplete, but the following have been suggested or seen to have an association.

- Increasing age.
- Lower level of pre-existing educational attainment.
- History of previous stroke.
- Possibly, general anaesthesia (rather than regional or local anaesthesia), increased duration of anaesthesia, excessive depth of anaesthesia (*depth of anaesthesia monitoring has been found to have a protective effect, which is independent of actual depth of anaesthesia*).
- Pre-existing cognitive impairment.
- Postoperative pulmonary complications.
- Postoperative infection.
- Need for re-operation.
- Possibly, use of inhalational agents.

REFERENCES

Brodier E, Cibelli M. Postoperative cognitive dysfunction in clinical practice. *BJA Educ.* 2021: 21: 75–82.

Murray D, Dodds C. Perioperative care of the elderly. *Contin Educ Anaesth Crit Care Pain.* 2004: 4: 193–196.

Pang C, Gooneratne M, Partridge J. Preoperative assessment of the older patient. *BJA Educ.* 2021: 21: 314–320.

24.12 September 2020 Obesity

a) Give the World Health Organization (WHO) classification of obesity, according to patient body mass index (BMI). (3 marks)
b) What is meant by the term lean body mass (LBM)? (1 mark)
c) What dose of rocuronium would you use in an obese patient for rapid sequence induction, how do you calculate it, and why is it calculated in this way? (3 marks)
d) Describe four effects of obesity on respiratory physiology, giving an implication for the provision of anaesthesia for each. (8 marks)
e) Give five approaches to maximising the efficiency of ventilation of obese patients perioperatively. (5 marks)

The Chairs' Report for the original CRQ on this topic said that "for a condition that is extremely prevalent, the scores for this question were disappointing. This question showed familiar failings in basic sciences. Less than half the candidates knew the correct dose of rocuronium and the reasons why. Similarly, the [subsection on] effects of obesity on the respiratory system was poorly answered." The pass rate was 46%. Have a look at the references for this question below – an article about anaesthesia for the obese patient featured in the BJA Education the month before the exam.

a) **Give the World Health Organization (WHO) classification of obesity, according to patient body mass index (BMI). (3 marks)**

Perioperative risk increases above BMI 40 kg/m² and is also increased in patients who are underweight (BMI < 18.5 kg/m²).

Obese class 1	BMI > 30 kg/m².
Obese class 2	BMI > 35 kg/m².
Obese class 3 *(previously called "morbid obesity")*	BMI > 40 kg/m².

b) **What is meant by the term lean body mass (LBM)? (1 mark)**

- The difference between measured body mass and the mass deemed to be due to fat content.

From a pharmacokinetic perspective, lean body mass reflects "vessel rich" and metabolically active tissue and so is commonly used for drug dosing of anaesthetic medications (especially hydrophilic ones or ones where the initial effect is limited to the central compartment) including bolus induction agents, neuromuscular blocking drugs (except suxamethonium), opioids, and local anaesthetics. There are a number of formulae for calculating LBM, and they differ for males and females.

c) **What dose of rocuronium would you use in an obese patient for rapid sequence induction, how do you calculate it, and why is it calculated in this way? (3 marks)**

- 1.2 mg/kg.
- Calculated according to lean body mass.
- Rocuronium is a very polar molecule with a small volume of distribution limited to blood circulation (hence dosing by total body weight would result in overdose).

d) **Describe four effects of obesity on respiratory physiology, giving an implication for the provision of anaesthesia for each. (8 marks)**

The question has asked specifically for respiratory physiology, so you would not get marks for describing issues relating to airway or difficult airway management, even though these are valid concerns in the obese patient.

- Increased basal oxygen requirements results in elevated minute ventilation and tachypnoea. Risk of desaturation during airway management.
- Reduced expiratory reserve volume, functional residual capacity, and vital capacity due to intra-abdominal fat and diaphragmatic splinting. Tendency to desaturate at onset of apnoea.
- Adiposity within chest and abdomen causes closure of small airways leading to reduced lung compliance, V/Q mismatch, and increased airway resistance. Difficulty with intraoperative ventilation with risk of high airway pressures, risk of shunt, and postoperative atelectasis.
- Airway hyper-reactivity due to pro-inflammatory state of obesity. Further exacerbates risk of small airway obstruction, may be triggered by e.g. airway management, coughing, and is less responsive to β_2-agonist treatment compared to asthma so may be difficult to manage perioperatively.
- Reduced efficiency of respiratory mechanics as increased adipose tissue reduces chest wall compliance which increases the work of breathing. Increases risk of postoperative respiratory failure.
- Coexisting breathing disorder e.g. OSA or obesity hypoventilation syndrome which may be exacerbated by opioid and anaesthetic medications. Risk of hypopnoea and apnoeas is increased postoperatively with possible need for invasive or noninvasive ventilation and may have associated pulmonary hypertension, which may decompensate perioperatively.

e) **Give five approaches to maximising the efficiency of ventilation of obese patients perioperatively. (5 marks)**

- Lung protective ventilation with higher PEEP to counteract the effects of reduced lung compliance due to increased mass of chest and abdominal fat.
- Use of recruitment manoeuvres if derecruitment suspected e.g. after difficult airway management.
- Adequate intraoperative muscle relaxation and appropriate reversal before extubation.
- Intraoperative (where feasible) and postoperative head-up tilt to decrease effect of diaphragmatic splinting.
- Establishment on noninvasive ventilation (NIV) preoperatively of any patient diagnosed with OSA after preoperative screening, with extubation straight onto NIV.
- Consideration of use of NIV for obese patients without OSA who have additional risks for hypoventilation postoperatively e.g. significant abdominal surgery or need for ongoing intravenous opioids.
- Minimisation of opioid use by using multimodal analgesia and regional or neuraxial techniques where appropriate.

REFERENCES

Hebbes C, Thompson J. Pharmacokinetics of anaesthetic drugs at extremes of body weight. *BJA Educ.* 2018: 18: 364–370.

Lotia S, Bellamy M. Anaesthesia and morbid obesity. *Contin Educ Anaes Crit Care Pain.* 2008: 8: 151–156.

Wynn-Hebden A, Bouch D. Anaesthesia for the obese patient. *BJA Educ.* 2020: 20: 388–395.

24.13 March 2021 Venous thromboembolism

a) List the three underlying factors that cause venous thromboembolism (VTE). (3 marks)
b) List five patient risk factors for the development of VTE. (5 marks)
c) List three contraindications to the application of anti-embolic stockings. (3 marks)
d) How do intermittent pneumatic compression devices prevent VTE? (2 marks)
e) List the acceptable values of INR, APTT (s) and platelet count (x10⁹/l) for safe performance of spinal anaesthesia for elective surgery. (3 marks)
f) After what time interval can treatment dose low molecular weight heparin be given following removal of an epidural catheter? (1 mark)
g) Give one patient risk factor for the development of vertebral canal haematoma apart from pharmacological or pathological anticoagulation. (1 mark)
h) Give two indications for inferior vena caval filter placement. (2 marks)

The Chairs' Report following the original CRQ reflected that it was "an important clinical topic, but again the pass rate (44.3%) for this question was disappointing. Most candidates answered well in sections (a) and (b), being able to name pathophysiological factors that lead to venous thrombus formation and risk factors for venous thrombus formation. The rest of the question was poorly answered. Question (e) the safe practice of central neuraxial block, only had 20% of candidates achieving full marks."

a) List the three underlying factors that cause venous thromboembolism (VTE). (3 marks)

There are several risk factors for the development of venous thromboembolism, which all lead to one or more of the three elements of Virchow's triad.

- Blood stasis or turbulent flow.
- Endothelial injury.
- Hypercoagulability.

b) List five patient risk factors for the development of VTE. (5 marks)

I have listed non-patient factors here for completeness too and grouped them according to Virchow's triad.

	Patient factors	Other factors
Blood stasis	Trauma, prolonged immobility, venous abnormality e.g. valvular incompetence or varicosity.	Surgery, indwelling central line.
Endothelial injury	Increased age, cigarette smoking, history of VTE, medical comorbidities associated with a pro-inflammatory state, burns, trauma, inflammatory response to surgery.	Indwelling central line, trauma, surgery.
Hypercoagulability	Thrombophilia, malignancy, pregnancy, obesity, smoking, dehydration, stress response to surgery, medical comorbidities associated with a pro-inflammatory state.	Oral contraceptive pill, hormone replacement therapy, chemotherapy.

c) List three contraindications to the application of anti-embolic stockings. (3 marks)

Properly measured and applied, antiembolic stockings promote venous return and reduce venous stasis. They are graduated to maintain a pressure gradient from distal calf to the knees.

- Peripheral vascular disease.
- Severe peripheral neuropathy.
- Severe peripheral oedema.
- Open leg wounds, cellulitis, or burns.

d) How do intermittent pneumatic compression devices prevent VTE? (2 marks)

Intermittent pneumatic compression devices inflate 10 times per minute to a pressure of 35–40 mmHg.

- Prevents venous stasis by mimicking the effect of calf muscle pump.
- Promotes fibrinolysis.

e) List the acceptable values of INR, APTT (s) and platelet count (x10⁹/l) for safe performance of spinal anaesthesia for elective surgery. (3 marks)

These are the values given by the Association of Anaesthetists' guidance of 2013; however there is recognition within this guideline and subsequent ones that risk is a spectrum and other patient factors must be considered when deciding whether to perform a neuraxial technique. More recent guidance from the Association specifically regarding management of patients with hip fracture deems INR < 1.5 as an acceptable value for performance of spinal anaesthesia if the risks of general anaesthesia or delay of surgery are a greater risk.

- INR < 1.4.
- APTT within normal range (20–35 seconds, APTTR < 1.4).
- Platelets > 75 × 10⁹/l.

f) After what time interval can treatment dose low molecular weight heparin be given following removal of an epidural catheter? (1 mark)

As recommended by both the Association of Anaesthetists and American Society of Regional Anaesthesia (ASRA). The Association of Anaesthetists recommend increasing the time interval to 24 hours if there was recognised trauma during catheter placement.

- Four hours.

g) Give one patient risk factor for the development of vertebral canal haematoma apart from pharmacological or pathological anticoagulation. (1 mark)

- Increased age.
- Female sex.
- Spinal pathology e.g. scoliosis, spinal stenosis.

h) Give two indications for inferior vena caval filter placement. (2 marks)

- Proximal deep vein thrombosis (DVT) or pulmonary embolism (PE) in a patient in whom anticoagulation is contraindicated.
- Proximal DVT or PE development while on anticoagulation, after addressing any reasons for treatment failure.
- As part of a clinical trial.

REFERENCES

Ashken T, West S. Regional anaesthesia in patients at risk of bleeding. *BJA Educ.* 2021: 21: 84–94.
Barker R, Marval P. Venous thromboembolism: risks and prevention. *Contin Educ Anaesth Crit Care Pain.* 2011: 11: 18–23.
Griffiths R et al. Guideline for the management of hip fractures 2020: guideline by the Association of Anaesthetists. *Anaesthesia.* 2021: 76: 225–237.

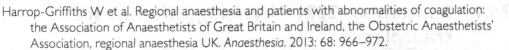

Harrop-Griffiths W et al. Regional anaesthesia and patients with abnormalities of coagulation: the Association of Anaesthetists of Great Britain and Ireland, the Obstetric Anaesthetists' Association, regional anaesthesia UK. *Anaesthesia*. 2013: 68: 966–972.

Horlocker T et al. Regional anesthesia in the patient receiving antithrombotic or thrombolytic therapy: American Society of Regional Anaesthesia and Pain Medicine evidence-based guidelines, 4th edition. *Reg Anesth Pain Med*. 2018: 43: 263–309.

Kearsley R, Stocks G. Venous thromboembolism in pregnancy – diagnosis, management and treatment. *BJA Educ*. 2021: 21: 117–123.

National Institute for Health and Care Excellence. *Thromboembolic diseases: diagnosis, management and thrombophilia testing: NG158*, March 2020.

24.14 September 2021 Physiology after heart transplant

A 56-year-old man is listed for elective surgery. He received an orthotopic heart transplant 12 years previously.
a) List four consequences of the immunosuppressant drugs tacrolimus and mycophenolate. (4 marks)
b) List four alterations in cardiac physiology following heart transplant. (4 marks)
c) List four comorbidities that this patient is at increased risk of following his heart transplant. (4 marks)
d) List four investigations that may be required to assist in the evaluation of cardiac function preoperatively. (4 marks)
e) State how the following drugs would affect cardiovascular physiology in a patient with an orthotopic heart transplant: adenosine, adrenaline, atropine, GTN. (4 marks)

This CRQ paper was withdrawn, and no Chairs' Report given. There appeared to be significant overlap in content with the March 2013 SAQ but the format, as one would expect with a CRQ, was more targeted.

a) List four consequences of the immunosuppressant drugs tacrolimus and mycophenolate. (4 marks)

A common combination for long-term immunosuppression = antimetabolite (azathioprine, mycophenolate mofetil) + calcineurin inhibitor (tacrolimus, ciclosporin) + steroid. Sometimes a TOR inhibitor (sirolimus, everolimus) is added to reduce the dose of or eliminate the need for a calcineurin inhibitor and its nephrotoxic effects, and steroids with their toxic metabolic effects. The side effects of these drugs are numerous, and so I have listed here the ones that are most significant. The general principles of managing this patient's immunosuppression perioperatively would include liaising with the transplant centre for advice, ensuring no interruption to immunosuppression perioperatively, having a plan to cover any time period where enteric absorption may not be feasible, management of PONV to maximise oral medication toleration, avoidance of other drugs that are nephrotoxic or may interact with the immunosuppressants, strict asepsis and removal of indwelling lines as soon as possible, maintaining a high index of suspicion for unusual infections, seeking advice from microbiology if infection is suspected or prophylaxis required. Steroid supplementation may be required for a patient still taking significant steroid doses.

Tacrolimus	• Renal toxicity with risk of acute renal failure.
	• Increased risk of malignancy long term.
	• Increased risk of infection.
	• Diabetes.
	• Electrolyte disruption.
	• Arrhythmias.
	• Reduced seizure threshold.
Mycophenolate mofetil	• Increased risk of malignancy long term.
	• Increased risk of infection.
	• Bone marrow failure.

b) List four alterations in cardiac physiology following heart transplant. (4 marks)

The underlying physiological changes relate to loss of autonomic innervation of the denervated heart. Intrinsic cardiac mechanisms remain; the Frank-Starling law will determine cardiac output in the absence of regulation of heart rate, and so it is imperative to avoid hypovolaemia.

- Loss of vagal tone but maintenance of effect of circulating catecholamines resulting in a resting heart rate of 90–100 beats per minute.
- Vagal reflex arcs (e.g. oculocardiac, response to peritoneal stretch, carotid massage) are lost.
- Blunted heart rate response to intraoperative triggers such as laryngoscopy, surgical stimulation, or light anaesthesia, as the effect is mediated via circulating catecholamines only.
- Slower heart rate response to postural changes leading to risk of exaggerated postural hypotension.
- Loss of baroreceptor reflex; if systemic vascular resistance drops due to anaesthetic drugs or spinal anaesthesia, there is no compensatory heart rate increase.

c) **List four comorbidities that this patient is at increased risk of following his heart transplant. (4 marks)**

Avoid repeating yourself from your answer regarding immunosuppression.

Cardiovascular comorbidities:

- Cardiac allograft vasculopathy; immunological and non-immunological mechanisms (hyperlipidaemia, hypertension, hyperglycaemia due to the diabetogenic effects of immunosuppression) leading to atherosclerotic obstruction of donor coronary arteries and late death after transplant.
- Rejection causing reduction in graft function (rare after the first year after transplant if on stable therapy).
- Hypertension and diabetes due to immunosuppression causing organ damage, including heart, kidney, brain.
- Symptomatic arrhythmias and conduction disorders.

Non-cardiovascular comorbidities:

- Epilepsy (associated with stroke at the time of the surgery in addition to the reduced seizure threshold with tacrolimus and ciclosporin).
- Cholelithiasis and pancreatitis.
- Ongoing consequences of systemic disease that originally necessitated the transplant e.g. sarcoid, amyloid, atherosclerosis.

d) **List four investigations that may be required to assist in the evaluation of cardiac function preoperatively. (4 marks)**

- ECG to assess for resting heart rate and rhythm.
- Chest X-ray to assess for evidence of pulmonary oedema.
- Echocardiography to assess graft function.
- Pacemaker interrogation if present.
- Functional assessments of heart function including cardiopulmonary exercise testing.
- Coronary or CT coronary angiogram if there are concerns about coronary atheroma.
- Endomyocardial biopsy is undertaken by the transplant team as surveillance in the early stages after transplant but also if there are concerns regarding rejection.

e) State how the following drugs would affect cardiovascular physiology in a patient with an orthotopic heart transplant: adenosine, adrenaline, atropine, GTN. (4 marks)

Denervation of the transplanted heart leads to "supersensitivity" to directly acting agents and loss of effect of drugs that act via the cholinergic pathways such as atropine, glycopyrrolate, neostigmine, and suxamethonium.

Adenosine	Exaggerated reduction in heart rate with risk of asystole due to supersensitivity.
Adrenaline	Exaggerated increase in heart rate and contractility due to supersensitivity.
Atropine	No effect on heart rate or blood pressure *(this is the case for glycopyrrolate too)*.
GTN	Causes vasodilation to reduce blood pressure, but there will be no (sympathetically mediated) reflex tachycardia.

REFERENCES

Morgan-Hughes N, Hood G. Anaesthesia for a patient with a cardiac transplant. *BJA CEPD Rev.* 2002: 2: 74–78.

Navas-Blanco JR, Modak RK. Perioperative care of heart transplant recipients undergoing non-cardiac surgery. *Ann Card Anaesthesia.* 2021: 24: 140–148.

Velleca A et al. The International Society for Heart and Lung Transplantation (ISHLT) guidelines for the care of heart transplant recipients. *J Heart Lung Transplant.* 2023. https://doi.org/10.1016/j.healun.2022.09.023.

24.15 September 2021 Hypothermia

a) State four mechanisms by which heat is lost during anaesthesia and surgery. (4 marks)
b) Describe two physiological methods of temperature conservation in response to heat loss. (2 marks)
c) List three patient factors in adults that increase the risk of development of inadvertent perioperative hypothermia or its consequences. (3 marks)
d) Why does regional anaesthesia increase the risk of perioperative hypothermia? (2 marks)
e) Give two reasons why neonates are at higher risk of developing inadvertent perioperative hypothermia. (2 marks)
f) List two haematological consequences of hypothermia. (2 marks)
g) Why does hypothermia increase the risk of postoperative wound infection? (1 mark)
h) State how hypothermia affects duration of neuromuscular blockade. (2 mark)
i) List two medications that can be used to treat postoperative shivering. (2 mark)

I would have felt quite fortunate to be given this topic in my Final, particularly given the BJA article, referenced, which was published a few years previously that reflected the content of the NICE guideline from 2008 on the topic and contained the majority of the answers! Are you getting the hang of it by now?

a) State four mechanisms by which heat is lost during anaesthesia and surgery. (4 marks)

- Radiation *(40% of heat loss. Limited by raising theatre temperature, covering the patient).*
- Convection *(30% of heat loss. Exacerbated by laminar flow and the rapid air changes in theatre).*
- Evaporation *(25% of heat loss. Limited by minimally invasive surgery, avoiding alcohol skin preparation, using humidification devices for the airway and low flows, limiting duration of body cavities being open, maintaining ambient humidity in theatre).*
- Conduction *(5% of heat loss. Limited by using forced air warming blankets, heated mattresses, warmed intravenous and irrigation fluids).*

Under anaesthesia, there are three phases in the development of hypothermia:

- *Initial rapid fall in temperature is due to vasodilation caused by anaesthetic agents with redistribution of core (warm) blood to the periphery.*
- *Second stage occurs at a reduced rate as compensatory mechanisms begin to reduce heat loss but are insufficient, so temperature still falls by the above four mechanisms.*
- *Third stage is a plateau where vasoconstriction leads to a balance between heat loss and production – temperature stays constant in this phase.*

b) Describe two physiological methods of temperature conservation in response to heat loss. (2 marks)

The thermoregulator centres in the hypothalamus create thermogenic responses via the sympathetic nervous system. Higher responses (moving to a warm area) are part of the physiological response but not relevant to a patient under anaesthesia.

- Peripheral vasoconstriction mediated by sympathetic stimulation of α_1 adrenergic receptors.
- Piloerection, sympathetically mediated but via acetylcholine as the final neurotransmitter.
- Shivering.
- Non-shivering thermogenesis, the generation of heat within brown adipose tissues (more relevant in neonates and infants).
- Endocrine responses e.g. increased thyroid hormone activity.

c) List three patient factors in adults that increase the risk of development of inadvertent perioperative hypothermia or its consequences. (3 marks)

Inadvertent perioperative hypothermia is defined as core body temperature < 36°C in the hour before, during, or 24 hours after surgery. Pathological hypothermia, as taught in resuscitation courses, or in association with cardiopulmonary bypass, is core body temperature < 35°C.

- Unmanaged patient preoperative hypothermia < 36°C.
- High ASA score.
- Low BMI.
- Advanced age.
- Cardiovascular comorbidities.

d) Why does regional anaesthesia increase the risk of perioperative hypothermia? (2 marks)

Patients receiving combined general and regional anaesthesia are at greater risk of hypothermia.

- Sensory or spinothalamic blockade reduces the sensation of cold below the level of the block (in awake patients).
- Motor blockade leads to reduced shivering below the level of the block.
- Sympathetic blockade causes vasodilation, which increases heat loss.

e) Give two reasons why neonates are at higher risk of developing inadvertent perioperative hypothermia. (2 marks)

- Higher surface area to volume ratio leads to greater heat loss via conduction and radiation.
- Less subcutaneous adipose tissue means poorer insulation.
- Immature hypothalamus means that thermoregulation responses are inefficient.
- Higher resting vagal tone reduces ability to vasoconstrict.
- Inability to communicate need for or create for themselves a warmer environment *(this is obviously relevant to the 1 hour before and 24 hours after surgery rather than the intraoperative time).*

f) List two haematological consequences of hypothermia. (2 marks)

- Impaired platelet function.
- Impaired clotting factor function.
- Hyperfibrinolysis.

g) Why does hypothermia increase the risk of postoperative wound infection? (1 mark)

- The vasoconstriction response to hypothermia reduces blood flow and thus oxygen and nutrient delivery to peripheral tissues.
- Impaired immune function at low temperature.

h) State how hypothermia affects duration of neuromuscular blockade. (2 mark)

- Reduced hepatic blood flow and hepatic metabolism causes prolonged action of aminosteroids.
- Reduced rate of Hoffman degradation causes prolonged action of atracurium and cis-atracurium.

i) List two medications that can be used to treat postoperative shivering. (2 mark)

Shivering is unpleasant for the patient but also increases myocardial and systemic oxygen demand (increased systemic vascular resistance due to vasoconstriction and increased metabolic demand due to muscle activity) with the risk of causing perioperative ischaemic cardiac events. The patient should always be warmed, if hypothermic (a forced air warmer being most efficient), and drug treatment used if shivering persists beyond rewarming. Drug treatment alone will exacerbate hypothermia by abolishing the physiological compensation of shivering.

- Pethidine.
- Clonidine.
- Doxapram.

REFERENCES

National Institute for Health and Care Excellence. *Hypothermia: prevention and management in adults having surgery: CG65*, April 2008, updated December 2016.
Riley C andrzejowski J. Inadvertent perioperative hypothermia. *BJA Educ.* 2018: 18: 227–233.

24.16 March 2022 Hyperoxia

a) Give two respiratory complications of hyperoxia. (2 marks)
b) Give two vascular complications of hyperoxia. (2 marks)
c) Give two neurological manifestations of hyperbaric hyperoxia. (2 marks)
d) List three conditions in which hyperoxia for non-hypoxaemic patients may be beneficial. (3 marks)
e) Give three cellular mechanisms of damage in hyperoxia. (3 marks)
f) State two dangers of hyperoxia during neonatal resuscitation. (2 marks)
g) Give two anaesthetic considerations in managing a patient with previous bleomycin chemotherapy. (2 marks)
h) State the British Thoracic Society guidelines for target oxygen saturations in patients admitted to intensive care. (2 marks)
i) List two approaches to avoid unintentional hyperoxia. (2 marks)

The Chairs' Report following the original CRQ acknowledged that this question was deemed "to be one of the harder questions on the paper but reassuringly it was answered well [pass rate 59.9%]. Overall, candidates were aware of the risks of hyperoxia but less clear as to how that manifest in the clinical setting and its pathophysiology."

Even though this topic appears to be difficult, relax, it is still very possible to pick up the 10–12 marks needed to pass the question. This particular topic was almost entirely based on the recent BJA article, referenced, stressing once again the importance of using these as a focus for exam preparation.

a) Give two respiratory complications of hyperoxia. (2 marks)

In the electron transport chain during metabolism, oxygen eventually combines with hydrogen to form water and to release ATP. However, along the way, some reactive oxygen species "leak out." These have unpaired electrons which make them reactive, which is what gives them the ability to cause damage. Oxygen in excess of what is required will lead to an increase in generation of these reactive oxygen species and an imbalance with the antioxidant chemicals which counteract their effects.

- Pulmonary oxygen toxicity causing acute lung injury or ARDS (with the stages of inflammation, proliferation, and fibrosis).
- Absorption (or diffusion) atelectasis where high alveolar-arterial oxygen concentration gradient results in rapid volume loss from the alveoli causing their collapse.
- Abolishment of hypoxic pulmonary vasoconstriction by high inspired oxygen concentration can lead to perfusion of still poorly ventilated areas of the lung with the consequence of impairing CO_2 clearance.

b) Give two vascular complications of hyperoxia. (2 marks)

- Systemic vasoconstriction including cerebral and coronary circulation. *Alongside the issue of creation of more reactive oxygen species at a time of already great oxidative stress, this is another reason to avoid hyperoxia after stroke or myocardial infarction. BTS guidelines advise against oxygen unless there is hypoxaemia.*
- Prothrombotic state can lead to thromboembolic disease.

c) Give two neurological manifestations of hyperbaric hyperoxia. (2 marks)

- Headache.
- Dizziness.

- Visual disturbances.
- Seizures.
- Disorientation.
- Ischaemic stroke.
- Coma.

d) List three conditions for which hyperoxia for non-hypoxaemic patients may be beneficial. (3 marks)

The BTS guideline discusses situations where high concentrations of oxygen are given while awaiting the ability to monitor its effects e.g. during adult resuscitation, severe illness, seizures, and traumatic head injury, but this question requires a list of the circumstances in which there may be a benefit of continuing with intentional hyperoxia (as opposed to hyperbaric oxygen therapy). We also frequently knowingly give oxygen in excess of requirements just before an airway intervention to provide a reservoir in the event of a complication.

- Carbon monoxide poisoning. *100% oxygen reduces the half-life of carbon monoxide from 4–5 hours, when breathing air, to 30–90 minutes.*
- Cyanide poisoning.
- Spontaneous pneumothorax, to accelerate the rate of pneumothorax resolution.
- Cluster headache.
- Perioperatively to reduce risk of anastomotic breakdown.
- Possibly, perioperatively to reduce the risk of surgical site infections.

e) Give three cellular mechanisms of damage in hyperoxia. (3 marks)

Reactive oxygen species (superoxide anion and hydrogen peroxide) can cause cellular harm:

- Damage to DNA and impairment of DNA repair causing cell abnormality or death.
- Damage of RNA and impairment of transcription, impairing protein synthesis.
- Lipid peroxidation causing damage to cell membranes.
- Oxidation of amino acids affecting protein function.
- Oxidation of enzymes causing loss of enzymatically mediated reactions.

f) State two dangers of hyperoxia during neonatal resuscitation. (2 marks)

Neonatal resuscitation guidelines advise titration of oxygen use to oxygen saturations, ideally using air for these very reasons:

- Retinopathy *(vasoconstriction in the retina, particularly in preterm babies, increases risk of retinopathy of prematurity)*.
- Bronchopulmonary dysplasia.

g) Give two anaesthetic considerations in managing a patient with previous bleomycin chemotherapy. (2 marks)

Bleomycin is used to treat germ cell tumours, squamous cell carcinoma, and non-Hodgkin's lymphoma. Treatment may have been in the patient's childhood, and they may not recall the importance of informing their anaesthetist. It acts by causing DNA damage by facilitating reactive oxygen species generation. It results in pulmonary fibrosis and a lifelong risk of further damage on exposure to oxygen.

- Consider avoidance of need for oxygen therapy with neuraxial or regional technique if feasible.

- Tolerate oxygen saturation > 85% in the case of known bleomycin lung injury and > 88–92% in patients with possible bleomycin lung injury.
- If general anaesthesia required, aim for lung protective ventilation strategy and minimisation of airway pressures if significant pre-existing fibrosis.
- Consider need for cardiac evaluation in patients with significant long-standing lung fibrosis.

h) **State the British Thoracic Society guidelines for target oxygen saturations in patients admitted to intensive care. (2 marks)**

Even if you didn't know the guidelines, an educated guess would likely have scored one mark.

- Initiate resuscitative treatment with a reservoir mask at 15 l/min and target oxygen saturations 94–98%.
- Once stabilised, titrate oxygen therapy targeting saturations 94–98%.
- If the patient is at risk of hypercapnic respiratory failure, target 88–92%.

i) **List two approaches to avoid unintentional hyperoxia. (2 marks)**

- Oxygen to be specifically prescribed like other drugs.
- Patients should have target oxygen saturations to guide titration of oxygen therapy.
- 15 l/min oxygen via non-rebreathe mask to be restricted to medical emergencies, cardiopulmonary resuscitation, and initial management of the critically ill.
- Arterial blood gas analysis for titration of oxygen therapy where feasible.

REFERENCES

Horncastle E, Lumb A. Hyperoxia in anaesthesia and intensive care. *BJA Educ.* 2019: 19: 176–182.
O'Driscoll BR et al. British Thoracic Society guideline for oxygen use in adults in healthcare and emergency settings. *Thorax.* 2017: 72(suppl 1).

25 NUTRITION

25.1 September 2012 Enteral nutrition

A 45-year-old man with a history of ulcerative colitis and excessive alcohol use is admitted to the intensive care unit for inotropic and ventilatory support following a laparotomy and bowel resection for toxic megacolon. His body mass index is 18 kg/m².

a) Give three aspects of this patient's history that would suggest he is malnourished. (3 marks)
b) List three perioperative benefits of nutritional support in this patient. (3 marks)
c) List four components of a standard nutritional regimen, giving the standard daily requirement for each and explaining how it would need to be adjusted for this patient. (8 marks)
d) List three advantages of enteral nutrition. (3 marks)
e) List three disadvantages of enteral nutrition. (3 marks)

The Chair's Report of the original SAQ on this topic stated that it was "answered poorly," with a pass rate of 44.9%, going on to say that "The provision of enteral and parenteral nutrition in critically ill patients is very important and a detailed knowledge of the specific components of a feeding regimen is essential. . . . Many candidates failed to be specific enough. Leaving the prescribing to the 'nutrition team' or 'intensive care dietician' are not appropriate answers."

Assessment of a patient's nutritional status is a common question and comprises aspects of their medical history, specific scoring systems (such as BMI, MUST, and NUTRIC) and specific calculations of energy expenditure (Harris-Benedict equation). These are explained in the referenced article on nutrition in critical care.

a) **Give three aspects of this patient's history that would suggest he is malnourished. (3 marks)**

- Low BMI.
- Long-term gastrointestinal disease is associated with malnutrition.
- Inflammatory condition, recent surgery, sepsis, and critical illness all contribute to a catabolic state.
- Chronic alcohol excess is associated with malnutrition.

b) **List three perioperative benefits of nutritional support in this patient. (3 marks)**

- Improved wound healing.
- Improved weaning from ventilator, reduced risk of respiratory infection, and maintenance of respiratory muscle strength all contribute to fewer ventilator-dependent days.
- Improved immune function.
- Improved rehabilitation due to maintenance of skeletal muscle strength.
- Reduced ICU length of stay.

DOI: 10.1201/9781003388494-25

c) **List four components of a standard nutritional regimen, giving the standard daily requirement for each and explaining how it would need to be adjusted for this patient. (8 marks)**

The components that the examiners were looking for were stated in the Chair's Report of the original SAQ. After adjusting for changes in the approach to enteral feeding since 2012, I have listed them below alongside the normal daily requirements. The precise ranges of normal requirements vary between guidelines and, where this is the case, I have given a value that is easy to remember. A specialist dietician should be involved in the management of this patient as he is at risk of refeeding syndrome due to the following:

- *Low BMI.*
- *Alcohol abuse.*
- *Low recent oral intake likely due to illness.*
- *Toxic megacolon and ulcerative colitis may have resulted in electrolyte imbalance.*

Component	Normal daily requirement	Potential adjustments in this case
Water	25–30 ml/kg/day	Increased requirement due to insensible losses perioperatively and intravascular replacement following "third-spacing" related to the patient's stress response to severe illness and major surgery.
Energy	25–30 kcal/kg/day	Reduction to one-third of normal calorie intake in the first four to seven days due to the risk of refeeding syndrome.
Carbohydrate	2 g/kg/day (~50% intake)	
Fat	1 g/kg/day (~25% intake)	
Protein	1 g/kg/day (~25% intake)	
Sodium	1–2 mmol/kg/day	Additional replacement on top of standard regimen would be guided by blood tests, but is likely in the case of refeeding syndrome, especially for potassium, phosphate, and magnesium. Hypernatraemic patients may be switched to a low sodium feed.
Potassium	0.8–1.2 mmol/kg/day	
Calcium	0.1 mmol/kg/day	
Magnesium	0.1 mmol/kg/day	
Phosphate	0.2–0.5 mmol/kg/day	
Vitamins	Balanced multivitamin intake to include B vitamins, A, D, E, K, and C	Intravenous thiamine (vitamin B1) and riboflavin (vitamin B2) as well as other B vitamins in the form of one to two pairs Pabrinex twice daily started 30 minutes *before* starting feeding and continued for 10 days.
Trace elements	Balanced trace element intake to include copper, zinc, selenium, and manganese	

d) List the three advantages of enteral nutrition. (3 marks)

e) List three disadvantages of enteral nutrition. (3 marks)

Advantages	Disadvantages
Cheaper (than TPN).	May not be absorbed, causing high aspirate volumes or vomiting.
Avoidance of line infections and the complications of line insertion.	May therefore result in malnutrition.
Reduced risk of stress ulceration.	Risk of aspiration and pneumonia.
Maintenance of gut integrity, absorptive and immune function.	Necrosis and bleeding of nose or small bowel due to erosion by feeding tube (nasogastric, PEG or PEJ).
Lower risk of hyperglycaemia.	
Reduced risk of abnormal liver function test results, hypertriglyceridaemia, metabolic acidosis, electrolyte imbalance and uraemia associated with parenteral feeding.	

REFERENCES

Chowdhury R, Lobaz S. Nutrition in critical care. *BJA Educ.* 2019: 19: 90–95.

Macdonald K, Page K, Brown L, Bryden D. Parenteral nutrition in critical care. *Contin Educ Anaesth Crit Care Pain.* 2013: 13: 1–5.

National Institute for Health and Care Excellence. *Nutrition support for adults: oral nutrition support, enteral tube feeding and parenteral nutrition: CG32,* February 2006, updated August 2017.

25.2 March 2019 Refeeding syndrome

a) Give the daily energy requirement (kcal/day) of a healthy 70 kg adult. (1 mark)
b) Give the recommended daily proportions of carbohydrate, fat, and protein in a healthy adult. (3 marks)
c) Define refeeding syndrome. (2 marks)
d) Explain the underlying pathophysiology of refeeding syndrome. (5 marks)
e) List the three major electrolyte abnormalities seen in refeeding syndrome. (3 marks)
f) What is the commonest nutritional deficiency in refeeding syndrome? (1 mark)
g) List five risk factors for refeeding syndrome. (5 marks)

The pass rate for the original SAQ was the second lowest of the paper, at 37.4%. The Chairs' Report commented that it was "another example of candidates disadvantaging themselves by failing to answer the question asked. [Candidates were] clearly asked for proportions of carbohydrate etc., but many candidates gave actual daily values rather than a proportion. . . The section on patients at risk of refeeding syndrome was poorly answered with many candidates listing a series of illnesses, rather than showing that they knew the underlying problem."

a) Give the daily energy requirement (kcal/day) of a healthy 70 kg adult. (1 mark)

There is a range which would depend upon energy expenditure and the age of the adult, with more being required for sick patients. However, 25–30 kcal/kg/day features in many guidelines as a range for well adults and matches water requirements.

- 1750–2100 kcal/day.

b) Give the recommended daily proportions of carbohydrate, fat, and protein in a healthy adult. (3 marks)

Again, different sources have slightly different quoted ranges but this approach is easy to remember:

- Carbohydrates 50%.
- Fat 25%.
- Protein 25%.

c) Define refeeding syndrome. (2 marks)

- Potentially fatal <u>shifts in electrolytes and fluids</u> that may occur upon <u>feeding after a period of malnourishment.</u>

d) Explain the underlying pathophysiology of refeeding syndrome. (5 marks)

- Chronic malnutrition causes depletion of electrolytes through reduced intake.
- Serum concentrations are maintained better than intracellular concentrations as much ionic movement across cell membranes is energy dependent, and the intracellular compartment becomes contracted.
- Upon refeeding, the sudden availability of glucose causes insulin-driven movement of potassium into cells and provides an energy source for other active electrolyte transport mechanisms.
- Water moves into cells by osmosis, depleting the intravascular space.
- There is a rapid increase in basal metabolic rate with utilisation of electrolytes that have reached the intracellular space but now with a depleted intravascular reserve resulting in dysfunctional cellular activity.
- Altered serum electrolyte levels will affect electrochemical membrane potentials resulting in arrhythmias and seizures.

- Reintroduction of carbohydrate results in reduced renal sodium and water excretion. Iatrogenic fluid overload due to attempts to maintain urine output may result in congestive cardiac failure (especially as heart muscle has been weakened by the preceding malnutrition).
- Weakened respiratory muscles must now cope with increased carbon dioxide production as the body reverts to carbohydrate-based metabolism and therefore a higher respiratory quotient, risking respiratory failure.

e) List the three major electrolyte abnormalities seen in refeeding syndrome. (3 marks)

- Hypophosphataemia.
- Hypokalaemia.
- Hypomagnesaemia.

f) What is the commonest nutritional deficiency in refeeding syndrome? (1 mark)

- Vitamin B1 (thiamine) deficiency *(thiamine is a coenzyme in glycolysis, and humans have low thiamine stores. Upon refeeding, there may be a lack of thiamine for metabolism of the sudden carbohydrate load resulting in lactic acidosis and formation of reactive oxygen species causing neuronal death leading to Wernicke's encephalopathy, which may progress to irreversible Korsakoff's syndrome).*

g) List five risk factors for refeeding syndrome. (5 marks)

NICE has published guidance regarding the at-risk patient groups:

- Low BMI.
- Unintentional weight loss >10–15% in the preceding three to six months.
- Poor or absent nutritional intake for at least five to ten days (for whatever reason e.g. malabsorptive states, intentional reduction in intake due to anorexia nervosa, following surgery).
- Low serum potassium, magnesium or phosphate prior to resuming nutrition.
- History of alcohol misuse.
- Administration of drugs including chemotherapy, insulin, antacids, and diuretics.

REFERENCES

Chowdhury R, Lobaz S. Nutrition in critical care. *BJA Educ.* 2019: 19: 90–95.

Macdonald K, Page K, Brown L, Bryden D. Parenteral nutrition in critical care. *Contin Educ Anaesth Crit Care Pain.* 2013: 13: 1–5.

National Institute for Health and Care Excellence. *Nutrition support for adults: oral nutrition support, enteral tube feeding and parenteral nutrition: CG32,* February 2006, updated August 2017.

25.3 September 2022 Fluid management

a) Give three constituents of daily fluid maintenance for an otherwise well adult who is having a short period without oral intake. (3 marks)
b) List three ways in which you would assess the hydration status of a patient. (3 marks)
c) List three causes of perioperative hypovolaemia. (3 marks)
d) Complete the following table to give the osmolality (mOsm/kg), sodium (mmol/l), chloride (mmol/l), and potassium concentrations (mmol/l) in a litre of each of Hartmann's, sodium chloride 0.9%, and sodium chloride 0.18% with 4% glucose. (9 marks)
e) State the metabolic disturbance associated with infusion of large quantities of 0.9% sodium chloride. (1 mark)
f) Plasma-Lyte 148 and Hartmann's are considered "balanced" intravenous fluids. State what is meant by the term "balanced" in this context. (1 mark)

The Chairs' Report commented that the original CRQ was "very relevant to anaesthetic practice and yet candidates performed surprisingly poorly [pass rate 51.3%]. The sections . . . requiring the factual recall of numerical values were the worst answered sections. The more practical aspects of fluid management were generally answered well."

a) **Give three constituents of daily fluid maintenance for an otherwise well adult who is having a short period without oral intake. (3 marks)**

The figures listed below are from NICE guidance. 5% glucose contains 5 g glucose per 100 ml.

- 25–30 ml/kg/day water.
- 1 mmol/kg/day of sodium, potassium, and chloride.
- 50–100 g/day of glucose.

b) **List three ways in which you would assess the hydration status of a patient. (3 marks)**

Don't overcomplicate it – list the things you do day-to-day as part of your job.

- History:
  - Risk factors for dehydration e.g. fever, physical activity, comorbidities, inability to maintain own hydration levels.
  - Presence of thirst.
- Clinical examination:
  - Skin turgor, mucous membranes, central and peripheral capillary refill gradient, pulse volume, urine output, peripheral or pulmonary oedema.
  - Response of heart rate, blood pressure, peripheral perfusion and, in children, fontanelle and liver edge to a fluid challenge.
- Simple investigations:
  - Dehydration may be indicated by raised haematocrit, metabolic acidosis, hypernatraemia, high urinary sodium, uraemia.
- Invasive or special investigations:
  - Changes in haemodynamic variables, e.g. stroke volume, measured with cardiac output monitoring after a fluid challenge.
  - Serial central venous pressure measurements.

c) **List three causes of perioperative hypovolaemia. (3 marks)**

- Preoperative:
  - Excessive starvation times.

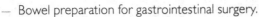

— Bowel preparation for gastrointestinal surgery.
— Effects of acute illness e.g. pyrexia, tachypnoea, diarrhoea, vomiting.
— Gastrointestinal losses due to bowel obstruction or toxic megacolon.
- Intraoperative:
  — Blood loss.
  — Insensible loss via open body cavities (may be 10 ml/kg/h).
  — "Third spacing" due to endothelial dysfunction due to the inflammatory response to major surgery and associated critical illness.
- Postoperative:
  — Delayed return to oral intake due to postoperative nausea and vomiting, reduced level of consciousness, failure to absorb, contraindication due to nature of surgery.
  — Ongoing endothelial dysfunction.

d) Complete the following table to give the osmolality (mOsm/kg), sodium (mmol/l), chloride (mmol/l), and potassium concentrations (mmol/l) in a litre of each of Hartmann's, sodium chloride 0.9%, and sodium chloride 0.18% with 4% glucose. (9 marks)

Normal plasma osmolality is 275–295 mOsm/kg; most crystalloids, except for sodium chloride 0.9%, are equivalent to this. 5% glucose is also iso-osmolar, but rapid metabolism of the glucose means that it behaves as a hypotonic fluid. These figures are taken from NICE guidance, but some do vary according to source.

	Osmolality (mOsm/kg)	Sodium (mmol/l)	Chloride (mmol/l)	Potassium (mmol/l)
Hartmann's	278	131	111	5
Sodium chloride 0.9%	308	154	154	
Sodium chloride 0.18% with 4% glucose	284	31		

e) State the metabolic disturbance associated with infusion of large quantities of 0.9% sodium chloride. (1 mark)

- Hyperchloraemic metabolic acidosis.

f) Plasma-Lyte 148 and Hartmann's are considered "balanced" intravenous fluids. State what is meant by the term "balanced" in this context. (1 mark)

- Reduced chloride content compared to 0.9% sodium chloride with alternative anions used e.g. increased quantity of potassium, to balance the quantity of sodium.

REFERENCES

Al-Khafaji A, Webb A. Fluid resuscitation. *Contin Educ Anaesth Crit Care Pain.* 2004: 4: 127–131.

Boer C, Bossers S, Koning N. Choice of fluid type: physiological concepts and perioperative indications. *BJA.* 2018: 120: 384–396.

Dunn J, Grocott M, Mythen G. The place of goal directed haemodynamic therapy in the 21st century. *BJA Educ.* 2016: 21: 179–185.

National Institute for Health and Care Excellence. *Intravenous fluid therapy in adults in hospital: CG174,* December 2013, updated May 2017.

Rassam S, Counsell D. Perioperative fluid therapy. *Contin Educ Anaesth Crit Care Pain.* 2005: 5: 176–178.

PHYSICS AND CLINICAL MEASUREMENT

26.1 September 2011 Equipment used in total intravenous anaesthesia

a) List three types of infusion control devices used in clinical settings. (3 marks)
b) List three general and three specific characteristics of pumps used for target-controlled infusion (TCI) anaesthesia. (6 marks)
c) List three specific indications for total intravenous anaesthesia (TIVA). (3 marks)
d) List four features of an intravenous giving set designed for use with TIVA that help ensure drug delivery. (4 marks)
e) List four other precautions that should be undertaken to help guarantee drug delivery when administering TIVA. (4 marks)

a) List three types of infusion control devices used in clinical settings. (3 marks)

Non-electrical:

- Gravity driven with manually adjustable clamp e.g. roller clamp on standard fluid administration set.
- Elastomeric pump.

Electrical:

- Volumetric pump.
- Syringe driver.

b) List three general and three specific characteristics of pumps used for target-controlled infusion (TCI) anaesthesia. (6 marks)

General:

- Mains and rechargeable battery powered with alarm if threat of power loss.
- Clear user interface, control buttons and screen.
- Clamp or other fixing device to position pump close to the level of the patient.
- Short- and long-term accuracy in infusion rate.
- Able to deliver a bolus with accuracy of volume.
- Able to be purged.
- High-pressure detection with alarm in the event of occlusion.
- Minimal post-occlusion bolus ("back-off" facility).
- Alarm/notification of user in event of incorrectly inserted syringe.
- Alarm in the event of infusion nearing end.
- Ability to programme small variations in flow rate over a wide range of rates.
- Secure fitting of syringe into driver mechanism.

DOI: 10.1201/9781003388494-26

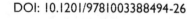

Specific:

- Programmed with TCI algorithms (some only programmed for a specific drug, others have a range of algorithms).
- Ability to input patient's weight, sex, height, and age.
- Screen that clearly shows the drug and algorithm in use as well as other key information such as effect site or plasma concentration.
- Specific syringe compatibilities (some only work with specific syringes e.g. the Diprifusor with propofol in pre-prepared syringes with magnetic strip).

c) **List three specific indications for total intravenous anaesthesia (TIVA). (3 marks)**

Patient indications:

- Patients at risk of or with a diagnosis of malignant hyperthermia.
- Patients with neuromuscular diseases (in whom neuromuscular blocking drugs may be potentially avoided with TIVA).
- Patient history of severe PONV with volatile anaesthesia.
- Anticipated difficult airway (to ensure anaesthesia).
- Long QT.

Equipment indications:

- Intra- or interhospital transfer of an anaesthetised patient.
- Remote site anaesthesia or surgery in non-theatre environments.
- Non-availability of scavenging or anaesthetic machine.

Procedure indications:

- Neurosurgery (inhalational agents may cause more uncoupling of cerebral metabolism and cerebral blood flow at high MAC values).
- Separates anaesthesia from oxygenation, so useful in "tubeless" ENT or thoracic surgery.
- Surgery requiring peripheral nerve or neurophysiological monitoring.
- Potentially quicker, smoother emergence profile compared to volatile which may be preferable in the obese, in patients in whom rises in intracranial and intraocular pressure should be minimised, head and neck surgery where coughing may impair haemostasis, long operative times.

d) **List four features of an intravenous giving set designed for use with TIVA that help ensure drug delivery. (4 marks)**

- Luer-lock connections at each end to reduce the risk of accidental disconnection.
- Anti-siphon valve at drug syringe connector points to reduce risk of uncontrolled drug infusion.
- Anti-reflux valve at fluid line connector point to reduce the risk of backward flow of drug up infusion tubing resulting in failure to deliver the drug or delivery of a bolus of the drug subsequently.
- Drug and fluid lines should join together as close as possible to the patient to minimise dead space in which a drug may accumulate.
- Connection points may be colour-coded.
- Extra connections or three-way taps should not be added to the drug delivery lines.

e) List four other precautions that should be undertaken to help guarantee drug delivery when administering TIVA. (4 marks)

Guaranteeing drug delivery in TIVA was the focus of a Safe Anaesthesia Liaison Group publication in 2009. However, even if you hadn't read the report, if you have used TIVA and have attended M&M meetings, you should be able to pick up many of the points.

Organisational:

- Pumps should undergo regular maintenance checks.
- Staff should be trained in pump use.
- Anaesthetist should have adequate training in TIVA prior to using TIVA solo.
- Pumps to be plugged in to charge when not in use.
- Pumps should be standardised within each trust.

Prior to use:

- Check that the pump is functioning and has run self-check.
- Correct entry of patient data.
- Correct drug in syringe, correctly drawn up (check with second person), and correct algorithm entered.
- Syringe intact and correctly seated in the mechanism to avoid siphoning.
- Priming of line to minimise "backlash" and to eliminate air bubbles.

During use:

- Cannula visible at all times to check for disconnection or extravasation.
- Pump at similar height to the patient to minimise risk of siphoning or under-delivery of drug.
- Pump to be kept plugged in when possible.
- Intermittent check that the expected volume of drug has been infused.
- Respond appropriately to pump alarms.

REFERENCES

Al-Rifai Z, Mulvey D. Principles of total intravenous anaesthesia: practical aspects of using total intravenous anaesthesia. *BJA Educ.* 2016: 16: 276–280.

Keay S, Callander C. The safe use of infusion devices. *Contin Educ Anaesth Crit Care Pain.* 2004: 4: 81–85.

Safe Anaesthesia Liaison Group. *Guaranteeing drug delivery in total intravenous anaesthesia,* 2009. www.rcoa.ac.uk/system/files/CSQ-PS-2-Safety-notification-TIVA.pdf. Accessed 20th December 2017.

26.2 September 2011 Ultrasound

a) State the frequency of ultrasound probe most commonly used for the purposes of vascular access in adults. (1 mark)
b) List eight other indications for the use of ultrasound in anaesthetic and critical care practice. (8 marks)
c) List five pieces of information that transthoracic echocardiography can provide in a haemodynamically unstable patient. (5 marks)
d) What is the Doppler effect? (1 mark)
e) What is the Doppler equation? (1 mark)
f) Give four echocardiographic assessments that are facilitated by the Doppler effect. (4 marks)

The College loves ultrasound. There were four SAQ questions based on its use between 2011 and 2017. Maybe it's time for a new appearance as a CRQ? It continues to be a common topic in the viva.

a) **State the frequency of ultrasound probe most commonly used for the purposes of vascular access in adults. (1 mark)**

- Approximately 5–15 MHz.

b) **List eight other indications for the use of ultrasound in anaesthetic and critical care practice. (8 marks)**

I have used my alphabet approach to dredge my brain. Having a structure really does help.

- Airway:
  - Check for anterior vessels prior to percutaneous tracheostomy.
  - Identification of cricothyroid membrane prior to anaesthesia of patient with potentially difficult to manage airway.
- Respiratory:
  - Locate pleural effusions to guide insertion of pleural drains.
  - Identify areas of consolidation or oedema.
  - Identification of pneumothorax.
- Cardiovascular:
  - Transoesophageal/transthoracic echo; to guide fluid management, assess ejection fraction, detect air embolism, assess valvular function, detect tamponade, or even complete echocardiographic assessment of the heart.
  - Oesophageal Doppler; optimise filling, inotrope and vasopressor use.
  - FAST (focused assessment with sonography for trauma) scanning; assessment of bleeding in thorax or abdomen.
- Neurological:
  - Identification of nerves for peripheral nerve blocks.
  - Identification of planes for nerve blocks.
  - Identification of epidural space.
  - Transcranial Doppler ultrasonography.
- Gastrointestinal:
  - To guide insertion of drain for an abdominal collection.
  - Identification of ascites for drainage.
  - Assessment of degree of gastric emptying prior to anaesthesia.

c) List five pieces of information that transthoracic echocardiography can provide in a haemodynamically unstable patient. (5 marks)

In reality, this list is endless with echocardiography techniques becoming more advanced.

- Evidence of left ventricular failure; reduced longitudinal and radial contraction and chamber dilatation.
- Evidence of right ventricular failure; reduced longitudinal and radial contraction and chamber dilatation, approaching size of left ventricle. D-shaped left ventricle due to increased pressure in right ventricle on interventricular septum. Tricuspid valve may be regurgitant.
- Evidence of hypovolaemia; narrow and excessively collapsing inferior vena cava, small chambers, hyperdynamic left ventricle (raised ejection fraction).
- Evidence of reduced afterload; hyperdynamic left ventricle.
- Specific diagnoses:
  - Evidence of tamponade; pericardial effusion, dilated inferior vena cava, collapse of right and then all heart chambers, "swinging heart."
  - Evidence of aortic root dissection; dilated root with aortic regurgitation and pericardial effusion.
  - Evidence of myocardial ischaemia or infarction; evidence of heart failure with regional wall motion abnormalities.
  - Evidence of pulmonary embolism; evidence of right heart failure, rarely thrombus can be visualised in the right heart.
  - Evidence of valve disease; regurgitant jet on colour Doppler or thickened, calcified immobile leaflets.

d) What is the Doppler effect? (1 mark)

- The Doppler effect is the change in perceived frequency of a sound wave when the source is moving in relation to the observer. The frequency, and therefore pitch, increases as the distance between observer and source reduces.

e) What is the Doppler equation? (1 mark)

$$V = \frac{\Delta F.c}{2\,F_0.\cos\theta}$$

V = velocity of object
ΔF = frequency shift ($F_R - F_0$)
c = speed of sound in blood
F_0 = frequency of emitted sound
θ = angle between sound and object

f) Give four echocardiographic assessments that are facilitated by the Doppler effect. (4 marks)

Ultrasound provides the image of the structure of the heart itself, but Doppler provides the information about all moving aspects of the echocardiography study, including blood flow. The transmitted wave is reflected off moving red blood cells, causing a frequency shift of the reflected wave. This can be used to measure the following:

- Assessment of valve function, direction of flow, turbulent flow due to stenosis.
- Cardiac output by measurement of the velocity time integral through the left ventricular outflow tract.
- Degree and direction of shunt in structural or congenital heart diseases.

- Dynamic obstructions.
- Coronary artery flow.
- Diastolic function; E/A ratio is an assessment of peak blood flow entering the left ventricle during early diastole compared to late diastole caused by atrial contraction, a measure of diastolic function.

REFERENCES

Cross M, Plunkett E. *Physics, pharmacology and physiology for anaesthetists key concepts for the FRCA.* Cambridge: Cambridge Medicine, 2008.

Magee P. Essential notes on the physics of Doppler ultrasound. *BJA Educ.* 2020: 20: 112–113.

Roscoe A, Strang T. Echocardiography in intensive care. *Contin Educ Anaesth Crit Care Pain.* 2008: 8: 46–49.

Walley P et al. A practical approach to goal-directed echocardiography in the critical care setting. *Crit Care.* 2014: 18: 681.

26.3 March 2012 Ultrasound

a) How may ultrasound techniques be used in anaesthetic and critical care practice? (6 marks)
b) What information can echocardiography provide in a haemodynamically unstable patient? (10 marks)
c) What is the Doppler effect? How may this be used in clinical practice? (4 marks)

The Chair's Report for the SAQ, reproduced here as it appeared in the exam, found that "candidates demonstrated sound knowledge but had greater difficulty in explaining the Doppler effect and how the principle is applied." This question is very similar to that from just six months earlier. Parts (a) and (b) were identical except that the weighting of points changed slightly. This time, part (c) asked about all clinical applications of Doppler, not just about its use in echocardiography.

c) What is the Doppler effect? How may this be used in clinical practice? (4 marks)

The first part of this answer is as written in the September 2011 question. The second part of the question highlights the importance of being observant in your day-to-day practice.

- Echocardiography; flow across valves, cardiac output, dynamic obstructions, coronary artery flow, diastolic function.
- Fetal wellbeing; umbilical artery flow, fetal heart rate.
- Transcranial Doppler; assessment of cerebral perfusion e.g. intraoperatively, in patients with vascular abnormalities, in young patients with sickle cell anaemia.
- Oesophageal Doppler; blood velocity in descending aorta to indicate cardiac output and guide fluid and vasopressor use.
- Assessment of arterial flow when assessing for peripheral arterial disease.
- Assessment of venous flow in legs when assessing for venous thrombo-embolism.

26.4 March 2012 Capnography

a) State the reason why carbon dioxide absorbs infrared radiation. (1 mark)
b) Give one other expired gas that can be measured by infrared absorption. (1 mark)
c) State the reason why the measuring chamber windows of the capnograph are made of crystal. (1 mark)
d) State the physical laws that underpin the ability of a capnograph to measure carbon dioxide. (4 marks)
e) List three diagnoses that can be made when continuous capnography is used in an anaesthetised patient. For each diagnosis, state how the value of end-tidal carbon dioxide and the capnograph waveform would change. (9 marks)
e) Name four clinical situations and locations where continuous capnography should be available for use. (4 marks)

There was a 60.8% pass rate for the original SAQ on this topic.

a) State the reason why carbon dioxide absorbs infrared radiation. (1 mark)

- Molecules containing dissimilar atoms absorb infrared light. *The covalent bond between carbon and oxygen maximally absorbs infrared radiation at a wavelength of 4.3 micrometres.*

b) Give one other expired gas that can be measured by infrared absorption. (1 mark)

Oxygen is measured by paramagnetic analysis.

- Nitrous oxide.
- Volatile anaesthetic agents.

c) State the reason why the measuring chamber windows of the capnograph are made of crystal. (1 mark)

- This will allow only the specific wavelength of light through to the measurement chamber that is maximally absorbed by the gas being measured.

d) State the physical laws that underpin the ability of a capnograph to measure carbon dioxide. (4 marks)

A small proportion of the patient's expired gas is diverted to the capnography sample chamber. Infrared (generated by a heated wire) is passed through a crystal window into the sample chamber and a reference chamber. The radiation is attenuated proportionally to the amount of carbon dioxide in the chamber, but that which passes all of the way through is focused onto a photodetector and an electronic monitor displays the quantity, of exhaled carbon dioxide concentration and the waveform. A range of different filters are used in order to be able to measure the concentration of volatile agents as well.

- Beer's law; absorption (of the infrared) is proportional to the concentration of the sample (and therefore variable according to how much exhaled carbon dioxide there is).
- Lambert's law; absorption (of the infrared) will be proportional to the path length (which is the distance within the chamber and is therefore fixed).

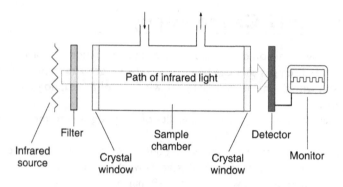

Capnograph monitor.

e) List three diagnoses that can be made when continuous capnography is used in an anaesthetised patient. For each diagnosis, state how the value of end-tidal carbon dioxide and the capnograph waveform would change. (9 marks)

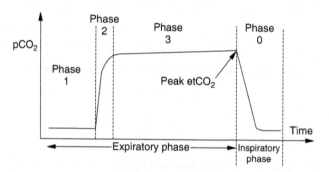

Capnograph waveform.

Information is gained from the absolute value of end-tidal carbon dioxide ($etCO_2$) and the waveform.

Diagnosis	Value of $etCO_2$	Waveform
Ventilatory sufficiency.	High if underventilated, low if overventilated.	Normal waveform, but height proportional to value of $etCO_2$. Rate will be demonstrated by the number of waveforms per unit time.
Respiratory disease, ranging from stable chronic obstructive pulmonary disease to acute bronchospasm under anaesthesia.	May be normal or elevated.	Gradually upsloping phase 3, failure to achieve plateau.
Acute reduction or loss of cardiac output.	Rapidly reducing $etCO_2$ value.	Normal morphology but waveform rapidly reducing in size with sequential breaths.
Soda lime exhaustion or inadequate fresh gas flow rate.	Elevated $etCO_2$.	Baseline not returning to zero between breaths.
Disconnection of breathing system/accidental extubation/dislodgement of tracheostomy tube.	No $etCO_2$.	Sudden loss of trace.
Inadequate paralysis.	If inadequate paralysis interferes with effective ventilation, $etCO_2$ will rise.	Clefts in the plateau phase of the trace. Extra, small waveforms interspersed in the overall trace.

Diagnosis	Value of etCO$_2$	Waveform
Incorrect tube placement.	Reducing value of etCO$_2$, if any at all.	It is possible that there may be approximately three smaller-than-usual waveforms after oesophageal intubation (as carbon dioxide present in the stomach is expelled), or there may be no trace at all.
Malignant hyperthermia.	Rapidly rising etCO$_2$ value.	Morphology of the trace will remain normal, but the height of the waveform will rise with successive breaths.

e) **Name four clinical situations and locations where continuous capnography should be available for use. (4 marks)**

This question featured a year after the updated statement from the Association of Anaesthetists concerning when and where capnography should be used. The statement quoted NAP4 (then recently published), which stated that 80% of deaths from airway complications in the ICU and 50% of deaths from airway complications in ED were caused by absence of, or failure of proper use of capnography.

- All anaesthetised patients, regardless of the airway device used or the location of the patient.
- All intubated patients, regardless of location.
- All patients undergoing moderate or deep sedation.
- All patients undergoing advanced life support.
- Continuous capnography should be available wherever patients are recovered from anaesthesia and moderate or deep sedation.

REFERENCES

Association of Anaesthetists of Great Britain and Ireland. *The use of capnography outside the operating theatre: updated statement from the Association of Anesthetists of Great Britain and Ireland, 2011.*

Cook T, Woodall N, Frerk C (eds.). *4th National Audit Project of the Royal College of Anaesthetists and the Difficult Airway Society: major complications of airway management in the United Kingdom.* London: The Royal College of Anaesthetists and Association of Anaesthetists of Great Britain and Ireland, 2011.

Kerslake I, Kelly F. Uses of capnography in the critical care unit. *BJA Educ.* 2017: 17: 178–183.

Langton J, Hutton A. Respiratory gas analysis. *Contin Educ Anaesth Crit Care Pain.* 2009: 9: 19–23.

26.5 March 2013 Circle breathing system

a) List three advantages of using low-flow anaesthesia. (3 marks)
b) List four disadvantages of using low-flow anaesthesia. (4 marks)
c) What is the theoretical minimal fresh gas flow that may be used in a circle system for a 70 kg adult patient? (1 mark)
d) List two components of soda lime. (2 marks)
e) List two advantages of use of soda lime in a circle system apart from carbon dioxide absorption. (2 marks)
f) Describe the stages in performing a two-bag test when checking an adult circle breathing system. (4 marks)
g) List the components of the anaesthetic equipment that must be checked before the start of each case. (4 marks)

The Chair was clearly displeased with the pass rate of only 35.3% for the original SAQ, saying, "Candidates should have far better knowledge of a breathing system that most would use every day. There is no excuse for the apparent ignorance of a safety checking system that should be performed many times a week, particularly when the Association of Anaesthetists of Great Britain and Ireland have recently published a safety guideline on checking anaesthetic equipment (2012). These new guidelines emphasise that checks of equipment should be undertaken before each operating session and then a shorter set of checks before each case." The marks should have been easy to pick up for anyone who had kept up to date with important guidelines in the years leading up to the exam.

a) List three advantages of using low-flow anaesthesia. (3 marks)

- Economy (reduced volatile use, reduced oxygen use).
- Heat and moisture conservation (less relevant when HME used).
- Pollution reduction (chlorine-containing volatiles cause ozone destruction).

b) List four disadvantages of using low-flow anaesthesia. (4 marks)

- Carbon dioxide absorber required.
- Overall larger size of equipment needed, not suitable for e.g. transfer.
- Increasing difference between inspired gas concentrations and rotameter levels as anaesthesia continues, difficult to predict inhaled concentrations at very low flows.
- Leak-free circle system required (so not suitable for mask anaesthesia or if LMA poorly fitting or if uncuffed tube with large leak).
- Slow response to changed setting on vaporiser.
- Accumulation of unwanted gases:
  - Substances exhaled by patient: alcohol, methane, carbon monoxide, acetone, therefore contraindicated in intoxication, diabetic ketoacidosis, carbon monoxide poisoning.
  - Products of reaction with absorbents e.g. carbon monoxide production resulting from reaction of desflurane and dry baralyme.
- Multiple components which could fail; a degree of expertise is required to train staff in its use.

c) What is the theoretical minimal fresh gas flow that may be used in a circle system for a 70 kg adult patient? (1 mark)

- Theoretically this would equal the basal metabolic oxygen requirements, 250 ml/min, although this assumes no leaks in the circuit.

d) **List two components of soda lime. (2 marks)**

- Calcium hydroxide (the majority).
- Sodium hydroxide (4%).
- Potassium hydroxide (1%).
- Water (~20%).

You should also refamiliarise yourself with the reactions that occur in soda lime:

$CO_2 + H_2O \Leftrightarrow H_2CO_3$

$2NaOH + H_2CO_3 \Rightarrow Na_2CO_3 + 2H_2O + heat$

$Ca(OH)_2 + Na_2CO_3 \Rightarrow CaCO_3 + 2NaOH + heat$

e) **List two advantages of use of soda lime in a circle system apart from carbon dioxide absorption. (2 marks)**

- Heat generation.
- Water generation.

f) **Describe the stages in performing a two-bag test when checking an adult circle breathing system. (4 marks)**

A circle system comprises the fresh gas supply, the carbon dioxide absorption canister, the reservoir bag, unidirectional inspiratory and expiratory valves, and the pressure relief valve.

- Two-bag test is performed after breathing system, ventilator, and vaporisers have been checked.
- Attach a second bag/test lung on patient end (ensure angle piece and filter attached).
- Set fresh gas flow to 5 l/min and manually ventilate – check whole breathing system patent and unidirectional valves are moving appropriately.
- Check function of APL by squeezing both bags together.
- Turn on ventilator. Turn off fresh gas flow. Turn on and off each vaporiser in turn – there should be no loss of volume.

g) **List the components of the anaesthetic equipment that must be checked before the start of each case. (4 marks)**

- Breathing system (system patent, leak-free, two-bag test. Vaporisers correctly fitted, filled, leak free, plugged in if necessary. Alternative systems (Bain, T-piece) checked. Correct gas outlet selected).
- Ventilator; functioning and correctly configured.
- Airway equipment; full range required, working, with spares.
- Suction; clean, functioning.

REFERENCES

Association of Anaesthetists of Great Britain and Ireland. Checking anaesthetic equipment 2012. *Anaesthesia.* 2012: 67: 660–668.

Herbert L, Magee P. Circle systems and low-flow anaesthesia. *BJA Educ.* 2017: 17: 301–305.

26.6 September 2013 Invasive arterial monitoring

a) List three measurement or diagnostic indications for arterial cannulation apart from blood pressure monitoring. (3 marks)
b) List three therapeutic indications for arterial cannulation. (3 marks)
c) Explain what is meant by gauge pressure in relation to invasive blood pressure monitoring. (1 mark)
d) How may an invasive arterial pressure measuring system be calibrated? (3 marks)
e) Define damping with reference to clinical measurement. (2 marks)
f) State two causes of damping within an invasive arterial blood pressure measuring system. (2 marks)
g) State how an under-damped invasive arterial blood pressure measuring system would affect the measured blood pressure. (3 marks)
h) State three other sources of error when measuring invasive arterial pressure. (3 marks)

The Chair's Report following the original SAQ stated this question was "poorly answered [pass rate 35.8%] despite a low pass mark being set. Many candidates wrongly interpreted the question as 'indications for intra-aortic balloon pump.' The indications for arterial cannulation were for measurement (continuous blood pressure; cardiac output; blood gases), diagnostic (angiography) and therapeutic purposes (thrombolysis, vasodilators chemotherapy, EVAR, ECMO, stenting, renal replacement therapy). Many candidates focused on aspects of measurement only. All transducers are calibrated in the factory, but calibration is carried out in the clinical environment using static and dynamic testing methods: a short description was all that was required. Sources of error included transducer drift, the causes of damping/ resonance and incorrect transducer height. There appeared to be a lack of understanding of the physical principles of transducers and confusion between damping and resonance. The ODP might well calibrate the transducer for you, but this fact was not included in the model answer as it is important that anaesthetists understand the methods and principles of calibration even if they do not carry them out themselves."

A "low" pass mark implies that this would have been viewed as a difficult question. The pass mark for these is 10–11/20. I think that it is unsurprising that anaesthetists did not come up with the range of indications for arterial cannulation as listed in the Chair's Report, but with 7 marks attributed to that section of the question (which asked, "What are the indications for arterial cannulation?") it should have been clear that they wanted more than just what we normally use arterial cannulation for.

a) **List three measurement or diagnostic indications for arterial cannulation apart from blood pressure monitoring. (3 marks)**

- Arterial blood gas analysis.
- Cardiac output monitoring.
- Diagnostic angiography (e.g. coronary or cerebral).

b) **List three therapeutic indications for arterial cannulation. (3 marks)**

- Thrombolysis.
- Vasodilator administration.
- Chemotherapy administration.
- EVAR.
- ECMO.
- Cardiopulmonary bypass.
- Percutaneous coronary intervention.
- Intra-arterial balloon pump insertion.

- Arterial embolisation (e.g. upper GI bleeding, obstetric haemorrhage).
- Interventional neurosurgical procedures (e.g. cerebral aneurysm coiling).
- Renal replacement therapy.

c) **Explain what is meant by gauge pressure in relation to invasive blood pressure monitoring. (1 mark)**

- Gauge pressure is pressure relative to atmospheric pressure (hence the requirement to be zero-referenced to ambient pressure) as opposed to absolute pressure.

d) **How may an invasive arterial pressure measuring system be calibrated? (3 marks)**

Calibration: to set or check the graduations by comparison with a standard. I don't believe we truly calibrate the system clinically, but we do zero it, level it, and then check that it gives roughly the same reading as noninvasive blood pressure monitoring.

- Zero: aseptic technique, turn stopcock "off" to patient, open cap to air, press "zero" on invasive pressure measurement module, check the trace is at zero and the monitor states zero, replace cap, open three-way tap between patient and transducer. Atmospheric pressure is therefore set as zero, and blood pressure is measured against that pressure.
- Level: once zeroed, the transducer must be placed level with the heart to ensure that the hydrostatic pressure of blood is not included in the blood pressure recording (fourth intercostal space midaxillary line).
- Calibrate clinically: compare invasive with noninvasive blood pressure. Invasive systolic blood pressure is usually 5–10 mmHg higher than NIBP, diastolic BP usually 5–10 mmHg lower, mean should be the same.

e) **Define damping with reference to clinical measurement. (2 marks)**

- Damping is a decrease in the amplitude of oscillation and increase in response time, as a result of energy losses (due to frictional or other forces) within a measuring system.

f) **State two causes of damping within an invasive arterial blood pressure measuring system. (2 marks)**

- Overly compliant tubing.
- Excessive length of tubing.
- Air bubbles in the column of fluid between patient and transducer.
- Clots in the cannula.
- Excess of three-way taps.

g) **State how an under-damped invasive arterial blood pressure measuring system would affect the measured blood pressure. (3 marks)**

- Over-read the systolic blood pressure.
- Under-read the diastolic blood pressure.
- No change in mean arterial pressure.

The opposite changes would occur in an over-damped system. In addition, an over-damped system would be slow to respond to real-time changes in blood pressure.

h) State three other sources of error when measuring invasive arterial pressure. (3 marks)

- Failure to zero.
- Failure to keep transducer level with heart (a 10 cm error in positioning height will lead to a 7.4 mmHg error in blood pressure recording).
- Transducer drift (repeated exposure of the transducer to pressure causes distortion of the materials with which it is made, causing sensed value to gradually drift away from actual value).
- Resonance. *All objects have a natural frequency, a frequency at which the object will readily oscillate if force is applied to it at a frequency close to the natural frequency. This is resonance. If the natural frequency of the invasive blood pressure measuring system was similar to the frequencies of the sine waves that make up the arterial pressure waveform, then the system would resonate, causing the output of the system to be greater than it should be. So the natural frequency of the measuring system is intentionally made higher than the frequencies of the waveforms that make up the arterial pulse. It is important that a short, rigid-walled cannula is used and that the tubing does not exceed 120 cm in length in order to maintain the high natural frequency of the measuring system.*

REFERENCE

Jones A, Pratt O. Physical principles of intra-arterial blood pressure measurement. *ATOTW.* 2009: 137.

26.7 March 2014 Implantable cardiac defibrillators

a) List three indications for insertion of an implantable cardiac defibrillator (ICD). (3 marks)
b) State three ways in which surgical diathermy may affect the ICD. (3 marks)
c) With reference to ICD nomenclature, state the meaning of three of the letters. (3 marks)
d) State four specific preoperative preparations that may be required for a patient with an ICD listed for elective surgery. (4 marks)
e) State four specific intraoperative preparations that may be required for a patient with an ICD having elective surgery. (4 marks)
f) List two postoperative considerations for a patient with an ICD following surgery. (2 marks)
g) How does the management differ if this patient requires emergency surgery? (1 mark)

The Chair's Report of the original SAQ stated a 67.1% pass rate. They said that "some candidates gave generalised answers and failed to focus on the specifics of how the risk of an ICD working inappropriately, or failing to work when necessary, would influence anaesthetic practice. In an emergency situation, deactivation of the ICD would be a reasonable 'balance of risks' action."

a) List three indications for insertion of an implantable cardiac defibrillator (ICD). (3 marks)

When this was questioned back in 2014, the range of indications was smaller. Recent guidance has extended the range of conditions for which ICD is indicated or should be considered. However, this being an anaesthetic exam and not a cardiology exam, I suspect full recall of the slightly abridged list below would not be required. However, I think it is useful to have an appreciation of the range of patients who will now be presenting for surgery with an ICD.

- Secondary prevention in patients with a history of VF/VT who have survived a cardiac arrest or have had significant haemodynamic compromise or syncope, or who have left ventricular ejection fraction (LVEF) < 35% but no worse than class III New York Heart Association (NYHA) function.
- Secondary prevention in patients who have survived a cardiac arrest due to coronary artery spasm.
- A range of cardiomyopathies e.g. sarcoid, amyloid, dilated cardiomyopathy, hypokinetic non-dilated cardiomyopathy, Chaga's, chronic myocarditis, or hypertrophic cardiomyopathy in conjunction with poor prognostic indicators such as destabilising VT/VF, reduced ejection fraction, NYHA II-III, or gene mutations.
- Documented VF or haemodynamically destabilising VT more than 48 hours after myocardial infarction in the absence of ongoing ischaemia.
- Patients with familial arrhythmogenic conditions e.g. long QT, Brugada, arrhythmogenic right ventricular cardiomyopathy in conjunction with a range of poor prognostic indicators such as systolic dysfunction or VF/VT.
- Following surgical correction of congenital heart disease with NYHA II-III and LVEF < 35%.
- Patients with coronary artery disease and low LVEF despite best medical therapy (EF < 30% and asymptomatic or < 35% and NHYA II-III).
- Patients with coronary artery disease with LVEF < 40% despite best medical therapy and inducible sustained monomorphic VT.

b) State three ways in which surgical diathermy may affect the ICD. (3 marks)

- Damage to and, therefore, malfunction of device.
- Sensing of diathermy by ICD as arrhythmia, resulting in inappropriate shock delivery.
- Energy induction in cardiac leads, resulting in tip heating and tissue damage. Scar development around the lead tips can cause changes in resistance and failure of the device to work.

c) With reference to ICD nomenclature, state the meaning of three of the letters. (3 marks)

- First letter: chambers that can be shocked in the event of significant arrhythmia.
- Second letter: chambers that can be paced in the event of tachycardia.
- Third letter: method of detecting tachycardia.
- Fourth letter: chambers with pacing in the event of bradycardia.

d) State four specific preoperative preparations that may be required for a patient with an ICD listed for elective surgery. (4 marks)

- Patient history and examination focusing on cardiac conditions and symptoms that may indicate device failure (dizziness, syncope, worsening cardiac function, excessive shocking) or deterioration of cardiac disease.
- Electrolytes; increased risk of arrhythmia if abnormal.
- Device registration card or other method of ascertaining nature of device, indication for insertion, follow-up, remaining battery and device life.
- Satisfactory ICD check within the past six months.
- Discussion with surgeon regarding need for use of diathermy or any other possible risk of interference that may be interpreted as arrhythmia by ICD.
- Reprogramming of device to stop shock capability (and maybe change pacing mode to fixed mode) if diathermy is to be used or other interference likely.

e) State four specific intraoperative preparations that may be required for a patient with an ICD having elective surgery. (4 marks)

- ECG monitoring and external defibrillator pads to be applied from the point of deactivation of ICD. Anterior-posterior positioning recommended to minimise current passage through device.
- Ensure availability of appropriate cardiac personnel especially cardiac physiologist.
- Avoid diathermy use if possible. If diathermy is needed, ideally use bipolar, keeping the cables away from the ICD as much as possible. If monopolar essential, ensure the return electrode is anatomically positioned so that the current pathway between the diathermy electrode and return electrode is as far away from the ICD (and leads) as possible. Limit use to short bursts.
- Avoid precipitants of arrhythmia; hypoxia, hypercapnia, acidosis, electrolyte abnormalities.
- Consider cardiac output monitoring.

f) List two postoperative considerations for a patient with an ICD following surgery. (2 marks)

- Patient to remain fully monitored in a high-observation area with ECG monitoring and immediate access to defibrillation until ICD reactivated.
- ICD to be reactivated and checked for functionality.

g) How does the management differ if this patient requires emergency surgery? (1 mark)

- If the emergency surgery is during normal working hours with usual staffing, aim to follow the same approach as for elective surgery.
- If out-of-hours, or time not permitting, a clinical magnet secured over the implant site with surgical tape will deactivate shock mode. Any subsequent VT/VF will need to be treated using external defibrillation (although magnet can be removed and functionality should return within seconds if problems with external defibrillation). The pacemaker component would usually be put into a fixed mode by the application of a magnet.

REFERENCES

British Heart Rhythm Society. *British Heart Rhythm Society guidelines for the management of patients with cardiac implantable electrical devices (CIEDs) around the time of surgery,* January 2016, revised February 2019. https://bhrs.com/wp-content/uploads/2019/05/Revised-guideline-CIED-and-surgery-Feb-19.pdf. Last accessed 24th January 2023.

Bryant H, Roberts P, Diprose P. Perioperative management of patients with cardiac implantable electronic devices. *BJA Educ.* 2016: 16: 388–396.

Medicines and Healthcare Products Regulatory Agency. *Perioperative management of pacemakers/ICDs: guidelines for the perioperative management of patients with implantable pacemakers or implantable cardioverter defibrillators, where the use of surgical diathermy/electrocautery is anticipated,* 2006.

National Institute for Health and Care Excellence. *Implantable cardioverter defibrillators and cardiac resynchronisation therapy for arrhythmias and heart failure: TA314,* June 2014.

Zeppenfeld K et al. 2022 ESC Guidelines for the management of patients with ventricular arrhythmias and the prevention of sudden cardiac death: developed by the task force for the management of patients with ventricular arrhythmias and the prevention of sudden cardiac death of the European Society of Cardiology (ESC) endorsed by the Association for European Paediatric and Congenital Cardiology (AEPC). *Eur Heart J.* 2022: 40: 3997–4126.

26.8 September 2014 Ultrasound

a) Outline the basic principles of ultrasound signal and image generation. (6 marks)
b) How may physical factors influence the image quality of an ultrasound device? (6 marks)
c) Which two needling techniques are commonly used in ultrasound-guided nerve blocks and what are the advantages and disadvantages of each? (8 marks)

The Chair's Report of the SAQ, reproduced here in its original form, said that the pass rate was just 5.7%. Here is the full comment from the Chair: "The very poor scores for this question were surprising given the widespread use of ultrasound imaging in current clinical practice. Eight marks were attainable for discussing two types of needling technique, hence this question was deemed to be moderately difficult [therefore 12–13/20 required to pass] and not hard. Despite this, many candidates failed to score more than five marks. A 'black box' approach was evident in the written answers and examiners questioned whether the candidates had any knowledge of the factors which affect the generation of a good quality ultrasound image. Previous reports from the SAQ Group Chair have emphasised that knowledge acquired in preparation for the Primary FRCA examination can be tested in any element of the Final FRCA process. This advice seems to have been largely ignored. The question was of moderate discriminatory value as ignorance of the topic was widespread within the candidate cohort." Clearly not impressed. As often happens, this question was repeated in an almost identical manner in September 2017 and so I will address the content there.

26.9 September 2017 Ultrasound

a) Outline the basic physical principles involved in the formation of an ultrasound image. (5 marks)
b) Give three patient factors that may influence the ultrasound image quality. (3 marks)
c) Give four acoustic artefacts that may influence the ultrasound image quality. (4 marks)
d) Which two needling techniques are commonly used in ultrasound-guided nerve blocks? (2 marks)
e) List the advantages and disadvantages of these needling techniques. (6 marks)

The original SAQ was almost a replica of the poorly answered question from 2014, reiterating the need to look at past questions. This time, the pass rate was 58.9%, and the Chairs' Report stated, "Most marks were scored in [the part asking about the advantages and disadvantages of the two needling approaches] with candidates still demonstrating a lack of knowledge of the basic scientific principles involved in generation of an image." I have changed the question minimally to turn it into a CRQ.

a) Outline the basic physical principles involved in the formation of an ultrasound image. (5 marks)

- The transducer contains an array of piezoelectric crystals; when current is applied across it, the crystals expand and contract as the polarity of the voltage changes, thus emitting sound waves with ultrasonic frequency.
- The ultrasound waves are reflected at interfaces between structures of different acoustic impedance.
- The crystals are an emitter and receiver all-in-one; the reflected sound wave causes squeezing and stretching of the crystal, which in turn generates a voltage change across the surface.
- Electrical signals are filtered and processed to ultimately produce to a two-dimensional image on a monitor composed of pixels representing the ultrasound waves.
- The higher the intensity of the returning sound wave, the greater the mechanical and thus electrical energy generated, causing a brighter pixel on the monitor.
- Sound waves reflecting off more distant tissues take a longer time to return, allowing a microprocessor to formulate a cross-sectional image to assess depth of the structure being imaged.

b) Give three patient factors that may influence the ultrasound image quality. (3 marks)

- Obesity; increased thickness of fat results in greater attenuation of ultrasound beam.
- Positioning; optimum imaging for some techniques requires specific patient positioning which may not be feasible e.g. arm abduction for axillary nerve block, left lateral positioning during cardiac echo.
- Ability to comply with the study; patient will need to remain still to ensure best possible image generation, may not be feasible due to dementia, tremor, delirium.
- Previous surgical or traumatic disruption of the tissue to be imaged.

c) Give four acoustic artefacts that may influence the ultrasound image quality. (4 marks)

- Contact artefact; where the probe is not in contact with the skin (via ultrasound gel), the image will be lost.
- Acoustic shadowing; much of the ultrasound beam is reflected back at interfaces between lesser and highly attenuating tissues. Tissues deep to these will therefore not be seen.
- Post-cystic enhancement; ultrasound passes readily through fluid-filled structures, resulting in enhancement of structures deep to them.

- Lateral shadowing; when ultrasound beam hits the curved edges of a rounded structure, the beam is refracted and so does not bounce back to the ultrasound probe. Imaging of these parts of the structure is therefore lost.
- Reverberation artefact; reflection of the ultrasound beam from a highly reflective interface back to the probe, back to the interface, back to the probe, resulting in multiple representations of the same structure.
- Insufficient resolution; use of an ultrasound wavelength that is greater than the size of the structures being imaged may result in failure of the image to demonstrate the separation of those structures.
- Scattering; use of an ultrasound frequency of similar size or smaller than the structure being imaged will result in scattering of the reflected ultrasound beam rather than reflection of it back to the probe.
- Refraction; when the ultrasound beam hits an interface at an angle that is not 90°, the path of the ongoing beam deviates resulting in artefact.
- Anisotropy; the image of tissues is dependent on the angle to the ultrasound beam at which they are viewed, with better resolution when the emitted and received ultrasound beams follow the same trajectory but in reverse. The image quality of a structure becomes poorer and disappears altogether as the angle between the probe and the skin becomes more acute.

d) Which two needling techniques are commonly used in ultrasound-guided nerve blocks? (2 marks)

e) List the advantages and disadvantages of these needling techniques. (6 marks)

Technique	Advantages	Disadvantages
Long axis, in-plane.	Needle visualised along full length. Good visualisation of needle tip near nerve.	Difficult to keep full length of needle in view. Longer distance from skin to nerve, increased potential for pain (and possibly damage) as the needle passes through more structures.
Short axis, out-of-plane.	Uses familiar entry points, comparable to non-ultrasound-guided nerve block techniques. Shortest skin-nerve distance. Less painful as the needle doesn't pass through muscle.	Needle seen only as a bright dot when in the ultrasound beam. May be more difficult to visualise the proximity of the needle tip to the nerve.

REFERENCES

Carty S, Nichols B. Ultrasound-guided regional anaesthesia. *Contin Educ Anaesth Crit Care Pain.* 2007: 7: 20–24.

Magee P. Essential notes on the physics of Doppler ultrasound. *BJA Educ.* 2020: 20: 112–113.

Ng A, Swanevelder J. Resolution in ultrasound imaging. *Contin Educ Anaesth Crit Care Pain.* 2011: 11: 186–192.

26.10 March 2018 Total intravenous anaesthesia

a) What are the indications for total intravenous anaesthesia (TIVA)? (7 marks)
b) What are the main components of a target-controlled infusion (TCI) system? (3 marks)
c) What are the potential technical problems with TIVA (4 marks) and how might each be prevented? (4 marks)
d) What are the potential patient complications with this technique? (2 marks)

The Chairs' Report of this SAQ, reproduced here as it appeared in the exam, acknowledged it had a "good pass rate [74%] . . . A few candidates misread the question and gave answers about the pharmacokinetics rather than the components of a target-controlled infusion system." This is the fourth appearance of TIVA or TCI in this book, two questions in applied clinical pharmacology and two in this chapter. Subsections (a) and (b) were asked in the September 2011 SAQ. Subsection (c) is a slightly reworded version of what has been asked before, and (d) was new; I have given answers for these below. TIVA is heavily emphasised in the RCoA curriculum and candidates should be confident in their knowledge of practical and safety aspects of its use.

c) What are the potential technical problems with TIVA (4 marks) and how might each be prevented? (4 marks)

Potential problem	Prevention
Electrical failure leading to pump failure.	Mains and rechargeable battery powered with alarm if threat of power loss, regular checking and maintenance of pumps.
Incorrect drug concentration prepared, wrong pump with wrong syringe.	Standardised setup, one strength of drug only available within hospital trust, labelling, two-person check when preparing medications.
Failed drug delivery due to problem with giving set or disconnection.	Specific TIVA giving set with anti-siphon and anti-reflux valves, low dead space, Luer-lock connectors.
Tissued cannula.	Cannula visible ideally, large bore access to minimise risk of tissuing, depth of anaesthesia monitoring, high pressure alarms on pumps.
Drug remaining (e.g. remifentanil) in cannula at end of case.	Flush cannula at end of case
Incorrect drug infusion rate due to wrong patient data inputted.	Up-to-date measurements made on admission, two-person check of data entry.

d) What are the potential patient complications with this technique? (2 marks)

- Accidental awareness under anaesthesia (either due to technical problems as above, or difficulty in drug dosing for patients at the extremes of weight or human error).
- Hyperalgesia following remifentanil infusion, or inadequate analgesia if other opioids not given after cessation of remifentanil infusion.
- Risk of excessive dosing with haemodynamic consequences in the elderly or obese, depending on model used.
- Propofol infusion syndrome (rare in theatre settings, but may be an issue when prolonged propofol infusions are administered at doses of > 4 mg/kg/h).

REFERENCE

Al-Rifai Z, Mulvey D. Principles of total intravenous anaesthesia: practical aspects of using total intravenous anaesthesia. *BJA Educ.* 2016: 16: 276–280.

26.11 March 2020 Oesophageal Doppler

a) List four noninvasive methods of cardiac output monitoring. (4 marks)
b) What is the gold standard cardiac output monitoring device? (1 mark)
c) What is the Doppler effect and equation? (2 marks)
d) Describe how an oesophageal Doppler probe measures cardiac output. (4 marks)
e) Give four limitations of use or sources of error when using an oesophageal Doppler probe to measure cardiac output. (4 marks)
f) List the physiological parameters that are reflected by peak velocity, corrected flow time, and stroke distance when using oesophageal Doppler. (3 marks)
g) State what happens to corrected flow time in a patient with sepsis. (1 mark)
h) State what happens to corrected flow time in a hypovolaemic patient. (1 mark)

The Chairs' Report following the original CRQ commented that the pass rate for this question was 39.1%, the second lowest overall for the paper. The original CRQ included a Doppler waveform with questions based on it, and the Report said, "This type of question would have been unfamiliar to candidates but illustrates what can be tested with CRQs. Components of this question such as diagrams may not have been anticipated by candidates. This was reflected in the poor answers. The stems featuring diagrams . . . were the worst answered parts of this question."

Cardiac output monitors can be classified as noninvasive (see part (a) of the question below), minimally invasive (e.g. oesophageal Doppler, pulsed contour analysis) or invasive (transoesophageal echocardiography, pulmonary artery catheterisation). Invasive methods carry disadvantages relating to the invasive procedure but have increased accuracy and allow assessment of more sophisticated haemodynamic parameters.

a) List four noninvasive methods of cardiac output monitoring. (4 marks)

- Transthoracic echocardiogram; *can allow visual estimation of ejection fraction, or calculation of stroke volume (and thus cardiac output) by Doppler assessment of the velocity time integral. Major disadvantages related to user skill required, user variability, difficulty in obtaining images due to body habitus, and non-continuous measurements.*
- Finapres (Finger arterial pressure); *uses a finger cuff to maintain a fixed arterial diameter by applying external pressure to counteract detected intra-arterial pressure. Computerised software can then calculate cardiac output. Can give continuous measurements but would be inaccurate in patients who are severely vasoconstricted.*
- Partial gas rebreathing; *utilises the Fick principle to measure changes in expired and end-tidal CO_2 after a period of rebreathing to determine cardiac output. Offers continuous measurements but may be of limited use in patients with chronic lung disease.*
- Externally placed Doppler measurement e.g. in the suprasternal notch; *inaccuracy related to positioning.*
- Bioimpedance/bioelectrance; *uses surface electrodes on the chest to measure intrathoracic resistance to a low current. Resistance is inversely proportional to thoracic fluid volume, which changes with the cardiac cycle. Disadvantages include interference from other electrical devices and inaccuracies due to movement, arrhythmias, and poor contact from electrodes.*

b) What is the gold standard cardiac output monitoring device? (1 mark)

- Pulmonary artery (PA) catheterisation *(new cardiac output monitors are still compared against the accuracy of PA measurement of cardiac output via the thermodilution technique, which uses the area under a thermodilution curve to calculate cardiac output using the Stewart Hamilton equation: cardiac output is inversely proportional to area under the curve).*

c) **What is the Doppler effect and equation? (2 marks)**

- The Doppler effect is the change in perceived frequency of a sound wave when the source is moving in relation to the observer. The frequency, and therefore pitch, increases as the distance between observer and source reduces.

- Doppler equation:

$$V = \frac{\Delta F.\, c}{2F_0.\, \cos\theta}$$

V = velocity of object
ΔF = frequency shift $(F_R - F_0)$
c = speed of sound in blood
F_0 = frequency of emitted sound
θ = angle between sound and object

d) **Describe how an oesophageal Doppler probe measures cardiac output. (4 marks)**

- An oesophageal probe is placed so that its tip faces towards the descending aorta (to which it is approximately parallel) at approximately T5–6 (35–40 cm from teeth).
- The Doppler equation allows calculation of the velocity of red blood cells in the descending aorta moving away from the probe, by measuring the change in frequency of sound waves that reflect off them.
- The cross-sectional area of the descending aorta is assumed from nomograms by using patient characteristics such as age, mass, and height.
- The velocity-time integral gives the stroke distance, the distance moved by a column of blood per heartbeat, and is determined by the area under the curve.
- Cardiac output is the product of the stroke distance of the blood, cross-sectional area (CSA) of the aorta, and heart rate.
- A correction factor is applied because 70% of total cardiac output is assumed to enter the descending thoracic aorta at rest.

e) **Give four limitations of use or sources of error when using an oesophageal Doppler probe to measure cardiac output. (4 marks)**

- Probe placement normally requires a sedated or anaesthetised patient.
- Small changes in probe placement can lead to significantly different readings.
- Arrhythmias such as atrial fibrillation will give beat-to-beat variability in measurements.
- Measurement is based on a number of assumptions which may be inaccurate:
  - Laminar flow in the aorta; however, flow may become turbulent in the elderly, or in the presence of atherosclerosis.
  - 70% of cardiac output entering the descending aorta; this may change in disease states when circulation is redistributed (e.g. shock).
  - Diameter of aorta does not vary; in reality it may decrease in hypotension and may have aneurysmal segments.
  - Negligible blood flow in diastole; but reverse flow may occur in aortic regurgitation.
  - Assumption of aortic CSA based on age, weight, and height; does not account for inter-individual variation or presence of atherosclerosis, which would reduce CSA.
  - Parallel positioning of descending aorta compared to oesophagus; in reality, this may not be the case.
- Contraindications include patients with intra-aortic balloon pump, coarctation, oesophageal pathology (varices, stricture, or malignant disease).

f) List the physiological parameters that are reflected by peak velocity, corrected flow time and stroke distance, when using oesophageal Doppler. (3 marks)

This is very similar to an arterial pressure waveform analysis.

- Peak velocity; the peak of the waveform correlates with <u>myocardial contractility.</u>
- Corrected flow time; the width of each individual curve which is a measure of <u>systemic vascular resistance or afterload,</u> it being the duration of forward flow (corrected to a heart rate of 60 bpm).
- Stroke distance; the area under the curve which, when multiplied by cross-sectional area, correlates with stroke volume.

g) State what happens to corrected flow time in a patient with sepsis. (1 mark)

- Becomes longer; *more time is spent in forward flow when vasodilated (sepsis, general or neuraxial anaesthesia). Healthy patients compensate by increasing peak velocity and stroke distance but in patients with concomitant septic cardiomyopathy peak velocity and stroke distance may reduce (and this may subsequently "normalise" flow time).*

h) State what happens to corrected flow time in a hypovolaemic patient. (1 mark)

- Becomes shorter; *reduced ejection causes a shorter time spent in forward flow. Hypovolaemic states are also associated with lower stroke distances (due to reduced preload giving reduced stroke volume) and may be associated with reduced or normal peak velocity.*

REFERENCES

Drummond K, Murphy E. Minimally invasive cardiac output monitors. *Contin Educ Anaesth Crit Care Pain.* 2012: 12: 5–10.

King S, Lim M. The use of the oesophageal Doppler monitor in the intensive care unit. *Crit Care Resusc.* 2004: 6: 113–122.

Wigfull J, Cohen A. Critical assessment of haemodynamic data. *Contin Educ Anaesth Crit Care Pain.* 2005: 5: 84–88.

STATISTICAL BASIS FOR TRIAL MANAGEMENT

27.1 September 2014 Meta-analysis

A recent meta-analysis of studies of the utility of the Mallampati score in the prediction of a difficult airway found that it had a sensitivity of 60% and a specificity of 70%.
a) Outline what is meant by meta-analysis and the factors that ensure a high-quality conclusion from the process. (10 marks)
b) Explain what is meant by sensitivity and specificity as applied to the interpretation of the Mallampati data given above. (6 marks)
c) Rank the levels of scientific proof used to grade medical evidence. (4 marks)

The Chair's Report following the original SAQ, reproduced here as it was in the exam, said that "It was anticipated that candidates would find this subject matter to be difficult. Surprisingly, the question generated the highest overall pass rate [72.8%] and the majority of candidates scored in excess of the pass mark. Weak candidates were unable to indicate how a high-quality conclusion can be ensured from a meta-analysis or to interpret the data for Mallampati studies in a meaningful way." This question was repeated in 2018 with a couple of additional subsections.

DOI: 10.1201/9781003388494-27

27.2 September 2018 Meta-analysis

A recent meta-analysis of Mallampati scoring of the airway found that it had a sensitivity of 60% and a specificity of 70%.

a) Briefly define the terms systematic review (1 mark) and meta-analysis. (1 mark)
b) List four factors that help to ensure a high-quality conclusion from a meta-analysis. (4 marks)
c) Explain what is meant by sensitivity (2 marks) and specificity (2 marks) as applied to the interpretation of the Mallampati data given above, and give the equations by which they are calculated.
d) State how the positive predictive value (1 mark) and negative predictive value (1 mark) of a test can be calculated.
e) When interpreting a forest plot, what is represented by the central vertical line, the diamond at the bottom of the plot, and the size of each rectangular block? (3 marks)
f) Rank the five levels of scientific proof used to grade medical evidence. (5 marks)

The Chairs' Report acknowledged that the original SAQ on this topic had been used before. "This question divided candidates more than any other and showed very good correlation with overall performance. However, some candidates confused systematic review with meta-analysis." The pass rate this time was only 46.6%. The CEACCP and BJA Education journals have a number of reasonably concise articles on statistics, addressing the key concepts and definitions that are included on the RCoA syllabus (see references below).

a) **Briefly define the terms systematic review (1 mark) and meta-analysis. (1 mark)**

- Meta-analysis: a <u>quantitative</u> review of data from all available primary studies that are similar in nature, in order to reach a valid statistical conclusion to a specific question. *(Studies have to be sufficiently similar to be analysed together in this way. Results are normally portrayed as a forest plot.)*
- Systematic review: a <u>qualitative</u> review of the data of all available similar studies in response to a specific research question. *(Differs from a "literature review" because search criteria and study selection [to avoid bias] follows the same methodology and protocol as when designing a randomised control trial.)*

b) **List four factors that help to ensure a high-quality conclusion from a meta-analysis. (4 marks)**

- Clearly defined question as the basis of the analysis.
- Clear and reproducible methodology.
- Comprehensive search of all available electronic databases based on appropriate search terms, ensuring studies reported in languages other than English are included.
- Clear and valid criteria for inclusion or exclusion of studies from the analysis, ensuring only studies of sufficient quality included.
- Consideration of publication bias to avoid risk of over-representation of studies with a positive outcome.

c) **Explain what is meant by sensitivity (2 marks) and specificity (2 marks) as applied to the interpretation of the Mallampati data given above, and give the equations by which they are calculated.**

Make sure you answer this question with reference to the data provided in the question about Mallampati scoring!

- The sensitivity of a clinical test refers to its ability to correctly identify patients with the disease or issue in question, the true positives i.e. the Mallampati score's ability to correctly identify patients with a difficult airway – the meta-analysis shows that 60% of the people who have a difficult airway can be predicted as difficult by using the Mallampati test.

$$Sensitivity = \frac{True\ Positives}{True\ Positives + False\ Negatives}$$

- The specificity of a clinical test refers to its ability to correctly identify those patients without the disease or issue in question, the true negatives i.e. the Mallampati score's ability to correctly identify patients with a straightforward airway – the meta-analysis shows 70% of the patients assessed as having a straightforward airway will indeed have a straightforward airway.

$$Specificity = \frac{True\ Negatives}{True\ Negatives + False\ Positives}$$

d) State how the positive predictive value (1 mark) and negative predictive value (1 mark) of a test can be calculated.

It is important to note that the actual numbers of false and true positives and negatives are needed to calculate these values: it cannot be done with the percentage sensitivity and specificity. The positive and negative predictive values of two different tests with identical sensitivities and specificities will vary greatly depending on the background prevalence of the disease or issue that each are testing for. Try putting some imaginary numbers into the equations and see for yourself.

- Positive predictive value: proportion of people with a positive test result who actually have the disease or issue (or how "reliable" a positive test result is).

$$Positive\ predicted\ value = \frac{True\ Positives}{True\ Positives + False\ Positives}$$

- Negative predictive value: proportion of people with a negative test result who truly do not have the disease (or how "reliable" a negative test result is).

$$Negative\ predictive\ value = \frac{True\ Negatives}{True\ Negatives + False\ Negatives}$$

e) When interpreting a forest plot, what is represented by the central vertical line, the diamond at the bottom of the plot, and the size of each rectangular block? (3 marks)

Forest plots (also called "blobbograms") are how results of a meta-analysis are displayed. The x-axis demonstrates strength of clinical effect and may be in the form of odds ratio or relative risk, for example. Each study is then displayed as an individual box (study weight) and whisker (95% confidence interval) plot parallel to the x-axis.

- Central vertical line: the line of equality, or the line of no effect (odds ratio or relative risk = 1). Any study which has a 95% confidence interval that crosses the line did not demonstrate a significant difference.
- Diamond at the bottom of the plot: represents the pooled analysis ("average") of all studies in the meta-analysis, and gives a representation of overall effect.
- Size of each rectangular block: represents the weight of that particular study on the overall meta-analysis (largely determined by the study's sample size).

f) Rank the five levels of scientific proof used to grade medical evidence. (5 marks)

1. Meta-analyses, or systematic reviews of randomised controlled trials (RCTs), or large high-quality RCTs.
2. RCTs.
3. Non-randomised trials, cohort studies or matched case-control studies
4. Case series, case reports, non-experimental studies.
5. Expert opinion, formal consensus.

REFERENCES

Lalkhen A, McCluskey A. Clinical tests: sensitivity and specificity. *Contin Educ Anaesth Crit Care Pain.* 2008a: 8: 221–223.

Lalkhen A, McCluskey A. Statistics V: introduction to clinical trials and systematic reviews. *Contin Educ Anaesth Crit Care Pain.* 2008b: 8: 143–146.

Newport M, Smith A. Implementation of evidence-based practice in anaesthesia. *BJA Educ.* 2015: 15: 311–315.

INDEX

G

H

I

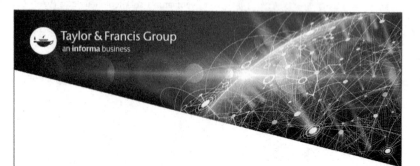